Nutrition and Diet Factors in Type 2 Diabetes

Special Issue Editors

Peter Pribis
Hana Kahleova

MDPI • Basel • Beijing • Wuhan • Barcelona • Belgrade

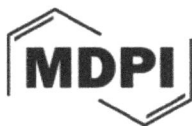

MDPI

Special Issue Editors
Peter Pribis
University of New Mexico
USA

Hana Kahleova
Clinical Research, Physicians Committee for Responsible Medicine
USA

Editorial Office
MDPI
St. Alban-Anlage 66
Basel, Switzerland

This edition is a reprint of the Special Issue published online in the open access journal *Nutrients* (ISSN 2072-6643) from 2016–2017 (available at: http://www.mdpi.com/journal/nutrients/special_issues/type_2_diabetes).

For citation purposes, cite each article independently as indicated on the article page online and as indicated below:

Lastname, F.M.; Lastname, F.M. Article title. *Journal Name* **Year**, *Article number*, page range.

First Edition 2018

ISBN 978-3-03842-916-6 (Pbk)
ISBN 978-3-03842-915-9 (PDF)

Table of contents

About the Special Issue Editors

Peter Pribis, Dr., M.D., DR.P.H., is an Associate Professor of Nutrition and Dietetics in the Department of Individual, Family & Community Education at the University of New Mexico. He graduated from the School of Medicine at King Charles University in Prague, Czech Republic and from Loma Linda University, School of Public Health with Dr. P.H. He is a Registered Dietitian and a member of the Academy of Nutrition and Dietetics. He worked for nine years as the Director of the Master of Science Program in Nutrition and Wellness at Andrews University in Michigan before moving to New Mexico. Dr. Pribis has authored more than 20 articles for different health publications, one book chapter for a nutrition book, 12 research articles for scholarly peer-reviewed journals, and co-authored two cookery books. His research expertise is studying the potential of plant-based diets in preventing chronic diseases and nutritional neuroscience. He is an enthusiastic speaker on the benefits of healthy nutrition and a promoter of evidence-based lifestyle medicine.

Hana Kahleova, Dr., M.D., Ph.D., is a medical doctor specializing in internal medicine and endocrinology and has a PhD in nutrition and diabetes. She has done several research studies on the beneficial effects of plant-based diets in type 2 diabetes. Dr. Kahleova enjoys studying how metabolic function works in regard to diet composition, meal timing, and frequency. She is the director of clinical research at the Physicians Committee for Responsible Medicine in Washington, DC.

Preface to "Nutrition and Diet Factors in Type 2 Diabetes"

Diabetes can be rightly called the new plague of the 21st century. It follows the pandemic of obesity, usually with a delay of 5–10 years. Approximately seven million people develop diabetes in both developed and developing countries every year, with the most dramatic increases occurring in Type 2 Diabetes (DM2). Global prevalence of DM2 is approximately 8% presently, and it is likely to grow substantially in the next few decades. Especially alarming, is the rising incidence of DM2 in obese children before puberty. Diabetes mellitus has become a major global public health problem. In April 2017, a Special Issue of Nutrients entitled "Nutrition and Diet Factors in Type 2 Diabetes" closed with 19 published papers—eight original studies on humans, five on animals, one brief report and five reviews. The focus of the issue was on nutrition, diet factors, whole foods, broad dietary and lifestyle strategies, dietary patterns, intensive personalized treatments, nutritional prevention programs, and food policies that can be used in the development, treatment, and prevention of DM2.

The five animal studies presented covered a wide array of topics. Xiao et al. provided novel evidence that maternal low-protein diet may be associated with chronic inflammation in the offspring. Pelgrim et al. suggested that butyrate, Liu et al. suggested that leucine, and Almomen et al. suggested that grape powder might be beneficial and attenuate diabetes risk factors. Burgeiro et al. described the liver glucose and lipid dysmetabolism in an animal prediabetes model induced by high-sucrose diet.

As for the human studies: Jablonska et al.'s study suggests that selenium may affect glycemic control at different levels of gene regulation, linked to insulin signaling, glycolysis and pyruvate metabolism. Jacobo-Cejudo et al. reported that n-3 PUFA supplementation had a beneficial effect on some selective DM2 risk factors. A descriptive study of Canadians by Bertinato et al. discovered that a substantial portion of the population is hypomagnesaemic which can be negatively associated with diabetes, glycemic control and insulin resistance.

Simple interventions such as the inclusion of fiber-rich functional bread into the diet (Tessari et al.) or avoidance of large amounts of carbohydrates from high-glycemic index sources in the evening (Diederichs et al.), as reported by the DONALD study, should be considered as preventive dietary strategies. Studying the black South African population, Chikowore et al. concluded that plant driven nutrient patterns are associated with low fasting glucose and glycated hemoglobin levels. Veleba et al.'s study suggests that in DM2 patients, a vegetarian diet led to more effective improvement in physical fitness than a conventional diet.

There are two reports from large European-based cohorts. Fogelholm et al. described the design, methodology and baseline characteristics of the PREVIEW project that was initiated to find the most effective lifestyle for the prevention of DM2; while Gant at al. reported results from the DIALECT project that suggest that incorporating nutrition management in routine care would greatly improve the treatment quality.

As for the five reviews: Fang et al. concluded that combined data support the role for magnesium in reducing risk of DM2; Luo et al. concluded that there is evidence for an association between vitamin D deficiency and an increased risk of diabetic retinopathy in DM2 patients; and Hernández-Alonso et al. suggest that nuts and dried fruits could play a significant role in the prevention and treatment of insulin resistance and DM2; Kosinski et al. discussed the role and safety of ketogenic diets in animals and humans; while Vaiserman summarized recent research regarding early-life nutrition programing of DM2.

Nutrition and Diet Factors in Type 2 Diabetes is written for clinical and academic nutritionists, for registered dietitians, health professionals, graduate students, and for everybody with a deeper interest in diabetes care. Studies and reviews presented here demonstrate that diabetes research is extensive and vibrant and the prevention, treatment and reversal of diabetes are achievable, economical, powerful, and possible.

Peter Pribis, Hana Kahleova
Special Issue Editors

nutrients

MDPI

Brief Report

"A Vegetarian vs. Conventional Hypocaloric Diet: The Effect on Physical Fitness in Response to Aerobic Exercise in Patients with Type 2 Diabetes." A Parallel Randomized Study

Jiri Veleba [1], Martin Matoulek [2], Martin Hill [3], Terezie Pelikanova [1] and Hana Kahleova [1,*]

[1] Institute for Clinical and Experimental Medicine, Videnska 1958/9, 14021 Prague, Czech Republic; jivb@ikem.cz (J.V.); tepe@ikem.cz (T.P.)
[2] General University Hospital, 3rd Internal Clinic of Endocrinology and Metabolism, 12808 Prague, Czech Republic; mmato@vstj.cz
[3] Institute of Endocrinology, Narodni 8, 11394 Prague, Czech Republic; mhill@endo.cz
* Correspondence: hana.kahleova@gmail.com; Tel.: +420-261-362-150; Fax: +420-261-362-820

Received: 26 July 2016; Accepted: 17 October 2016; Published: 26 October 2016

Abstract: It has been shown that it is possible to modify macronutrient oxidation, physical fitness and resting energy expenditure (REE) by changes in diet composition. Furthermore, mitochondrial oxidation can be significantly increased by a diet with a low glycemic index. The purpose of our trial was to compare the effects of a vegetarian (V) and conventional diet (C) with the same caloric restriction (-500 kcal/day) on physical fitness and REE after 12 weeks of diet plus aerobic exercise in 74 patients with type 2 diabetes (T2D). An open, parallel, randomized study design was used. All meals were provided for the whole study duration. An individualized exercise program was prescribed to the participants and was conducted under supervision. Physical fitness was measured by spiroergometry and indirect calorimetry was performed at the start and after 12 weeks Repeated-measures ANOVA (Analysis of variance) models with between-subject (group) and within-subject (time) factors and interactions were used for evaluation of the relationships between continuous variables and factors. Maximal oxygen consumption (VO_{2max}) increased by 12% in vegetarian group (V) (F = 13.1, $p < 0.001$, partial $\eta^2 = 0.171$), whereas no significant change was observed in C (F = 0.7, $p = 0.667$; group $\times$ time F = 9.3, $p = 0.004$, partial $\eta^2 = 0.209$). Maximal performance (Watt max) increased by 21% in V (F = 8.3, $p < 0.001$, partial $\eta^2 = 0.192$), whereas it did not change in C (F = 1.0, $p = 0.334$; group $\times$ time F = 4.2, $p = 0.048$, partial $\eta^2 = 0.116$). Our results indicate that V leads more effectively to improvement in physical fitness than C after aerobic exercise program.

Keywords: insulin sensitivity; maximal oxygen consumption; maximal performance; physical fitness; type 2 diabetes; vegetarian diet

1. Introduction

Dietary intervention and physical exercise are both cornerstones in the treatment of type 2 diabetes (T2D) patients [1]. A vegetarian diet is a promising way to reduce energy intake by consuming foods with a low energy density, with a fair degree of patient adherence [2,3].

The superior effects of a vegetarian diet on body weight, glycemic control, blood lipids, insulin sensitivity and oxidative stress markers compared with a conventional diet have been shown by us and others previously [2–4]. A vegetarian diet was also reported to reduce the content of intramuscular lipids [5].

Physical activity combats insulin resistance by several different mechanisms: by influencing changes in body composition such as reducing fat mass and volume of visceral fat and increasing fat-free mass, by enhancing insulin-stimulated glucose disposal in skeletal muscle, morphological changes in muscle, and by decreased glucose production in the liver [6]. To the best of our knowledge, a direct comparison between the effect of a vegetarian diet and a conventional hypocaloric diet on physical fitness and resting energy expenditure (REE) in subjects with T2D during aerobic exercise training has not yet been performed.

It has been shown that it is possible to modify macronutrient oxidation, physical fitness and resting energy expenditure (REE) by changes in diet composition. Furthermore, mitochondrial oxidation can be significantly increased by a diet with a low glycemic index. The aim of this secondary analysis was to compare the effects of vegetarian (V) and conventional diabetic diet (C) with the same caloric restriction (-500 kcal/day) on physical fitness and REE after 12 weeks of diet plus aerobic exercise in patients with type 2 diabetes (T2D).

2. Experimental Section

The characteristics of our study population and the methods can be found elsewhere [3]. Briefly: In the context of a randomized, open, parallel design, 74 patients with T2D treated by oral hypoglycemic agents, both men (47%) and women (53%) were randomly assigned either into the vegetarian group (V, $n = 37$) or the control group (C, $n = 37$) treated by conventional diet. Both diets were calorie-restricted (-500 kcal/day) according to the indirect calorimetry measurement [7]. The dietary interventions were combined with aerobic exercise for 12 weeks, performed under professional supervision. All meals were provided for the whole study duration. The study protocol was approved by the Institutional Ethics Committee of the Thomayer Hospital and Institute for Clinical and Experimental Medicine, Prague, Czech Republic. (The approval code is G-08-08-22.)

2.1. Diet

The vegetarian diet (~60% of energy from carbohydrates, 15% protein, and 25% fat) was based on whole plant foods (whole grains, legumes, vegetables, fruits and nuts). Animal products were rectricted to one portion of low-fat dairy a day. The composition of the conventional diabetic diet met the dietary guidelines of the Diabetes and Nutrition Study Group (DNSG) of the European Association for the Study of Diabetes (EASD) [8]. It derived 50% of energy from carbohydrates, 20% protein, less than 30% fat (≤7% energy from saturated fat, less than 200 mg/day of cholesterol/day).

2.2. Exercise

An individualized exercise program was prescribed to the participantsbased on previous physical activity and spiroergometry. Aerobic exercise was performed twice a week at 60% of maximal heart rate for 1 h under professional supervision at the sports center, and the third weekly session took place either at the sports center or at home. The participants used a sport-tester and a pedometer.

2.3. Medication

No changes in medication use were made, except for the case of repeated hypoglycemia (plasma glucose determined at the laboratory <4.4 mmol·L^{-1} or capillary glucose reading <3.4 mmol·L^{-1} accompanied by hypoglycemic symptoms). In this case, medications were reduced by a study physician following a standard protocol. All participants used an Accu-Chek Go glucometer (Roche, Basel, Switzerland).

2.4. Adherence

All visits to pick up meals were recorded. Three-day dietary records (two weekdays and one weekend day) were completed by each participant at baseline and at week 12, and analyzed by a registered dietician. High adherence was defined as the average daily energy intake being no more than 100 kcal in excess of the prescribed, medium adherence was less than 200 kcal in excess.

Additional criteria for high adherence to vegetarian diet were the average daily cholesterol intake ≤ 50 mg, for medium adherence less than 100 mg. In the control group, the average daily cholesterol limit was ≤ 200 mg for high adherence, and less than 300 mg for medium adherence.

Adherence to the exercise program was defined as more than 75% of prescribed visits at the sports center (18/24).

2.5. Hunger and Depressive Symptoms

Hunger and depressive symptoms were assessed using the Three-Factor Eating Questionnaire [9] and the Beck Depression Inventory [10], respectively.

2.6. Statistical Analysis

The intention-to-treat analysis was used, and all participants were included. To eliminate skewed data distribution and heteroscedasticity, the original data was transformed to a Gaussian distribution before further processing by a power transformation using the statistical software Statgraphics Centurion, version XV from Statpoint Inc. (Herndon, Virginia, VA, USA). Non-homogeneities in the data were detected using residual analysis. Repeated-measures ANOVA (Analysis of variance) models with between-subject (group) and within-subject (time) factors and interactions were used. Factors of treatment group, subject and time were included in the model. Interactions between group and time (group $\times$ time) were calculated for each variable.

Paired *t*-tests were calculated within each group, to check the significance of changes from baseline. Bonferroni post-hoc correction for seven variables implies that *p*-values < 0.007 can be considered significant.

3. Results

Data are presented as means with 95% confidence intervals. Maximal performance (Watt max) increased by 21% in vegetarian group (V) (F = 8.3, $p < 0.001$, partial $\eta^2 = 0.192$), whereas it did not change in control group (C) (F = 1.0, $p = 0.334$; group $\times$ time F = 4.2, $p = 0.048$, partial $\eta^2 = 0.116$; Figure 1A). Maximal oxygen consumption (VO_{2max}) increased by 12% in V (F = 13.1, $p < 0.001$, partial $\eta^2 = 0.171$), whereas it did not change significantly in C (F = 0.7, $p = 0.667$; group $\times$ time F = 9.3, $p = 0.004$, partial $\eta^2 = 0.209$; Figure 1B). REE remained constant in V (F = 0.6, $p = 0.556$), whereas it decreased in C (F = 4.1, $p = 0.032$, partial $\eta^2 = 0.113$; group $\times$ time F = 2.8, $p = 0.067$; Figure 1C). The respiratory quotient did not change significantly in either group (F = 2.7, $p = 0.0673$ for V, and F = 1.5, $p = 0.224$ for C; group $\times$ time F = 0.4, $p = 0.666$; Figure 1D). No change in fasting oxidation of fat was observed in either group (F = 0.3, $p = 0.742$ for V, and F = 1.1, $p = 0.318$ for C; group $\times$ time F = 0.4, $p = 0.658$; Figure 1E). Fasting oxidation of carbohydrates decreased in C by 89% (F = 3.8, $p = 0.01$, partial $\eta^2 = 0.029$), while it did not change in V (F = 0.2, $p = 0.865$; group $\times$ time F = 4.0, $p = 0.024$; partial $\eta^2 = 0.139$; Figure 1F). Fasting oxidation of protein did not change in either group (F = 0.3, $p = 0.742$ for V, and F = 1.4, $p = 0.259$ for C; group $\times$ time F = 2.6, $p = 0.082$; Figure 1G).

Adherence

The diet adherence was high among 55% of participants in V and 32% in C, medium among 22.5% in V and 39% in C, and low among 22.5% in V and 29% in C. Adherence to the exercise program was 90.3% in V and 80.6 in C.

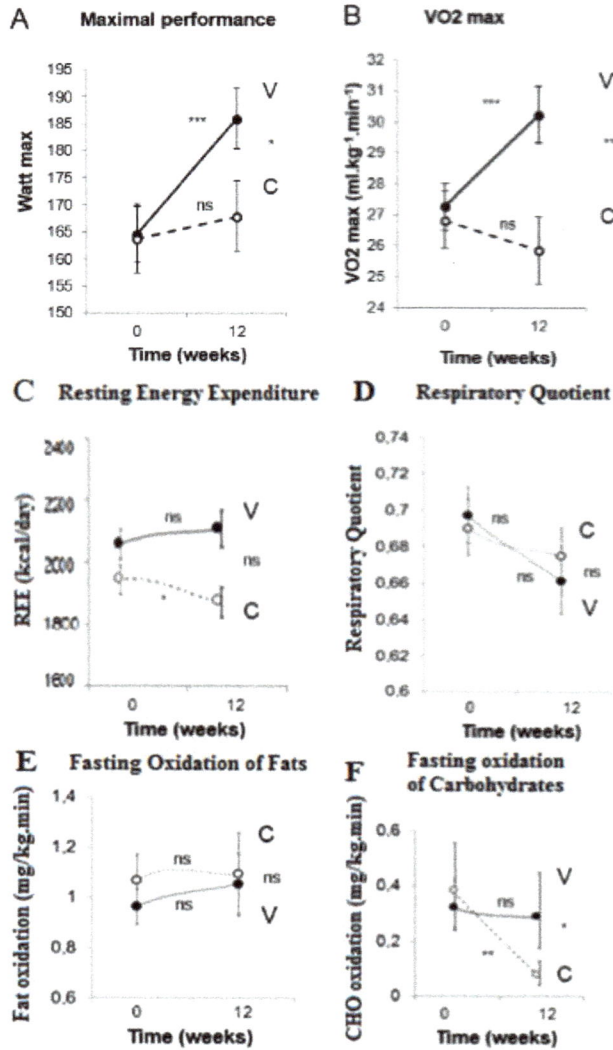

Figure 1. *Cont.*

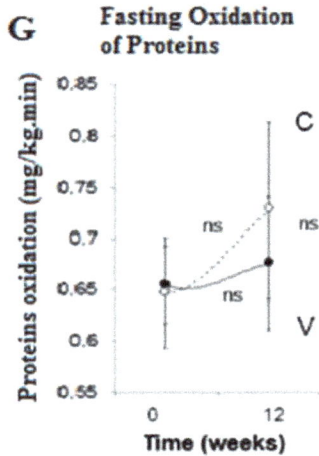

Figure 1. Changes in physical fitness in response to a vegetarian (V, full line and full circles) and conventional diet (C, dashed line and empty circles). Data are means ± 95% confidence intervals. Significant changes from baseline to 12 weeks within groups assessed by paired comparison *t*-tests are indicated by * for $p < 0.05$, ** for $p < 0.01$, and *** for $p < 0.001$. *p*-values for the interaction between factors group (vegetarian and control group) and time (0 and 12 weeks) assessed by repeated measures. ANOVA are: $p = 0.048$ for maximal performance (**A**), $p = 0.004$ for maximal oxygen consumption, VO_{2max} (**B**), $p = 0.067$ for resting energy expenditure (**C**), $p = 0.666$ for respiratory quotient (**D**), $p = 0.793$ for fasting oxidation of fats (**E**), $p = 0.024$ for fasting oxidation of carbohydrates (**F**), and $p = 0.082$ for fasting oxidation of protein (**G**).

4. Discussion

Our results show a slight improvement in physical fitness after a 12-week aerobic training program with a vegetarian diet compared with a conventional hypocaloric diet. David Nieman demonstrated in his review in 1999 [11] that vegetarianism and veganism do not diminish physical fitness. Several studies showed that endurance athletes and marathon runners might benefit from plant-based diets with an emphasis on high-carbohydrate and antioxidant-rich foods such as pasta, grains, cereals, legumes, vegetables, and dried fruits [12,13].

Numerous comparative studies reveal no fundamental differences in morphological or enzymatic equipment of skeletal muscle in vegetarians/vegans compared to omnivores [14,15]. In our study, we showed that visceral fat decreased more in V compared to C [3]. This might suggest the possible decrease of ectopic fat in the muscle, potentially related to improved physical fitness. Several studies reported lower levels of intramyocellular fat in vegetarians/vegans, implying their improved insulin sensitivity. However, the impact of this finding on physical fitness is unclear. Given the described athlete's paradox [6], where trained athletes have more intramyocellular fat than healthy subjects, and even more than those with type 2 diabetes, it is questionable if lower intramyocellular fat content can be expected to be related to better fitness.

Abete et al. showed that a diet with a lower glycemic index increases mitochondrial oxidation [16], which corresponds with our findings. Plant-based diets with an emphasis on whole plant foods have a low glycemic index due to the high fiber content [17]. In addition, it seems that participants in V were able to better utilize carbohydrates compared to the control group. Together with the increased insulin sensitivity demonstrated previously [3], these are markers of improved metabolic flexibility, which may partly explain the increased maximal performance and VO_{2max} in V.

Besides physiological mechanisms, we need to mention the potential role of psychological factors. We observed reduced hunger and a reduced Beck depressive score in V [18], pointing to a higher executive potential including a positive attitude toward exercise. This hypothesis is also supported by lower levels of leptin in V [3], which may potentiate readiness for physical activity through the central nervous system [19].

The strengths of the study are represented by the randomized, parallel design, providing all meals, and exercising under professional supervision. The study duration was reasonably long, allowing sufficient time for tracking the changes in response to the diet and exercise. However, the number of subjects and study duration preclude generalizing our study for free-living conditions. Further larger-scale, long-term studies are essential before offering recommendations in terms of vegetarian diet during aerobic exercise.

5. Conclusions

In conclusion, our results indicate that V leads more effectively to improvement in physical fitness than C after an aerobic exercise program. We have also observed a decrease in REE only in C in response to aerobic exercise. The lower glycemic index of V, the higher fasting oxidation of carbohydrates, and the possible increase in mitochondrial oxidation may be partly responsible for a trend toward greater REE with V after aerobic exercise. V might be a more convenient alternative in the nutritional treatment of T2D during an aerobic exercise program.

Acknowledgments: This work was supported by the project grant AZV15-27431A from Ministry of Health, Prague, Czech Republic, and Institutional Support MZCR 00023001 (IKEM, Prague, Czech Republic). We thank David Warren Hardekopf for great help with text corrections.

Author Contributions: J.V., H.K. and T.P. designed the study, wrote the grant application, recruited the patients, collected the data and wrote the manuscript. M.M. was involved in acquisition and analyses of data. M.H. carried out the statistical analyses and interpretation of data. All authors had full access to the data and revised and approved the manuscript for publication. The guarantor is H.K.

Conflicts of Interest: The author declares no conflict of interest.

References

1. American Diabetes Association. Nutrition Recommendations and Interventions for Diabetes: A position statement of the American Diabetes Association. *Diabetes Care* **2008**, *31*, S61–S78.
2. Barnard, N.D.; Cohen, J.; Jenkins, D.J.; Turner-McGrievy, G.; Gloede, L.; Jaster, B.; Seidl, K.; Green, A.A.; Talpers, S. A low-fat vegan diet improves glycemic control and cardiovascular risk factors in a randomized clinical trial in individuals with type 2 diabetes. *Diabetes Care* **2006**, *29*, 1777–1783. [CrossRef] [PubMed]
3. Kahleova, H.; Matoulek, M.; Malinska, H.; Oliyarnik, O.; Kazdova, L.; Neskudla, T.; Skoch, A.; Hajek, M.; Hill, M.; Kahle, M.; et al. Vegetarian diet improves insulin resistance and oxidative stress markers more than conventional diet in subjects with Type 2 diabetes. *Diabet Med.* **2011**, *28*, 549–559. [CrossRef] [PubMed]
4. Nicholson, A.S.; Sklar, M.; Barnard, N.D.; Gore, S.; Sullivan, R.; Browning, S. Toward improved management of NIDDM: A randomized, controlled, pilot intervention using a lowfat, vegetarian diet. *Prev. Med.* **1999**, *29*, 87–91. [CrossRef] [PubMed]
5. Goff, L.M.; Bell, J.D.; So, P.W.; Dornhorst, A.; Frost, G.S. Veganism and its relationship with insulin resistance and intramyocellular lipid. *Eur. J. Clin. Nutr.* **2005**, *59*, 291–298. [CrossRef] [PubMed]
6. Dubé, J.J.; Amati, F.; Stefanovic-Racic, M.; Toledo, F.G.; Sauers, S.E.; Goodpaster, B.H. Exercise-induced alterations in intramyocellular lipids and insulin resistance: The athlete's paradox revisited. *Am. J. Physiol. Endocrinol. Metab.* **2008**, *294*, E882–E888. [CrossRef] [PubMed]
7. Ferrannini, E. The theoretical bases of indirect calorimetry: A review. *Metabolism* **1988**, *37*, 287–301. [CrossRef]
8. Mann, J.I.; De Leeuw, I.; Hermansen, K.; Karamanos, B.; Karlström, B.; Katsilambros, N.; Riccardi, G.; Rivellese, A.A.; Rizkalla, S.; Slama, G.; et al. Evidence-based nutritional approaches to the treatment and prevention of diabetes mellitus. *Nutr. Metab. Cardiovasc. Dis.* **2004**, *14*, 373–394. [CrossRef]
9. Stunkard, A.J.; Messick, S. The three-factor eating questionnaire to measure dietary restraint, disinhibition and hunger. *J. Psychosom. Res.* **1985**, *29*, 71–83. [CrossRef]

10. Steer, R.A.; Cavalieri, T.A.; Leonard, D.M.; Beck, A.T. Use of the Beck depression inventory for primary care to screen for major depression disorders. *Gen. Hosp. Psychiatry* **1999**, *21*, 106–111. [CrossRef]
11. Nieman, D.C. Physical fitness and vegetarian diets: Is there a relation? *Am. J. Clin. Nutr.* **1999**, *70*, 570S–575S. [PubMed]
12. Eisinger, M.; Plath, M.; Jung, K.; Leitymann, C. Nutrient intake of endurance runners with ovo-lacto-vegetarian diet and regular western diet. *Z. Ernahrung.* **1994**, *33*, 217–229. [CrossRef]
13. Nieman, D.C.; Butler, J.V.; Pollett, L.M.; Dietrich, S.J.; Lutz, R.D. Nutrient intake of marathon runners. *J. Am. Diet Assoc.* **1989**, *89*, 1273–1278. [PubMed]
14. Haub, M.D.; Wells, A.M.; Tarnopolsky, M.A.; Campbell, W.W. Effect of protein source on resistive-training-induced changes in body composition and muscle size in older men. *Am. J. Clin. Nutr.* **2002**, *76*, 511–517. [PubMed]
15. Gojda, J.; Patková, J.; Jaček, M.; Potočková, J.; Trnka, J.; Kraml, P.; Anděl, M. Higher insulin sensitivity in vegans is not associated with higher mitochondrial density. *Eur. J. Clin. Nutr.* **2013**, *67*, 1310–1315. [CrossRef] [PubMed]
16. Abete, I.; Parra, D.; Martinez, J.A. Energy-restricted diets based on a distinct food selection affecting the glycemic index induce different weight loss and oxidative response. *Clin. Nutr.* **2008**, *27*, 545–551. [CrossRef] [PubMed]
17. Kahleova, H.; Pelikanova, T. Vegetarian diets in the prevention and treatment of type 2 diabetes. *J. Am. Coll. Nutr.* **2015**, *34*, 448–458. [CrossRef] [PubMed]
18. Kahleova, H.; Hrachovinova, T.; Hill, M.; Pelikanova, T. Vegetarian diet in type 2 diabetes—Improvement in quality of life, mood and eating behaviour. *Diabet. Med.* **2013**, *30*, 127–129. [CrossRef] [PubMed]
19. Hsuchou, H.; Wang, Y.; Cornelissen-Guillaume, G.G.; Kastin, A.J.; Jang, E.; Halberg, F.; Pan, W. Diminished leptin signaling can alter circadian rhythm of metabolic activity and feeding. *J. Appl. Physiol.* **2013**, *115*, 995–1003. [CrossRef] [PubMed]

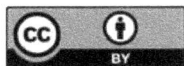

nutrients

Article

Dose-Response Relationship between Dietary Magnesium Intake and Risk of Type 2 Diabetes Mellitus: A Systematic Review and Meta-Regression Analysis of Prospective Cohort Studies

Xin Fang [1,*,†], Hedong Han [2,†], Mei Li [3], Chun Liang [3], Zhongjie Fan [4], Jan Aaseth [5,6], Jia He [2,*], Scott Montgomery [7,8,9] and Yang Cao [1,7]

[1]   Unit of Biostatistics, Institute of Environmental Medicine, Karolinska Institutet, Stockholm 17177, Sweden; yang.cao@ki.se
[2]   Department of Health Statistics, Second Military Medical University, Shanghai 200433, China; he_dong1102@126.com
[3]   Department of Cardiology, Shanghai Changzheng Hospital, Second Military Medical University, Shanghai 200003, China; happyxiaoant@126.com (M.L.); chunliangliang@hotmail.com (C.L.)
[4]   Department of Cardiology, Peking Union Medical College Hospital, Peking Union Medical College, Chinese Academy of Medical Sciences, Beijing 100730, China; Fan@pumch.cn
[5]   Faculty of Public Health, Hedmark University of Applied Sciences, Elverum 2411, Norway; jaol-aas@online.no
[6]   Innlandet Hospital Trust, Kongsvinger Hospital Division, Kongsvinger 2226, Norway
[7]   Clinical Epidemiology and Biostatistics, School of Medical Sciences, Örebro University, Örebro 70182, Sweden; scott.montgomery@regionorebrolan.se
[8]   Clinical Epidemiology Unit, Karolinska University Hospital, Karolinska Institutet, Stockholm 17177, Sweden
[9]   Department of Epidemiology and Public Health, University College London, London WC1E 6BT, UK
*   Correspondence: xin.fang@ki.se (X.F.); hejia63@yeah.net (J.H.); Tel.: +46-700-972-639 (X.F.); +86-21-8187-1441 (J.H.)
†   These authors contributed equally to this work.

Received: 12 October 2016; Accepted: 14 November 2016; Published: 19 November 2016

Abstract: The epidemiological evidence for a dose-response relationship between magnesium intake and risk of type 2 diabetes mellitus (T2D) is sparse. The aim of the study was to summarize the evidence for the association of dietary magnesium intake with risk of T2D and evaluate the dose-response relationship. We conducted a systematic review and meta-analysis of prospective cohort studies that reported dietary magnesium intake and risk of incident T2D. We identified relevant studies by searching major scientific literature databases and grey literature resources from their inception to February 2016. We included cohort studies that provided risk ratios, i.e., relative risks (RRs), odds ratios (ORs) or hazard ratios (HRs), for T2D. Linear dose-response relationships were assessed using random-effects meta-regression. Potential nonlinear associations were evaluated using restricted cubic splines. A total of 25 studies met the eligibility criteria. These studies comprised 637,922 individuals including 26,828 with a T2D diagnosis. Compared with the lowest magnesium consumption group in the population, the risk of T2D was reduced by 17% across all the studies; 19% in women and 16% in men. A statistically significant linear dose-response relationship was found between incremental magnesium intake and T2D risk. After adjusting for age and body mass index, the risk of T2D incidence was reduced by 8%–13% for per 100 mg/day increment in dietary magnesium intake. There was no evidence to support a nonlinear dose-response relationship between dietary magnesium intake and T2D risk. The combined data supports a role for magnesium in reducing risk of T2D, with a statistically significant linear dose-response pattern within the reference dose range of dietary intake among Asian and US populations. The evidence from Europe and black people is limited and more prospective studies are needed for the two subgroups.

Nutrients **2016**, *8*, 739

Keywords: magnesium; dietary intake; type 2 diabetes; prospective study; cohort study; meta-analysis

1. Introduction

Type 2 diabetes mellitus (T2D) represents a growing public health burden across the world and is a leading cause of death. In 2013, an estimated 340 million people worldwide had T2D and this number is expected to increase to 400 million or more by 2030 [1,2]. Obesity and diet are widely believed to play an important role in the development of T2D [3,4]. Magnesium is the most abundant divalent intracellular cation, the second most abundant cellular ion next to potassium and the fourth cation in general in the human body. Of the 21–28 g of magnesium present in the adult human body, 99% is distributed in the intracellular compartment, and only 1% in the extracellular fluid [5]. Magnesium has received considerable interest for its potential in improving insulin sensitivity and preventing diabetes [6–9]. T2D is often accompanied by altered magnesium status. An increased prevalence of magnesium deficit has been identified in T2D patients, especially in those with poorly controlled glycemic profiles, longer duration of disease and the presence of micro- and macro-vascular chronic complications [10–12]. A number of prospective cohort studies of magnesium intake and diabetes incidence have been conducted [7,13–24] and statistically significant negative associations between magnesium intake and risk of T2D were reported in previous meta-analyses [25–27]. However, these meta-analyses did not examine whether the association was confounded by other established risk factors such as being overweight and other factors highly associated with magnesium intake, such as amount of cereal fiber, and whether the relationship is linear.

During the past few years, the number of studies on this topic has increased. With mounting evidence, we conducted a meta-analysis of prospective cohort studies for the following purpose: (1) to update the epidemiological evidence on the association between magnesium intake and T2D risk; (2) to evaluate the association according to characteristics of study designs and population; and (3) to examine the linear and nonlinear dose-response pattern of magnesium intake and T2D risk.

2. Materials and Methods

The protocol for this systematic review was registered in the PROSPERO database of prospectively registered systematic reviews in February 2016 (www.crd.york.ac.uk/PROSPERO; CRD42016033519). The completed review conforms to the standard criteria PRISMA (Preferred Reporting Items for Systematic Reviews and Meta-Analysis) and MOOSE (Meta-analysis of Observational Studies in Epidemiology) [28,29].

2.1. Data Sources and Searches

We conducted a systematic review for all population-based studies that evaluated the association of magnesium intake with T2D. We searched Pubmed (http://www.ncbi.nlm.nih.gov/), Web of Science (http://webofscience.com/), ScienceDirect (http://www.sciencedirect.com/) and China Knowledge Resource Integrated Database (http://oversea.cnki.net/kns55/default.aspx) and the Cochrane Library (http://www.cochranelibrary.com/) from their inception to 29 February, 2016. The later cut-off date to 30 June 2016 was subsequently revised to include the latest published studies. To avoid publication bias, we also used the National Library of Medicine Gateway (https://gateway.nlm.nih.gov/), Virtual Health Library (http://pesquisa.bvsalud.org/portal/), the System for Information on Grey Literature in Europe (http://www.opengrey.eu/), the National Academic Research and Collaborations Information System (http://www.narcis.nl/?Language=en) and Grey Literature Report (www.greylit.org) to find potential unpublished relevant studies. Key search terms included magnesium intake, type 2 diabetes, diabetes mellitus, prospective study, longitudinal study, cohort study, and nested case-control study, combined with incidence or risk. These searches were supplemented by hand-searching of the reference lists of identified research articles or relevant reviews. No language restrictions were imposed.

2.2. Inclusion Criteria

We only included original research in this meta-analysis. Reviews, editorials, commentaries and letters were not eligible. All population-based cohort studies (including nested case-control studies) were included if they fulfilled the following criteria: (1) had a prospective study design; (2) the doses of magnesium intake (dietary and supplemental) were reported; (3) the endpoint of interest was incidence of T2D; (4) the risk ratio was reported such as relative risk (RR), odds ratio (OR) or hazard ratio (HR), as well as the associated 95% confidence interval (CI) or other data to estimate the variance or accuracy (standard deviation or standard error) were reported; (5) the risk assessment had to be adjusted for potential confounding factors or by other forms of standardization (if applicable). For multiple studies using the same population, only the study with the largest number of events or with adjustment for additional potential confounders was included. Studies were excluded if they: (1) focused on the populations with disrupted mineral homeostasis (such as patients with heart failure or kidney disease); (2) were narrative reviews, editorial papers, methodological papers, experimental studies, case control or cross-sectional; (3) assessed type 1 diabetes; (4) identified a dietary pattern that did not fit into healthy or unhealthy dietary pattern categories; (5) evaluated magnesium only in drinking water or had no reliable magnesium estimates. For included studies only in abstract form, we tried to contact authors to obtain the necessary estimates or risks and relevant accuracy.

2.3. Quality Assessment and Data Extraction

Computerized bibliographic searches of pre-determined literature databases used an optimized version of the Cochrane Collaboration search strategy [30]. Three investigators (X.F., C.L. and M.L.) screened all the identified titles and abstracts for relevance (n = 2858). Full papers were downloaded for all the abstracts judged potentially relevant (n = 60). No new studies were identified among the cited references of all included articles. Of 60 full-text articles reviewed independently, we excluded 35 studies for the following reasons: they were not prospective studies (n = 14); outcomes were not T2D (n = 9); did not report dietary magnesium (n = 7); did not assess the risk (n = 3); or duplicated another study (n = 1). All papers identified through the screening process were assessed for relevance independently by two investigators (C.L. and M.L.) using standardized study assessment and a sorting form. The studies were evaluated and scored based on the guidelines adapted from the tools for assessing quality and susceptibility to bias in observational studies in epidemiology [31]. Inter-rater agreement was substantial (Cohen κ > 0.6) [32]. No studies were excluded by the quality assessment. In total, 25 studies met the inclusion criteria and were included in the meta-analysis.

Full papers were obtained for all abstracts judged potentially relevant. Data extraction was conducted independently by two investigators (X.F. and M.L.) with the use of a standardized electronic form in Microsoft Excel. The following data were extracted from each study: first author's surname; study design; location; year the study started, finished and was published; age; sex; ethnicity; sample size (number of those with T2D and the total number of participants); diseases present at baseline (hypertension or hypercholesterolemia, etc.); magnesium intake modes (dietary or supplemental) and dose; as well as covariates adjusted for in the multivariable analysis. For magnesium intake, data on assessment method used (food frequency questionnaire, dietary recall, other) and whether the data were energy-adjusted (yes, no) were obtained. For each study, the median magnesium intake for each quantile (tertile, quartile or quintile) of magnesium intake was assigned as the representative dose. When the median intake per quantile was not provided, we assigned the midpoint of lower and upper boundaries in each quantile as the average intake. If the lower or upper boundary for the lowest or highest quantile, respectively, was not reported, we assumed that the boundary has the same amplitude as the closest quantile. The increment of dietary magnesium intake was calculated as the difference between the representative dose of the higher quantiles and the representative dose of the control quantile.

For each dose quantile, we extracted RR, OR or HR with their measure of uncertainty (standard error) or variance (95% CI). Risk estimates for continuous exposure were also extracted. If estimates were presented for more than one multivariate model, we only extracted estimates from the model maximally adjusted for potential confounding variables to ensure a conservative conclusion. Because there are studies based on the same cohort but conducted at different times, they shared the T2D patients. When we calculated the total participants and T2D cases, we only used the studies with the largest numbers.

2.4. Statistical Analysis

We used OR and HR as RR in our pooled analysis because when event rates are small, the OR, HR and RR approximate one another [33]. We estimated a pooled risk with 95% CI for a 100 mg/day increase in daily magnesium intake for the studies. To maximize all the data for calculating the pooled dose-response, the restricted maximum likelihood (REML) approach proposed by Harbord [34], which provides improved estimation of the between-study variance, was used to compute the linear trend of the log transformed risk estimates across magnesium intake doses. We also performed subgroup analysis by level of magnesium intake increment, sex, geographic area and adjustment.

The Higgins's I^2 statistic, a quantitative measure of inconsistency, was calculated to evaluate the statistical heterogeneity across the studies [35]. $I^2 > 30\%$ was considered as at least moderate heterogeneity. In view of substantial heterogeneity being detected, we presented the pooled estimates based on the random-effects model.

Potential publication bias was assessed by Egger's test [36]. Because the sample sizes of reference groups and comparative groups were balanced in all the studies, we used Harbord's modification to Egger's test to reduce the false-positive rate [37]. The results were also confirmed by Begg's test [38] and Peters's test [39].

Potential nonlinear associations were assessed using restricted cubic splines; we used four knots at fixed percentiles 5%, 35%, 65% and 95% of the distribution [40]. The study-specific estimates were pooled by using the REML method in a random-effects meta-analysis [41].

We also conducted a sensitivity analysis to investigate the influence of a single study on the overall risk estimate by dropping one study in each turn. We performed all analyses in Stata (version 14.1; Stata Corp., College Station, TX, USA). A p value < 0.05 was considered statistically significant, except where otherwise specified.

3. Results

3.1. Eligible Studies and Characteristics

Our literature search identified 25 studies from 17 cohorts that met the eligibility criteria (Figure 1). These studies were published between 1997 and 2014 and comprised 637,922 individuals and 26,828 T2D cases after excluding duplicated cohorts (Table 1). There were 16 studies conducted in the U.S. (including Hawaii), two in Europe (Italy and Germany), and seven in Asia (five in Japan and two in China). Studies treated dietary calcium [42–44], red/processed meat [45,46], whole grain [47], fiber [14,15,48], vitamin D [43,44], carbohydrates [14], coffee [49] or glycemic load [15,48,50] as main exposures, but also reported dietary magnesium intakes which were included in our meta-analysis. The main endpoints of two studies were impaired insulin metabolism [7] and insulin resistance [22], but both studies also reported the incidence of T2D. Participants were predominately middle-aged at baseline, with a mean age of 51.2 years and a mean BMI of 25.0 kg/m^2 across the studies. The length of the follow-up period ranged from four to 20 years.

Dietary intake of magnesium was evaluated by food frequency questionnaires (FFQs) in all the studies and 13 studies indicated that the questionnaires were validated. The median magnesium intake of the different dose groups ranged from 115 mg/day in U.S. black women [18] (much lower than the US Recommended Dietary Allowance of 400 mg/day for men and 310 magnesium for women >30 years [51]) to 478 mg/day in a U.S. population [22]. T2D was ascertained by self-report and 21 studies indicated that the self-reported diagnoses were validated.

For the 16 studies with the magnesium as the main exposure, although the degree of covariate and confounder adjustment varied in the multivariate models, most studies adjusted for age, body mass index (BMI), total energy intake, smoking, physical activity, family history of diabetes and hypertension; fewer studies adjusted for intake of calcium or other nutrition supplement and education attainment. For the nine studies with other nutrients as main exposure, only crude RRs were extracted.

Table 1. Characteristics of 25 cohort studies providing risk estimates for dietary magnesium intake and T2D incidence.

First Author, Year, Study, Country	No. of Case (Cohort Size)	Years of Follow-Up	Dietary Assessment Method	Case Ascertainment	Sex, Mean Age at Baseline (Years)	Magnesium Intake (Magnesium/Day) for Highest vs. the Lowest Quantile [RR (95% CI)]	Confounders Adjusted for
Hruby, 2014, FHSO, U.S. [7]	179 (2582)	7	Validated FFQ	Validated self-report	M and F, 53.9	395 vs. 236 (0.49 (0.27, 0.88))	Age, sex, energy intake, family history of diabetes, BMI, physical activity, smoking, alcohol, hypertension, dietary fiber
Oba, 2013, JPHCPS, Japan [50]	Men: 690 (27,769)	5	Validated FFQ	Validated self-report	M: 56.5	349 vs. 232 (0.85 (0.69, 1.06))	Crude *
	Women: 500 (36,864)				F: 56.9	356 vs. 211 (0.69 (0.54, 0.88))	
Hata, 2013, Hisayama, Japan [52]	417 (1999)	15.6	FFQ	Self-report	M and F, 57.0	215 vs. 133 (0.63 (0.44, 0.90))	Age, sex, family history of diabetes, BMI, HDL-cholesterol, triglycerides, hypertension, smoking, alcohol, physical activity, total energy intake, carbohydrate, crude fiber, saturated fatty acid, polyunsaturated fatty acid and vitamin C
Weng, 2012, CVDFACTS, Taiwan [53]	141 (1604)	4.6	Validated FFQ	Self-report	M and F, 50.0	406 vs. 212 (0.38 (0.21, 0.70))	Age, sex, caloric intake, residential area, family history of diabetes, BMI, education, smoking, alcohol, physical activity, hypertension, hypercholesterolemia, hypertriglyceridemia, low HDL-cholesterol
Hopping, 2010, MEC, Hawaii [21]	Men: 4555 (36,255)	14	FFQ	Validated self-report	M: 57.4	185 vs. 129 (0.77 (0.70, 0.85))	Ethnicity, BMI, physical activity, education, calories
	Women: 4032 (39,255)				F: 57.2	200 vs. 139 (0.84 (0.76, 0.93))	
Kirii, 2010, JACC, Japan [23]	Men: 237 (6480)	5	Validated FFQ	Validated self-report	M: 53.3	323 vs. 156 (0.64 (0.44, 0.91))	Age, BMI, family history of diabetes, smoking, alcohol, physical activity, green tea, coffee, total energy intake
	Women: 222 (11,112)				F: 53.1	298 vs. 159 (0.68 (0.33, 0.75))	
Nanri, 2010, JPHCPS, Japan [24]	Men: 634 (25,872)	5	FFQ	Validated self-report	M: 56.5	348 vs. 213 (0.86 (0.63, 1.16))	Age, study area, BMI, smoking, alcohol, family history of diabetes, physical activity, hypertension, coffee, calcium intake, total energy intake
	Women: 480 (33,919)				F: 57.3	333 vs. 213 (0.92 (0.66, 1.28))	
Kim, 2010, CARDIA, U.S. [22]	330 (4497)	20	Validated FFQ	Validated self-report	M and F, 24.9	478 vs. 362 (0.53 (0.32, 0.86))	Age, sex, ethnicity, study center, education, smoking, alcohol, physical activity, family history of diabetes, BMI, blood pressure, total energy intake, saturated fat, crude fiber
Kirii, 2009, JPHCPS, Japan [43]	Men: 634 (25,877)	5	FFQ	Validated self-report	M: 56.5	331 vs. 245 (0.89 (0.72, 1.10))	Crude
	Women: 480 (33,919)				F: 57.3	314 vs. 248 (0.76 (0.59, 0.98))	
Villegas, 2009, SWHS, China [20]	2270 (64,190)	7	Validated FFQ	Self-report	F: 51.0	318 vs. 214 (0.86 (0.75, 0.97))	Age, energy intake, WHR, smoking, alcohol, physical activity, income, education level, occupation, hypertension
Schulze, 2007, EPIC, Germany [19]	844 (27,550)	7	Validated FFQ	Validated self-report	M and F, 49.6	359 vs. 298 (0.75 (0.60, 0.94))	Crude
Liu, 2006, WHS, U.S. [42]	651 (14,874)	10	Validated FFQ	Validated self-report	F: 54.5	340 vs. 307 (0.88 (0.76, 1.04))	Crude
Pereira, 2006, IWHS, U.S. [49]	1415 (28,812)	11	FFQ	Validated self-report	F: 61.3	334 vs. 281 (0.60 (0.47, 0.76))	Crude

Table 1. *Cont.*

First Author, Year, Study, Country	No. of Case (Cohort Size)	Years of Follow-Up	Dietary Assessment Method	Case Ascertainment	Sex, Mean Age at Baseline (Years)	Magnesium Intake (Magnesium/Day) for Highest vs. the Lowest Quantile [RR (95% CI)]	Confounders Adjusted for
van Dam, 2006, BWHS, U.S. [18]	1964 (41,186)	8	Validated FFQ	Validated self-report	F: 38.7	244 vs. 115 (0.65 (0.54, 0.78))	Age, energy intake, BMI, smoking, alcohol, physical activity, family diabetes history, education level, calcium, coffee, sugar, soft drink, processed meat, red meat
Pittas, 2006, NHS, U.S. [44]	4843 (83,779)	20	FFQ	Validated self-report	F: 46.1	313 vs. 281 (0.79 (0.64, 0.96))	Crude
Song, 2004, WHS, U.S. [45]	708 (14,924)	8.8	Validated FFQ	Validated self-report	F: 53.9	377 vs. 305 (0.47 (0.41, 0.55))	Crude
Song 2004, WHS, U.S. [17]	918 (38,025)	6	Validated FFQ	Validated self-report	F: 53.9	399 vs. 252 (0.88 (0.71, 1.1))	Age, smoking, BMI, exercise, alcohol, family history of diabetes and total calories
Lopez-Ridaura, 2004, NHS, U.S. [16]	4085 (85,060)	18	FFQ	Validated self-report	F: 46.1	373 vs. 222 ((0.73 (0.65, 0.82))	Age, energy, family history of diabetes, BMI, physical activity, smoking, alcohol, hypertension, hypercholesterolemia, other dietary variables
Lopez-Ridaura, 2004, HPFS, U.S. [16]	1333 (42,872)	12	FFQ	Validated self-report	M: 53.3	457 vs. 270 (0.72 (0.58, 0.89))	Age, energy, family history of diabetes, BMI, physical activity, smoking, alcohol, hypertension, hypercholesterolemia, other dietary variables
Hodge, 2004, MCCS, Italy [15]	365 (31,641)	4	FFQ	Validated self-report	M and F: 54.5	Per 500 magnesium increment (0.73 (0.51, 1.04))	Age, sex, country of birth, physical activity, family history of diabetes, alcohol, education, weight change, energy intake, BMI and WHR
Schulze, 2003, NHS II, U.S. [46]	741 (92,146)	8	Validated FFQ	Validated self-report	F: 36.0	341 vs. 281 [0.26 (0.20, 0.36)]	Crude
Liu, 2000, NHS, U.S. [47]	1879 (75,521)	10	Validated FFQ	Validated self-report	F: 56.5	342 vs. 248 (1.04 (0.90, 1.19))	Crude
Meyer, 2000, IWHS, U.S. [14]	1141 (35,988)	6	FFQ	Validated self-report	F: 61.5	362 vs. 220 (0.67 (0.55, 0.82))	Age, total energy intake, BMI, WTH ratio, education, smoking, alcohol intake, physical activity
Kao, 1999, ARIC, U.S. [13]	White people: 739 (9506)	6	FFQ	Validated self-report	M and F: 54.2	418 vs. 308 (1.25 (0.88, 0.1.78))	Age, sex education, family history of diabetes, BMI, WHR, physical activity, alcohol, diuretic use, dietary calcium, potassium, fasting insulin and glucose
Kao, 1999, ARIC, U.S. [13]	Black people: 367 (2622)				M and F: 53.0	374 vs. 264 (1.05 (0.58, 1.93))	
Salmeron, 1997, HPFS, U.S. [48]	523 (42,759)	6	FFQ	Validated self-report	M: 53.3	461 vs. 262 (0.72 (0.54, 0.96))	Age, BMI, alcohol, smoking, physical activity, family history of diabetes
Salmeron, 1997, NHS, U.S. [54]	915 (65,173)	6	FFQ	Validated self-report	F: 46.1	338 vs. 222 (0.62 (0.50, 0.78))	Age, BMI, alcohol, smoking, physical activity, family history of diabetes

* Simple risk ratio without any adjustment.

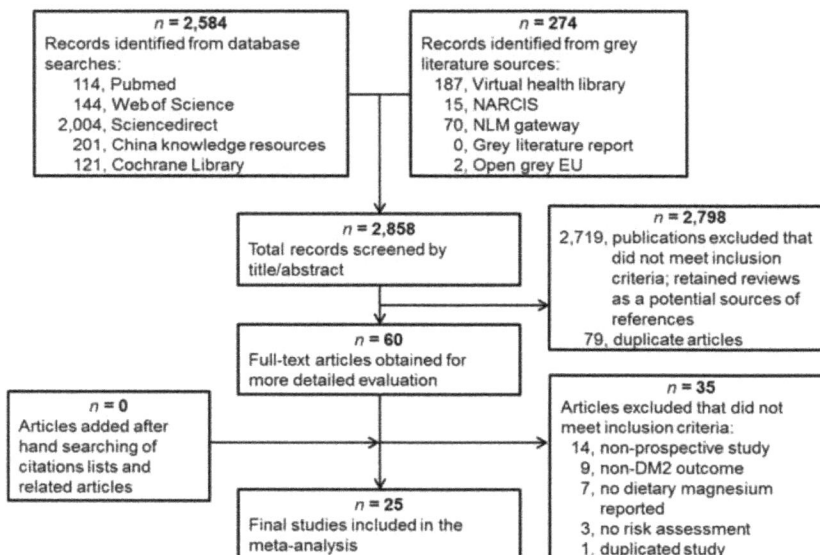

Figure 1. Screening and selection of articles on dietary magnesium intake and risk of type 2 diabetes mellitus.

3.2. Dietary Magnesium Intake and Type 2 Diabetes Mellitus (T2D) Incidence

We divided the increment of dietary magnesium intake into four categories, i.e., <50 mg/day, 50–99 mg/day, 100–149 mg/day and ≥150 mg/day, by subtracting the reference doses from the compared doses. Heterogeneity was found by Higgins's test, with I^2 = 73.3% ($p < 0.001$) for all compared doses, and 67.2% ($p < 0.001$), 75.0% ($p < 0.001$), 52.3% ($p = 0.005$) and 54.5% ($p = 0.031$) for four increment categories, respectively. However, the approximately symmetric funnel plot of all but four doses suggests a moderate homogeneity among the studies (Figure 2). Although there is evidence of publication bias among all compared doses for Egger's test ($p = 0.002$), Begg's, Harbord's and Peters's tests show no evidence of publication bias ($p = 0.170, 0.401$ and 0.105, respectively).

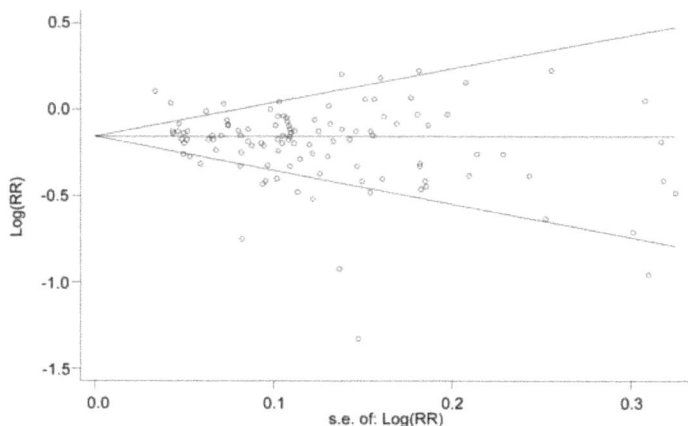

Figure 2. Funnel plot with pseudo 95% confidence limits.

The overall combined RR for T2D incidence is 0.83 (95% CI: 0.80, 0.86; $p < 0.001$) for all compared doses. The results of subgroup analysis are presented in Table 2. A statistically significant negative association between dietary magnesium and risk of T2D incidence was observed across sexes and the pooled RRs are 0.81 (95% CI: 0.77, 0.86) for women, 0.84 (95% CI: 0.80, 0.88) for men, and 0.85 (95% CI: 0.78, 0.94) for the studies that only reported sex-combined risk estimates. The association was statistically significant in all the study areas and the largest magnitude association was found among U.S. studies (pooled RR = 0.82 in U.S. vs. 0.86 in Europe and 0.85 in Asia), compared with the unadjusted associations (pooled RR = 0.81; 95% CI: 0.74, 0.88), with lower magnitude after adjustment (pooled RR = 0.83; 95% CI: 0.81, 0.86). Two studies investigated the association specially in black people and showed a statistically significant association (pooled RR = 0.82; 95% CI: 0.71, 0.94), however, it seems this is mainly observed among black women [18] rather than black men [13].

Table 2. Pooled RRs * for T2D incidence of increased dietary magnesium intake by sex, area and adjustment.

Subgroup	No. of Studies (Dose Quantiles)	RR (95% CI)	I^2 (%)	Heterogeneity-p
Sex				
Women	17 (58)	0.814 (0.774, 0.856)	82.4	<0.001
Men	7 (25)	0.838 (0.803, 0.876)	25.7	0.120
Both	7 (26)	0.854 (0.775, 0.941)	46.7	0.005
Area				
U.S.	16 (67)	0.817 (0.780, 0.857)	81.7	<0.001
Europe	2 (5)	0.858 (0.774, 0.951)	0	0.498
Asia	7 (37)	0.846 (0.811, 0.883)	10.2	0.294
Adjustment				
Adjusted [†]	16 (76)	0.830 (0.806, 0.855)	39.6	<0.001
Crude [‡]	9 (33)	0.808 (0.741, 0.881)	87.8	<0.001
Black people	2 (7)	0.815 (0.711, 0.935)	59.3	0.022

* Random-effects model was used; † Adjusted for age, BMI, energy intake, smoking, alcohol, physical activity, calcium, sugar, soft drink, red meat family and/or other dietary intakes, and/or family history, sociodemographic factors; ‡ Simple risk ratio without any adjustment.

The dose-category-specific pooled RRs for T2D incidence from the included studies are shown in Figure 3a–d, which are 0.88 (95% CI: 0.85, 0.92), 0.81 (95% CI: 0.76, 0.86), 0.77 (95% CI: 0.70, 0.83) and 0.72 (95% CI: 0.61, 0.84) for increment <50 mg/day, 50–99 mg/day, 100–149 mg/day and ≥150 mg/day, respectively. In general, the RR decreases 4% to 7% per 50 mg/day increment (equivalent to 8% to 14% per 100 mg/day increment) in dietary magnesium intake.

3.3. Linear Dose-Response Relationship

After adjusting for age and BMI in random-effects meta-regression models, a statistically significant linear dose-response relationship between incremental dietary magnesium intake and T2D incidence was found across all the studies (see Table 3 and Figure 4). The RRs (95% CI) for the association of a 100 mg/day increment in dietary magnesium intake with T2D incidence are 0.92 (95% CI: 0.85, 0.99) and 0.88 (0.80, 0.97) for including and excluding one extreme dose, respectively. The statistically significant linear dose-response relationship was also found for men (RR = 0.87; 95% CI: 0.77, 0.98) but not for women (RR = 0.88; 95% CI = 0.76, 1.02). Regarding study areas, significantly linear dose-response relationship was only found in Asia (RR = 0.87; 95% CI: 0.77, 0.98). No significant linear dose-response relationship was found in black people (RR = 0.75; 95% CI = 0.23, 2.41).

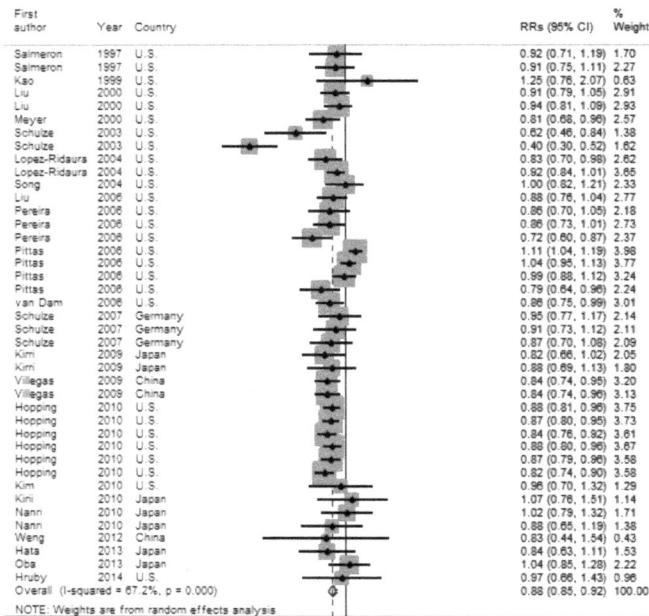

(a) Increment<50 mg/d

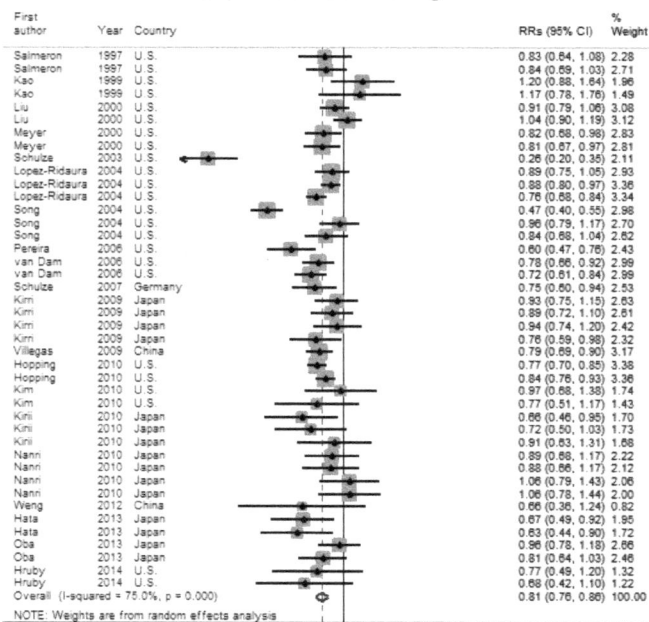

(b) Increment >=50 and <100 mg/d

Figure 3. *Cont.*

First author	Year	Country		RRs (95% CI)	% Weight
Salmeron	1997	U.S.		0.66 (0.49, 0.88)	5.01
Salmeron	1997	U.S.		0.82 (0.67, 1.01)	7.09
Salmeron	1997	U.S.		0.62 (0.50, 0.77)	6.83
Kao	1999	U.S.		1.23 (0.93, 1.61)	5.46
Kao	1999	U.S.		1.05 (0.58, 1.93)	1.74
Meyer	2000	U.S.		0.67 (0.55, 0.82)	7.25
Lopez-Ridaura	2004	U.S.		0.66 (0.55, 0.80)	7.60
Song	2004	U.S.		0.88 (0.71, 1.10)	6.72
van Dam	2006	U.S.		0.65 (0.54, 0.78)	7.70
Villegas	2009	China		0.86 (0.76, 0.98)	9.38
Kim	2010	U.S.		0.53 (0.32, 0.87)	2.42
Kirii	2010	Japan		0.68 (0.45, 1.03)	3.22
Nanri	2010	Japan		0.86 (0.63, 1.17)	4.77
Nanri	2010	Japan		0.92 (0.66, 1.28)	4.31
Weng	2012	China		0.62 (0.33, 1.17)	1.59
Oba	2013	Japan		0.85 (0.69, 1.06)	6.86
Oba	2013	Japan		0.77 (0.61, 0.98)	6.22
Oba	2013	Japan		0.69 (0.54, 0.88)	6.02
Overall (I-squared = 52.3%, p = 0.005)				0.77 (0.70, 0.83)	100.00

NOTE: Weights are from random effects analysis

(c) Increment >=100 and <150 mg/d

First author	Year	Country		RRs (95% CI) Weight
Salmeron	1997	U.S.		0.72 (0.54, 0.96) 14.13
Kao	1999	U.S.		1.25 (0.88, 1.78) 11.32
Hodge	2004	Italy		0.73 (0.51, 1.04) 11.28
Lopez-Ridaura	2004	U.S.		0.72 (0.58, 0.89) 17.90
Lopez-Ridaura	2004	U.S.		0.73 (0.65, 0.82) 23.37
Kirii	2010	Japan		0.64 (0.45, 0.92) 11.03
Weng	2012	China		0.38 (0.21, 0.70) 5.36
Hruby	2014	U.S.		0.49 (0.27, 0.88) 5.61
Overall (I-squared = 54.5%, p = 0.031)				0.72 (0.61, 0.84) 100.00

NOTE: Weights are from random effects analysis

(d) Increment >=150 mg/d

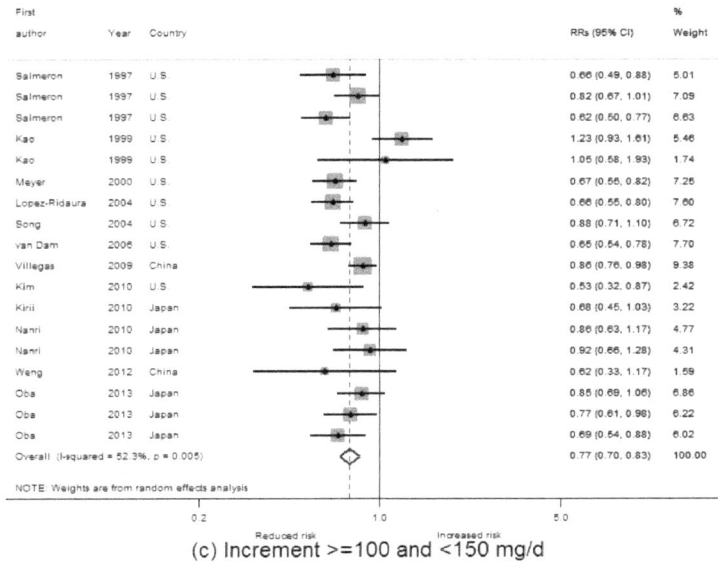

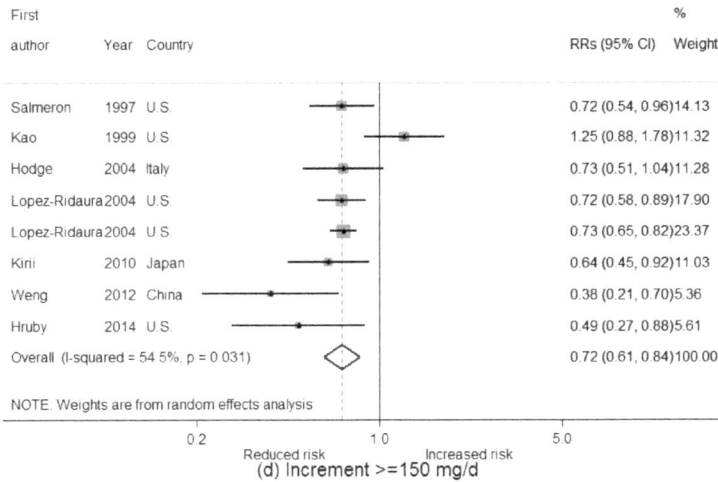

Figure 3. Relative risks (RRs) for risk of T2D incidence for different dietary magnesium increment categories: (**a**) <50 mg/day; (**b**) 50–99 mg/day; (**c**) 100–159 mg/day; (**d**) ≥150 mg/day.

Table 3. Estimated RRs for T2D incidence per 100 mg/day increment in dietary magnesium intake, adjusted for age and BMI.

	No. of Studies (Doses)	I^2 (%)	RR (95% CI)	*p*-Value
All studies	25 (105)	69.72	0.916 (0.852, 0.985)	0.018
All studies *	24 (104)	69.13	0.882 (0.803, 0.969)	0.010
Sex				
Women	17 (56)	78.87	0.879 (0.756, 1.023)	0.094
Men	7 (23)	0	0.865 (0.767, 0.975)	0.020
Both	7 (26)	26.51	0.935 (0.853, 1.026)	0.148
Both *	6 (25)	29.00	0.857 (0.695, 1.057)	0.141
Area				
U.S.	16 (63)	79.09	0.910 (0.796, 1.042)	0.169
Europe	2 (5)	0	1.071 (0.264, 4.351)	0.644
Europe *	1 (4)	-	-	-
Asia	7 (37)	0	0.867 (0.768, 0.978)	0.022
Adjustment				
Adjusted	16 (72)	25.73	0.911 (0.864, 0.961)	0.001
Adjusted *	15 (71)	24.09	0.885 (0.830, 0.944)	<0.001
Crude	9 (33)	85.14	0.653 (0.462, 0.924)	0.018
Black people	2 (7)	0	0.747 (0.232, 2.409)	0.486

* One extreme dose was excluded.

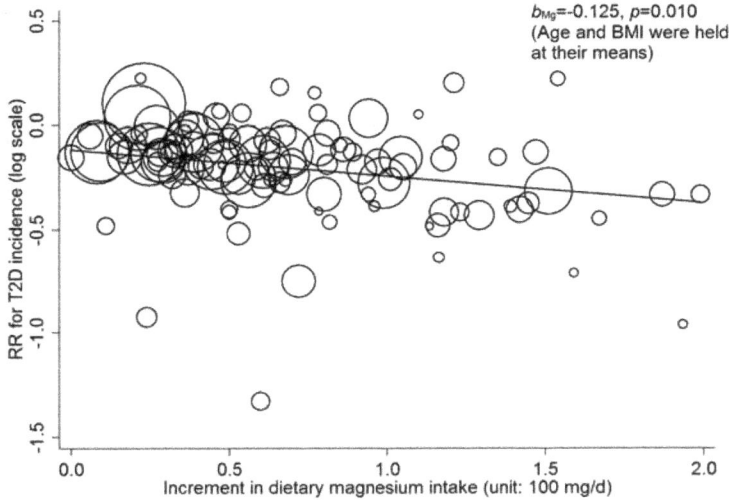

Figure 4. Dose-response relationship between risk of T2D incidence and incremental dietary magnesium intake (excluding one extreme dose). The size of the bubble reflects the study-specific analytical weight, i.e., the inverse of the variance.

In general, the risk of T2D incidence decreases by 8% (across all studies) to 13% (in the Asian population) per 100 mg/day increment in dietary magnesium intake, which is consistent with the result from dose-category-specific analysis.

3.4. Nonlinear Dose-Response Relationship

We found no evidence of nonlinear associations between dietary magnesium intake and T2D incidence across all the studies with ($p = 0.665$) or without ($p = 0.980$) one extreme dose (Figure 5), adjusting for age and BMI. For subgroup analysis, no evidence of nonlinear association was found for women ($p = 0.637$), men ($p = 0.790$), sex-combined ($p = 0.987$), black people ($p = 0.787$), U.S. population ($p = 0.686$), Asian population ($p = 0.519$), adjusted RRs ($p = 0.663$) and crude RRs ($p = 0.250$), which suggested that pooling the dose-response estimates from linear trend estimation for dietary magnesium intake and T2D incidence was appropriate. Because of insufficient dose observations, no nonlinear association was evaluated for European studies.

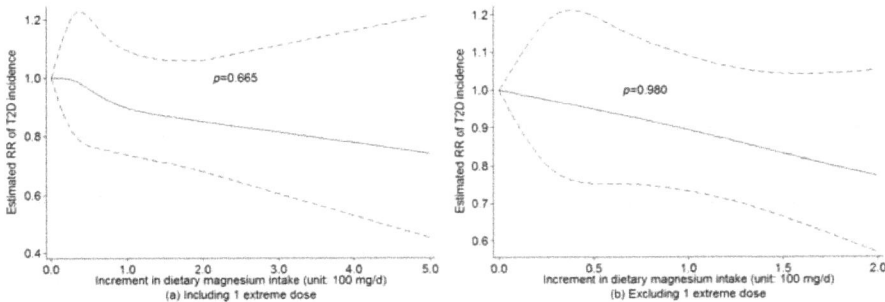

Figure 5. Examination of nonlinear association between increment in dietary magnesium intake and risk of T2D incidence by random-effects model with the use of restricted cubic splines.

3.5. Sensitivity Analysis

Regarding the combined risk of T2D incidence for all studies, the sensitivity analysis omitting one study at a time yielded statistically significant RRs within a very narrow range from 0.82 (95% CI: 0.79, 0.84) to 0.84 (95% CI: 0.81, 0.87). The subgroup analyses also showed robust results for women (RR range: 0.80, 0.84), men (RR range: 0.83, 0.85), sex-combined (RR range: 0.79, 0.88), U.S. population (RR range: 0.80, 0.84), Asian population (RR range: 0.83, 0.85), adjusted RRs (RR range: 0.82, 0.84) and crude RRs (RR range: 0.78, 0.86). However, because of a limited number of studies in Europe and black people, the sensitivity analysis generated relatively wide ranges for these two subgroups. The RR ranges were from 0.73 (95% CI: 0.51, 1.04) to 0.87 (95% CI: 0.78, 0.97) and from 0.76 (95% CI: 0.67, 0.85) to 1.17 (95% CI: 0.88, 1.54) for European studies and black people, respectively.

The sensitivity analyses for linear and nonlinear dose-response relationships between incremental dietary magnesium intake and the risk of T2D incidence show similar results. The RRs of linear dose-response relationship across all the studies are statistically significant and range from 0.88 (95% CI: 0.80, 0.97) to 0.93 (95% CI: 0.87, 1.00) when omitting one study at a time. The *p*-values for a nonlinear dose-response relationship across all studies range from 0.52 to 0.96 when omitting one study at a time. The results for subgroup analysis also change little except for European studies and black people (data not show). Overall, the results from sensitivity analyses indicate the robustness of our findings.

4. Discussion

This meta-analysis of 25 prospective studies showed a statistically significant negative association between dietary magnesium intake and T2D incidence. Compared with the lowest dietary magnesium consumption groups in the populations, the risk of T2D could be reduced by 19% in women and 16% in men (Table 2). The largest reduction of risk was observed for the U.S. population (18%). A statistically significant linear dose-response relationship was found between incremental dietary magnesium intake and T2D incidence across all the studies, in male and Asian populations, adjusting for age and BMI. The risk of T2D was associated with a reduction of 8%–13% per 100 g/day increment in dietary magnesium intake. After adjusting for age and BMI, we did not find a statistically significant nonlinear dose-response relationship of incremental dietary magnesium intake with T2D risk. The present systematic review, which includes a total of 637,922 participants and 26,828 T2D cases, provides the most robust evidence to date of the linear dose-response relationship between incremental dietary magnesium intake across its physiological range and risk of T2D.

4.1. Dose-Response Association of Dietary Magnesium Intake with T2D Incidence

A putative protective effect of magnesium intake against T2D incidence has been reported previously [13,14]. The negative association between magnesium intake and T2D incidence is biologically plausible and may be partially explained by its influence on glucose metabolism, insulin sensitivity and insulin action [5,6]. However, there is no conclusive evidence for the beneficial dose of dietary magnesium. For example, a meta-analysis indicated that 300 mg/day of magnesium intake was the essential dose for preventing T2D [27]. A cross-sectional study concluded that more than 300 mg/day of magnesium intake might not improve insulin sensitivity and have no influence [55]. Evidence from a prospective study showed that increased intake of magnesium might provide more benefit to participants with magnesium deficiency, as magnesium deficiency and hypomagnesaemia have been associated with the development of insulin resistance [18]. Meta-analyses of magnesium supplementation have also revealed conflicting results. A review including 12 randomized controlled trials (RCTs) assessing the efficacy of magnesium supplementation on insulin sensitivity and glucose levels included studies yielding inconsistent results [56]. However, concerning the effect of dietary magnesium intake on T2D incidence, the previous meta-analyses appeared to reach a consensus [19,25,27]. A meta-analysis of eight cohort studies showed a significant negative association (RR = 0.77; 95% CI: 0.72, 0.84). Another meta-analysis of 13 prospective cohort studies detected a significant negative association between magnesium intake and risk of T2D (RR = 0.78; 95% CI:

0.73, 0.84). A more recent meta-analysis with a total of 539,735 participants and 25,252 incident diabetes cases also indicated that magnesium intake was associated with a significant lower risk of T2D (RR = 0.77; 95% CI: 0.71, 0.82). However, there is less conclusive evidence of dose-response relationship between dietary magnesium intake and risk of T2D incidence [26]. By combining results of seven cohort studies, Larsson et al. observed a statistically significant lower risk of T2D for 100 mg/day increase in magnesium intake (RR = 0.85; 95% CI: 0.79, 0.92). Dong et al. also found a linear dose-response relationship for every 100 mg/day increment in magnesium intake (RR = 0.86; 95% CI: 0.82, 0.89) [25]. In contrast, a nonlinear relationship (p = 0.003) between magnesium intake and type 2 diabetes was reported by Xu et al. [27].

Our meta-analysis with a larger number of people with T2D did support existence of a statistically significant linear dose-response relationship between increased dose of dietary magnesium intake and T2D incidence among all the participants, especially in males and in Asian populations. In addition, we found no evidence of nonlinear associations between dietary magnesium intake and T2D incidence across all the studies (p = 0.665). The magnitude of the effect for 100 mg/day increment in magnesium intake in this meta-analysis (8%–13% reduction in risk of T2D) is comparable to those from other meta-analyses (8%–21% reduction in risk of T2D).

The discrepant findings between women and men might be due to the influence of other factors than magnesium intake. For example, the influence of magnesium on T2D incidence in women may be potentially attenuated by changed endogenous sex hormones in postmenopausal women [57,58]; which could accelerate T2D development and counteract the potentially protective influence of magnesium. The discrepancy between the Asian population and non-Asian population needs further research. However, because of the limited number of the included studies in Europe, the discrepancy may have been accidental and a chance finding cannot be ruled out.

It should be noted that our sensitivity analysis revealed robust associations for linear and nonlinear dose-response analyses among all the participants.

4.2. Implication for Practice

Magnesium is mainly consumed through diet, and low magnesium consumption is common worldwide. It has been estimated that magnesium intake in a normal Western diet is often inadequate for the body's needs; in the United States, 67% of women and 64% of men consume inadequate amounts of magnesium [59]. For people aged more than 30, the recommended dietary allowance (RDA) of magnesium for men and women is 350 mg/day and 420 mg/day, respectively [51]. On the basis of the studies we have reviewed, current evidence from population-based prospective cohort studies support the recommendation for increasing dietary magnesium intake.

4.3. Strengths and Limitations

The population-based evidence on whether increased magnesium intake may reduce T2D incidence is still sparse. To our knowledge, this study is the largest meta-analysis that investigated the dose-response relationship between dietary magnesium intake and T2D risk. It has several strengths. First, our data providing a systematic review of prospective studies represent the best available evidence of how dietary magnesium intake may influence risk of T2D incidence. Because of the lagged and cumulative effects of exposure on outcome of chronic diseases, the dose-response relationship without reversed causality would be revealed only by prospective studies rather than cross-sectional or retrospective studies. In addition, the prospective studies also minimized recall and selection bias. Second, by combining all available doses in included studies across a wide range of exposure, we increased the validity of the dose-response estimates. Our studies included 141 dietary magnesium doses and 108 risk estimates, which enabled us to estimate both linear and nonlinear dose-response relationship with a high statistical power. Third, age and BMI were adjusted for in our meta-regression model and stratified analyses were used for sex, study areas and adjustment, which reduced the potential confounding from demographic and other factors. Furthermore, the random-effects model considered the heterogeneity among studies, which resulted in a relatively conservative conclusion rather than an exaggerated one.

However, some limitations warrant consideration. First, although the majority of the studies adjusted for known risk factors for T2D incidence, such as age, BMI, smoking status, education, physical activity level and alcohol consumption, we could only retrieve age and BMI for all the studies and adjust only for them in our final model. The possible bias from residual confounders remained. Subgroup analyses that distinguish the studies with and without adjustment for these confounders would be informative. For example, we conducted the subgroup analysis for the studies adjusting for intake of cereal fiber; however, the overall RRs changed little, which were 0.892 (95% CI: 0.834, 0.954) and 0.916 (95% CI: 0.852, 0.985) for adjusted and unadjusted studies, respectively. Second, the magnesium intake in these studies were only assessed by FFQ, which do not capture the magnesium intake from drinking water and nutritional supplementation, and thereby might underestimate total magnesium intake and result in potential misclassification. However, the misclassification would most likely lead to an underestimated association. Third, influence of other nutrients or dietary components such as coffee [49], red meat [45], calcium [43] and fiber [14,19] that are correlated with dietary magnesium could not be excluded; other nutrients may have been responsible for the observed association partly or completely. Finally, publication bias may be a problem in our pooling analysis. Although we tried as much as possible to search for potential unpublished studies, no valid studies were identified from the available grey literature resources. However, the evidence (Harbord's $p = 0.401$) did not indicate notable publication bias in our meta-analysis.

5. Conclusions

In conclusion, results from this meta-analysis indicate that dietary magnesium intake is associated with a reduced risk of type 2 diabetes (T2D). The greatest magnitude in risk reduction was found in the US population. A statistically significant linear dose-response relationship was identified across all the studies, and the largest magnitude association was found in the Asian population. A 100 mg/day increment in dietary magnesium intake was associated with an 8%–13% reduction in risk of T2D. No nonlinear dose-response relationship was found between incremental dietary magnesium intake and T2D incidence. Regarding the dose-response relationship between dietary magnesium intake and T2D in populations in Africa and Europe, more evidence is needed.

Acknowledgments: X.F. is supported by the Karolinska Institutet doctoral research grant (KID-funds). Y.C. is supported by the Junior Faculty Research Grants (C62412022) of the Institute of Environmental Medicine, Karolinska Institutet, Sweden.

Author Contributions: Y.C. and J.A. designed the research; X.F. and J.H. provided study oversight and took primary responsibility for the final content of the manuscript; X.F., C.L. and M.L. undertook literature search, screening and data extraction; X.F. and H.H. performed statistical analysis; X.F. drafted the manuscript; Z.F. and S.M. revised the article critically; and all authors contributed to the manuscript writing, made critical revision, read and approved the final manuscript.

Conflicts of Interest: The authors declare no conflict of interest.

Abbreviations

CI	Confidence interval
FFQ	Food frequency questionnaires
HR	Hazard ratio
OR	Odds ratio
RCT	Randomized controlled trial
REML	Restricted maximum likelihood
RR	Relative risk
T2D	Type 2 diabetes
US	United States

References

1. Shaw, J.E.; Sicree, R.A.; Zimmet, P.Z. Global estimates of the prevalence of diabetes for 2010 and 2030. *Diabetes Res. Clin. Pract.* **2010**, *87*, 4–14. [CrossRef] [PubMed]
2. Shi, Y.; Hu, F.B. The global implications of diabetes and cancer. *Lancet* **2014**, *383*, 1947–1948. [CrossRef]
3. Colditz, G.A.; Manson, J.E.; Stampfer, M.J.; Rosner, B.; Willett, W.C.; Speizer, F.E. Diet and risk of clinical diabetes in women. *Am. J. Clin. Nutr.* **1992**, *55*, 1018–1023. [PubMed]
4. Knowler, W.C.; Barrett-Connor, E.; Fowler, S.E.; Hamman, R.F.; Lachin, J.M.; Walker, E.A.; Nathan, D.M. Reduction in the incidence of type 2 diabetes with lifestyle intervention or metformin. *N. Engl. J. Med.* **2002**, *346*, 393–403. [PubMed]
5. Barbagallo, M.; Dominguez, L.J. Magnesium metabolism in type 2 diabetes mellitus, metabolic syndrome and insulin resistance. *Arch. Biochem. Biophys.* **2007**, *458*, 40–47. [CrossRef] [PubMed]
6. Balon, T.W.; Jasman, A.; Scott, S.; Meehan, W.P.; Rude, R.K.; Nadler, J.L. Dietary magnesium prevents fructose-induced insulin insensitivity in rats. *Hypertension* **1994**, *23*, 1036–1039. [CrossRef] [PubMed]
7. Hruby, A.; Meigs, J.B.; O'Donnell, C.J.; Jacques, P.F.; McKeown, N.M. Higher magnesium intake reduces risk of impaired glucose and insulin metabolism and progression from prediabetes to diabetes in middle-aged Americans. *Diabetes Care* **2014**, *37*, 419–427. [CrossRef] [PubMed]
8. Bo, S.; Pisu, E. Role of dietary magnesium in cardiovascular disease prevention, insulin sensitivity and diabetes. *Curr. Opin. Lipidol.* **2008**, *19*, 50–56. [CrossRef] [PubMed]
9. Barbagallo, M.; Dominguez, L.J.; Galioto, A.; Ferlisi, A.; Cani, C.; Malfa, L.; Pineo, A.; Busardo, A.; Paolisso, G. Role of magnesium in insulin action, diabetes and cardio-metabolic syndrome X. *Mol. Asp. Med.* **2003**, *24*, 39–52. [CrossRef]
10. Ramadass, S.; Basu, S.; Srinivasan, A.R. Serum magnesium levels as an indicator of status of diabetes mellitus type 2. *Diabetes Metab. Syndr.* **2015**, *9*, 42–45. [CrossRef] [PubMed]
11. Ma, J.; Folsom, A.R.; Melnick, S.L.; Eckfeldt, J.H.; Sharrett, A.R.; Nabulsi, A.A.; Hutchinson, R.G.; Metcalf, P.A. Associations of serum and dietary magnesium with cardiovascular disease, hypertension, diabetes, insulin, and carotid arterial wall thickness: The aric study. Atherosclerosis risk in communities study. *J. Clin. Epidemiol.* **1995**, *48*, 927–940. [CrossRef]
12. Del Gobbo, L.C.; Song, Y.; Poirier, P.; Dewailly, E.; Elin, R.J.; Egeland, G.M. Low serum magnesium concentrations are associated with a high prevalence of premature ventricular complexes in obese adults with type 2 diabetes. *Cardiovasc. Diabetol.* **2012**, *11*, 23. [CrossRef] [PubMed]
13. Kao, W.H.; Folsom, A.R.; Nieto, F.J.; Mo, J.P.; Watson, R.L.; Brancati, F.L. Serum and dietary magnesium and the risk for type 2 diabetes mellitus: The atherosclerosis risk in communities study. *Arch. Intern. Med.* **1999**, *159*, 2151–2159. [CrossRef] [PubMed]
14. Meyer, K.A.; Kushi, L.H.; Jacobs, D.R., Jr.; Slavin, J.; Sellers, T.A.; Folsom, A.R. Carbohydrates, dietary fiber, and incident type 2 diabetes in older women. *Am. J. Clin. Nutr.* **2000**, *71*, 921–930. [PubMed]
15. Hodge, A.M.; English, D.R.; O'Dea, K.; Giles, G.G. Glycemic index and dietary fiber and the risk of type 2 diabetes. *Diabetes Care* **2004**, *27*, 2701–2706. [CrossRef] [PubMed]
16. Lopez-Ridaura, R.; Willett, W.C.; Rimm, E.B.; Liu, S.; Stampfer, M.J.; Manson, J.E.; Hu, F.B. Magnesium intake and risk of type 2 diabetes in men and women. *Diabetes Care* **2004**, *27*, 134–140. [CrossRef] [PubMed]
17. Song, Y.; Manson, J.E.; Buring, J.E.; Liu, S. Dietary magnesium intake in relation to plasma insulin levels and risk of type 2 diabetes in women. *Diabetes Care* **2004**, *27*, 59–65. [CrossRef] [PubMed]
18. Van Dam, R.M.; Hu, F.B.; Rosenberg, L.; Krishnan, S.; Palmer, J.R. Dietary calcium and magnesium, major food sources, and risk of type 2 diabetes in U.S. black women. *Diabetes Care* **2006**, *29*, 2238–2243. [CrossRef] [PubMed]
19. Schulze, M.B.; Schulz, M.; Heidemann, C.; Schienkiewitz, A.; Hoffmann, K.; Boeing, H. Fiber and magnesium intake and incidence of type 2 diabetes: A prospective study and meta-analysis. *Arch. Intern. Med.* **2007**, *167*, 956–965. [CrossRef] [PubMed]
20. Villegas, R.; Gao, Y.T.; Dai, Q.; Yang, G.; Cai, H.; Li, H.; Zheng, W.; Shu, X.O. Dietary calcium and magnesium intakes and the risk of type 2 diabetes: The Shanghai women's health study. *Am. J. Clin. Nutr.* **2009**, *89*, 1059–1067. [CrossRef] [PubMed]

21. Hopping, B.N.; Erber, E.; Grandinetti, A.; Verheus, M.; Kolonel, L.N.; Maskarinec, G. Dietary fiber, magnesium, and glycemic load alter risk of type 2 diabetes in a multiethnic cohort in Hawaii. *J. Nutr.* **2010**, *140*, 68–74. [CrossRef] [PubMed]

22. Kim, D.J.; Xun, P.; Liu, K.; Loria, C.; Yokota, K.; Jacobs, D.R., Jr.; He, K. Magnesium intake in relation to systemic inflammation, insulin resistance, and the incidence of diabetes. *Diabetes Care* **2010**, *33*, 2604–2610. [CrossRef] [PubMed]

23. Kirii, K.; Iso, H.; Date, C.; Fukui, M.; Tamakoshi, A. Magnesium intake and risk of self-reported type 2 diabetes among Japanese. *J. Am. Coll. Nutr.* **2010**, *29*, 99–106. [CrossRef] [PubMed]

24. Nanri, A.; Mizoue, T.; Noda, M.; Takahashi, Y.; Kirii, K.; Inoue, M.; Tsugane, S.; Japan Public Health Center-based Prospective Study Group. Magnesium intake and type ii diabetes in japanese men and women: The Japan public health center-based prospective study. *Eur. J. Clin. Nutr.* **2010**, *64*, 1244–1247. [CrossRef] [PubMed]

25. Dong, J.Y.; Xun, P.; He, K.; Qin, L.Q. Magnesium intake and risk of type 2 diabetes: Meta-analysis of prospective cohort studies. *Diabetes Care* **2011**, *34*, 2116–2122. [CrossRef] [PubMed]

26. Larsson, S.C.; Wolk, A. Magnesium intake and risk of type 2 diabetes: A meta-analysis. *J. Intern. Med.* **2007**, *262*, 208–214. [CrossRef] [PubMed]

27. Xu, T.; Chen, G.C.; Zhai, L.; Ke, K.F. Nonlinear reduction in risk for type 2 diabetes by magnesium intake: An updated meta-analysis of prospective cohort studies. *Biomed. Environ. Sci.* **2015**, *28*, 527–534. [PubMed]

28. Liberati, A.; Altman, D.G.; Tetzlaff, J.; Mulrow, C.; Gotzsche, P.C.; Ioannidis, J.P.A.; Clarke, M.; Devereaux, P.J.; Kleijnen, J.; Moher, D. The PRISMA statement for reporting systematic reviews and meta-analyses of studies that evaluate health care interventions: Explanation and elaboration. *PLoS Med.* **2009**, *6*, e1000100. [CrossRef] [PubMed]

29. Stroup, D.F.; Berlin, J.A.; Morton, S.C.; Olkin, I.; Williamson, G.D.; Rennie, D.; Moher, D.; Becker, B.J.; Sipe, T.A.; Thacker, S.B. Meta-analysis of observational studies in epidemiology: A proposal for reporting. Meta-analysis of observational studies in epidemiology (MOOSE) group. *JAMA* **2000**, *283*, 2008–2012. [CrossRef] [PubMed]

30. Gargon, E.; Williamson, P.R.; Clarke, M. Collating the knowledge base for core outcome set development: Developing and appraising the search strategy for a systematic review. *BMC Med. Res. Methodol.* **2015**, *15*, 26. [CrossRef] [PubMed]

31. Sanderson, S.; Tatt, I.D.; Higgins, J.P. Tools for assessing quality and susceptibility to bias in observational studies in epidemiology: A systematic review and annotated bibliography. *Int. J. Epidemiol.* **2007**, *36*, 666–676. [CrossRef] [PubMed]

32. Carletta, J. Assessing agreement on classification tasks: The kappa statistic. *Comput. Linguist.* **1996**, *22*, 249–254.

33. Rothman, K.J.; Greenland, S.; Lash, T.L. *Modern Epidemiology*; Lippincott Williams & Wilkins: Philadelphia, PA, USA, 2008.

34. Harbord, R.M.; Higgins, J.P.T. Meta-regression in Stata. *Stata J.* **2008**, *8*, 493–519.

35. Higgins, J.P.; Thompson, S.G. Quantifying heterogeneity in a meta-analysis. *Stat. Med.* **2002**, *21*, 1539–1558. [CrossRef] [PubMed]

36. Egger, M.; Davey, S.G.; Schneider, M.; Minder, C. Bias in meta-analysis detected by a simple, graphical test. *BMJ* **1997**, *315*, 629–634. [CrossRef] [PubMed]

37. Harbord, R.M.; Egger, M.; Sterne, J.A. A modified test for small-study effects in meta-analyses of controlled trials with binary endpoints. *Stat. Med.* **2006**, *25*, 3443–3457. [CrossRef] [PubMed]

38. Begg, C.B.; Mazumdar, M. Operating characteristics of a rank correlation test for publication bias. *Biometrics* **1994**, *50*, 1088–1101. [CrossRef] [PubMed]

39. Peters, J.L.; Sutton, A.J.; Jones, D.R.; Abrams, K.R.; Rushton, L. Comparison of two methods to detect publication bias in meta-analysis. *JAMA* **2006**, *295*, 676–680. [CrossRef] [PubMed]

40. Harrell, F.E., Jr.; Lee, K.L.; Pollock, B.G. Regression models in clinical studies: Determining relationships between predictors and response. *J. Natl. Cancer Inst.* **1988**, *80*, 1198–1202. [CrossRef] [PubMed]

41. Jackson, D.; White, I.R.; Thompson, S.G. Extending dersimonian and laird's methodology to perform multivariate random effects meta-analyses. *Stat. Med.* **2010**, *29*, 1282–1297. [CrossRef] [PubMed]

42. Liu, S.; Choi, H.K.; Ford, E.; Song, Y.; Klevak, A.; Buring, J.E.; Manson, J.E. A prospective study of dairy intake and the risk of type 2 diabetes in women. *Diabetes Care* **2006**, *29*, 1579–1584. [CrossRef] [PubMed]

43. Kirii, K.; Mizoue, T.; Iso, H.; Takahashi, Y.; Kato, M.; Inoue, M.; Noda, M.; Tsugane, S. Calcium, vitamin D and dairy intake in relation to type 2 diabetes risk in a Japanese cohort. *Diabetologia* **2009**, *52*, 2542–2550. [CrossRef] [PubMed]
44. Pittas, A.G.; Dawson-Hughes, B.; Li, T.; Van Dam, R.M.; Willett, W.C.; Manson, J.E.; Hu, F.B. Vitamin D and calcium intake in relation to type 2 diabetes in women. *Diabetes Care* **2006**, *29*, 650–656. [CrossRef] [PubMed]
45. Song, Y.; Manson, J.E.; Buring, J.E.; Liu, S. A prospective study of red meat consumption and type 2 diabetes in middle-aged and elderly women: The women's health study. *Diabetes Care* **2004**, *27*, 2108–2115. [CrossRef] [PubMed]
46. Schulze, M.B.; Manson, J.E.; Willett, W.C.; Hu, F.B. Processed meat intake and incidence of type 2 diabetes in younger and middle-aged women. *Diabetologia* **2003**, *46*, 1465–1473. [CrossRef] [PubMed]
47. Liu, S.; Manson, J.E.; Stampfer, M.J.; Hu, F.B.; Giovannucci, E.; Colditz, G.A.; Hennekens, C.H.; Willett, W.C. A prospective study of whole-grain intake and risk of type 2 diabetes mellitus in US women. *Am. J. Public Health* **2000**, *90*, 1409–1415. [PubMed]
48. Salmeron, J.; Ascherio, A.; Rimm, E.B.; Colditz, G.A.; Spiegelman, D.; Jenkins, D.J.; Stampfer, M.J.; Wing, A.L.; Willett, W.C. Dietary fiber, glycemic load, and risk of NIDDM in men. *Diabetes Care* **1997**, *20*, 545–550. [CrossRef] [PubMed]
49. Pereira, M.A.; Parker, E.D.; Folsom, A.R. Coffee consumption and risk of type 2 diabetes mellitus: An 11-year prospective study of 28,812 postmenopausal women. *Arch. Intern. Med.* **2006**, *166*, 1311–1316. [CrossRef] [PubMed]
50. Oba, S.; Nanri, A.; Kurotani, K.; Goto, A.; Kato, M.; Mizoue, T.; Noda, M.; Inoue, M.; Tsugane, S. Dietary glycemic index, glycemic load and incidence of type 2 diabetes in japanese men and women: The Japan public health center-based prospective study. *Nutr. J.* **2013**, *12*, 165. [CrossRef] [PubMed]
51. He, K.; Song, Y.; Belin, R.J.; Chen, Y. Magnesium intake and the metabolic syndrome: Epidemiologic evidence to date. *J. Cardiometab. Syndr.* **2006**, *1*, 351–355. [CrossRef] [PubMed]
52. Hata, A.; Doi, Y.; Ninomiya, T.; Mukai, N.; Hirakawa, Y.; Hata, J.; Ozawa, M.; Uchida, K.; Shirota, T.; Kitazono, T.; et al. Magnesium intake decreases type 2 diabetes risk through the improvement of insulin resistance and inflammation: The Hisayama study. *Diabet. Med.* **2013**, *30*, 1487–1494. [CrossRef] [PubMed]
53. Weng, L.C.; Lee, N.J.; Yeh, W.T.; Ho, L.T.; Pan, W.H. Lower intake of magnesium and dietary fiber increases the incidence of type 2 diabetes in Taiwanese. *J. Formos. Med. Assoc.* **2012**, *111*, 651–659. [CrossRef] [PubMed]
54. Salmeron, J.; Manson, J.E.; Stampfer, M.J.; Colditz, G.A.; Wing, A.L.; Willett, W.C. Dietary fiber, glycemic load, and risk of non-insulin-dependent diabetes mellitus in women. *JAMA* **1997**, *277*, 472–477. [CrossRef] [PubMed]
55. Ma, B.; Lawson, A.B.; Liese, A.D.; Bell, R.A.; Mayer-Davis, E.J. Dairy, magnesium, and calcium intake in relation to insulin sensitivity: Approaches to modeling a dose-dependent association. *Am. J. Epidemiol.* **2006**, *164*, 449–458. [CrossRef] [PubMed]
56. Rodriguez-Moran, M.; Simental, M.L.; Zambrano, G.G.; Guerrero-Romero, F. The role of magnesium in type 2 diabetes: A brief based-clinical review. *Magnes. Res.* **2011**, *24*, 156–162. [PubMed]
57. Meisinger, C.; Thorand, B.; Schneider, A.; Stieber, J.; Doring, A.; Lowel, H. Sex differences in risk factors for incident type 2 diabetes mellitus: The MONICA Augsburg cohort study. *Arch. Intern. Med.* **2002**, *162*, 82–89. [CrossRef] [PubMed]
58. Kalyani, R.R.; Franco, M.; Dobs, A.S.; Ouyang, P.; Vaidya, D.; Bertoni, A.; Gapstur, S.M.; Golden, S.H. The association of endogenous sex hormones, adiposity, and insulin resistance with incident diabetes in postmenopausal women. *J. Clin. Endocrinol. Metab.* **2009**, *94*, 4127–4135. [CrossRef] [PubMed]
59. Moshfegh, A.; Goldman, J.; Cleveland, L. *What We Eat in America, NHANES 2001–2002: Usual Nutrient Intakes from Food Compared to Dietary References Intake*; Agricultural Research Service, U.S. Department of Agriculture: Washington, DC, USA, 2005; pp. 1–56.

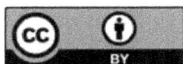

nutrients

MDPI

Article

The Effect of Selenium Supplementation on Glucose Homeostasis and the Expression of Genes Related to Glucose Metabolism

Ewa Jablonska [1,*], Edyta Reszka [1], Jolanta Gromadzinska [2], Edyta Wieczorek [1], Magdalena B. Krol [2], Sara Raimondi [3], Katarzyna Socha [4], Maria H. Borawska [4] and Wojciech Wasowicz [2]

[1] Nofer Institute of Occupational Medicine, Department of Toxicology and Carcinogenesis, Sw. Teresy 8 Street, 91-348 Lodz, Poland; edyta.reszka@imp.lodz.pl (E.R.); edyta.wieczorek@imp.lodz.pl (E.W.)
[2] Nofer Institute of Occupational Medicine, Department of Biological and Environmental Monitoring, Sw. Teresy 8 Street, 91-348 Lodz, Poland; jolanta.gromadzinska@imp.lodz.pl (J.G.); magdalena.krol@imp.lodz.pl (M.B.K.); wojciech.wasowicz@imp.lodz.pl (W.W.)
[3] European Institute of Oncology, Division of Epidemiology and Biostatistics, via Ripamonti 435, Milan 20139, Italy; sara.raimondi@ieo.it
[4] The Medical University of Bialystok, Department of Bromatoloy, A. Mickiewicza 2D Street, 15-222 Bialystok, Poland; sara.raimondi@ieo.it (K.S.); borawska@umb.edu.pl (M.H.B.)
* Correspondence: ewa.jablonska@imp.lodz.pl; Tel.: +48-42-631-4612

Received: 10 October 2016; Accepted: 24 November 2016; Published: 13 December 2016

Abstract: The aim of the study was to evaluate the effect of selenium supplementation on the expression of genes associated with glucose metabolism in humans, in order to explain the unclear relationship between selenium and the risk of diabetes. For gene expression analysis we used archival samples of cDNA from 76 non-diabetic subjects supplemented with selenium in the previous study. The supplementation period was six weeks and the daily dose of selenium was 200 µg (as selenium yeast). Blood for mRNA isolation was collected at four time points: before supplementation, after two and four weeks of supplementation, and after four weeks of washout. The analysis included 15 genes encoding selected proteins involved in insulin signaling and glucose metabolism. In addition, HbA1c and fasting plasma glucose were measured at three and four time points, respectively. Selenium supplementation was associated with a significantly decreased level of HbA1c but not fasting plasma glucose (FPG) and significant down-regulation of seven genes: *INSR, ADIPOR1, LDHA, PDHA, PDHB, MYC,* and *HIF1AN.* These results suggest that selenium may affect glycemic control at different levels of regulation, linked to insulin signaling, glycolysis, and pyruvate metabolism. Further research is needed to investigate mechanisms of such transcriptional regulation and its potential implication in direct metabolic effects.

Keywords: selenium; gene expression; insulin signaling; glucose metabolism; glycolysis; pyruvate metabolism; energy metabolism; glycated hemoglobin; fasting plasma glucose

1. Introduction

Selenium (Se) is a trace element with multiple biological functions. The majority of studies related to this nutrient and human health were devoted to its potential anticancer activity and chemoprevention based on Se supplementation [1–3]. However recent scientific focus has been switched towards possible harmful effects of Se supplementation, especially in terms of its unclear link with glucose metabolism and diabetes [4–6]. The increased risk of diabetes type II (T2DM) in humans associated with elevated Se status has been suggested for the first time on the basis of reanalysis of a placebo-controlled randomized trial (NPC, Nutritional Prevention of Cancer) conducted in the USA in the years 1983–1991 in a group of 1312 subjects. In that study, there was a significant increase in the risk of diabetes among Se-supplemented subjects who had the highest Se status (plasma concentration >121.6 ng/mL) before supplementation (Risk Ratio (RR) = 2.40; p = 0.01) [7]. In another American study (SELECT, Selenium and Vitamin E Cancer Prevention Trial) conducted in 35,533 individuals, there was a non-significant increase in the risk of diabetes among Se- supplemented arm (RR = 1.07%, p = 0.16) [8]. Results of this large and well-designed, randomized, placebo-controlled trial generated much controversy and up to now, no clear conclusion have been made with respect to the potentially diabetogenic properties of Se. Several observational studies, as well as Se supplementation trials, in which the association between Se status/Se intake and the risk of diabetes or markers of glucose metabolism has been investigated, generated inconsistent results [4,9–12]. On the other hand, animal studies indicated that Se supplementation may lead to hyperinsulinemia, insulin resistance, and glucose intolerance [13]. To complicate this, previous in vivo studies indicated protective role of Se in diabetes [14,15]. The link between Se and glucose seems very complex and is supposed to be reflected by a non-linear U-shaped dose-response relationship [16].

The insights from experimental studies in animals indicate that Se is involved in glucose metabolism via Se-dependent proteins (selenoproteins), which possess redox properties. It is assumed that they may influence the insulin-dependent metabolic pathways, because both insulin release and insulin signaling are regulated by the cellular redox potential [17]. In particular, the essential role in the regulation of both processes is attributed to hydrogen peroxide, which is one of the reactive oxygen species produced inter alia by dismutation of superoxide anion radical (catalyzed by superoxide dismutase, SOD). Hydrogen peroxide is reduced to water with the participation of enzymes, such as Se-dependent glutathione peroxidase (GPx) and catalase (CAT). The role of GPx in the metabolism of insulin appears to be significant and complex, which is reflected by a relatively low expression of mRNA for GPx1 and its low enzymatic activity in the pancreas (1%–5% of the value observed in the liver; the study in mice) [18]. Moreover, it was shown that global overexpression of GPx1 mRNA in mice fed with a normal Se diet (0.4 mg/kg) was associated with hyperglycemia, hyperinsulinemia, and an increase in plasma leptin concentrations [19]. Another selenoprotein potentially important in the etiology of diabetes is selenoprotein P (Sepp1) which is produced mainly in the liver and secreted into plasma, acting as a Se transporter, and having also antioxidant properties. Misu et al. observed a positive correlation between the level of Sepp1 mRNA and insulin resistance in humans [20]. The same authors also demonstrated in vitro that cells stimulated exogenously with purified Sepp1 were characterized by impaired insulin signaling and impaired glucose metabolism [20]. Recently it has been also observed that serum concentration of Sepp1 was positively correlated with fasting plasma glucose (FPG) concentration (r = 0.35, p = 0.037) and negatively correlated with serum adiponectin levels (r = -0.355, p = 0.034; r = -0.367, p = 0.028) in patients with T2DM [21].

Altogether, mechanisms of action of Se in humans at the level of glucose metabolism and its potential role in the etiology of diabetes are unknown and point to the need for more studies relevant to human metabolism. The aim of this study was to assess the effect of Se supplementation on the expression of genes related to glucose metabolism, including genes encoding hormones responsible for glycemic control (insulin, glucagon, leptin, and adiponectin), receptors for these hormones, enzymes involved in glycolysis, as well as key transcription factors involved in the regulation of glycolysis. To our knowledge this is the first study conducted in humans, which aimed to investigate more in-depth molecular effects of Se with respect to glucose homeostasis.

2. Materials and Methods

2.1. Study Design

For the purpose of this study we used archival samples of cDNA obtained from subjects who were supplemented with Se during the trial conducted by us previously. Details of the trial, as well as subjects' exclusion criteria, were described elsewhere [22]. The exclusion criteria for subjects' recruitment included inter alia current smoking and self-reported prevalence of diabetes. Briefly, the 95 non-smoking and non-diabetic individuals were supplemented with 200 µg of Se/day (in the form of Se yeast) for six weeks and fasting blood was collected at four time points: at baseline, after two weeks of supplementation, after six weeks of supplementation, and after four weeks of washout. In the present study, gene expression analysis was performed with the use of cDNA obtained from 76 subjects, randomly selected out of the entire study group, including 36 males and 40 females. Table 1 presents basic characteristics of the subjects. Plasma Se concentration was measured previously (as described in [22]) and mean plasma Se levels calculated for 76 subjects at each time points are presented also in Table 1.

Written informed consent was obtained from all the study participants and the study was approved by the Local Ethics Committee (Ethical Institutional Review Board at the Nofer Institute of Occupational Medicine, Lodz, Poland, Resolution No. 3/2010).

Table 1. Basic characteristics of the study group (76 subjects supplemented with selenium).

Variable	All (*n* = 76)	Males (*n* = 36)	Females (*n* = 40)	*p* (Males vs. Females)
Age (years)	34.8 ± 10.4	35 ± 18	36 ± 18	0.7549 [a]
BMI (kg/m^2)	24.0 ± 2.9	25.0 ± 2.7	23.0 ± 2.9	**0.0009** [a]
Smoking, *n* (%)				
Current	0 (0)	0 (0)	0 (0)	
Ever	18 (24)	8 (23)	10 (24)	
Never	58 (76)	27 (77)	31 (76)	ns
Use of Se-containing supplements in the past 6 months, *n* (%)				
Yes	5 (7)	3 (9)	2 (5)	
No	71 (93)	32 (91)	39 (95)	ns
Mean plasma Se ± SD (µg/L)				
Baseline	65.2 ± 16.5	65.2 ± 16.6	65.3 ± 16.5	0.9729 [b]
After two weeks	101.1 ± 24.5	98.7 ± 22.8	103.3 ± 26.1	0.3907 [a]
After six weeks	99.1 ± 20.3	95.0 ± 16.9	102.7 ± 22.4	0.0928 [b]
After four weeks of washout	76.5 ± 15.6	75.3 ± 15.3	77.6 ± 16.1	0.7777 [b]
p (ANOVA)	<0.0001	<0.0001	<0.0001	

[a]—Mann-Whitney U test; [b]—Student's *t*-test. Significant *p* values are in bold.

2.2. Gene Expression Experiment

mRNA for gene expression analysis was isolated from white blood cells (WBC). The description of material preservation, mRNA isolation, quantification, and quality assessment were described previously [22]. For reverse transcription we used a QuantiTect Kit (Qiagen, Hilden, Germany). Gene expression was analyzed by means of qPCR and conducted on a QuantStudioTM 12K Flex Real-Time PCR System (Thermo Fisher Scienific, Waltham, MA, USA), using Custom Taqman® array cards and TaqMan® Universal Master Mix (Thermo Fisher Scienific, Waltham, MA, USA). For each array card 6 µg of cDNA was taken. Reaction conditions were as follows: 95 °C of initial denaturation for 10 min followed by 50 cycles of 95 °C for 15 s and 60 °C for 60 s. The analysis included 15 genes encoding selected proteins involved in insulin signaling and glucose metabolism. The expression was normalized against *GAPDH*. The list of all targets is presented in Table 2. The genes were divided into four groups according to the type of encoded protein: (1) hormones: insulin (*INS*), glucagon (*GCG*), adiponectin (*ADIPOQ*), and leptin (*LEP*); (2) hormone receptors: insulin receptor (*INSR*), glucagon receptor (*GCGR*), adiponectin receptors (*ADIPOR1*, *ADIPOR2*), and leptin receptor (*LEPR*); (3) enzymes involved in pyruvate metabolism: lactic acid dehydrogenase (*LDHA*), pyruvate dehydrogenase, alpha subunit (*PDHA1*) and beta subunit (*PDHB*); (4) transcription factors or their inhibitors driving glycolysis: transcription factor HIF1 (*HIF1A*), HIF1A inhibitor (*HIF1AN*), and nuclear transcription factor MYC (*MYC*).

Table 2. Genes of interest selected for the study.

Gene	Locus	Gene Product	Protein Group
INS	11p15.5	insulin	
GCG	2q36-q37	glucagon	hormones
ADIPOQ	3q27	adiponectin	
LEP	1p31	leptin	
INSR	19p13.3-p13.2	insulin receptor	
GCGR	17q25	glucagon receptor	
ADIPOR1	1q32.1	adiponectin receptor 1	hormone receptors
ADIPOR2	12p13.31	adiponectin receptor 2	
LEPR	7q31.3	leptin receptor	
LDHA	11p15.4	lactate dehydrogenase	enzymes involved in
PDHA1	Xp22.1	pyruvate dehydrogenase (lipoamide) alpha 1 subunit	pyruvate metabolism
PDHB	3p21.1-p14.2	pyruvate dehydrogenase (lipoamide) beta subunit	
HIF1A	14q23.2	hypoxia inducible factor 1, alpha subunit	transcription factors and their
HIF1AN	10q24	hypoxia inducible factor 1, alpha subunit inhibitor	inhibitors, involved in the
MYC	8q24.21	v-myc avian myelocytomatosis viral oncogene homolog	regulation of glycolysis

2.3. HbA1c, Fasting Plasma Glucose

Levels of HbA1c (glycated hemoglobin) were determined in 10 µL of whole blood (heparinized tube) immediately after the blood was collected. The analysis was performed commercially in the certified laboratory of clinical diagnostics, using immunoturbidimetric assay on an INTEGRA 400 system (Roche Diagnostics, Rotkreuz, Switzerland). The enzymic colorimetric method was based on an oxidase/peroxidase method and the respective commercial kit (Alpha Diagnostics, Warsaw, Poland) was used to analyze FPG. All absorbance values were measured on a UV4 Unicam UV-VIS spectrophotometer (Cambridge, UK). Intra- and inter-assay coefficients of variation for FPG analyses were 2.52% (n = 10) and 4.57% (n = 32), respectively.

2.4. Statistical Analysis

The analysis on gene expression data was performed on the log-transformed values in order to have a normal distribution. Repeated measures analysis of variance (MANCOVA) with an unstructured covariance matrix was carried out to test the effects of time on FPG, HbA1c, and gene expression. With this analysis, markers (FPG, HbA1c, gene expression) at different time points were considered as dependent variables, while covariates (age, sex, BMI, and baseline Se) were included in the models as independent variables. The possible correlation between variation of Se and of gene expression values at different time points was investigated by a linear regression model with the difference of gene expression at two time points as the dependent variable, and the difference of Se, age, sex, BMI, baseline Se, and baseline gene expression as independent variables. All of the analyses were carried out in the whole group of subjects and separately in women and men. Post-hoc comparisons between pairwise time points were performed by contrast tests, using Bonferroni correction. All of the other statistical tests were performed at a significance level of α = 0.05. To adjust the results for multiple comparisons, we performed a false discovery rate (FDR) analysis. Statistical analyses were conducted using SAS software, version 9.2 (SAS Institute, Cary, NC, USA).

3. Results

3.1. The Effect of Se Supplementation on HbA1c and Fasting Plasma Glucose

Significant changes in HbA1c levels were observed upon Se supplementation (p < 0.0001), with post hoc tests indicating a significant decrease both after six weeks of supplementation and after four weeks of washout (p < 0.0001 and p = 0.02 vs. baseline, respectively) (Table 3). On the contrary, FPG concentration remained unaffected upon supplementation trial (p = 0.553).

Table 3. The effect of Se supplementation on fasting plasma glucose concentration, HbA1c levels and gene expression. Data for all study subjects ($n = 76$).

Marker	Time Points				p (MANCOVA *)
	Baseline	Two Weeks	Six Weeks	Washout	
FPG (mg/dL)	91.96 ± 13.94	90.55 ± 14.07	91.00 ± 14.15	91.56 ± 13.79	0.55
HbA1c (%)	4.74 ± 0.80	na	4.44 ± 0.63 [c]	4.57± 0.65 [a]	<0.05
INSR	1.23 ± 0.67	**0.98 ± 0.25** [b]	**1.02 ± 0.27** [b]	**0.95 ± 0.25** [c]	0.005
ADIPOR1	2.05 ± 0.23	**2.00 ± 0.18** [a]	2.07 ± 0.21	2.04 ± 0.23	0.002
ADIPOR2	1.88 ± 0.23	1.84 ± 0.18	1.84 ± 0.19	1.80 ± 0.19	0.08
LEPR	0.87 ± 0.35	0.80 ± 0.34	0.80 ± 0.29	0.82 ± 0.38	0.26
LDHA	2.74 ± 0.30	**2.59 ± 0.26** [c]	**2.49 ± 0.21** [c]	**2.51 ± 0.27** [c]	<0.0001
PDHA	2.03 ± 0.29	**1.93 ± 0.24** [a]	**1.90 ± 0.20** [c]	**1.90 ± 0.26** [b]	0.0002
PDHB	1.92 ± 0.25	1.86 ± 0.20	**1.81 ± 0.18** [c]	**1.81 ± 0.21** [b]	0.0008
HIF1A	2.37 ± 0.26	2.29 ± 0.23	2.29 ± 0.24	2.30 ± 0.27	0.16
HIF1AN	1.71 ± 0.32	**1.61 ± 0.19** [b]	1.70 ± 0.20	1.67 ± 0.21	0.0001
MYC	2.31 ± 0.29	**2.22 ± 0.26** [a]	**2.14 ± 0.22** [c]	**2.18 ± 0.25** [a]	<0.0001

Values significantly different as compared to baseline are in bold, [a]—$p < 0.05$, [b]—$p < 0.01$, [c]—$p < 0.001$; *—Multivariate analysis of covariance, model included age, sex, BMI and baseline selenium; na—not analyzed (HbA1c was not analyzed after two weeks of supplementation).

3.2. The Effect on Gene Expression

In the first step of analysis, we excluded genes which were not expressed or which had very low expression. These were five genes: *INS, GCG, GCGR, ADIPOQ*, and *LEP*. Further analysis of the remaining 10 genes indicated a significant reduction in mRNA expression of seven targets, including *INSR, ADIPOR1, LDHA, PDHA, PDHB, MYC*, and *HIF1AN*. In the case of *INSR, LDHA, PDHA*, and *MYC*, a significant decrease was observed at all measurement points as indicated by contrast tests (during supplementation and the washout period). For genes *ADIPOR2, LEPR*, and *HIF1A* there was no statistically significant changes over time (Table 3).

Further analysis aimed to test whether the variation of gene expression depended on the variation of Se. We conducted this analysis for all 10 genes and all time points regardless of the fact whether the overall effect was significant or not. Significant correlations between Se status and gene expression were found in the case of *ADIPOR1* after six weeks of supplementation ($p = 0.012$) and in the case of *HIF1AN* after two weeks ($p = 0.045$) and six weeks ($p = 0.002$) of supplementation. All data are shown in Table S3.

3.3. Sex Differences

At baseline, males had significantly higher levels of FPG ($p = 0.01$) as compared to females, however, both sexes did not differ significantly in the level of HbA1c ($p = 0.175$). No modifying effect of sex was observed at the level of both markers upon time (during supplementation and after washout period, as assessed in the MANCOVA model; $p = 0.55$ and $p = 0.09$ for time interaction with sex for FPG and HbA1c, respectively). Data on FPG, HbA1c, and on gene expression analyzed separately for males and females are presented in the supplementary materials (Tables S1 and S2). The results of analysis stratified by sex were less powered and some p-values were no more significant. However, general trends were similar. Analogically to the analyses conducted in the whole group, we tested the correlation between variations in plasma Se levels and in gene expression. In males significant correlation was found for *HIF1AN* after six weeks of supplementation ($p = 0.038$). In females significant correlations were observed for four genes after six weeks of supplementation: *ADIPOR1* ($p = 0.047$), *PDHB* ($p = 0.034$), *HIF1AN* ($p = 0.035$), and *MYC* ($p = 0.048$). Regression analysis data are shown in Tables S4 (for males) and S5 (for females).

3.4. False Discovery Rate Analysis

P-values for the effect on gene expression (Table 3, Tables S1 and S2) were still statistically significant after FDR adjustment for multiple comparisons, except for two genes in women: *ADIPOR1* and *HIF1AN* (in both cases the FDR-adjusted *p*-value was 0.06).

4. Discussion

In this study we observed that six weeks of supplementation with 200 µg of Se in the form of Se yeast had significantly decreased the level of HbA1c in the subjects with relatively low baseline Se status. On the other hand we did not observe any changes at the level of FPG. However, FPG reflects the glycemic status at the time of measurement. HbA1c is regarded as a more reliable marker since it indicates long-term changes in the glycemic control. Thus, the impact of Se supplementation on HbA1c levels observed in this study confirms that Se is involved in the metabolism of glucose. Moreover, significant decrease in HbA1c levels was maintained four weeks after supplementation discontinuation, which clearly shows that the effect of Se on the glycemic control was relatively strong. There are only a few other studies reporting the effect of Se supplementation on glucose homeostasis in humans. Three of them, being all randomized, placebo-controlled trials (RCTs), have shown beneficial effect of short-term Se supplementation in specific groups of women. In the first study, 70 women with gestational diabetes were supplemented with Se at a dose of 200 µg per day for six weeks. Improved glucose homeostasis was observed as reflected by decreased levels of FPG and serum insulin as well as decreased HOMA-IR values (homeostasis model of assessment of insulin resistance) [23]. The second study was conducted in 70 women with polycystic ovary syndrome. After eight weeks of supplementation with Se at 200 µg per day, there was a significant decrease in serum insulin levels, HOMA-IR, HOMA-B (homeostatic model of assessment of beta-cell function) values, and an increase in QUICKI (quantitative insulin sensitivity check index), whereas FPG remained unchanged [24]. The last study investigated the effect of Se supplementation in women with central obesity. After six weeks of Se supplementation (200 µg/day), significant decrease in serum insulin levels and HOMA-IR values was observed [25]. Another study which was conducted in 60 subjects of both sexes (20 males and 40 females) diagnosed with T2DM and coronary heart disease also showed beneficial effects of Se supplementation (200 µg/day for eight weeks) in terms of decreased insulin, HOMA-IR, HOMA-B parameters, and increased QUICKI [26]. On the contrary, only one RCT, conducted in patients with T2DM (n = 60, including 34 males and 26 females), indicated that three months of Se supplementation (200 µg/day) led to the increased FPG levels [27]. To compare with short term supplementation, long-term RCTs did not indicate any effects on glucose homeostasis upon Se supplementation, as shown at the level of serum glucose concentration in 140 men with prostate cancer (supplemented with Se at dose 200 µg/day for five years) or at the level of FPG in 3146 participants of the SU.VI.MAX trial (supplemented with 100 µg of Se in combination with zinc (Zn) and vitamins C, E, and beta-carotene, for 7.5 years) [28,29]. Overall, the inconsistent results of the above RCTs coincide with a lack of compliance in the observational studies investigating the link between Se and diabetes. These studies also suggest that Se-induced effects may largely depend on specific health conditions (notably none of them has been conducted in the general population). A similar conclusion has been drawn from recent studies in mice, which were fed with a high-fat diet in order to induce insulin resistance [30]. It was observed that pre-treatment with Se protected animals against developing insulin resistance, whereas post-treatment with Se exacerbated this metabolic disorder. The effects of pre-treatment and post-treatment with Se were different in the context of adipogenesis and lipolysis, showing increased adipocyte differentiation and fat accumulation in adipose tissue in pre-treated mice, whereas post-treated mice were characterized by increased lipolysis and ectopic lipid deposition [30]. The above study clearly shows that Se exerts differential effects under different health conditions.

Along with HbA1c decrease upon Se supplementation, we have observed in this study a significant decrease of leukocyte mRNA levels for seven genes involved in different steps of glucose metabolism regulation. The first group of mRNA targets (*INSR* and *ADIPOR1*) concerned receptors for endocrine hormones: insulin and adiponectin, which are key players in insulin signaling responsible for cellular glucose uptake. Suppressive effects of Se on insulin receptors was observed previously in a study of gestating rats and their offspring [31]. In that experiment, decreased mRNA expression for *Insr*, as well as other insulin signaling genes, including *Irs-1* (insulin receptor substrate 1), *Irs-2* (insulin receptor substrate 2), and *Akt2* (serine/threonine protean kinase 2), was observed in the liver of dams supplemented with 3 mg Se/kg diet (as compared to dams fed basal diet). Importantly, similar changes in the liver, additionally accompanied by decreased protein levels of insulin receptors, were observed in the offspring of dams also receiving a high Se diet. At the same time, high Se diet was associated in both dams and the offspring with hyperinsulinemia, insulin resistance and glucose intolerance [31]. The impact of a high Se diet on protein levels for insulin receptors was also investigated in pigs, showing tissue-specific changes, with up-regulation in the liver and down-regulation in the muscle. However, no changes in both tissues were observed for insulin receptors at the level of mRNA [32]. Similarly, another study conducted in pigs also failed to show any effect of supranutritional intake of Se on insulin receptor mRNA levels, analyzed in liver, muscle, and visceral adipose tissue [33]. Significant reduction of mRNA expression for the adiponectin receptor, *ADIPOR1*, observed in our study after two weeks of supplementation, was accompanied by a borderline significant decrease in *ADIPOR2* ($p = 0.08$). AdipoR2 is expressed mainly in the liver; thus, in blood leukocytes it was more probable to observe a significant effect in the case of AdipoR1, which is expressed ubiquitously [34]. Both receptors bind adiponectin, a hormone produced by adipocytes and involved in glucose metabolism via modulating insulin sensitivity [34]. Though our study may suggest some effect of Se on adiponectin signaling, two supplementation trials failed to show any effect of Se administration on plasma adiponectin levels in humans [35,36]. Nevertheless, the suppressive effect on *INSR* and *ADIPOR1* indicated in this study deserves further research, as decreased expression of mRNA levels for these receptors has been linked to insulin resistance and diabetes in humans and animals [37–39]. Decreased expression of essential genes involved in glucose metabolism, such as those encoding receptors for insulin and adiponectin, may indicate rather detrimental effects of Se supplementation in the study group. On the other hand, the effect at the level of HbA1c was somewhat positive. The hypothetical explanation for these contradictory observations may be that the potentially beneficial decrease in HbA1c level reflects an adaptive response which counteracts the adverse effects of the metalloid on glucose homeostasis and that this response is rather short-term. This adaptive mechanism when induced in a constant manner (by introducing the factor day by day for several weeks) may be strong enough to influence the level of HbA1c, however, not in the long-term. The hypothesis about short-term adaptive response is in line with overall observations from Se supplementation trials, indicating mainly beneficial effects of Se on glucose metabolism in the case of short-term administration and, on the other hand, null or negative effects upon long-term supplementation with this nutrient. Alternative explanation for decreased levels of HbA1c upon Se is the possibility that Se may prevent the process of hemoglobin glycation. This may be suggested on the basis of a recent study by Yu and colleagues, showing Se nanoparticles prevent protein glycation in vitro [40]. Nevertheless, it is not clear whether changes observed in our study at the level of leukocyte gene expression reflect changes in insulin-sensitive tissues. If they do, down-regulation of *INSR* and *ADIPOR1* in blood leukocytes could serve as an early biomarker of adverse health effects of Se supranutrition in humans, leading to impaired glucose homeostasis.

The second group of down-regulated genes in this study included *LDH*, *PDHA*, and *PDHB*, all three encoding enzymes involved in pyruvate metabolism. Pyruvate is the end product of glycolysis and its further metabolism depends on cellular oxygen concentration. Under anaerobic conditions, it is transformed by lactate dehydrogenase (LDH) to lactic acid whereas, under normal aerobic conditions, it is metabolized by pyruvate dehydrogenase complex (PDC) to acetyl coenzyme A (acetyl CoA). The latter reaction links glycolysis to the Krebs cycle. Importantly, pyruvate recycling (occurring across mitochondrial membranes) is an important regulator of insulin secretion due to the generation of NADPH (the reduced form of nicotinamide adenine dinucleotide phosphate), the pivotal molecule required for insulin granule exocytosis in beta cells [41]. Pyruvate metabolism was shown to be implicated in diabetes, as reflected by increased activity of pyruvate dehydrogenase kinase (PDK) in diabetic subjects (PDK plays significant role in glucose disposal as it decreases the activity of PDC) [42]. In general, glycolytic pathway was shown to be dysregulated in diabetes [43]. A study in rats showed, for example, that an alloxan-induced diabetic state significantly altered the activities of glycolytic enzymes in lymphocytes [44]. Importantly, recent animal studies suggest that Se interferes with glycolytic targets and pyruvate metabolism, supporting our observation. Pigs fed with a supranutritional dose of Se exhibited decreased expression of mRNA for pyruvate kinase (enzyme responsible for pyruvate synthesis in the last step of glycolysis) [33]. Interestingly, increased pyruvate levels in the liver and increased expression of pyruvate metabolizing enzymes (pyruvate carboxylase (Pcx) and pyruvate dehydrogenase (Pdh)) were shown in mice with a knocked out gene for selenocysteine lyase (SCLY, the enzyme catalyzing conversion of selenocysteine into alanine and selenide, an important step in Se metabolism, as selenide is a substrate for selenoprotein biosynthesis) [45]. Recently it has been also shown that Se affects glycolysis in cancer cells, suggesting that down-regulation of glycolytic enzymes is a novel mechanism of Se toxicity in cancer and that this mechanism targets the well-known metabolic hallmark of cancer cells associated with enhanced glycolysis, which is called the Warburg effect [46]. In our study we have observed, additionally that Se may affect also transcriptional regulation of glycolysis, leading to significantly decreased expression of *MYC*. c-MYC protein, encoded by *MYC* gene, is responsible for transcriptional regulation of all glycolytic targets, including pyruvate kinase, pyruvate kinase dehydrogenase and lactate dehydrogenase [47]. Importantly, it was also shown to regulate the expression of glucose transporter 2 (GLUT2) and 4 (GLUT4) [47]. mRNA expression of the second major transcriptional regulator of glycolytic targets, HIF1 [47] was not affected upon Se supplementation in our study, whereas a significant decrease was observed for its inhibitor (but only after two weeks of supplementation). Altogether, these results suggest the need for a more in-depth investigation of the link between Se and glycolysis in humans.

We were not able to detect the expression of genes encoding: insulin (*INS*), glucagon (*GCG*), adiponectin (*ADIPOQ*), and leptin (*LEP*) in leukocytes. This was not surprising as all of these hormones are produced either by pancreas (insulin, glucagon) or by adipocytes (adiponectin, leptin). Similarly, *GCGR* levels were not detectable in leukocytes, which was also expected, as the glucagon receptor is expressed mainly in the liver, in which it mediates glucagon effects: glycogen breakdown and glucose release into the bloodstream.

The last analysis in this study concerned the correlation between the variation in gene expression and variation in plasma Se concentrations at a particular time point. There were only a few significant correlations and those that were significant were very small, indicating that changes in gene expression were not high enough to correlate with changes in Se.

Since this report presents secondary outcomes of the supplementation trial, it has several weaknesses. First of all, due to the short-term supplementation (six weeks) we were not able to assess changes in HbA1c levels after the whole life span of erythrocytes (which is about 120 days). HbA1c levels reflect the cumulative history of glycemic control in the past two to three months [48]. After this period the measurement of HbA1c levels is most indicative. However it is possible to observe changes earlier, as shown by studies investigating the effects of glucose-lowering drugs [49]. Since erythrocytes are produced constantly (meaning that the whole pool of erythrocytes contains cells of different ages) the effect observed in our study resulted from HbA1c reduction in the youngest erythrocytes. Nevertheless, one could speculate that these changes might have occurred due to some potential confounders present in the study during several weeks before the beginning of the trial, such as pharmacological or dietary factors. However, none of the supplemented subjects declared to be taking any drugs or supplements that could affect glucose metabolism (we asked all subjects about their use of glucose-lowering drugs or supplements before and during the trial). As for the influence of diet, none of the individuals reported a change to his/her dietary habits during the trial.

The second major weakness of this study is attributable to the fact that the trial was not randomized (subjects were selected for the study according to genotype) and not placebo controlled (for details see [22]). Since no separate control group was investigated, we compared all data with respect to baseline values, measured on the first day of the trial, before taking the first pill with the supplement. Finally, gene expression was analyzed in this study in blood leukocytes and it is not clear whether these changes reflect general reactions to Se at the molecular level in humans or if they are tissue specific. In addition we did not analyze the protein levels for genes of interest; thus, we were unable to show any correspondence between transcriptomic and proteomic expression and elucidate whether observed subtle changes in mRNA have any further consequences.

To conclude, results of this study suggest that Se may affect glycemic control at different levels of regulation, linked not only to insulin signaling, but also to glycolytic pathway and pyruvate metabolism. Further research is needed to investigate mechanisms of negative transcriptional regulation in blood leukocytes upon Se treatment, its relevance to other tissues, correspondence to protein levels and, finally, potential implications in direct metabolic and cellular effects. Overall, findings of this study added more insight into the controversial topic of possible diabetogenic effects of Se supplementation in humans. What is the exact impact of Se supplementation on glucose homeostasis and the risk of diabetes remains still an open question. The answer will not be obtained without studies unraveling the underlying mechanisms, as well as factors which may modify Se effects with respect to glucose homeostasis, in addition to these already suggested, such as sex and genotype [50,51], as well as Se speciation [52,53]. Explaining the link between Se, glucose metabolism, and diabetes is currently one of the priority goals in Se research because it will determine the further direction of studies focusing on Se as a potential chemopreventive agent.

Supplementary Materials: The following are available online at http://www.mdpi.com/2072-6643/8/12/772/s1, Table S1: The effect of Se supplementation on fasting plasma glucose concentration, HbA1c levels and gene expression. Data for male subjects ($n = 36$); Table S2: The effect of Se supplementation on fasting plasma glucose concentration, HbA1c levels and gene expression. Data for female subjects ($n = 40$); Table S3: Correlation between changes in Se and changes in gene expression measured between two different time points. Data for all subjects ($n = 76$); Table S4: Correlation between changes in Se and changes in gene expression measured between two different time points in male subjects (calculated only for genes which were shown to be significantly changed upon Se supplementation). Data for male subjects ($n = 36$); Table S5: Correlation between changes in Se and changes in gene expression measured between two different time points in all subjects (calculated only for genes which were shown to be significantly changed upon Se supplementation). Data for female subjects ($n = 40$).

Acknowledgments: This study was supported by The Polish Ministry of Science and Higher Education (grant 1666/B/P01/2011/40) and NIOM Internal Grant IMP 1.36/2015-2016.

Author Contributions: E.J. designed the study, performed data analysis and wrote the manuscript, E.R. and E.W. performed gene expression experiments, S.R. performed statistical analysis, M.B.K. collected blood and questionnaire data from the subjects and performed biochemical analyses, K.S. analyzed plasma for selenium concentration, J.G., M.H.B. and W.W. supplied materials and reagents, E.R. revised the manuscript. All authors have read and accepted the final version of the manuscript.

Conflicts of Interest: The authors declare no conflict of interest.

References

1. Labunskyy, V.M.; Hatfield, D.L.; Gladyshev, V.N. Selenoproteins: Molecular pathways and physiological roles. *Physiol. Rev.* **2014**, *94*, 739–777. [CrossRef] [PubMed]
2. Hatfield, D.L.; Tsuji, P.A.; Carlson, B.A.; Gladyshev, V.N. Selenium and selenocysteine: Roles in cancer, health, and development. *Trends Biochem. Sci.* **2014**, *39*, 112–120. [CrossRef] [PubMed]
3. Vinceti, M.; Dennert, G.; Crespi, C.M.; Zwahlen, M.; Brinkman, M.; Zeegers, M.P.A.; Horneber, M.; D'Amico, R.; Del Giovane, C. Selenium for preventing cancer. *Cochrane Database Syst. Rev.* **2014**, *3*, CD005195.
4. Rayman, M.P.; Stranges, S. Epidemiology of selenium and type2 diabetes: Can we make sense of it? *Free Radic. Biol. Med.* **2013**, *65*, 1557–1564. [CrossRef] [PubMed]
5. Mueller, A.S.; Mueller, K.; Wolf, N.M.; Pallauf, J. Selenium and diabetes: An enigma? *Free Radic. Res.* **2009**, *43*, 1029–1059. [CrossRef] [PubMed]

6. Rocourt, C.R.; Cheng, W.H. Selenium supranutrition: Are the potential benefits of chemoprevention outweighed by the promotion of diabetes and insulin resistance? *Nutrients* **2013**, *5*, 1349–1365. [CrossRef] [PubMed]

7. Stranges, S.; Marshall, J.R.; Natarajan, R.; Donahue, R.P.; Trevisan, M.; Combs, G.F.; Cappuccio, F.P.; Ceriello, A.; Reid, M.E. Effects of long-term selenium supplementation on the incidence of type 2 diabetes: A randomized trial. *Ann. Intern. Med.* **2007**, *147*, 217–223. [CrossRef] [PubMed]

8. Lippman, S.M.; Klein, E.A.; Goodman, P.J.; Lucia, M.S.; Thompson, I.M.; Ford, L.G.; Parnes, H.L.; Minasian, L.M.; Gaziano, J.M.; Hartline, J.A.; et al. Effect of selenium and vitamin e on risk of prostate cancer and other cancers: The selenium and vitamin e cancer prevention trial (select). *JAMA* **2009**, *301*, 39–51. [CrossRef] [PubMed]

9. Gao, H.; Hagg, S.; Sjogren, P.; Lambert, P.C.; Ingelsson, E.; van Dam, R.M. Serum selenium in relation to measures of glucose metabolism and incidence of type 2 diabetes in an older swedish population. *Diabet. Med. A J. Br. Diabet. Assoc.* **2014**, *31*, 787–793. [CrossRef] [PubMed]

10. Wei, J.; Zeng, C.; Gong, Q.Y.; Yang, H.B.; Li, X.X.; Lei, G.H.; Yang, T.B. The association between dietary selenium intake and diabetes: A cross-sectional study among middle-aged and older adults. *Nutr. J.* **2015**, *14*, 18. [CrossRef] [PubMed]

11. Yuan, Z.; Xu, X.; Ye, H.; Jin, L.; Zhang, X.; Zhu, Y. High levels of plasma selenium are associated with metabolic syndrome and elevated fasting plasma glucose in a chinese population: A case-control study. *J. Trace Elem. Med. Biol.* **2015**, *32*, 189–194. [CrossRef] [PubMed]

12. Thompson, P.A.; Ashbeck, E.L.; Roe, D.J.; Fales, L.; Buckmeier, J.; Wang, F.; Bhattacharyya, A.; Hsu, C.H.; Chow, H.H.; Ahnen, D.J.; et al. Selenium supplementation for prevention of colorectal adenomas and risk of associated type 2 diabetes. *J. Natl. Cancer Inst.* **2016**, *108*. [CrossRef] [PubMed]

13. Zhou, J.; Huang, K.; Lei, X.G. Selenium and diabetes-evidence from animal studies. *Free Radic. Biol. Med.* **2013**, *65*, 1548–1556. [CrossRef] [PubMed]

14. Ezaki, O. The insulin-like effects of selenate in rat adipocytes. *J. Biol. Chem.* **1990**, *265*, 1124–1128. [PubMed]

15. Müller, A.S.; Most, E.; Pallauf, J. Effects of a supranutritional dose of selenate compared with selenite on insulin sensitivity in type II diabetic dbdb mice. *J. Anim. Physiol. Anim. Nutr.* **2005**, *89*, 94–104. [CrossRef] [PubMed]

16. Wang, X.L.; Yang, T.B.; Wei, J.; Lei, G.H.; Zeng, C. Association between serum selenium level and type 2 diabetes mellitus: A non-linear dose-response meta-analysis of observational studies. *Nutr. J.* **2016**, *15*, 48. [CrossRef] [PubMed]

17. Steinbrenner, H. Interference of selenium and selenoproteins with the insulin-regulated carbohydrate and lipid metabolism. *Free Radic. Biol. Med.* **2013**, *65*, 1538–1547. [CrossRef] [PubMed]

18. Lenzen, S.; Drinkgern, J.; Tiedge, M. Low antioxidant enzyme gene expression in pancreatic islets compared with various other mouse tissues. *Free Radic. Biol. Med.* **1996**, *20*, 463–466. [CrossRef]

19. McClung, J.P.; Roneker, C.A.; Mu, W.; Lisk, D.J.; Langlais, P.; Liu, F.; Lei, X.G. Development of insulin resistance and obesity in mice overexpressing cellular glutathione peroxidase. *Proc. Natl. Acad. Sci. USA* **2004**, *101*, 8852–8857. [CrossRef] [PubMed]

20. Misu, H.; Takamura, T.; Takayama, H.; Hayashi, H.; Matsuzawa-Nagata, N.; Kurita, S.; Ishikura, K.; Ando, H.; Takeshita, Y.; Ota, T.; et al. A liver-derived secretory protein, selenoprotein p, causes insulin resistance. *Cell Metab.* **2010**, *12*, 483–495. [CrossRef] [PubMed]

21. Misu, H.; Ishikura, K.; Kurita, S.; Takeshita, Y.; Ota, T.; Saito, Y.; Takahashi, K.; Kaneko, S.; Takamura, T. Inverse correlation between serum levels of selenoprotein p and adiponectin in patients with type 2 diabetes. *PLoS ONE* **2012**, *7*, e34952. [CrossRef] [PubMed]

22. Jablonska, E.; Raimondi, S.; Gromadzinska, J.; Reszka, E.; Wieczorek, E.; Krol, M.B.; Smok-Pieniazek, A.; Nocun, M.; Stepnik, M.; Socha, K.; et al. DNA damage and oxidative stress response to selenium yeast in the non-smoking individuals: A short-term supplementation trial with respect to gpx1 and sepp1 polymorphism. *Eur. J. Nutr.* **2015**, *55*, 2469–2484. [CrossRef] [PubMed]

23. Asemi, Z.; Jamilian, M.; Mesdaghinia, E.; Esmaillzadeh, A. Effects of selenium supplementation on glucose homeostasis, inflammation, and oxidative stress in gestational diabetes: Randomized, double-blind, placebo-controlled trial. *Nutrition* **2015**, *31*, 1235–1242. [CrossRef] [PubMed]

24. Jamilian, M.; Razavi, M.; Fakhrie Kashan, Z.; Ghandi, Y.; Bagherian, T.; Asemi, Z. Metabolic response to selenium supplementation in women with polycystic ovary syndrome: A randomized, double-blind, placebo-controlled trial. *Clin. Endocrinol. (Oxf.)* **2015**, *82*, 885–891. [CrossRef] [PubMed]

25. Alizadeh, M.; Safaeiyan, A.; Ostadrahimi, A.; Estakhri, R.; Daneghian, S.; Ghaffari, A.; Gargari, B.P. Effect of L-arginine and selenium added to a hypocaloric diet enriched with legumes on cardiovascular disease risk factors in women with central obesity: A randomized, double-blind, placebo-controlled trial. *Ann. Nutr. Metab.* **2012**, *60*, 157–168. [CrossRef] [PubMed]

26. Farrokhian, A.; Bahmani, F.; Taghizadeh, M.; Mirhashemi, S.M.; Aarabi, M.H.; Raygan, F.; Aghadavod, E.; Asemi, Z. Selenium supplementation affects insulin resistance and serum hs-crp in patients with type 2 diabetes and coronary heart disease. *Horm. Metab. Res.* **2016**, *48*, 263–268. [CrossRef] [PubMed]

27. Faghihi, T.; Radfar, M.; Barmal, M.; Amini, P.; Qorbani, M.; Abdollahi, M.; Larijani, B. A randomized, placebo-controlled trial of selenium supplementation in patients with type 2 diabetes: Effects on glucose homeostasis, oxidative stress, and lipid profile. *Am. J. Ther.* **2014**, *21*, 491–495. [CrossRef] [PubMed]

28. Algotar, A.M.; Stratton, M.S.; Stratton, S.P.; Hsu, C.H.; Ahmann, F.R. No effect of selenium supplementation on serum glucose levels in men with prostate cancer. *Am. J. Med.* **2010**, *123*, 765–768. [CrossRef] [PubMed]

29. Czernichow, S.; Couthouis, A.; Bertrais, S.; Vergnaud, A.C.; Dauchet, L.; Galan, P.; Hercberg, S. Antioxidant supplementation does not affect fasting plasma glucose in the supplementation with antioxidant vitamins and minerals (Su.Vi.Max) study in France: Association with dietary intake and plasma concentrations. *Am. J. Clin. Nutr.* **2006**, *84*, 395–399. [PubMed]

30. Wang, X.; Wu, H.; Long, Z.; Sun, Q.; Liu, J.; Liu, Y.; Hai, C. Differential effect of Se on insulin resistance: Regulation of adipogenesis and lipolysis. *Mol. Cell Biochem.* **2016**, *415*, 89–102. [CrossRef] [PubMed]

31. Zeng, M.-S.; Li, X.; Liu, Y.; Zhao, H.; Zhou, J.-C.; Li, K.; Huang, J.-Q.; Sun, L.-H.; Tang, J.-Y.; Xia, X.-J.; et al. A high-selenium diet induces insulin resistance in gestating rats and their offspring. *Free Radic. Biol. Med.* **2012**, *52*, 1335–1342. [CrossRef] [PubMed]

32. Zhao, Z.; Barcus, M.; Kim, J.; Lum, K.L.; Mills, C.; Lei, X.G. High dietary selenium intake alters lipid metabolism and protein synthesis in liver and muscle of pigs. *J. Nutr.* **2016**, *146*, 1625–1633. [CrossRef] [PubMed]

33. Pinto, A.; Juniper, D.T.; Sanil, M.; Morgan, L.; Clark, L.; Sies, H.; Rayman, M.P.; Steinbrenner, H. Supranutritional selenium induces alterations in molecular targets related to energy metabolism in skeletal muscle and visceral adipose tissue of pigs. *J. Inorg. Biochem.* **2012**, *114*, 47–54. [CrossRef] [PubMed]

34. Freitas Lima, L.C.; Braga, V.A.; do Socorro de Franca Silva, M.; Cruz, J.C.; Sousa Santos, S.H.; de Oliveira Monteiro, M.M.; Balarini, C.M. Adipokines, diabetes and atherosclerosis: An inflammatory association. *Front. Physiol.* **2015**, *6*, 304. [CrossRef] [PubMed]

35. Rayman, M.P.; Blundell-Pound, G.; Pastor-Barriuso, R.; Guallar, E.; Steinbrenner, H.; Stranges, S. A randomized trial of selenium supplementation and risk of type-2 diabetes, as assessed by plasma adiponectin. *PLoS ONE* **2012**, *7*, e45269. [CrossRef] [PubMed]

36. Mao, J.; Bath, S.C.; Vanderlelie, J.J.; Perkins, A.V.; Redman, C.W.; Rayman, M.P. No effect of modest selenium supplementation on insulin resistance in UK pregnant women, as assessed by plasma adiponectin concentration. *Br. J. Nutr.* **2016**, *115*, 32–38. [CrossRef] [PubMed]

37. Kadowaki, T.; Yamauchi, T.; Kubota, N.; Hara, K.; Ueki, K.; Tobe, K. Adiponectin and adiponectin receptors in insulin resistance, diabetes, and the metabolic syndrome. *J. Clin. Investig.* **2006**, *116*, 1784–1792. [CrossRef] [PubMed]

38. Foti, D.; Chiefari, E.; Fedele, M.; Iuliano, R.; Brunetti, L.; Paonessa, F.; Manfioletti, G.; Barbetti, F.; Brunetti, A.; Croce, C.M.; et al. Lack of the architectural factor hmga1 causes insulin resistance and diabetes in humans and mice. *Nat. Med.* **2005**, *11*, 765–773. [CrossRef] [PubMed]

39. Boucher, J.; Kleinridders, A.; Kahn, C.R. Insulin receptor signaling in normal and insulin-resistant states. *Cold Spring Harb. Perspect. Biol.* **2014**, *6*, a009191. [CrossRef] [PubMed]

40. Yu, S.X.; Zhang, W.T.; Liu, W.; Zhu, W.X.; Guo, R.C.; Wang, Y.S.; Zhang, D.H.; Wang, J.L. The inhibitory effect of selenium nanoparticles on protein glycation in vitro. *Nanotechnology* **2015**, *26*, 145703. [CrossRef] [PubMed]

41. Luo, X.; Li, R.; Yan, L.J. Roles of pyruvate, NADH, and mitochondrial complex I in redox balance and imbalance in beta cell function and dysfunction. *J. Diabetes Res.* **2015**, *2015*, 512618. [CrossRef] [PubMed]

42. Jeoung, N.H. Pyruvate dehydrogenase kinases: Therapeutic targets for diabetes and cancers. *Diabetes Metab. J.* **2015**, *39*, 188–197. [CrossRef] [PubMed]
43. Guo, X.; Li, H.; Xu, H.; Woo, S.; Dong, H.; Lu, F.; Lange, A.J.; Wu, C. Glycolysis in the control of blood glucose homeostasis. *Acta Pharm. Sin. B* **2012**, *2*, 358–367. [CrossRef]
44. Otton, R.; Mendonca, J.R.; Curi, R. Diabetes causes marked changes in lymphocyte metabolism. *J. Endocrinol.* **2002**, *174*, 55–61. [CrossRef] [PubMed]
45. Seale, L.A.; Gilman, C.L.; Hashimoto, A.C.; Ogawa-Wong, A.N.; Berry, M.J. Diet-induced obesity in the selenocysteine lyase knockout mouse. *Antioxid. Redox Signal.* **2015**, *23*, 761–774. [CrossRef] [PubMed]
46. Bao, P.; Chen, Z.; Tai, R.Z.; Shen, H.M.; Martin, F.L.; Zhu, Y.G. Selenite-induced toxicity in cancer cells is mediated by metabolic generation of endogenous selenium nanoparticles. *J. Proteome Res.* **2015**, *14*, 1127–1136. [CrossRef] [PubMed]
47. Yeung, S.J.; Pan, J.; Lee, M.H. Roles of p53, myc and hif-1 in regulating glycolysis—The seventh hallmark of cancer. *Cell Mol. Life Sci.* **2008**, *65*, 3981–3999. [CrossRef] [PubMed]
48. Sherwani, S.I.; Khan, H.A.; Ekhzaimy, A.; Masood, A.; Sakharkar, M.K. Significance of hba1c test in diagnosis and prognosis of diabetic patients. *Biomark. Insights* **2016**, *11*, 95–104. [PubMed]
49. Hirst, J.A.; Stevens, R.J.; Farmer, A.J. Changes in hba1c level over a 12-week follow-up in patients with type 2 diabetes following a medication change. *PLoS ONE* **2014**, *9*, e92458. [CrossRef] [PubMed]
50. Ogawa-Wong, A.N.; Berry, M.J.; Seale, L.A. Selenium and metabolic disorders: An emphasis on type 2 diabetes risk. *Nutrients* **2016**, *8*, 80. [CrossRef] [PubMed]
51. Hellwege, J.N.; Palmer, N.D.; Ziegler, J.T.; Langefeld, C.D.; Lorenzo, C.; Norris, J.M.; Takamura, T.; Bowden, D.W. Genetic variants in selenoprotein p plasma 1 gene (sepp1) are associated with fasting insulin and first phase insulin response in hispanics. *Gene* **2014**, *534*, 33–39. [CrossRef] [PubMed]
52. Mueller, A.S.; Pallauf, J.; Rafael, J. The chemical form of selenium affects insulinomimetic properties of the trace element: Investigations in type ii diabetic dbdb mice. *J. Nutr. Biochem.* **2003**, *14*, 637–647. [CrossRef] [PubMed]
53. Kiersztan, A.; Lukasinska, I.; Baranska, A.; Lebiedzinska, M.; Nagalski, A.; Derlacz, R.A.; Bryla, J. Differential effects of selenium compounds on glucose synthesis in rabbit kidney-cortex tubules and hepatocytes. In vitro and in vivo studies. *J. Inorg. Biochem.* **2007**, *101*, 493–505. [CrossRef] [PubMed]

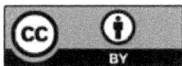

nutrients

MDPI

Article

Nutrient Patterns Associated with Fasting Glucose and Glycated Haemoglobin Levels in a Black South African Population

Tinashe Chikowore [1,*], Pedro T. Pisa [2], Tertia van Zyl [1], Edith J. M. Feskens [3], Edelweiss Wentzel-Viljoen [1,4] and Karin R. Conradie [1]

[1] Centre for Excellence in Nutrition, North-West University, Potchefstroom 2520, North West Province, South Africa; tertia.vanzyl@nwu.ac.za (T.v.Z.); edelweiss-wentzel-viljoen@nwu.ac.za (E.W.-V.); karin.conradie@nwu.ac.za (K.R.C.)
[2] Wits Reproductive Health and HIV Institute, University of the Witwatersrand, Johannesburg 2000, South Africa; ppisa@wrhi.ac.za
[3] Division of Human Nutrition, Wageningen University, P.O. Box 17, 6700 AA Wageningen, The Netherlands; edith.feskens@wur.nl
[4] Medical Research Council Research Unit for Hypertension and Cardiovascular Disease, Faculty of Health Sciences, North-West University, Potchefstroom 2520, South Africa
* Correspondence: tinashedoc@gmail.com; Tel.: +27-7-8116-9789

Received: 27 September 2016; Accepted: 19 December 2016; Published: 19 January 2017

Abstract: Type 2 diabetes (T2D) burden is increasing globally. However, evidence regarding nutrient patterns associated with the biomarkers of T2D is limited. This study set out to determine the nutrient patterns associated with fasting glucose and glycated haemoglobin the biomarkers of T2D. Factor analysis was used to derive nutrient patterns of 2010 participants stratified by urban/rural status and gender. Principal Component Analysis (PCA) was applied to 25 nutrients, computed from the quantified food frequency questionnaires (QFFQ). Three nutrient patterns per stratum, which accounted for 73% of the variation of the selected nutrients, were identified. Multivariate linear regression models adjusted for age, BMI, smoking, physical activity, education attained, alcohol intake, seasonality and total energy intake were computed. Starch, dietary fibre and B vitamins driven nutrient pattern was significantly associated with fasting glucose ($\beta = -0.236$ (-0.458; -0.014); $p = 0.037$) and glycated haemoglobin levels ($\beta = -0.175$ (-0.303; -0.047); $p = 0.007$) in rural women. Thiamine, zinc and plant protein driven nutrient pattern was associated with significant reductions in glycated haemoglobin and fasting glucose (($\beta = -0.288$ (-0.543; -0.033); $p = 0.027$) and ($\beta = -0.382$ (-0.752; -0.012); $p = 0.043$), respectively) in rural men. Our results indicate that plant driven nutrient patterns are associated with low fasting glucose and glycated haemoglobin levels.

Keywords: plant based; fasting glucose and glycated haemoglobin; T2D; dietary patterns

1. Introduction

Type 2 diabetes (T2D) prevalence and the burden it places on populations is increasing globally, thereby making it a public health challenge which requires urgent attention [1]. For instance, the global prevalence of T2D among women increased from 5% to 7.9% from 1980 to 2014 [2]. The diabetes prevalence in Africa is projected to have the largest increase of 109% compared to other regions in the world by 2035 [3]. Urban black South Africans have not been spared from the T2D burden. The highest prevalence of T2D in Sub Saharan Africa was reported among urban black South Africans, with 60% of these cases being reported amongst women [4]. Black South African women also have the highest prevalence of obesity, which has been reported to be rising together with T2D in this population [5].

The adoption of Westernised lifestyles by urban dwellers is suggested to be among the leading factors resulting in the increase in non-communicable diseases (NCDs) such as T2D in developing countries [6]. The migration of populations from rural to urban areas has been accompanied by an increase in meat consumption as well as an increase in the consumption of sugary foods in South Africa [7]. Both of these foods are recognised as dietary risk factors for T2D [6]. However, improvements in micronutrient intake among black South African women in urban areas is suggested to be a result of the increased consumption of fruits and vegetables which are protective of T2D risk [8–10]. Thus, the role of diet as a risk factor for T2D is complex among the black South African women. In addition, people eat meals with a variety of nutrients which have interactive and synergistic effects on health [11]. Therefore, it is difficult to determine the separate effect of a food or nutrient on disease development as it is highly interrelated with other nutrients [11]. There is need of dietary pattern analysis methods which are able to evaluate the diet as a whole and clarify the effects of the consumption of sugary foods and meat products, together with improved intakes of fruits and vegetables, related to T2D risk amongst this population group.

Dietary pattern (or food pattern) approaches comprise data driven methods such as factor analysis, which allow the dietary information (or food intake) at hand to determine the unique dietary pattern for the population group being evaluated [10]. Although dietary patterns have been associated with disease risk, their effect is considered to be through nutrient intake; therefore, it is pivotal to determine nutrient patterns that are associated with T2D risk [12]. This information will aid in the understanding of the aetiology of T2D. The foods that people eat are governed by their cultural norms and beliefs, which vary amongst ethnic groups, making dietary patterns limited and not applicable across divergent population groups [12]. Evidence exists that the Western dietary pattern association with fasting glucose varies among different ethnic groups [13]. However, nutrients are universal, thereby making nutrient patterns associations with disease risk applicable for multiple population groups [14]. To the best of our knowledge, no study has reported on the association of the nutrient patterns with fasting glucose and glycated haemoglobin levels among apparently healthy individuals. T2D is a complex and multifactorial diseases, however glycated haemoglobin and fasting glucose levels are proxies for the development of this disease which are affected by diet [15]. Fasting glucose levels are indicative of the short term changes in glucose metabolism, while glycated haemoglobin depicts the long term changes [15]. This study seeks to evaluate the association of nutrient patterns derived by factor analysis with fasting glucose and glycated haemoglobin levels among apparently healthy black South Africans.

2. Materials and Methods

2.1. Study Population

The study participants (*n* = 2010) were recruited from two urban and rural areas of the North West Province into the South African arm of the Prospective urban and rural epidemiological (PURE) study using a population based sampling strategy. Apparently healthy male and female volunteers between the ages of 35 and 60 years were recruited by the fieldworkers. Individuals were considered to be apparently healthy if they were not using any medication for chronic disease and if they were not diagnosed with a chronic medical condition/disease. The international PURE study is a large-scale epidemiological study, which comprises research participants recruited from 17 low, middle, and high income countries [16]. The South African arm of the PURE study was initiated in 2005 with initial five-year follow-up intervals up to 2015. At baseline in 2005 and at the five-year intervals during the course of the study, medical history, lifestyle behaviour (physical activity and dietary intake), blood collection (for both genetic and biochemical analyses), an electrocardiogram, and anthropometric assessments were performed to determine the role of risk factors in the development of cardiovascular diseases [16]. Our study was nested in the 2005 PURE study baseline data. Stratified nutrient pattern analysis was conducted according to gender and urban/rural status among the 2010 participants of the PURE study. However, significant associations of the nutrient patterns with fasting glucose and glycated haemoglobin were noted only among the rural women and rural men. Therefore, the detailed nutrient pattern and association results of the rural participants are elaborated in the main text while results of the urban men and women are illustrated in the Supplementary Materials.

2.2. Ethical Approval

The participants gave written informed consent before participating in the study and the study was conducted according to the Declaration of Helsinki principles [17]. Ethical approval was granted by the Ethics Committee of the North-West University, Potchefstroom Campus, with ethics number NWU-00016-10-A1.

2.3. Dietary, Anthropometric and Physical Activity Assessments

The trained fieldworkers captured the dietary intake of the participants using a standardised quantitative food frequency questionnaire (QFFQ) which had been validated for the same ethnic population group of the study participants [18,19]. The reproducibility of the QFFQ was also assessed and found to be good in this specific study population [20]. The dietary intake data were coded, analysed and nutrient intakes were computed using the South African Food Composition Database [21]. Body weight measurements were performed in duplicate by the PURE research team members using a portable electronic scale (Precision Health Scale, A & D Company, Tokyo, Japan), after which the mean was recorded. The heights of the subjects were determined by the PURE study research team members using a stadiometer (IP 1465, Invicta, and London, UK). The BMI of the participants was computed using the formula: BMI = weight (kg/height (m^2)). The Baecke physical activity questionnaire (BPAQ) which was validated for South Africa was used to collect the physical activity information of the participants [22]. The questionnaire was used to compute a physical activity index score as described elsewhere [22,23]. This physical activity index scores were used in the multivariate regression analysis to adjust for physical activity.

2.4. Biochemical Measurements

The research participants were required to fast (at least 8 h with no food or beverages, including water before measurements) and their blood glucose levels were measured by the PURE research team. These fasting glucose levels were measured using the SYNCHRON® System from fluoride plasma. The Bio-Rad D-10™, HbA1c kit (Bio-Rad Laboratories, Inc., Hercules, France), which operates via cation exchange high performance liquid chromatography was used to assess HbA1c levels from whole blood ethylenediaminetetraacetic acid (EDTA) treated samples. The coefficient of variation of the glycated haemoglobin and fasting glucose tests were 1.16% and 2.1%, respectively.

2.5. Statistical Analysis

The statistical analysis was performed using the statistical package for social scientists (SPSS) version 23. Normality tests for the continuous variables were performed using the Q-Q plots. Twenty-five nutrients were used to determine the nutrient patterns as has been reported previously by Pisa et al. [24]. Among these 25 nutrients, total protein was split into animal protein and plant protein; total carbohydrates were divided into total sugar, starch, and total dietary fibre; and total fat was categorised into saturated fat, monounsaturated fat and polyunsaturated fat. The total dietary fibre comprised soluble and insoluble dietary fibre. Alcohol was not regarded as a nutrient and not included in deriving the nutrient pattern analysis. However, in view of the reported association of alcohol intake with glycated haemoglobin, it was adjusted for in the multivariate linear models for the association of the derived nutrient patterns with glycated haemoglobin and fasting glucose [25]. The nutrient intake variables from the quantitative food frequency questionnaire (QFFQ) were log transformed to remove bias due to variance as a result of the different measures of scale used to quantify the nutrients. These nutrients were adjusted for log alcohol free energy using the multivariate (standard) method [11]. The multivariate method was selected as it yielded more cumulative variance and interpretable nutrient patterns compared to the standard nutrient density method of adjusting for total energy intake [11]. Principal component analysis (PCA) was the factor reduction tool used to determine the nutrient patterns from the 25 selected nutrients. The PCA was performed with the variance based on the covariance matrix and Varimax rotation. The retained principal components (PC) were used to identify the nutrient patterns. The scree plot (Figure 1) was used to determine the number of PCs to retain. The nutrient patterns were named using the nutrients with loadings greater than ±0.47 on the PCs. The total variances explained by the retained PCs were also evaluated to determine the relevance of the extracted PCs. The PCA was a suitable data reduction approach for the nutrient data in this study as was indicated by a Kaiser–Meyer–Olkin measure of sampling adequacy of 0.911, and a Bartlett's test of sphericity which was significant at $p < 0.001$. The PCs were categorised into tertiles and analysis of variance ANOVA (for continuous variables) and Chi-square (for categorical variables) tests were used to determine the descriptive characteristics of the study participants across the tertiles of the extracted PCs.

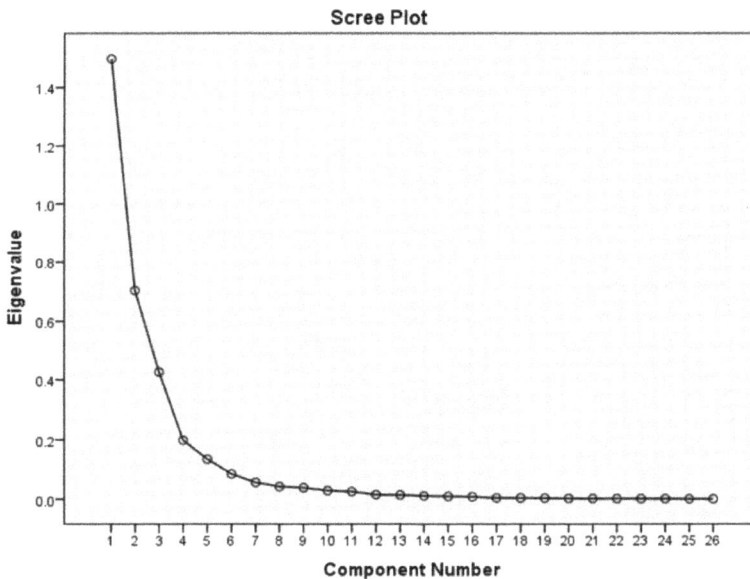

Figure 1. Scree plot of the nutrients and the extracted principal components among rural women.

Crude and adjusted multiple linear regression models were computed to assess the association between the extracted PCs with glycated haemoglobin and fasting glucose as dependent variables separately through varied models. In these models, regression coefficients for 1 standard deviation (SD) increase in the PC scores (and their 95% confidence intervals) were computed for four models: M1: (crude); M2: (adjusted for M1 plus Log Total Energy); M3: (adjusted for M2 plus Body Mass Index); and M4: (adjusted for M3 plus age, smoking, physical activity, education level, seasonality, alcohol intake and other PCs). Seasonality was adjusted based on the months in which the dietary assessments were conducted. Thus, for the rural participants, seasonality was adjusted basing on August and September; and the months of October and November were used to adjust for seasonality in the urban participants. Partial R^2 values were computed to express the variance explained by each model. Statistical significance was regarded at p value less than 0.05.

3. Results

3.1. Nutrient Patterns

Three nutrient patterns (Table S1) were extracted from the PCA, which explained 73% of the total variation of the selected nutrient factors among the rural women. The first nutrient pattern was depicted as "Magnesium, phosphorus and plant protein driven nutrients". This pattern consisted of higher loadings for magnesium, phosphorus and plant protein. The second nutrient pattern was termed "Fat and animal protein driven nutrients" as it had higher loadings of cholesterol, monounsaturated fat, animal protein, polyunsaturated fat and saturated fat. The "Starch, dietary fibre and B vitamins driven" based nutrient pattern was the third extracted nutrient pattern. This nutrient pattern had high loadings of starch, folate, vitamin B6, dietary fibre and thiamine as illustrated in Table S1.

Three nutrient patterns were extracted among rural men and named according to the nutrients with the highest loadings as indicated in Table S1. These were the "Thiamine, zinc and plant protein driven nutrients", "Fat and animal protein driven nutrients", and "Retinol and vitamin B12 driven nutrients". Three similar nutrients patterns were extracted among the rural men, urban men and urban women, which explained 76%, 77% and 76% (Tables S1 and S2) variance of the nutrients, respectively. However, some considerable differences were noted in the plant driven nutrient patterns, which accounted for the greater variation of the nutrients among the urban and rural participants (Table S3).

3.2. Descriptive Characteristics of the Study Population

The study participants included 659 rural women, 347 rural men, 605 urban women and 399 urban men. The mean fasting glucose levels and glycated haemoglobin were 4.96 ± 1.57 mmol·L^{-1} and $5.64\% \pm 0.88\%$, respectively [26]. The women had a mean BMI of 26.73 ± 7.21, which signified that a considerable proportion of the women were overweight. Overall, in the whole study population, 39.4% of the participants were overweight and 87.3% of these were women. The mean total energy intake was 7707.13 ± 3692.36 KJ. The high scores of magnesium, phosphorus and plant protein driven nutrient pattern were associated with high total energy intake and energy from alcohol in rural women, as indicated in Table 1. The high scores for the fat and animal protein driven nutrient pattern was significantly associated with tertiary education status, as indicated in Table 1.

High scores for the thiamine, zinc and plant protein nutrient pattern were associated with higher energy and alcohol intake compared to other nutrient patterns among the rural men (Table 2).

3.3. Nutrient Patterns Associations with Fasting and Glycated Haemoglobin Levels

The association results of glycated haemoglobin and fasting glucose levels with 1 SD increases in the extracted nutrient patterns are shown in Tables 3–6 for the rural women and rural men. The magnesium, phosphorus and plant protein driven nutrient pattern was associated with a consistent trend of increases in fasting glucose and glycated haemoglobin among rural women, as illustrated in Table 3.

Conversely, the starch, dietary fibre and B vitamins nutrient pattern was consistently associated with reduced glycated haemoglobin and fasting glucose levels in all evaluated linear models, for instance the M4 model: -0.175% (-0.303; -0.047); $p = 0.007$) and -0.236 mmol·L^{-1} (-0.458; -0.014); $p = 0.037$), respectively, as indicated in Tables 3 and 4 among rural women.

The thiamine, zinc and plant protein nutrient pattern was associated with reduced glycated haemoglobin and fasting glucose levels in rural men as illustrated in Tables 5 and 6. For instance, the M4 models, which explained the highest variances of the fasting glucose and glycated haemoglobin, indicated reductions of these outcome variables to be -0.382 mmol·L^{-1} (-0.752; -0.012; $p = 0.043$) and -0.288% (-0.543; -0.033; $p = 0.027$), respectively, as illustrated in Tables 5 and 6.

Table 1. Descriptive characteristics for the rural women of the study population according to the lowest and highest tertiles of the three nutrient patterns (PC).

	Magnesium, Phosphorus and Plant Protein Driven Nutrients			Fat and Animal Protein Driven Nutrients			Starch, Dietary Fibre and B Vitamin Driven Nutrients		
	T1	T3	p	T1	T3	p	T1	T3	p
Age	48.72 ± 10.23	47.51 ± 9.57	0.247	47.94 ± 8.89	47.73 ± 10.16	0.837	49.15 ± 10.40	46.94 ± 8.99	0.036
Body Mass Index	25.28 ± 6.63	25.27 ± 6.58	0.988	25.31 ± 6.75	26.13 ± 6.85	0.262	25.26 ± 6.41	25.65 ± 7.11	0.605
Total energy	4322.96 ± 1217.30	8365.01 ± 2476.92	<0.001	5631.33 ± 2816.62	6883.88 ± 2189.38	<0.001	5893.08 ± 2645.21	6567.51 ± 2425.60	0.013
Alcohol (%TE)	0.76 ± 2.56	7.42 ± 12.56	<0.001	5.54 ± 11.70	1.47 ± 4.40	<0.001	5.36 ± 11.91	1.69 ± 5.01	<0.001
Protein (%TE)	11.26 ± 1.96	10.77 ± 1.64	0.008	10.27 ± 1.33	11.67 ± 1.81	<0.001	11.23 ± 2.05	10.91 ± 1.31	0.092
Current Smokers (%)	33.5	36.8	0.168	38.0	34.7	0.005	30.6	36.4	0.595
Physical Activity Index	8.19 ± 1.42	8.28 ± 1.42	0.593	8.29 ± 1.29	8.32 ± 1.55	0.854	8.23 ± 1.37	8.44 ± 1.45	0.205
Tertiary education (%)	33.7	24.5	0.058	26.5	42.9	0.028	28.6	38.8	0.854
Fasting glucose (mmol·L^{-1})	4.73 ± 0.78	4.93 ± 1.47	0.219	4.91 ± 1.18	4.87 ± 1.02	0.784	5.12 ± 2.41	4.88 ± 0.83	0.160
HbA1C (%)	5.64 ± 0.53	5.67 ± 0.93	0.785	5.68 ± 0.91	5.69 ± 0.58	0.843	5.84 ± 1.23	5.62 ± 0.55	0.027

p = p value based on ANOVA or Chi-square test where appropriate; Alcohol (%TE) = percentage of total energy due to alcohol intake; Protein (%TE) = percentage of total energy due to protein intake; T1 = lowest tertile; T3 = highest tertile; TE = total energy; HbA1C = glycated haemoglobin.

Table 2. Descriptive characteristics for the rural men of the study population according to the lowest and highest tertiles of the three nutrient patterns (PC).

	Thiamine, Zinc and Plant Protein Driven Nutrients			Fat and Animal Protein Driven Nutrients			Retinol and Vitamin B12 Driven Nutrients		
	T1	T3	p	T1	T3	p	T1	T3	p
Age	47.95 ± 9.99	50.19 ± 10.69	0.156	48.43 ± 9.97	51.42 ± 11.45	0.057	49.66 ± 10.01	49.57 ± 9.95	0.954
Body Mass Index	20.86 ± 4.15	20.54 ± 4.31	0.606	20.86 ± 3.99	20.94 ± 4.65	0.894	20.30 ± 3.57	20.95 ± 4.19	0.297
Total energy	4693.60 ± 1584.26	10,637.00 ± 2887.76	<0.001	6319.63 ± 3228.51	8220.85 ± 3228.51	<0.001	7164.14 ± 2975.31	7855.83 ± 3672.65	0.159
Alcohol (%TE)	5.98 ± 9.40	13.82 ± 13.70	<0.001	11.19 ± 13.41	5.70 ± 9.16	0.002	6.65 ± 11.23	9.19 ± 11.79	0.159
Protein (%TE)	11.51 ± 2.69	10.76 ± 1.53	0.014	10.09 ± 1.43	12.19 ± 2.33	<0.001	10.64 ± 1.69	11.50 ± 2.48	0.005
Current Smokers (%)	32.4	35.9	0.636	40.0	26.2	0.003	31.7	31.7	0.577
Physical Activity Index	8.25 ± 1.64	8.02 ± 1.44	0.380	8.03 ± 1.65	7.99 ± 1.79	0.861	7.92 ± 1.61	7.97 ± 1.63	0.847
Tertiary education (%)	44.2	20.9	0.141	23.3	37.2	0.514	27.9	37.2	0.451
Fasting glucose (mmol·L^{-1})	4.90 ± 0.93	4.68 ± 0.90	0.113	4.75 ± 0.79	4.96 ± 1.24	0.138	4.94 ± 2.41	4.75 ± 0.78	0.190
HbA1C (%)	5.59 ± 0.52	5.51 ± 0.81	0.386	5.49 ± 0.34	5.62 ± 0.97	0.169	5.57 ± 0.83	5.53 ± 0.49	0.678

p = p value based on ANOVA or Chi-square test where appropriate; Alcohol (%TE) = percentage of total energy due to alcohol intake; Protein (%TE) = percentage of total energy due to protein intake; T1 = lowest tertile; T3 = highest tertile; TE = total energy; HbA1C = glycated haemoglobin.

Table 3. Regression coefficients for fasting glucose for 1 SD increase in the derived nutrient pattern scores among rural black South African women.

	Magnesium, Phosphorus and Plant Protein Driven Nutrients			Fat and Animal Protein Driven Nutrients			Starch, Dietary Fibre and B Vitamin Driven Nutrients		
	B (95% CI)	*p* Value	R^2	B (95% CI)	*p* Value	R^2	B (95% CI)	*p* Value	R^2
M1	0.129 (−0.014; 0.271)	0.077	0.007	0.009 (−0.141; 0.160)	0.902	0.000	−0.164 (−0.311; −0.018)	0.027	0.008
M2	0.196 (−0.063; 0.455)	0.138	0.007	−0.020 (−0.183; 0.143)	0.813	0.003	−0.197 (−0.349; −0.049)	0.011	0.016
M3	0.278 (−0.001; 0.280)	0.034	0.045	−0.038 (−0.198; 0.123)	0.645	0.037	−0.203 (−0.351; −0.054)	0.008	0.051
M4	0.147 (−0.360; 0.655)	0.569	0.086	−0.004 (−0.290; 0.281)	0.976	0.086	−0.236 (−0.458; −0.014)	0.037	0.086

M1: (crude); M2: (adjusted for M1 plus Log Total Energy); M3: (adjusted for M2 plus Body Mass Index); M4: (adjusted for M3 plus age, smoking, physical activity, alcohol intake, seasonality, education level, PC1, PC2 and PC3); M1 = model 1; M2 = model 2; M3 = model 3; M4 = model 4; PC1 = Magnesium, phosphorus and plant protein driven nutrients; PC2 = Fat and animal protein driven nutrients; PC3 = Starch, dietary fibre and B vitamin driven nutrients Fasting glucose units mmol·L^{-1} = millimoles per litre; SD = standard deviation; CI = confidence interval.

Table 4. Regression coefficients for glycated haemoglobin for 1 SD increase in the derived nutrient pattern scores among rural black South African women.

	Magnesium, Phosphorus and Plant Protein Driven Nutrients			Fat and Animal Protein Driven Nutrients			Starch, Dietary Fibre and B Vitamin Driven Nutrients		
	B (95% CI)	*p* Value	R^2	B (95% CI)	*p* Value	R^2	B (95% CI)	*p* Value	R^2
M1	0.029 (−0.055; 0.112)	0.502	0.001	0.032 (−0.056; 0.120)	0.477	0.001	−0.138 (−0.224; −0.053)	0.002	0.020
M2	0.048 (−0.104; 0.199)	0.538	0.001	0.028 (−0.067; 0.123)	0.563	0.001	−0.145 (−0.234; −0.056)	0.001	0.021
M3	0.112 (−0.036; 0.260)	0.139	0.069	0.014 (−0.078; 0.106)	0.766	0.065	−0.151 (−0.237; −0.065)	0.001	0.087
M4	0.107 (−0.188; 0.401)	0.478	0.150	−0.011 (−0.175; 0.154)	0.478	0.150	−0.175 (−0.303; −0.047)	0.007	0.150

M1: (crude); M2: (adjusted for M1 plus Log Total Energy); M3: (adjusted for M2 plus Body Mass Index); M4: (adjusted for M3 plus age, smoking, physical activity, alcohol intake, seasonality, education level, PC1, PC2 and PC3); M1 = model 1; M2 = model 2; M3 = model 3; M4 = model 4; PC1 = Magnesium, phosphorus and plant protein driven nutrients; PC2 = Fat and animal protein driven nutrients; PC3 = Starch, dietary fibre and B vitamin driven nutrients. Glycated haemoglobin unit = per cent; SD = standard deviation; CI = confidence interval.

Table 5. Regression coefficients for fasting glucose for 1 SD increase in the derived nutrient pattern scores among rural black South African men.

	Thiamine, Zinc and Plant Protein Driven Nutrients			Fat and Animal Protein Driven Nutrients			Retinol and Vitamin B12 Driven Nutrients		
	B (95% CI)	p Value	R^2	B (95% CI)	p Value	R^2	B (95% CI)	p Value	R^2
M1	−0.057 (−0.172; 0.057)	0.326	0.004	0.054 (−0.061; 0.169)	0.355	0.003	−0.039 (−0.156; 0.077)	0.504	0.002
M2	−0.237 (−0.492; 0.019)	0.069	0.013	0.061 (−0.064; 0.186)	0.335	0.004	−0.055 (−0.173; 0.064)	0.363	0.003
M3	−0.255 (−0.496; 0.014)	0.038	0.117	0.055 (−0.063; 0.172)	0.363	0.115	−0.082 (−0.194; 0.030)	0.153	0.120
M4	−0.382 (−0.752; −0.012)	0.043	0.182	−0.051 (−0.241; 0.139)	0.596	0.182	−0.109 (−0.229; 0.032)	0.074	0.182

M1: (crude); M2: (adjusted for M1 plus Log Total Energy); M3: (adjusted for M2 plus Body Mass Index); M4: (adjusted for M3 plus age, smoking, physical activity, alcohol intake, seasonality, education level, PC1, PC2 and PC3); M1 = model 1; M2 = model 2; M3 = model 3; M4 = model 4; PC1 = Magnesium, phosphorus and plant protein driven nutrients; PC2 = Fat and animal protein driven nutrients; PC3 = Starch, dietary fibre and B vitamin driven nutrients Fasting glucose units mmol·L^{-1} = millimoles per litre; SD = standard deviation; CI = confidence interval.

Table 6. Regression coefficients for glycated haemoglobin for 1 SD increase in the derived nutrient pattern scores among rural black South African women.

	Thiamine, Zinc and Plant Protein Driven Nutrients			Fat and Animal Protein Driven Nutrients			Retinol and Vitamin B12 Driven Nutrients		
	B (95% CI)	p Value	R^2	B (95% CI)	p Value	R^2	B (95% CI)	p Value	R^2
M1	−0.039 (−0.117; 0.038)	0.320	0.000	0.046 (−0.031; 0.123)	0.241	0.005	0.012 (−0.065; 0.090)	0.754	0.000
M2	−0.214 (−0.384; 0.044)	0.014	0.024	0.053 (−0.031; 0.138)	0.213	0.006	0.015 (−0.065; 0.094)	0.713	0.001
M3	−0.230 (−0.392; −0.067)	0.006	0.113	0.050 (−0.030; 0.131)	0.219	0.092	0.001 (−0.075; 0.077)	0.975	0.086
M4	−0.288 (−0.543; −0.033)	0.027	0.174	−0.057 (−0.189; 0.075)	0.396	0.174	−0.018 (−0.100; 0.064)	0.662	0.174

M1: (crude); M2: (adjusted for M1 plus Log Total Energy); M3: (adjusted for M2 plus Body Mass Index); M4: (adjusted for M3 plus age, smoking, physical activity, alcohol intake, seasonality, education level, PC1, PC2 and PC3); M1 = model 1; M2 = model 2; M3 = model 3; M4 = model 4; PC1 = Magnesium, phosphorus and plant protein driven nutrients; PC2 = Fat and animal protein driven nutrients; PC3 = Starch, dietary fibre and B vitamin driven nutrients. Glycated haemoglobin unit = per cent; SD = standard deviation; CI = confidence interval.

The plant driven nutrient patterns had significant results as has been shown above among the urban and rural participants. However, some notable differences were depicted in the plant driven nutrient patterns illustrated in Table S3. The following nutrient patterns, "thiamine, zinc and plant protein driven nutrients", "thiamine, starch and folate driven nutrients", and "magnesium, phosphorus and plant protein driven nutrients" extracted from the urban men, urban women and rural women, respectively, had higher loadings for animal protein, saturated fat, mono-saturated fat and sugar compared to the "thiamine, zinc and plant protein driven nutrients" and "the starch, dietary fibre and B vitamin driven nutrients patterns", which were associated with significant reductions in fasting and glycated haemoglobin among the rural men and women respectively (see factor loadings in bold in Table S3). These two nutrient patterns that had significant associations with fasting glucose and glycated haemoglobin had very low cholesterol and saturated fat as illustrated in Table S3.

4. Discussion

We set out to determine the nutrient patterns associated with fasting glucose and glycated haemoglobin levels among apparently healthy volunteers. The principal component analysis method enabled the extraction of three nutrient patterns among a black South African population which explained about 73% of the variation of the nutrient factors in the urban/rural and gender stratifications. The magnesium, phosphorus and plant protein driven nutrient pattern was associated with a trend of increasing fasting glucose and glycated haemoglobin levels per 1 SD increase in the pattern in the rural women while the thiamine, zinc and plant protein nutrient pattern was associated with a positive trend of increasing glycated haemoglobin among urban men. Notably, the starch, dietary fibre and B vitamin nutrient pattern was associated with decreases in glycated haemoglobin and fasting glucose levels, -0.175% $((-0.303; -0.047); p = 0.007)$ and -0.236 mmol·L^{-1} $((-0.458; -0.014);$ $p = 0.037)$, respectively, among rural women. The thiamine, zinc and plant protein driven nutrient pattern was associated with significant reductions in fasting glucose and glycated haemoglobin of -0.382 mmol·L^{-1} $(-0.752; -0.012; p = 0.043)$ and -0.288% $(-0.543; -0.033; p = 0.027)$ in rural men. These associations were significantly maintained after adjusting for age, BMI, log total energy intake, smoking, physical activity, alcohol intake, seasonality and education level attained thus indicating an independent association of the starch, dietary fibre and B vitamin nutrient pattern and the thiamine, zinc and plant protein driven nutrient pattern with fasting glucose and glycated haemoglobin in the rural women and rural men strata's, respectively.

Comparable studies evaluating the associations of nutrients patterns with fasting glucose and glycated haemoglobin are scarce. However, evidence exists of dietary patterns which have evaluated this phenomenon [10]. The Health/Prudent dietary pattern has been associated with decreases in fasting glucose and glycated haemoglobin levels while the Western dietary pattern has been associated with increases in these biomarkers of T2D [27,28]. However, the association of the Western dietary pattern, which is characterised with high intakes of animal proteins and snacks, with fasting glucose levels was noted to vary among ethnic groups [13]. The Western dietary pattern was reported in one study to be only significantly associated with high fasting glucose levels and glycated haemoglobin levels among Dutch and not among the Moroccans and Turkish groups [13]. Dietary patterns are known to vary among different ethnic groups, therefore nutrient patterns that were considered in our study are considered helpful in indicating a non-ethnic insight into this phenomenon.

In our study, we noted that fat and animal protein driven nutrients were also not associated with fasting glucose and glycated levels, as had been depicted in dietary pattern analysis studies among different ethnic groups [13]. This disparity from the Western populations where the animal based/Western dietary patterns are associated with increasing fasting glucose levels has been explained by the realisation that ethnic groups such as Asians may adopt the Western diets but their intake of animal products will remain lower as they also continue to consume traditional cereals and vegetables [29]. Similarly, in this study population, the intake of fat and animal protein nutrients were lower in the plant driven nutrients patterns that accounted for the greatest variance among the three nutrients patterns extracted per stratum as illustrated in Table S3. In other local studies, the protein and fat intakes as percentage of total energy intake for urban women from 1975 to 2005 did not change drastically though evidences of the adoption of Western dietary patterns were being noted and the greater proportion of the energy intake was still being contributed by the carbohydrate intake as had been noted in the Asians [6]. From 1975 to 2005, the percentage of energy of protein intake changed from 14% to 13%, while fat intake as percentage of energy changed from 21% to 30% and carbohydrate intake changed from 67% to 57% of total energy intake [6]. Thus, the intake of fat and animal protein driven nutrients in this population group might have been lower and thus not associated with increases in fasting glucose and glycated haemoglobin as was expected.

The magnesium, phosphorus and plant protein driven nutrient pattern indicated a positive trend association with increases in fasting glucose and glycated haemoglobin levels among rural women, while the thiamine, zinc and plant protein driven nutrient pattern was associated with a trend of increasing glycated haemoglobin levels in the urban men (Table S7). However, plant protein and zinc, which were high in these nutrient patterns, have been reported to independently lower fasting glucose levels [30–33]. In addition, the thiamine, zinc and plant protein driven nutrient pattern was associated with a trend of decreasing glycated haemoglobin and fasting glucose levels in the rural men. In view that the study population comprised people who consumed diets with both animal and plant based nutrients and not purely vegetarians, the discrepancies in the associations of the plant driven nutrients can be explained by the varied proportions of animal protein, saturated fat, mono-saturated fat, cholesterol and sugar among these plant driven nutrient patterns, as illustrated in Table S3. The magnesium, phosphorus and plant protein driven nutrient pattern in rural women and the thiamine, zinc and plant protein driven nutrient pattern in urban men had higher loadings of animal protein, saturated fat, mono-saturated fat, cholesterol and sugar compared to the other nutrient patterns discussed below such as the starch, dietary fibre and B vitamins driven nutrient pattern among rural women and the thiamine, zinc and plant protein nutrient pattern among rural men which associated with low fasting glucose and glycated haemoglobin levels. Animal protein, saturated fat, cholesterol and sugar are high in Western dietary patterns which have been previously associated with increased risk of T2D and this helps clarify the positive trend of association of the magnesium, phosphorus and plant protein driven nutrient pattern in rural women and the thiamine, zinc and plant protein driven nutrient pattern in urban men with the study outcome variables [34]. The comparisons of the varied constituents of the plant driven nutrients as discussed above and illustrated in Table S3 indicates the attractiveness of the PCA approach of nutrient pattern determination as it allows a whole based approach of the effect of nutrients to particular outcomes to be evaluated.

The starch, dietary fibre and B vitamins driven nutrient pattern was consistently associated with reduced fasting glucose and glycated haemoglobin levels in all the multivariate linear models which were considered in this study among rural women. The thiamine, zinc and plant protein nutrient pattern was also associated with significant reductions in glycated haemoglobin and fasting glucose among rural men. These findings are similar to the results of other studies on plant based dietary patterns and T2D risk [10,34]. It has been consistently reported that plant based diets are protective against T2D risk [10,34,35]. A number of mechanisms have been proposed to explain this phenomenon [10]. Plant based diets which are rich in dietary fibre are suggested to reduce T2D risk by reducing postprandial insulin demand, improving insulin sensitivity and the antioxidants found in these diets may help enhance β-cell function [36,37]. Dietary fibre from cereal foods which are also high in starch has been consistently shown across eight European countries to be associated with reduced T2D risk [38]. Maize meal fortified with iron, zinc and B vitamins which is largely consumed among the black South African population group is known to contain resistant starches that are partially digested and have been associated with improved insulin sensitivity which may then lead to reductions in fasting glucose levels [39,40]. Thiamine was also high in this nutrient pattern. Evidence exists that dietary fibre beneficial effects might also be due to its concomitant intake together with thiamine [41]. The results of this study suggest that starch, dietary fibre and B vitamins nutrients, zinc and plant protein consumed together may lead to the lowering of fasting and glycated haemoglobin levels as has been postulated elsewhere [35].

The strengths of the current study include the use of a validated QFFQ and recruitment criteria of selecting apparently healthy individuals who were not taking chronic medications or suffering from chronic diseases. This might have helped to prevent the confounding of drugs and T2D to the nutrient pattern association results with glycated haemoglobin and fasting glucose levels. The factor analysis approach used to derive the nutrient patterns is known for depicting real-world dietary behaviours [42]. However, this approach is based on a number of subjective decisions such as naming nutrient patterns, method of rotation and selection of food groups which can lead to an overall measurement error [10,42]. Since this approach is a posteriori analysis tool, it derives nutrient patterns based on data at hand and this makes comparisons with other studies difficult [10,42]. However, regardless of the differences in the constituents of the nutrient patterns due to the data driven approaches used to derive them, consistent similarities of the dietary factors associated with T2D risk as reported in this study, has been depicted in multiple populations [10,34,37]. It might be probable that the residual confounding effect of total energy intake might have led to distortions in the association of the nutrient patterns with fasting glucose and glycated haemoglobin levels. Residual confounding is a result of measurement error in a confounder included in the model [43]. Although the nutrient and total energy intake based on the QFFQs are not precisely measured, adjustment for total energy intake should control for total energy intake confounding [44]. However, evidence exists that the control of total energy intake is not complete in epidemiological studies involving QFFQs thereby leading to residual confounding [44,45]. Therefore, there is need to further explore the association of the nutrient patterns in isocaloric clinical trials which are better designed to control for confounding for total energy intake [45].

5. Conclusions

In summary, our results indicate the beneficial associations of plant driven nutrient patterns with reductions in fasting glucose and glycated haemoglobin levels. However, the small variances that were explained by the models explored in this study are suggestive of the presence of other factors that affect the variation of fasting glucose and glycated haemoglobin which were not accounted for in this study. Thus, more studies are required to further explore the association of nutrient patterns with fasting glucose and glycated haemoglobin.

Supplementary Materials: The following are available online at http://www.mdpi.com/2072-6643/9/1/9/s1, Table S1. Extracted nutrient patterns and factor loadings of rural women and rural men, Table S2. Nutrient patterns and factor loadings for urban participants, Table S3. Comparison of the factors loadings in the plant driven nutrient patterns among the urban and rural participants, Table S4. Regression coefficients for fasting glucose for 1 SD increase in the derived nutrient pattern scores among urban black South African women, Table S5. Regression coefficients for glycated haemoglobin for 1 SD increase in the derived nutrient pattern scores among urban black South African women, Table S6. Regression coefficients for fasting glucose for 1 SD increase in the derived nutrient pattern scores among urban black South African men, Table S7. Regression coefficients for glycated haemoglobin for 1 SD increase in the derived nutrient pattern scores among urban black South African men.

Acknowledgments: This research was supported by a grant National Research Foundation of South Africa (87970). Tinashe Chikowore is supported by the National Research Foundation of South Africa (89117). We would like to acknowledge A. Kruger and the PURE research team, funders and participants.

Author Contributions: T.C. conceptualized the paper, analysed the data and wrote the draft article. P.T.P. designed the data analysis plan and contributed to the writing of the paper. E.W.-V. designed the dietary data collection tools, coded and analysed the data for nutrients and contributed to the writing of the paper. T.v.Z., E.J.M.F. and K.R.C. supervised and contributed to the writing of the paper.

Conflicts of Interest: The authors declare no conflict of interest.

References

1. Chen, L.; Magliano, D.J.; Zimmet, P.Z. The worldwide epidemiology of type 2 diabetes mellitus—Present and future perspectives. *Nat. Rev. Endocrinol.* **2012**, *8*, 228–236. [CrossRef] [PubMed]
2. Collaboration, N.C.D.R.F. Worldwide trends in diabetes since 1980: A pooled analysis of 751 population-based studies with 4.4 million participants. *Lancet* **2016**, *387*, 1513–1530.
3. Guariguata, L.; Whiting, D.R.; Hambleton, I.; Beagley, J.; Linnenkamp, U.; Shaw, J.E. Global estimates of diabetes prevalence for 2013 and projections for 2035. *Diabetes Res. Clin. Pract.* **2014**, *103*, 137–149. [CrossRef] [PubMed]
4. Peer, N.; Steyn, K.; Lombard, C.; Lambert, E.V.; Vythilingum, B.; Levitt, N.S. Rising diabetes prevalence among urban-dwelling black South Africans. *PLoS ONE* **2012**, *7*, e43336. [CrossRef] [PubMed]
5. Sartorius, B.; Veerman, L.J.; Manyema, M.; Chola, L.; Hofman, K. Determinants of obesity and associated population attributability, South Africa: Empirical evidence from a national panel survey, 2008–2012. *PLoS ONE* **2015**, *10*, e0130218. [CrossRef] [PubMed]
6. Vorster, H.H.; Kruger, A.; Margetts, B.M. The nutrition transition in Africa: Can it be steered into a more positive direction? *Nutrients* **2011**, *3*, 429–441. [CrossRef] [PubMed]
7. Vorster, H.H.; Kruger, A.; Wentzel-Viljoen, E.; Kruger, H.S.; Margetts, B.M. Added sugar intake in South Africa: Findings from the adult prospective urban and rural epidemiology cohort study. *Am. J. Clin. Nutr.* **2014**, *99*, 1479–1486. [CrossRef] [PubMed]
8. Vorster, H.H.; Margetts, B.M.; Venter, C.S.; Wissing, M.P. Integrated nutrition science: From theory to practice in South Africa. *Public Health Nutr.* **2005**, *8*, 760–765. [CrossRef] [PubMed]
9. Hattingh, Z.; Walsh, C.M.; Bester, C.J.; Oguntibeju, O.O. Evaluation of energy and macronutrient intake of black women in Bloemfontein: A cross-sectional study. *Afr. J. Biotechnol.* **2008**, *7*, 4019–4024.
10. McEvoy, C.T.; Cardwell, C.R.; Woodside, J.V.; Young, I.S.; Hunter, S.J.; McKinley, M.C. A posteriori dietary patterns are related to risk of type 2 diabetes: Findings from a systematic review and meta-analysis. *J. Acad. Nutr. Diet.* **2014**, *114*, 1759–1775. [CrossRef] [PubMed]
11. Hu, F.B. Dietary pattern analysis: A new direction in nutritional epidemiology. *Curr. Opin. Lipidol.* **2002**, *13*, 3–9. [CrossRef] [PubMed]
12. Salehi-Abargouei, A.; Esmaillzadeh, A.; Azadbakht, L.; Keshteli, A.H.; Feizi, A.; Feinle-Bisset, C.; Adibi, P. Nutrient patterns and their relation to general and abdominal obesity in Iranian adults: Findings from the Sepahan study. *Eur. J. Nutr.* **2016**, *55*, 505–518. [CrossRef] [PubMed]
13. Dekker, L.H.; van Dam, R.M.; Snijder, M.B.; Peters, R.J.; Dekker, J.M.; de Vries, J.H.; de Boer, E.J.; Schulze, M.B.; Stronks, K.; Nicolaou, M. Comparable dietary patterns describe dietary behavior across ethnic groups in The Netherlands, but different elements in the diet are associated with glycated hemoglobin and fasting glucose concentrations. *J. Nutr.* **2015**, *145*, 1884–1891. [CrossRef] [PubMed]
14. Freisling, H.; Fahey, M.T.; Moskal, A.; Ocke, M.C.; Ferrari, P.; Jenab, M.; Norat, T.; Naska, A.; Welch, A.A.; Navarro, C.; et al. Region-specific nutrient intake patterns exhibit a geographical gradient within and between European countries. *J. Nutr.* **2010**, *140*, 1280–1286. [CrossRef] [PubMed]
15. Koenig, R.J.; Peterson, C.M.; Jones, R.L.; Saudek, C.; Lehrman, M.; Cerami, A. Correlation of glucose regulation and hemoglobin A$_{Ic}$ in diabetes mellitus. *N. Engl. J. Med.* **1976**, *295*, 417–420. [CrossRef] [PubMed]
16. Teo, K.; Chow, C.K.; Vaz, M.; Rangarajan, S.; Yusuf, S. The Prospective Urban Rural Epidemiology (PURE) study: Examining the impact of societal influences on chronic noncommunicable diseases in low-, middle-, and high-income countries. *Am. Heart J.* **2009**, *158*, 1–7. [CrossRef] [PubMed]
17. Arie, S. Revision of Helsinki declaration aims to prevent exploitation of study participants. *BMJ* **2013**, *347*, f6401. [CrossRef] [PubMed]
18. MacIntyre, U.E.; Venter, C.S.; Vorster, H.H.; Steyn, H.S. A combination of statistical methods for the analysis of the relative validation data of the quantitative food frequency questionnaire used in the THUSA study. *Public Health Nutr.* **2001**, *4*, 45–51. [CrossRef] [PubMed]
19. Wolmarans, P.; Danster, N.; Dalton, A.; Rossouw, K.; Schönfeldt, H. *Condensed Food Composition Tables for South Africa*; Medical Research Council: Cape Town, South Africa, 2010.
20. Wentzel-Viljoen, E.; Laubscher, R.; Kruger, A. Using different approaches to assess the reproducibility of a culturally sensitive quantified food frequency questionnaire. *S. Afr. J. Clin. Nutr.* **2011**, *24*, 143–148. [CrossRef]

21. Wolmarans, P.; Chetty, J.; Danster-Christians, N. Food composition activities in South Africa. *Food Chem.* **2013**, *140*, 447–450. [CrossRef] [PubMed]
22. Kruger, H.; Venter, C.; Steyn, H. A standardised physical activity questionnaire for a population in transition: The THUSA study. *Afr. J. Phys. Health Educ. Recreat. Dance* **2000**, *6*, 54–64.
23. Oyeyemi, A.L.; Moss, S.J.; Monyeki, M.A.; Kruger, H.S. Measurement of physical activity in urban and rural South African adults: A comparison of two self-report methods. *BMC Public Health* **2016**, *16*, 1004. [CrossRef] [PubMed]
24. Pisa, P.T.; Pedro, T.M.; Kahn, K.; Tollman, S.M.; Pettifor, J.M.; Norris, S.A. Nutrient patterns and their association with socio-demographic, lifestyle factors and obesity risk in rural South African adolescents. *Nutrients* **2015**, *7*, 3464–3482. [CrossRef] [PubMed]
25. Boeing, H.; Weisgerber, U.M.; Jeckel, A.; Rose, H.J.; Kroke, A. Association between glycated hemoglobin and diet and other lifestyle factors in a nondiabetic population: Cross-sectional evaluation of data from the Potsdam cohort of the European Prospective Investigation into Cancer and Nutrition Study. *Am. J. Clin. Nutr.* **2000**, *71*, 1115–1122. [PubMed]
26. Alberti, K.G.; Zimmet, P.Z. Definition, diagnosis and classification of diabetes mellitus and its complications. Part 1: Diagnosis and classification of diabetes mellitus provisional report of a who consultation. *Diabet. Med.* **1998**, *15*, 539–553. [CrossRef]
27. Kim, H.S.; Park, S.Y.; Grandinetti, A.; Holck, P.S.; Waslien, C. Major dietary patterns, ethnicity, and prevalence of type 2 diabetes in rural Hawaii. *Nutrition* **2008**, *24*, 1065–1072. [CrossRef] [PubMed]
28. Liese, A.D.; Weis, K.E.; Schulz, M.; Tooze, J.A. Food intake patterns associated with incident type 2 diabetes: The insulin resistance atherosclerosis study. *Diabetes Care* **2009**, *32*, 263–268. [CrossRef] [PubMed]
29. Gilbert, P.A.; Khokhar, S. Changing dietary habits of ethnic groups in Europe and implications for health. *Nutr. Rev.* **2008**, *66*, 203–215. [CrossRef] [PubMed]
30. Roberts-Toler, C.; O'Neill, B.T.; Cypess, A.M. Diet-induced obesity causes insulin resistance in mouse brown adipose tissue. *Obesity (Silver Spring)* **2015**, *23*, 1765–1770. [CrossRef] [PubMed]
31. Capdor, J.; Foster, M.; Petocz, P.; Samman, S. Zinc and glycemic control: A meta-analysis of randomised placebo controlled supplementation trials in humans. *J. Trace Elem. Med. Biol.* **2013**, *27*, 137–142. [CrossRef] [PubMed]
32. Hruby, A.; Ngwa, J.S.; Renstrom, F.; Wojczynski, M.K.; Ganna, A.; Hallmans, G.; Houston, D.K.; Jacques, P.F.; Kanoni, S.; Lehtimaki, T.; et al. Higher magnesium intake is associated with lower fasting glucose and insulin, with no evidence of interaction with select genetic loci, in a meta-analysis of 15 CHARGE Consortium Studies. *J. Nutr.* **2013**, *143*, 345–353. [CrossRef] [PubMed]
33. Khattab, M.; Abi-Rashed, C.; Ghattas, H.; Hlais, S.; Obeid, O. Phosphorus ingestion improves oral glucose tolerance of healthy male subjects: A crossover experiment. *Nutr. J.* **2015**, *14*, 112. [CrossRef] [PubMed]
34. Alhazmi, A.; Stojanovski, E.; McEvoy, M.; Garg, M.L. The association between dietary patterns and type 2 diabetes: A systematic review and meta-analysis of cohort studies. *J. Hum. Nutr. Diet.* **2014**, *27*, 251–260. [CrossRef] [PubMed]
35. Sabate, J.; Wien, M. A perspective on vegetarian dietary patterns and risk of metabolic syndrome. *Br. J. Nutr* **2015**, *113* (Suppl. 2), S136–143. [CrossRef] [PubMed]
36. Barclay, A.W.; Petocz, P.; McMillan-Price, J.; Flood, V.M.; Prvan, T.; Mitchell, P.; Brand-Miller, J.C. Glycemic index, glycemic load, and chronic disease risk—A meta-analysis of observational studies. *Am. J. Clin. Nutr.* **2008**, *87*, 627–637. [PubMed]
37. Montonen, J.; Knekt, P.; Harkanen, T.; Jarvinen, R.; Heliovaara, M.; Aromaa, A.; Reunanen, A. Dietary patterns and the incidence of type 2 diabetes. *Am. J. Epidemiol.* **2005**, *161*, 219–227. [CrossRef] [PubMed]
38. InterAct Consortium. Dietary fibre and incidence of type 2 diabetes in eight European countries: The epic-interact study and a meta-analysis of prospective studies. *Diabetologia*, **2015**; *58*, 1394–1408.
39. Brites, C.M.; Trigo, M.J.; Carrapico, B.; Alvina, M.; Bessa, R.J. Maize and resistant starch enriched breads reduce postprandial glycemic responses in rats. *Nutr. Res.* **2011**, *31*, 302–308. [CrossRef] [PubMed]
40. Gower, B.A.; Bergman, R.; Stefanovski, D.; Darnell, B.; Ovalle, F.; Fisher, G.; Sweatt, S.K.; Resuehr, H.S.; Pelkman, C. Baseline insulin sensitivity affects response to high-amylose maize resistant starch in women: A randomized, controlled trial. *Nutr. Metab. (Lond.)* **2016**, *13*, 2. [CrossRef] [PubMed]

41. Bakker, S.J.; Hoogeveen, E.K.; Nijpels, G.; Kostense, P.J.; Dekker, J.M.; Gans, R.O.; Heine, R.J. The association of dietary fibres with glucose tolerance is partly explained by concomitant intake of thiamine: The hoorn study. *Diabetologia* **1998**, *41*, 1168–1175. [CrossRef] [PubMed]

42. Moeller, S.M.; Reedy, J.; Millen, A.E.; Dixon, L.B.; Newby, P.K.; Tucker, K.L.; Krebs-Smith, S.M.; Guenther, P.M. Dietary patterns: Challenges and opportunities in dietary patterns research an experimental biology workshop, April 1, 2006. *J. Am. Diet. Assoc.* **2007**, *107*, 1233–1239. [CrossRef] [PubMed]

43. Fewell, Z.; Davey Smith, G.; Sterne, J.A. The impact of residual and unmeasured confounding in epidemiologic studies: A simulation study. *Am. J. Epidemiol.* **2007**, *166*, 646–655. [CrossRef] [PubMed]

44. Willett, W. *Nutritional Epidemiology*; Oxford University Press: New York, NY, USA, 1998.

45. Jakes, R.W.; Day, N.E.; Luben, R.; Welch, A.; Bingham, S.; Mitchell, J.; Hennings, S.; Rennie, K.; Wareham, N.J. Adjusting for energy intake—What measure to use in nutritional epidemiological studies? *Int. J. Epidemiol.* **2004**, *33*, 1382–1386. [CrossRef] [PubMed]

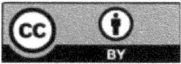

nutrients

MDPI

Article

Maternal Low-Protein Diet Modulates Glucose Metabolism and Hepatic MicroRNAs Expression in the Early Life of Offspring [†]

Jia Zheng, Xinhua Xiao *, Qian Zhang, Tong Wang, Miao Yu and Jianping Xu

Department of Endocrinology, Key Laboratory of Endocrinology, Ministry of Health, Peking Union Medical College Hospital, Diabetes Research Center of Chinese Academy of Medical Sciences & Peking Union Medical College, Beijing 100730, China; zhengjiapumc@163.com (J.Z.); rubiacordifolia@yahoo.com (Q.Z.); tongtong0716@sina.com (T.W.); yumiao@mendmail.com.cn (M.Y.); jpxuxh@163.com (J.X.)
* Correspondence: xiaoxinhua@medmail.com.cn; Tel./Fax: +86-10-6915-5073
† Parts of this study were presented in abstract form at the American Diabetes Association's 76th Scientific Sessions, 10–14 June 2016 in New Orleans, Louisiana.

Received: 28 December 2016; Accepted: 23 February 2017; Published: 27 February 2017

Abstract: Emerging studies revealed that maternal protein restriction was associated with increased risk of type 2 diabetes mellitus in adulthood. However, the mechanisms of its effects on offspring, especially during early life of offspring, are poorly understood. Here, it is hypothesized that impaired metabolic health in offspring from maternal low-protein diet (LPD) is associated with perturbed miRNAs expression in offspring as early as the weaning age. We examined the metabolic effects on the C57BL/6J mice male offspring at weaning from dams fed with LPD or normal chow diet (NCD) throughout pregnancy and lactation. Maternal LPD feeding impaired metabolic health in offspring. Microarray profiling indicated that mmu-miR-615, mmu-miR-124, mmu-miR-376b, and mmu-let-7e were significantly downregulated, while, mmu-miR-708 and mmu-miR-879 were upregulated in LPD offspring. Bioinformatic analysis showed target genes were mapped to inflammatory-related pathways. Serum tumor necrosis factor-α (TNF-α) levels were higher and interleukin 6 (IL-6) had a tendency to be elevated in the LPD group. Finally, both mRNA and protein levels of IL-6 and TNF-α were significantly increased in the LPD group. Our findings provide novel evidence that maternal LPD can regulate miRNAs expression, which may be associated with chronic inflammation status and metabolic health in offspring as early as the weaning age.

Keywords: maternal low-protein diet; metabolic health; microRNAs; inflammation; early life; offspring

1. Introduction

The prevalence of type 2 diabetes mellitus (T2DM) is increasing significantly throughout the world. However, the pathogenesis of diabetes has not been clearly demonstrated. Traditionally, it is generally believed that genes and adult lifestyle are critical factors of some metabolic diseases. Recently, several epidemiological studies of human populations highlighted that maternal nutrition, including over-nutrition and under-nutrition, may strongly influence the risks of developing metabolic diseases in adult life [1–3]. The mechanism underlying the increased susceptibility of T2DM in offspring of maternal malnutrition is poorly determined.

Recently, it seems as though epigenetic modifications may be one of the major mechanisms explaining the association between early life malnutrition and late-onset diseases, such as obesity, insulin resistance, impaired glucose tolerance, and T2DM [4–7]. MicroRNAs (miRNAs) have emerged as important epigenetic modifications in recent years. They are a major class of small non-coding RNAs with about 20–22 nucleotides, which can mediate posttranscriptional regulation of gene expressions.

miRNAs can specifically bind to the $3'$-untranslated regions ($3'$-UTR) of target genes, resulting in translation inhibition [8]. Numerous studies show that miRNAs play critical roles in the pathogenesis of diabetes, such as glucose uptake, transport, and insulin secretion [9].

Human studies have revealed that poor intrauterine environment elicited by maternal dietary insufficiency or imbalance increased the risk for intrauterine growth restriction (IUGR) and led to metabolic diseases in the offspring during adulthood, such as insulin resistance, impaired glucose tolerance, and T2DM [3,10]. The maternal protein restriction model, with 5%–9% protein, as compared to 20% protein in normal diet, has been one of the most extensively studied models [11]. However, these studies were confined to long-term influences in offspring of a maternal low-protein diet (LPD) with varying durations range from 1 to 18 months (adulthood to aging) [12–14], yet the metabolic health in the early life of offspring, such as at weaning, has not been well documented. Furthermore, little information is known about the role of miRNAs between maternal low-protein diet (LPD) and glucose metabolism in the early life of offspring, such as at weaning. It is noted that computational predictions of miRNA targets based on several databases exhibits that one single miRNA can affect a gamut of different genes, ranging from several to hundreds, suggesting that a large proportion of the transcriptome is subjected to miRNA modulation [15]. Thus, using a trans-generational mouse model of maternal protein restriction and microarray platform, we address the hypothesis that impaired metabolic health in offspring from LPD-fed dams is associated with perturbation of the programmed expression of key miRNAs in offspring as early as at weaning age.

2. Materials and Methods

2.1. Animals and Diets

The seven-week-old C57BL/6J female and male mice were purchased from the Institute of Laboratory Animal Science, Chinese Academy of Medical Sciences and Peking Union Medical College (Beijing, China). All of the mice were maintained under controlled conditions with room temperature at $22 \pm 2\,^{\circ}$C and 12-h light/dark cycle. The mice were fed a normal chow diet (NCD) (D02041001, Research Diets, New Brunswick, NJ, USA) for one week for acclimatization. Then, mating was performed by housing males with females together (male:female = 1:2) until a vaginal plug was detected, which was considered day 0.5 of pregnancy. Pregnant females were single-housed and were randomly assigned to either isocaloric LPD (9.6% protein, 80.2% carbohydrate, and 10.2% fat as kcal%, D02041002, Research Diets, New Brunswick, NJ, USA) or NCD (23.5% protein, 66.3% carbohydrate, and 10.2% fat as kcal%, D02041001, Research Diets, New Brunswick, NJ, USA) during pregnancy and lactation. Thus, offspring were divided into two groups according to maternal diets as the LPD group and the NCD group. At day 1 after birth, all of the litters were adjusted to six pups each to ensure no litter was nutritionally biased. Birth weight was measured by calculating the average of one litter. All offspring were weaned at 21 days postnatal. At weaning, only one male offspring was randomly selected from one litter and was sacrificed in each group (one mouse per litter, $n = 6$ to 8 per group). The female offspring were not examined in our present study in order to prevent confounding factors related to their hormone profile and estrus cycle. Blood samples were taken from the intraorbital retrobulbar plexus after 12-h of fasting in anesthetized mice, and the liver samples were quickly removed, snap frozen in liquid nitrogen, and stored at $-80\,^{\circ}$C for further analysis. Body weight in offspring and food intake of dams were monitored weekly. All of the animal experiments were conducted in accordance with the Guide of the Care and Use of Laboratory Animals (NIH Publication No. 86-23, revised 1996) and were approved by the Animal Care and Use Committee of the Peking Union Medical College Hospital (Beijing, China, MC-07-6004).

2.2. Glucose Tolerance Tests

The tolerance test was performed as described previously [16]. Mice were overnight-fasted (12–16 h) and fasted blood glucose was measured in tail vein blood samples. Mice were injected intraperitoneally with glucose (2 g/kg body weight), and blood glucose was measured at 30 min, 60 min, and 120 min following injection using a glucometer (Bayer, Beijing, China). Blood glucose response to glucose tolerance tests was calculated as the area under the glucose curve for each mouse according to the trapezoidal method, as previously described [17].

2.3. Measurement of Serum Insulin and Inflammatory Factors

Serum insulin levels were measured using the mouse ultrasensitive insulin enzyme-linked immunosorbent assay (ELISA) kit (80-INSMSU-E01, ALPCO Diagnostics, Salem, NH, USA). Serum interleukin 6 (IL-6) and tumor necrosis factor-α (TNF-α) concentrations were measured by mouse ELISA kits (ab100712 and ab108910, Abcam, MA, USA), respectively.

2.4. Microarray Profiling of MiRNAs in Offspring

Because of financial constraints, we could not perform a whole genome array for each mouse in the LPD and NCD groups. Thus, in order to obtain a relatively reliable estimate of the mean gene expression, each group contained three biological replicates, which were randomly selected from each group. We performed the microarray with pooled RNA samples, a method that has been shown to be appropriate and statistically valid for efficient microarray experiments, according to previous studies [18,19]. As our study previously described [20], total RNA was extracted from the liver tissues in LPD and NCD offspring using Trizol reagent (Life Technologies Inc., Carlsbad, CA, USA), according to the manufacturer's instructions. MiRNAs expressions in livers were detected by GeneChip microRNA 3.0 Array (Affymetrix, Inc., Santa, CA, USA), which provides for 100% miRBase v17 coverage [21,22].

2.5. Differential MiRNAs Expression Analysis in Offspring

Robust Multi-array Analysis (RMA) was utilized to convert raw data into recognizable miRNA expression data. Then it was followed by median normalization and $\log_2$ transformation using Affy package [23]. Differentially-expressed miRNAs between the LPD and NCD groups were analyzed by the Limma package of R language [23], which is based on the combined two criteria for true positive differences: (1) |FC (fold change)| ≥ 2 and (2) p value < 0.05 [21], which is a relatively robust cutoff point.

2.6. Bioinformatics Analysis of Predicted Targets for MiRNAs in Offspring

All of the microarray data were also pooled for further analysis. According to our previously published work [24], target genes of differentially expressed miRNAs between the two groups were identified using the miRWalk database [25], which can provide validated target genes information on miRNAs for mouse [26]. To further reveal the potential biological functions and pathways of the target genes, the target genes were analyzed with the Kyoto Encyclopedia of Genes and Genomes (KEGG) pathways [27] using Database for Annotation, Visualization and Integrated Discovery (DAVID) [28]. p value < 0.05 was the criterion for significant KEGG pathway terms.

2.7. Validation of Differentially Expressed MiRNAs in Offspring

In order to validate the expressions of differential miRNAs, quantitative real-time PCR (qRT-PCR) were utilized to detect the relative expression of differentially-expressed miRNAs, with samples enlarged in each group (n = 6 to 8 per group) using the TaqMan detection system (Life Technologies, Foster City, CA, USA). All of the mice in each group were included for the validation. Total RNA was reversely transcribed using the TaqMan MicroRNA Reverse Transcription kit (Applied Biosystems, Life Technologies, Foster City, CA, USA). All of the miRNA-specific reverse-transcription primers were provided with the TaqMan MicroRNA Assay and purchased from Life Technologies Corporation (Applied Biosystems, Life Technologies, Foster City, CA, USA). The primers were mmu-miR-615

(ID 2353), mmu-miR-124 (ID 2197), mmu-miR-376b (ID 2452), mmu-let-7e (ID 2407), mmu-miR-708 (ID 1643), and mmu-miR-879 (ID 2473). U6 small nuclear RNA (ID 1973) was used as an endogenous control. Gene expression was quantified by qRT-PCR and performed on an ABI prism Vii7 Sequence Detection System platform (ABI Prism® Vii7, Applied Biosystems, Life Technologies, Foster City, CA, USA). Data were analyzed and the fold change was calculated using the comparative Ct method. All reactions were carried out with three biological replicates, and each analysis consisted of three technical replicates.

2.8. Target Gene Expression by Quantitative Real-Time PCR

For the validation of miRNA target genes, mRNA expressions of target genes were performed using SYBR Green. Prior to PCR, total RNA of each sample was processed with Rnase-free Dnase (Qiagen, New York, NY, USA). The RNA was reverse transcribed by 1 µg of total RNA from each sample using the Power cDNA Synthesis kit (A3500, Promega BioSciences LLC, Sunnyvale, CA, USA). We used Oligo 7.0 software (Molecular Biology Insights, Inc., Cascade, CO, USA) to design the sequences of the primers for IL-6, TNF-α, and housekeeping gene β-actin. The sequences of the primers are as following: IL-6, forward 5'-CCAAGAGGTGAGTGCTTCCC-3', reverse 5'-CTGTTGTTCAGACTCTCTCCCT-3'; TNF-α, forward 5'-CCCACGTCGTAGCAAACCA-3', reverse 5'-ACAAGGTACAACCCATCGGC-3'; MAPK1, forward 5'-AATTGGTCAGGACAAGGGCT-3', reverse 5'-GAGTGGGTAAGCTGAGACGG-3'; β-actin, forward 5'-TGTTACCAACTGGGACGACA-3' reverse 5'-GGGGTGTTGAAGGTCTCAAA-3'. The reaction production was accurately measured by the ABI prism Vii7 Sequence Detection System (ABI Prism® Vii7, Applied Biosystems, Life Technologies, Foster City, CA, USA). Data were analyzed and quantified using the comparative Ct method, as described in the preceding section.

2.9. Immunohistochemical Staining

The liver tissues from offspring mice were rapidly dissected. Then, they were fixed overnight in a freshly-prepared 10% buffered formaldehyde solution. The tissue samples were ethanol-dehydrated and embedded in paraffin wax. Serial 5 µm paraffin embedded tissue sections were mounted on slides. Then, the slides were stained with the primary antibodies overnight at 4 °C, which were IL-6 (1:300; ab83339, Abcam, Cambridge, MA, USA) and TNF-α (1:50, ab6671, Abcam, Cambridge, MA, USA), while negative controls were incubated with phosphate-buffered saline (PBS). The slices were then washed and incubated for 1 h at 37 °C with secondary antibodies (1:1000, Cell Signaling, Danvers, MA, USA). Then, the slides were stained with 3, 3'-diaminobenzidine (DAB) and hematoxylin. Brownish yellow granular or linear deposits were identified as positive. Image-Pro Plus 5.0 (Media Cybernetics, Silver Spring, MD, USA) was used for semi-quantitative analysis.

2.10. Statistical Analysis

Results are expressed as the mean ± SEM. Statistical analyses were performed with Student's *t*-tests of unpaired samples. The comparisons of glucose tolerance tests were analyzed with a two-way ANOVA. Fisher's exact test was used for KEGG pathway analysis. A *p* value < 0.05 was considered statistically significant. Prism version 6.0 (GraphPad Software Inc., San Diego, CA, USA) was used for statistical analysis.

3. Results

3.1. Effects of Diets on Body Weight and Glucose Tolerance in Dams

By the end of lactation, there was no significant difference in maternal body weight between the dams (noted as F0) fed with LPD and NCD (Figure 1a). Glucose tolerance testing showed that blood glucose was indistinguishable between the two groups, as well as with the area under the curve (AUC) (Figure 2b,c). There was no significant difference in food intake between dams fed with LPD and NCD.

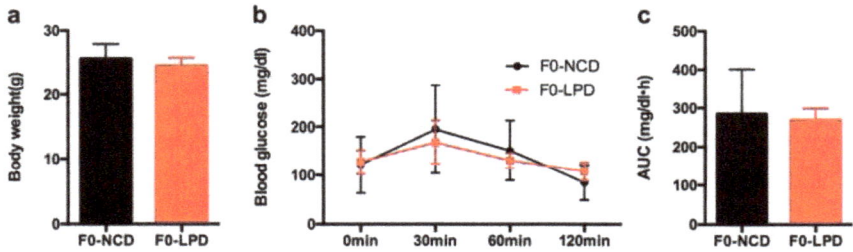

Figure 1. Effects of diets during pregnancy and lactation on metabolic phenotype in dams. (**a**) Body weight; (**b**) intraperitoneal glucose tolerance tests; and (**c**) area under the curve (AUC) of glucose tolerance tests. Data represented as the mean ± SEM (*n* = 6 to 8, per group). Dams were noted as F0; LPD, low-protein diet; NCD, normal chow diet.

3.2. Effects of Maternal Diet on Metabolic Profile in Offspring at Weaning

At birth, newborns whose mother was fed with LPD during pregnancy and lactation showed lower body weight compared to offspring of control diet mothers (*p* < 0.05, Figure 2a). No significant difference was found in litter size between LPD and NCD groups (Figure 2b). At weaning, the male offspring of LPD-fed dams exhibited significantly lower body weight, compared with the offspring of dams fed a control diet (*p* < 0.05, Figure 2c). There was no difference of fasted blood glucose in the LPD and NCD male offspring at weaning. However, the blood glucose of the male offspring in LPD group was higher at 30 min (*p* < 0.05) after intraperitoneal glucose administration (Figure 2d). Consistently, the area under the curve (AUC) of the glucose tolerance test was greater in LPD offspring (*p* < 0.05, Figure 2e). We further examined insulin concentration of the male offspring. As consistent with previous studies [15,29], LPD offspring showed lower fasted insulinemia at weaning, compared to control offspring (Figure 2f), which may be caused by aberrant insulin secretion due to intrauterine growth restriction.

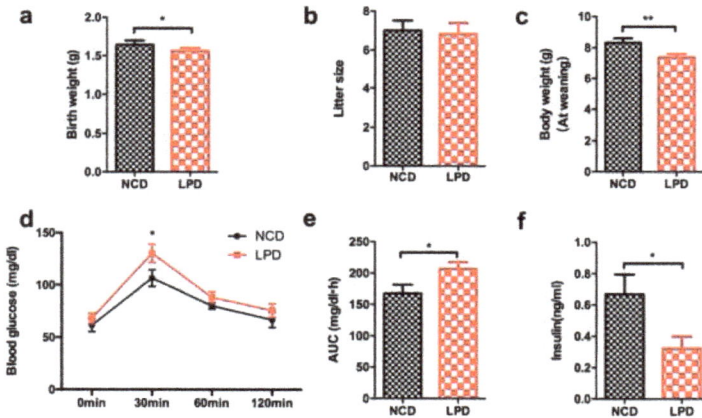

Figure 2. Metabolic profile and serum insulin concentration in offspring at weaning. (**a**) Birth weight; (**b**) litter size; (**c**) body weight at weaning; (**d**) intraperitoneal glucose tolerance test; (**e**) area under curve (AUC) of glucose tolerance test; and (**f**) serum insulin level. Data represented as the mean ± SEM (*n* = 6 to 8, per group). * *p* < 0.05, ** *p* < 0.01 vs. the NCD group. LPD, low-protein diet; NCD, normal chow diet.

3.3. Differential MiRNAs Expression in Offspring

Six miRNAs were shown to be significantly differentially expressed (|fold change| $\geq$ 2 and p value < 0.05) between LPD and NCD groups. In the livers of LPD offspring, mmu-miR-615, mmu-miR-124, mmu-miR-376b, and mmu-let-7e were significantly downregulated (fold change $\leq$ −2 and p value < 0.05). Meanwhile, mmu-miR-708 and mmu-miR-879 were significantly upregulated (fold change $\geq$ 2 and p value < 0.05) (Table 1, Figure 3).

Table 1. Differentially-expressed miRNA (|fold change| $\geq$ 2 and p-value < 0.05).

Probe Set ID	Fold Change	p Value	Sequence Length	Sequence
mmu-miR-615	−7.61	0.004	22	GGGGGUCCCCGGUGCUCGGAUC
mmu-miR-124	−4.37	0.014	22	CGUGUUCACAGCGGACCUUGAU
mmu-miR-376b	−3.81	0.016	21	AUCAUAGAGGAACAUCCACUU
mmu-let-7e	−2.60	0.000	22	CUAUACGGCCUCCUAGCUUUCC
mmu-miR-708	3.89	0.007	23	AAGGAGCUUACAAUCUAGCUGGG
mmu-miR-879	10.05	0.034	22	GCUUAUGGCUUCAAGCUUUCGG

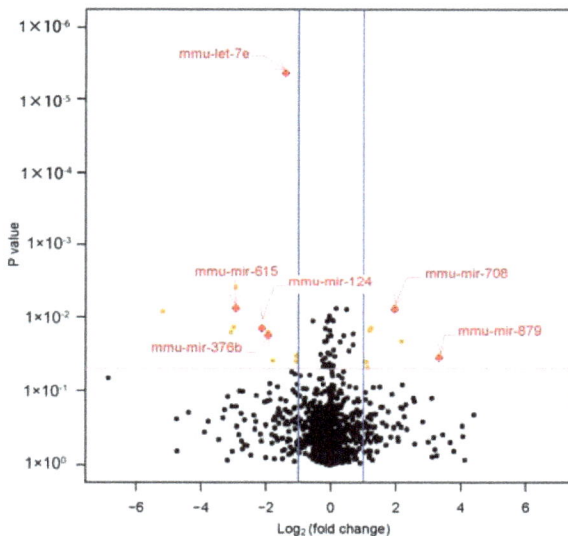

Figure 3. The volcano plot of the miRNA array. This graph shows $\log_2$ (fold change) in the expression miRNAs and p value from the t-test between LPD and NCD offspring. The vertical blue line indicates that the threshold of $|\log_2$ (fold change)$|$ is 1. The horizontal red line indicates that the p value threshold is 0.05. It showed six miRNAs were significantly differentially expressed (|fold change| $\geq$ 2 and p value < 0.05) between LPD and NCD offspring. LPD, Low-protein diet; NCD, normal chow diet.

3.4. Validation of Differentially Expressed MiRNAs

To verify the results of microRNA array, all the six differentially-expressed miRNAs were validated by increasing the quantity of samples in LPD and NCD groups using qRT-PCR (n = 6 to 8, per group). It showed that the expression levels of all the six miRNA were consistent with the results of microRNA array analysis, which were analyzed and quantified by qRT-PCR (Figure 4).

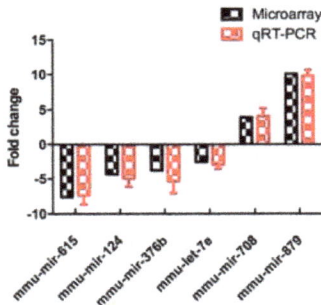

Figure 4. Differentially-expressed miRNAs were detected by miRNA array and validated by qRT-PCR. Data represented as the mean ± SEM (*n* = 6 to 8, per group). The fold change was calculated using the comparative Ct method. qRT-PCR: quantitative real time-PCR.

3.5. Functional Enrichment Analysis for Target Genes by Bioinformatics Analysis

Furthermore, target genes of these six differentially-expressed miRNAs were identified by the miRWalk database. The six miRNAs, including mmu-miR-615, mmu-miR-124, mmu-miR-376b, mmu-let-7e, mmu-miR-708, and mmu-miR-879 had a total of 349 validated target genes in the miRWalk database (Table 2). By utilizing the Database for Annotation, Visualization and Integrated Discovery (DAVID) and Kyoto Encyclopedia of Genes and Genomes (KEGG) databases, the functional enrichment analysis of these 349 validated genes were mapped in the MAPK signaling pathway, TGF-beta signaling pathway, Jak-STAT signaling pathway, cytokine-cytokine receptor interaction, chemokine signaling pathway, adipocytokine signaling pathway, and Toll-like receptor signaling pathway (Table 3), which are all associated with inflammation responses.

Table 2. Validated targeted genes for differentially-expressed miRNAs.

MiRNA	Count	Target Genes
mmu-miR-615	6	*Msx2, Hoxa7, Mbp, Lin28, Cdkn2a, Igf2*
mmu-miR-124	87	*Dll1, Sox9, Camk2g, Zic2, Fabp7, Hod, Pou5f1, Dicer1, Fgf8, Fgf10, H1foo, Bmp4, Lin28, Tcfap2b, Calb2, Btg2, Dcx, Pax6, Ifitm3, Dppa3, Mapk14, Evi1, Nr4a2, Mtpn, Nefm, Eomes, Cpeb1, Ctdspl, Mstn, Gata1, Stmn2, Rest, Trpm3, Mbp, Hprt1, Th, Oog4, Des, Uchl1, Foxp2, Rho, Eif2c3, Efnb1, Dnmt3b, Dbh ,H2afx, Npy, Med13, Prkca, Eif2c2, Fgf21, Phox2a, Mos, Gbx2, Emx1, Myh6, Mt1, Eif2c1, L1cam, Phox2b, Ctdsp1, Lmx1b, Tbr1, Nppa, Ccne1, Ccnb2, Eif2c4, Casp3, Tcfap2a, Sycp1, Gja1, Zp3, Rfpl4, Cdh1, Vax2, Slc6a3, Dlk1, Ntrk2, Pou3f3, Myh7, Sycp3, H2afz, Stat3, Wnt1, Foxa2, Ntrk3, Gja5*
mmu-miR-376b	28	*Hprt1, Oog4, Dnmt3b, H2afx, Fgf21, Mos, Dlk1, Mt1, Mbp, Ccne1, Ccnb2, Lin28, Zp3, Rfpl4, Gpr172b, Sycp3, H2afz, Timp4, Camk2g, Dicer1, Atg4c, Pou5f1, H1foo, Frap1, Ifitm3, Dppa3, Cpeb1, Ctdspl*
mmu-let-7e	217	*Lin28, Casp3, Ptch1, Zfp106, Mov10, Fgf16, E2f6, Fgf21, Ptges, Akt1, Scpep1, Rad52, Mgst1, Cdc34, Git1, Ebp, Mos, Kras, Il6, Capn10, Col1a1, Smad4, Hace1, Igfbp3, Fas, Hmga2, Fgfr1, Sox2, Irf4, Mt1, Kcnj16, Socs1, Mmp9, Prl, Nr2e1, Sp1, Il10, Trim71, Notch1, Nrip1, Lamc1, Acvr2a, Smox, Igf2, Cdkn1a, Egr1, Ccne1, Tagln, Akt1, Ccnb2, Vsnl1, Spp1, Egfr, Syne1, Mdk, Hnf4a, Msi1, Dnmt3a, Cd4, Sparcl1, Hspd1, Tppp3, Vim, Smad3, Tnf, Cyp2b10, Gtf2h4, Zp3, Hyou1, E2f2, Csf1r, Rfpl4, Akap6, Stat3, Golph3, Snai1, Arc, Scamp2, bp1, Mov10, Nanog, Clock, Acvr1, Wnt1, Bcl2l1, BC060632, Cdkn2a, Trp53, Fn1, Sycp3, Tpm1, Scpep1, Lpar1, H2afz, Gmfb, Pten, Arc, Snai1, Dync1i1, Mapre1, Dcn, Bcl2, Scpep1, Hras1, Igf1, E2f6, Grb2, Camk2g, Ogt, Pgc, Ctcf, Dicer1, Mapk1, Scpep1, Cxcr4, Rcan1, Clu, Dut, Piwil2, Ifng, Mtpn, Dclk1, Igfbp3, , Igf1r, Akt1, Kdr, Nanog, Hras1, Neurod1, Dppa3, H1foo, Bmpr2, Ebp, Hmox1, Gpd1, Cyp2b10, Socs3, Inha, Eif2c2, Epb4.1l3, Serpina1c, Ssr3, E2f2, Dicer1, Mstn, Pten, Ifitm3, Dhcr24, Racgap1, Dppa3, Gad1, Ccr4, Ddit3, Nr4a1, Hmga1, Ppargc1a, Bcl2, Nr6a1, Gadd45a, Scpep1, Ptp4a2, Nanog, Runx2, Zeb1, Bak1, Ghr, Birc2, Sall4, Cpeb1, Capn8, Il23r, Ctdspl, Ptges3, Ephb2, Rpe, Syt4, Trim32, Foxp1, Scpep1, Mmp14, Bcl2, Gnb1, Madd, Pgc, Gnrh1, Hmox1, Myc, Mycn, Socs1, Jarid1b, Hprt1, Cyp2b10, Oog4, Pdzd7, Cdkn1a, Cebpb, Aqp4, Rdx, Mbp, Hand1, Bcl2, Lancl1, Mapk3, Casp9, Fmr1, Klf15, Dnmt3b, Adora1, Stx1a, Kitl, Cd34, H2afx, Itgb1, Smad5, Pou5f1*
mmu-miR-708	9	*Foxo3, Cd34, Mbp, Lin28, Stat5a, Cd34, E2f6, Aqp1, Bmi1*
mmu-miR-879	2	*Mbp, Lin28*

Table 3. Validated target genes enriched by the Kyoto Encyclopedia of Genes and Genomes (KEGG) pathway.

KEGG ID	Term	Count	%	p Value	Genes
mmu04010	MAPK signaling pathway	24	9.7	2.8×10^{-8}	*Egfr, Prkca, Trp53, Fgfr1, Fgf8,* **Tnf**, *Grb2, Fgf16, Fgf10, Nr4a1, Fgf21, Ddit3, Hras1, Akt1, Mapk1, Casp3, Kras, Mapk14, Ntrk2, Mapk3, Mos, Fas, Myc, Gadd45a*
mmu04350	TGF-beta signaling pathway	14	5.7	7.3×10^{-8}	*Bmp4,* **Tnf**, *Smad5, Bmpr2, Smad4, Smad3, Dcn, Mapk1, Acvr2a, Sp1, Ifng, Mapk3, Myc, Acvr1*
mmu04630	Jak-STAT signaling pathway	14	5.7	4.4×10^{-5}	**Il6**, *Il23r, Socs3, Grb2, Stat5a, Socs1, Bcl2l1, Stat3, Il10, Akt1, Ifng, Myc, Prl, Ghr*
mmu04060	Cytokine-cytokine receptor interaction	17	6.9	1.4×10^{-4}	*Egfr,* **Il6**, **Tnf**, *Il23r, Bmpr2, Kitl, Il10, Kdr, Acvr2a, Ccr4, Cxcr4, Ifng, Fas, Prl, Acvr1, Ghr, Csf1r*
mmu04062	Chemokine signaling pathway	11	4.5	9.3×10^{-3}	*Akt1, Mapk1, Kras, Ccr4, Gnb1, Cxcr4, Grb2, Mapk3, Foxo3, Stat3, Hras1*
mmu04920	Adipocytokine signaling pathway	6	2.4	1.9×10^{-2}	*Akt1,* **Tnf**, *Npy, Socs3, Ppargc1a, Stat3*
mmu04620	Toll-like receptor signaling pathway	7	2.8	2.7×10^{-2}	*Akt1, Mapk1,* **Il6**, **Tnf**, *Mapk14, Mapk3, Spp1*

MAPK: mitogen-activated protein kinase; TGF: transforming growth factor; Jak-STAT: janus kinase-signal transducer and activator of transcription. *Il-6* and *Tnf* were marked as bold.

3.6. Effects of Maternal Diet on Serum Pro-Inflammatory Cytokines in Offspring

Our functional enrichment analysis indicated that target genes of our six differentially-expressed miRNAs were mapped in inflammatory pathways (Tables 2 and 3). *IL-6* and *Tnf* were two important target genes, which were located in several pathways (marked as bold in Table 3). Therefore, we first measured two important pro-inflammatory cytokines (serum IL-6 and TNF-α) in male offspring of dams fed with LPD and NCD, to determine whether maternal diets modulated the levels of inflammatory markers in the early life of offspring. It showed there was a tendency to be higher of serum IL-6 level in LPD male offspring ($p = 0.07$) (Figure 5a), and it also showed the level of serum TNF-α was significantly elevated in LPD male offspring at weaning ($p < 0.05$) (Figure 5b). However, no difference of MAPK1 expression was observed in offspring (data not shown).

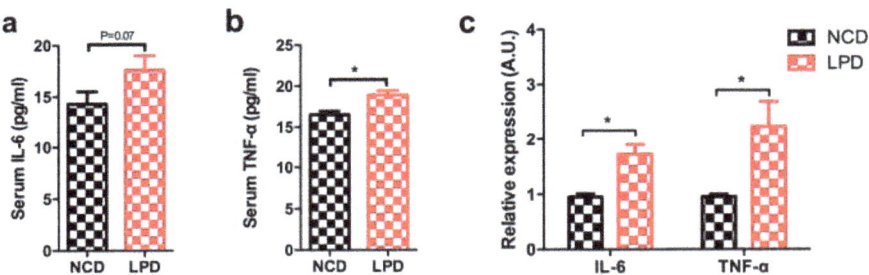

Figure 5. Effect of maternal LPD on serum IL-6 and TNF-α concentrations and mRNA expression in the offspring at weaning. (**a**) Serum IL-6; (**b**) serum TNF-α; and (**c**) IL-6 and TNF-α mRNA expression in the livers of offspring. Data represented as the mean ± SEM ($n = 6$ to 8, per group). * $p < 0.05$, vs. the NCD group. LPD, low-protein diet; NCD, normal chow diet; IL-6: interleukin-6; TNF-α: tumor necrosis factor-α.

3.7. Differential Expression of Pro-Inflammatory Markers in Offspring

Next, we measured *Il-6* and *TNF-α* expression in liver samples of male offspring of LPD- and NCD-fed dams using qRT-PCR. It indicated that *IL-6* and *TNF-α* expression were significantly increased in the LPD group, and the fold change of IL-6 and TNF-α expression is about 1.8 and 2.2, respectively ($p < 0.05$, Figure 5c). To further determine whether the protein expressions of *IL-6* and *TNF-α* in offspring were modulated by maternal LPD, the protein expressions of these two genes were examined by immunohistochemistry. As shown in Figure 6, there was a statistically significant increase in the immunoreactivities of *IL-6* and *TNF-α* in the early life of offspring exposed to maternal LPD during pregnancy and lactation, compared to offspring of NCD-fed dams ($p < 0.05$).

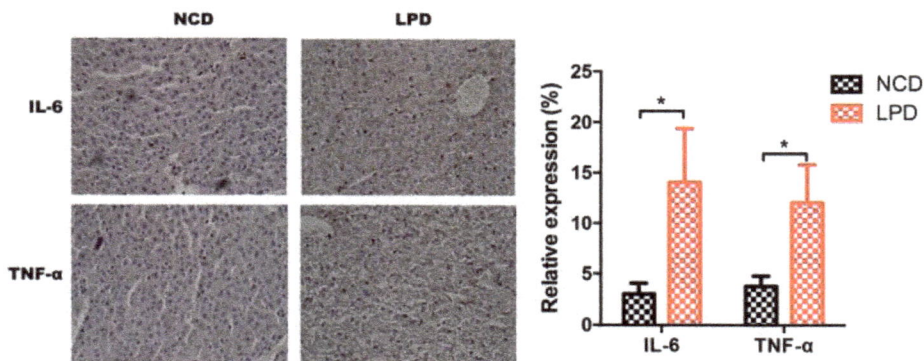

Figure 6. Immunohistochemistry for *IL-6* and *TNF-α* expression and semi-quantitative assessments. (**left**) *IL-6* and *TNF-α* staining in NCD and LPD groups. (**right**) Semi-quantitative scores of *IL-6* and *TNF-α*. Data represented as the mean ± SEM (*n* = 6 to 8, per group). * $p < 0.05$, vs. the NCD group. LPD, low-protein diet; NCD, normal chow diet; IL-6: interleukin-6; TNF-α: tumor necrosis factor-α.

4. Discussion

Epidemiological studies and animal experiments have indicated that adverse maternal nutriture influence organ development and metabolism of progeny, which may increase the susceptibility of developing diabetes in later life, and even in the following generation [30,31]. Maternal nutrition has long-term metabolic effects on offspring, which was known as the "fetal programming hypothesis" [32]. Here, our findings demonstrate that the exposure of LPD feeding during pregnancy and lactation resulted in low birth weight, impaired glucose tolerance, and lower insulin secretion in offspring, at as early as weaning age. We also observed that offspring from LPD-fed dams showed perturbation of the programmed expression of some key miRNAs in offspring at weaning. Thus, using microarray profiling, bioinformatics approaches, and functional enrichment analysis, all of the target genes of misexpressed miRNAs were mapped in seven inflammatory-related pathways. Finally, we showed that that serum levels of pro-inflammatory cytokines IL-6 and TNF-α were also increased in offspring from LPD-fed dams. Furthermore, the mRNA expression and protein levels of IL-6 and TNF-α were significantly increased in offspring from maternal LPD feeding. Therefore, these results show that maternal LPD consumption may regulate the expression of miRNAs, which may be associated with chronic inflammation status and glucose intolerance in offspring as early as weaning age (Figure 7).

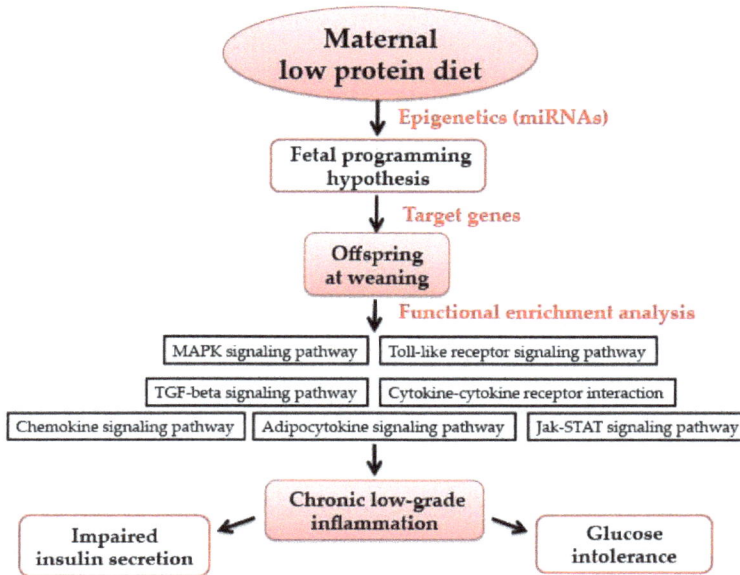

Figure 7. The possible mechanism of maternal low-protein diet during pregnancy and lactation on offspring at weaning. Maternal nutrition has long-term metabolic effects on offspring, which is known as the "fetal programming hypothesis". Epigenetics (such as miRNAs) has been deemed as an important molecular basis of maternal nutrition and metabolic health in offspring. Using functional enrichment analysis, the target genes of differentially-expressed miRNAs were mapped into seven pathways, which are all associated with inflammation. Thus, it may be related to chronic low-grade inflammation, which may cause impaired insulin secretion and glucose intolerance. MAPK: mitogen-activated protein kinase; TGF: transforming growth factor; Jak-STAT: Janus kinase-signal transducer and activator of transcription.

Obesity, insulin resistance, and diabetes mellitus are associated with chronic low-grade inflammation [33–35]. One recent review summarized that chronic inflammation is characterized by increased levels of pro-inflammatory cytokines in response to physiological and environmental stimuli that can arrest the immune system in a low-level activation state [36]. Our study demonstrates that maternal protein restriction diet during pregnancy and lactation may induce an inflammatory state in offspring at weaning age. Similar to our study, one recent study showed that male Wistar rats exposed to a low-protein (8%) diet in utero that had a low birth weight, but then underwent postnatal catch-up growth exhibited higher indexes of inflammatory, with increased hepatic expression of interleukin-6 (IL-6) levels, tumor necrosis factor α (TNF-α), and monocyte chemotactic protein-1 (MCP-1) at 12 months of age [37]. Sílvia et al. also showed that maternal low-protein (6%) diet during pregnancy and lactation showed increased transcription of nuclear factor kappa B (NF-κB) and IL-6, with reduced transcription of interleukin-6 (IL-10) (an anti-inflammatory cytokine) at 90 days of age in offspring [38]. However, the inflammatory state of offspring was examined at an adult or even older age in the aforementioned studies. Here our findings demonstrate that maternal LPD feeding during pregnancy and lactation can induce an inflammatory state in the offspring as early as weaning age. In our previous study, we found that a maternal high-calorie diet is associated with altered hepatic microRNA expression and impaired metabolic health in offspring at weaning age [20]. The composition of the high-calorie diet is 16.4% protein, 25.6% carbohydrate, and 58% fat as the kcal%. However, we found that both of the two studies showed that maternal nutrition are associated with inflammation in offspring. We cannot draw a conclusion that the same biological mechanisms are at play in these two studies because our study is very preliminary, which needs further experimentation and validation. However, we can speculate that maternal malnutrition (whether over-nutrition or under-nutrition) may be associated with aberrant metabolic health and inflammation status in offspring at weaning.

Increasing evidence showed that epigenetic information could be inherited as a trans-generational carrier between generations. It showed that nutrient-dependent regulation of miRNAs may trigger disease susceptibility and metabolic complications in offspring [39]. One clinical study indicated that placental expression of miR-210 increased in preeclampsia and was inversely related to birth weight and gestational age [40]. It showed that a maternal low-protein diet exhibited impaired glucose tolerance and suppressed pancreatic β-cell proliferation in mouse offspring via miR-15b at 12 weeks of age [41]. In addition to maternal nutrition, the advanced fetal programming hypothesis proposes that maternal genetic variants may influence the offspring's phenotype indirectly via epigenetic modification. Hocher et al. showed that altered expression of hepatic microRNA was observed in offspring of female eNOS −/+ mice, demonstrating that a maternal genetic defect can epigenetically alter the phenotype of the offspring, without inheritance of the defect itself [42]. Recently, inflammatory signaling has been identified as an epigenetic mediator and increasing evidence has shown the epigenetics can regulate inflammatory gene expression, which can ultimately result in multiple adverse physiological consequences [43]. Our study shows that validated target genes of differentially-expressed miRNAs in offspring from LPD-fed dams are part of inflammatory signaling pathways. *IL-6* and *TNF* are two validated target genes of let-7e. Recent findings offer a putative role of non-coding RNAs, especially miRNAs, in the progression and management of the inflammatory response [44]. The let-7 family of miRNAs is highly conserved across diverse animal species, and plays critical roles in the regulation of cell proliferation and differentiation [45]. In addition to cancer, an altered expression of let-7 has been reported in inflammation. Let-7 miRNAs demonstrated to be repressed in inflammation, which resulted in increased expression of pro-inflammatory cytokines and increased inflammatory status [46], which is consistent with our results. One clinical study showed that let-7e target genes were predicted to be associated with ulcerative colitis susceptibility [47]. In addition, several miRNAs, such as miR-126, miR-132, miR-146, miR-155, and miR-221 have also emerged as important transcriptional regulators of some inflammation-related mediators [44]. Therefore, we propose that maternal protein restriction diet induce altered hepatic microRNA expression, which may be associated with enhanced inflammatory responses in offspring as early as at weaning age.

To the best of our knowledge, our study provides the first evidence that maternal LPD feeding may regulate the expression of miRNA, which may be associated with chronic inflammation status and glucose intolerance in offspring as early as weaning age. However, some limitations should be considered in our study. First, we agree with the reviewer that our data is preliminary and cannot exclude the possibility that the association between miRNAs and markers of inflammation is due to a state of chronic systemic inflammation causing altered hepatic miRNA, rather than the other way around. Second, our present study focused on the mechanisms between maternal protein restriction and its detrimental effects on offspring during early life of offspring and there was no data on long-term effects in adulthood of our model. Our further research will be focused on the miRNAs expression and inflammation status in older mice offspring to examine the long-term effects in adulthood of our model. Third, the function of miRNA analysis, which showed to be related to inflammation, is mainly based on microarray profiling, bioinformatics analysis, and some preliminary molecular biology experiments. Therefore, using in vivo and in vitro experiments, further studies should be investigated to demonstrate the role of perturbed miRNA expression on glucose metabolism and inflammation status. A fourth limitation is that it is unknown when the critical time window of maternal LPD consumption is; during the gestation period or lactation period, or both periods. Our undergoing work aims to determine the effects of LPD in the dams on glucose metabolism in offspring in specific time window. Furthermore, recent reviews showed that paternal nutritional challenges can also cause programming of glucose impairment in the offspring and alterations of noncoding sperm micro-RNAs, histone acetylation, and targeted, as well as global, DNA methylation seem to be particularly involved in paternal programming of offspring's diseases in later life [48,49]. Therefore, our future study will be interested in examining the underlying epigenetic mechanism linking paternal nutrition and its programming effect on offspring.

In conclusion, here we demonstrated that maternal protein restriction diet with IUGR predisposes to impaired glucose tolerance in the offspring as early as weaning age. This study contributes to the current knowledge on the putative role of miRNAs between maternal low-protein diet and metabolic health in offspring, which are likely to be associated with inflammatory responses. A better understanding of the function of these miRNAs might open the way to the development of new strategies for the early prevention of diabetes. Thus, further studies in the field of trans-generational effects to clarify the underlying mechanisms are urgently warranted.

Acknowledgments: This work was supported by the National Natural Science Foundation of China (No. 81570715 and No. 81170736), National Key Research and Development Program of China (No. 2016YFA0101002), National Natural Science Foundation for Young Scholars of China (No. 81300649), and the National Key Program of Clinical Science and Peking Union Medical College Hospital.

Author Contributions: Xinhua Xiao conceived and designed the experiments. Qian Zhang, Jia Zheng and Tong Wang carried out the experiments. Miao Yu and Jianping Xu analysed data. All authors were involved in writing the paper and had final approval of the submitted and published versions.

Conflicts of Interest: The authors declare no conflict of interest.

References

1. Curhan, G.C.; Willett, W.C.; Rimm, E.B.; Spiegelman, D.; Ascherio, A.L.; Stampfer, M.J. Birth weight and adult hypertension, diabetes mellitus, and obesity in US men. *Circulation* **1996**, *94*, 3246–3250. [CrossRef] [PubMed]

2. Gniuli, D.; Calcagno, A.; Caristo, M.E.; Mancuso, A.; Macchi, V.; Mingrone, G.; Vettor, R. Effects of high-fat diet exposure during fetal life on type 2 diabetes development in the progeny. *J. Lipid Res.* **2008**, *49*, 1936–1945. [CrossRef] [PubMed]

3. De Rooij, S.R.; Painter, R.C.; Phillips, D.I.; Osmond, C.; Michels, R.P.; Godsland, I.F.; Roseboom, T.J. Impaired insulin secretion after prenatal exposure to the Dutch famine. *Diabetes Care* **2006**, *29*, 1897–1901. [CrossRef] [PubMed]

4. Gluckman, P.D.; Hanson, M.A.; Buklijas, T.; Low, F.M.; Beedle, A.S. Epigenetic mechanisms that underpin metabolic and cardiovascular diseases. *Nat. Rev. Endocrinol.* **2009**, *5*, 401–408. [CrossRef] [PubMed]

5. Stefan, M.; Zhang, W.; Concepcion, E.; Yi, Z.; Tomer, Y. DNA methylation profiles in type 1 diabetes twins point to strong epigenetic effects on etiology. *J. Autoimmun.* **2014**, *50*, 33–37. [CrossRef] [PubMed]

6. Waddington, C.H. The epigenotype. 1942. *Int. J. Epidemiol.* **2012**, *41*, 10–13. [CrossRef] [PubMed]

7. Januar, V.; Desoye, G.; Novakovic, B.; Cvitic, S.; Saffery, R. Epigenetic regulation of human placental function and pregnancy outcome: Considerations for causal inference. *Am. J. Obstet. Gynecol.* **2015**, *213* (Suppl. 4), S182–S196. [CrossRef]

8. Reddy, M.A.; Natarajan, R. Epigenetic mechanisms in diabetic vascular complications. *Cardiovasc. Res.* **2011**, *90*, 421–429. [CrossRef] [PubMed]

9. Deiuliis, J.A. MicroRNAs as regulators of metabolic disease: Pathophysiologic significance and emerging role as biomarkers and therapeutics. *Int. J. Obes. (Lond.)* **2016**, *40*, 88–101. [CrossRef] [PubMed]

10. Kahn, H.S. Glucose tolerance in adults after prenatal exposure to famine. *Lancet* **2001**, *357*, 1798–1799. [CrossRef]

11. Zohdi, V.; Lim, K.; Pearson, J.T.; Black, M.J. Developmental programming of cardiovascular disease following intrauterine growth restriction: Findings utilising a rat model of maternal protein restriction. *Nutrients* **2014**, *7*, 119–152. [CrossRef] [PubMed]

12. Jousse, C.; Parry, L.; Lambert-Langlais, S.; Maurin, A.C.; Averous, J.; Bruhat, A.; Jockers, R. Perinatal undernutrition affects the methylation and expression of the leptin gene in adults: Implication for the understanding of metabolic syndrome. *FASEB J.* **2011**, *25*, 3271–3278. [CrossRef] [PubMed]

13. Erhuma, A.; Salter, A.M.; Sculley, D.V.; Langley-Evans, S.C.; Bennett, A.J. Prenatal exposure to a low-protein diet programs disordered regulation of lipid metabolism in the aging rat. *Am. J. Physiol. Endocrinol. Metab.* **2007**, *292*, E1702–E1714. [CrossRef] [PubMed]

14. Watkins, A.J.; Ursell, E.; Panton, R.; Papenbrock, T.; Hollis, L.; Cunningham, C.; Eckert, J.J. Adaptive responses by mouse early embryos to maternal diet protect fetal growth but predispose to adult onset disease. *Biol. Reprod.* **2008**, *78*, 299–306. [CrossRef] [PubMed]

15. Dumortier, O.; Hinault, C.; Gautier, N.; Patouraux, S.; Casamento, V.; van Obberghen, E. Maternal protein restriction leads to pancreatic failure in offspring: Role of misexpressed microRNA-375. *Diabetes* **2014**, *63*, 3416–3427. [CrossRef] [PubMed]

16. Zheng, J.; Xiao, X.; Zhang, Q.; Yu, M.; Xu, J.; Wang, Z. Maternal high-fat diet modulates hepatic glucose, lipid homeostasis and gene expression in the PPAR pathway in the early life of offspring. *Int. J. Mol. Sci.* **2014**, *15*, 14967–14983. [CrossRef] [PubMed]

17. Purves, R.D. Optimum numerical integration methods for estimation of area-under-the-curve (AUC) and area-under-the-moment-curve (AUMC). *J. Pharmacokinet. Biopharm.* **1992**, *20*, 211–226. [CrossRef] [PubMed]

18. Peng, X.; Wood, C.L.; Blalock, E.M.; Chen, K.C.; Landfield, P.W.; Stromberg, A.J. Statistical implications of pooling RNA samples for microarray experiments. *BMC Bioinform.* **2003**, *4*, 26. [CrossRef] [PubMed]

19. Bruce, K.D.; Cagampang, F.R.; Argenton, M.; Zhang, J.; Ethirajan, P.L.; Burdge, G.C.; McConnell, J.M. Maternal high-fat feeding primes steatohepatitis in adult mice offspring, involving mitochondrial dysfunction and altered lipogenesis gene expression. *Hepatology* **2009**, *50*, 1796–1808. [CrossRef] [PubMed]

20. Zheng, J.; Zhang, Q.; Mul, J.D.; Yu, M.; Xu, J.; Qi, C.; Xiao, X. Maternal high-calorie diet is associated with altered hepatic microRNA expression and impaired metabolic health in offspring at weaning age. *Endocrine* **2016**, *54*, 70–80. [CrossRef] [PubMed]

21. Luo, Y.; Zhang, C.; Tang, F.; Zhao, J.; Shen, C.; Wang, C.; Chen, R. Bioinformatics identification of potentially involved microRNAs in Tibetan with gastric cancer based on microRNA profiling. *Cancer Cell Int.* **2015**, *15*, 115. [CrossRef] [PubMed]

22. The miRBase Sequence Database. Release 21. Available online: http://www.mirbase.org (accessed on 24 June 2014).

23. Methods for Affymetrix Oligonucleotide Arrays. Available online: http://www.bioconductor.org/packages/release/bioc/html/affy.html (accessed on 24 June 2015).

24. Zhang, Q.; Xiao, X.; Li, M.; Li, W.; Yu, M.; Zhang, H.; Xiang, H. Acarbose Reduces Blood Glucose by Activating miR-10a-5p and miR-664 in Diabetic Rats. *PLoS ONE* **2013**, *8*, e79697. [CrossRef] [PubMed]

25. MiRWalk2.0 Database. Available online: http://www.umm.uni-heidelberg.de/apps/zmf/mirwalk/ (accessed on 29 April 2015).

26. Dweep, H.; Gretz, N. miRWalk2.0: A comprehensive atlas of microRNA-target interactions. *Nat. Methods* **2015**, *12*, 697.

27. Kyoto Encyclopedia of Genes and Genomes (KEGG) Database. Release 74.0. Available online: http://www.kegg.jp/ (accessed on 1 April 2015).

28. Database for Annotation, Visualization and Integrated Discovery (DAVID) Database. Available online: https://david.ncifcrf.gov (accessed on 1 April 2015).

29. Petrik, J.; Reusens, B.; Arany, E.; Remacle, C.; Coelho, C.; Hoet, J.J.; Hill, D.J. A low protein diet alters the balance of islet cell replication and apoptosis in the fetal and neonatal rat and is associated with a reduced pancreatic expression of insulin-like growth factor-II. *Endocrinology* **1999**, *140*, 4861–4873. [CrossRef] [PubMed]

30. Hales, C.N.; Barker, D.J. Type 2 (non-insulin-dependent) diabetes mellitus: The thrifty phenotype hypothesis. *Diabetologia* **1992**, *35*, 595–601. [CrossRef] [PubMed]

31. Jimenez-Chillaron, J.C.; Isganaitis, E.; Charalambous, M.; Gesta, S.; Pentinat-Pelegrin, T.; Faucette, R.R.; Patti, M.E. Intergenerational transmission of glucose intolerance and obesity by in utero undernutrition in mice. *Diabetes* **2009**, *58*, 460–468. [CrossRef] [PubMed]

32. Kermack, A.J.; van Rijn, B.B.; Houghton, F.D.; Calder, P.C.; Cameron, I.T.; Macklon, N.S. The "Developmental Origins" Hypothesis: Relevance to the obstetrician and gynecologist. *J. Dev. Orig. Health Dis.* **2015**, *6*, 415–424. [CrossRef] [PubMed]

33. Verdile, G.; Keane, K.N.; Cruzat, V.F.; Medic, S.; Sabale, M.; Rowles, J.; Newsholme, P. Inflammation and Oxidative Stress: The Molecular Connectivity between Insulin Resistance, Obesity, and Alzheimer's Disease. *Mediat. Inflamm.* **2015**, *2015*, 105828. [CrossRef] [PubMed]
34. Chen, H. Cellular inflammatory responses: Novel insights for obesity and insulin resistance. *Pharmacol. Res.* **2006**, *53*, 469–477. [CrossRef] [PubMed]
35. Samuel, V.T.; Shulman, G.I. The pathogenesis of insulin resistance: Integrating signaling pathways and substrate flux. *J. Clin. Investig.* **2016**, *126*, 12–22. [CrossRef] [PubMed]
36. Davinelli, S.; Maes, M.; Corbi, G.; Zarrelli, A.; Willcox, D.C.; Scapagnini, G. Dietary phytochemicals and neuro-inflammaging: From mechanistic insights to translational challenges. *Immun. Ageing* **2016**, *13*, 16. [CrossRef] [PubMed]
37. Tarry-Adkins, J.L.; Fernandez-Twinn, D.S.; Hargreaves, I.P.; Neergheen, V.; Aiken, C.E.; Martin-Gronert, M.S.; Ozanne, S.E. Coenzyme Q10 prevents hepatic fibrosis, inflammation, and oxidative stress in a male rat model of poor maternal nutrition and accelerated postnatal growth. *Am. J. Clin. Nutr.* **2016**, *103*, 579–588. [CrossRef] [PubMed]
38. Reis, S.R.; Feres, N.H.; Ignacio-Souza, L.M.; Veloso, R.V.; Arantes, V.C.; Kawashita, N.H.; Latorraca, M.Q. Nutritional recovery with a soybean diet after weaning reduces lipogenesis but induces inflammation in the liver in adult rats exposed to protein restriction during intrauterine life and lactation. *Mediat. Inflamm.* **2015**, *2015*, 781703. [CrossRef] [PubMed]
39. Ferland-McCollough, D.; Fernandez-Twinn, D.S.; Cannell, I.G.; David, H.; Warner, M.; Vaag, A.A.; Siddle, K. Programming of adipose tissue miR-483-3p and GDF-3 expression by maternal diet in type 2 diabetes. *Cell Death Differ.* **2012**, *19*, 1003–1012. [CrossRef] [PubMed]
40. Lee, D.C.; Romero, R.; Kim, J.S.; Tarca, A.L.; Montenegro, D.; Pineles, B.L.; Mittal, P. miR-210 targets iron-sulfur cluster scaffold homologue in human trophoblast cell lines: Siderosis of interstitial trophoblasts as a novel pathology of preterm preeclampsia and small-for-gestational-age pregnancies. *Am. J. Pathol.* **2011**, *179*, 590–602. [CrossRef] [PubMed]
41. Su, Y.; Jiang, X.; Li, Y.; Li, F.; Cheng, Y.; Peng, Y.; Wang, W. Maternal Low Protein Isocaloric Diet Suppresses Pancreatic beta-Cell Proliferation in Mouse Offspring via miR-15b. *Endocrinology* **2016**, *157*, 4782–4793. [CrossRef] [PubMed]
42. Hocher, B.; Haumann, H.; Rahnenführer, J.; Reichetzeder, C.; Kalk, P.; Pfab, T.; Püschel, G.P. Maternal eNOS deficiency determines a fatty liver phenotype of the offspring in a sex dependent manner. *Epigenetics* **2016**, *11*, 539–552. [CrossRef] [PubMed]
43. Zhou, D.; Pan, Y.X. Pathophysiological basis for compromised health beyond generations: Role of maternal high-fat diet and low-grade chronic inflammation. *J. Nutr. Biochem.* **2015**, *26*, 1–8. [CrossRef] [PubMed]
44. Marques-Rocha, J.L.; Samblas, M.; Milagro, F.I.; Bressan, J.; Martínez, J.A.; Marti, A. Noncoding RNAs, cytokines, and inflammation-related diseases. *FASEB J.* **2015**, *29*, 3595–3611. [CrossRef] [PubMed]
45. Pasquinelli, A.E.; Reinhart, B.J.; Slack, F.; Martindale, M.Q.; Kuroda, M.I.; Maller, B.; Spring, J. Conservation of the sequence and temporal expression of let-7 heterochronic regulatory RNA. *Nature* **2000**, *408*, 86–89. [PubMed]
46. Iliopoulos, D.; Hirsch, H.A.; Struhl, K. An epigenetic switch involving NF-kappaB, Lin28, Let-7 MicroRNA, and IL6 links inflammation to cell transformation. *Cell* **2009**, *139*, 693–706. [CrossRef] [PubMed]
47. Coskun, M.; Bjerrum, J.T.; Seidelin, J.B.; Troelsen, J.T.; Olsen, J.; Nielsen, O.H. miR-20b, miR-98, miR-125b-1*, and let-7e* as new potential diagnostic biomarkers in ulcerative colitis. *World J. Gastroenterol.* **2013**, *19*, 4289–4299. [CrossRef] [PubMed]
48. Li, J.; Yang, X.; Hocher, B. Paternal programming of offspring cardiometabolic diseases in later life. *J. Hypertens.* **2016**, *34*, 2111–2126. [CrossRef] [PubMed]
49. Reichetzeder, C.; Dwi Putra, S.E.; Li, J.; Hocher, B. Developmental Origins of Disease—Crisis Precipitates Change. *Cell. Physiol. Biochem.* **2016**, *39*, 919–938. [CrossRef] [PubMed]

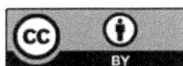

Review

Early-Life Nutritional Programming of Type 2 Diabetes: Experimental and Quasi-Experimental Evidence

Alexander M. Vaiserman

D.F. Chebotarev Institute of Gerontology, Kiev 04114, NAMS, Ukraine; vaiserman@geront.kiev.ua;
Tel.: +38-044-431-0558

Received: 11 February 2017; Accepted: 23 February 2017; Published: 5 March 2017

Abstract: Consistent evidence from both experimental and human studies suggest that inadequate nutrition in early life can contribute to risk of developing metabolic disorders including type 2 diabetes (T2D) in adult life. In human populations, most findings supporting a causative relationship between early-life malnutrition and subsequent risk of T2D were obtained from quasi-experimental studies ('natural experiments'). Prenatal and/or early postnatal exposures to famine were demonstrated to be associated with higher risk of T2D in many cohorts around the world. Recent studies have highlighted the importance of epigenetic regulation of gene expression as a possible major contributor to the link between the early-life famine exposure and T2D in adulthood. Findings from these studies suggest that prenatal exposure to the famine may result in induction of persistent epigenetic changes that have adaptive significance in postnatal development but can predispose to metabolic disorders including T2D at the late stages of life. In this review, quasi-experimental data on the developmental programming of T2D are summarized and recent research findings on changes in DNA methylation that mediate these effects are discussed.

Keywords: type 2 diabetes; famine; natural experiment; quasi-experimental design; epigenetics

1. Introduction

Type 2 diabetes (T2D) is one of most common chronic diseases, constituting a serious social and economic problem in modern societies, both developed and developing. It is caused by insulin resistance resulting from decreased activity and enhanced obesity levels that occur with increasing age. T2D is considered to be adult-onset disease, since it typically occurred in middle-age and old adults. Generally, T2D occurs after the age of 40, although it is now increasingly diagnosed in younger patients [1]. Over the last decades, a rapid increase in the prevalence of obesity arising from high caloric diet intake and sedentary lifestyle is driving a global pandemic of T2D. Currently, 415 million people (about 9% of whole adult population) across the world have T2D. During the next decade, the number of T2D patients is expected to rise to around 642 million persons [2]. Obviously, genetics plays a crucial role in driving this disease; however, the dramatic increase in T2D incidence across the globe cannot be explained by genetic factors alone but must involve environmental factors as well [3]. There is increasing experimental and epidemiological evidence that the risk of development of T2D can be influenced not only by actual adult-life environmental conditions (primarily, lifestyle ones) but also by conditions in early life [3]. Convincing evidence that risk of T2D cannot be completely attributable to genetic predisposition and/or adult-life environmental factors was obtained, e.g., in a study on Pima Indian nuclear families in which at least one sibling was born before and other after the mother was diagnosed with T2D [4]. In this research, those siblings conceived after the mother has been diagnosed with T2D were 3.7 times more likely to have T2D compared to siblings born before their mother developed diabetes, even though they lived in similar conditions the rest of their life.

In the present review, we have summarized and discussed findings on this topic from epidemiological studies conducted with quasi-experimental design ('natural experiments').

2. Conceptual Framework for Developmental Nutritional Programming of Type 2 Diabetes (T2D)

According to the developmental programming of health and disease (DOHaD) hypothesis, which has been confirmed by many research findings over the past decades, the physiology and structure of the developing organism may be adapted in response to unfavourable environmental conditions, thereby predisposing it to many pathological conditions in adult life [5]. In particular, poor nutritional environments in early life can induce structural and functional changes in key organs responsible for nutrient regulation, including brain, liver, adipose tissue, muscle and pancreas [6]. Presently, this view is commonly referred to as the 'predictive adaptive response (PAR)' concept [7]. Exposure to adverse environmental factors such as inadequate or unbalanced nutrient supply during in utero development may 'program' for the long term appetite regulation, feeding behaviour, as well as adipose tissue and pancreatic beta cell dysfunction in the developing foetus [3]. As a result of these processes, the foetus may be adapted to adverse nutritional conditions by reducing ability to produce insulin and by occurrence of insulin resistance. According to the 'thrifty phenotype' hypothesis [8], such metabolic adaptation may provide short-term survival benefit in a poor postnatal environment via enhanced capacity to store fat in conditions of irregular availability of food resources, but may predispose the child to T2D development in conditions of food abundance in postnatal life. More specifically, in malnourished conditions when the foetus exhibits poor growth in utero (commonly referred to as intrauterine growth restriction, IUGR), the foetal adaptation to undernutrition is realized by a variety of mechanisms responsible for the energy and glucose metabolism, such as enhanced peripheral insulin sensitivity for glucose utilization, increased hepatic glucose production, lowered insulin sensitivity for protein synthesis in muscle, and impaired pancreatic development [9]. All these mechanisms provide obvious survival benefit for the IUGR foetuses by promoting both energy uptake and utilization, reducing the demand for amino acids and anabolic hormone production, and elevating glucose production to maintain glucose supply to vital organs, primarily the heart and brain. These adaptations lead to asymmetrical growth restriction of the foetus. The muscle and subcutaneous tissues exhibit the most pronounced growth restriction, while the least pronounced growth restriction is peculiar to the growing brain. Collectively, such adaptations allow IUGR foetal tissues to maintain the energy-dependent basal metabolic functions at the expense of body growth in conditions of reduced nutrient supply. If these adaptive modifications persist, or are more readily inducible later in life, they have the potential to promote energy absorption beyond metabolic capability when energy supplies increase, thereby causing insulin resistance, obesity and T2D in adulthood [9]. Among the factors affecting the risk of metabolic dysfunctions, including T2D, in adulthood, the prenatal and early postnatal malnutrition (both under- and overnutrition) is currently believed to be most important [10,11]. It should be noted that in this review only one aspect of malnutrition i.e., undernutrition but not overnutrition will be discussed.

The majority of early population studies used birth weight as a proxy for foetal conditions. From the data obtained, it has been initially concluded that low birth weight is a risk factor for T2D and that birth weight is inversely related to the disease risk [12]. In addition to T2D, low birth weight is a predictor of other T2D-associated conditions and complications later in life, including the impaired body composition and fat distribution [13], fasting lipid profile, blood pressure and insulin resistance [14], life-long activation of the hypothalamic-pituitary-adrenal axis [15], as well as coronary heart disease in adulthood [16]. Several more recent studies, however, found that a relationship between birth weight and risk of T2D is not linear but rather U-shaped, and high birth weight (>4000 g) is associated with an increased risk of T2D to the same extent as low birth weight (<2500 g) [17].

An association between low birth weight and risk of T2D in later life is most thoroughly studied to date. This association is apparently mediated by catch-up growth early in life which is an important risk factor for later T2D. The catch-up growth leads to a disproportionately enhanced rate of fat gain in comparison with lean tissue gain [18]. Such preferential catch-up fat is partly driven by mechanisms of energy conservation operating through suppression of thermogenesis and resulting in the development of thrifty 'catch-up fat' phenotype generally characterized by insulin and leptin resistance. Abnormalities in the growth hormone/insulin-like growth factor-1 (GH/IGF-1) axis, known to play a central role in promoting human growth and development, have been repeatedly reported in children born small for gestational age (SGA) [19]. Such long-lasting abnormalities of IGF-1 in SGA children with catch-up growth are believed to be critically implicated in the association with metabolic disorders, including T2D, later in life.

Precise molecular mechanisms responsible for the nutritional developmental programming of T2D are not yet thoroughly characterized. In many recent studies, compelling evidence was provided that changes in epigenetic regulation of gene expression (heritable alterations in gene function without changes in the nucleotide sequence) is the most plausible mechanism for the link between unfavourable conditions in early development and adverse health outcomes in later life [20]. The main epigenetic mechanisms are DNA methylation and post-translational modifications of histone tails, as well as regulation by non-coding RNAs (microRNAs and long non-coding RNAs) [21]. Evidence for the key role of DNA methylation and other epigenetic mechanisms in mediating the risk of T2D and obesity has been repeatedly documented over the past years [22]. Initial evidence for the role of epigenetic regulation in obesity and T2D has been mainly provided by studies in animal models. These studies reported changes in epigenetic marks in key metabolic tissues following feeding with high-fat diet and by human investigation that demonstrated epigenetic alterations in T2D and obesity candidate genes in obese and/or diabetic persons. More recently, rapid technological advances and price reduction in epigenetic methodologies led to a rapid expansion of epigenome-wide association studies (EWAS) in human epidemiological examinations [22]. These studies clearly demonstrated epigenetic differences between diabetic and healthy control individuals, as well as epigenetic alterations associated with lifestyle interventions.

Within the DOHaD concept, an important point is that throughout embryonic and foetal development, intense epigenetic remodelling takes place that is necessary for the establishment of transcriptional programs responsible for cellular proliferation and differentiation. During these sensitive developmental periods, the epigenome is especially plastic and most sensitive to environmental disturbances [23]. Numerous research findings suggest that early-life adverse events (i.e., insufficient nutrition in utero) might be epigenetically 'imprinted' and 'remembered' decades later, thereby permanently influencing the metabolic phenotype [24]. There is convincing evidence that epigenetic alterations, including those triggered by early-life events and persisting through adulthood, is an important etiological factor in the development of T2D. Changes in DNA methylation and associated changes in patterns of expression of genes implicated in various aspects of glucose metabolism such as β-cell dysfunction, glucose intolerance and insulin resistance, have been shown to be critically involved in the pathogenesis of T2D [25]. The specific DNA methylation markers have been repeatedly identified in peripheral blood and pancreatic islets of the T2D patients (for review, see [26]).

A schematic representation of hypothetical regulatory pathways responsible for developmental nutritional programming of T2D is presented in Figure 1.

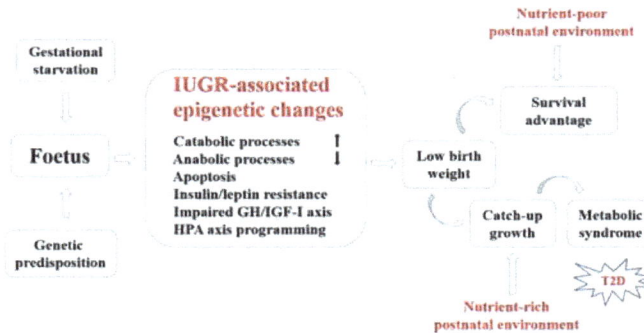

Figure 1. Schematic representation of hypothetical regulatory pathways responsible for developmental programming of type 2 diabetes (T2D) through prenatal undernutrition followed by catch-up growth in a nutrient-rich postnatal environment.

3. Evidence from Animal Models

The bulk of evidence linking intrauterine and/or early postnatal nutrient environment and predisposition to beta-cell failure and T2D in adulthood comes from animal models (for review, see [27–29]). Most of these studies have used rodent models of 50% maternal dietary restriction (DR) during pregnancy to examine the postnatal beta-cell mass development in pups exposed to either normal or restricted post-natal nutritional conditions. Rodents exposed to intrauterine DR and subsequent normal or restricted post-natal nutrition exhibited diminished beta-cell mass both at birth (30%–50% vs. control) and throughout the early postnatal development (50%–70% vs. control) [30–33]. In adulthood, these animals were unable to adaptively enhance beta-cell mass in response to rising metabolic demand and consequent insulin resistance. As a result, they developed diabetic phenotypes characterized by beta-cell failure due to insufficient expansion of beta-cell mass, impaired insulin secretion, glucose intolerance and fasting hyperglycaemia [34,35]. For example, in a study using cross-fostering methodology to isolate effects of selective pre- and postnatal 50% DR [36,37], prenatal DR resulted in a ~50% reduction in beta-cell mass whereas postnatal DR led to decreased body weight, but both beta-cell mass and beta-cell fractional area were increased compared with control animals. These findings indicate that prenatal DR largely determines endocrine cell development while postnatal DR primarily impacts development of the exocrine pancreas [37].

Currently, molecular mechanisms responsible for impaired formation of beta-cell mass in response to early-life DR have come under intensive investigation. Among them, mechanisms of epigenetic regulation of gene activity seem to play a dominant role [38–40]. Inadequate nutritional environment during intrauterine development suppressed transcription of key genes regulating beta-cell development in rats [39]. Feeding pregnant females with a low-protein diet led to hypomethylation of genes encoding glucocorticoid receptor and peroxisome proliferator-activated receptor gamma in the offspring livers. In a rat model, maternal DR also resulted in a significant reduction in the levels of expression of genes encoding key transcription factors regulating embryonic beta-cell development such as the pancreatic and duodenal homeobox 1 (PDX-1) [41,42]. Such changes on the epigenetic level were accompanied by reduced postnatal beta-cell formation and incapability to expand beta-cell mass in response to metabolic stress. Moreover, maternal DR diminished the postnatal expression of *Pdx-1* gene in pancreatic exocrine ducts which is suspected to harbor a putative pool of pancreatic beta-cell progenitor population in adult rodents [39]. Other factors potentially contributing to these effects are hormones that operate during foetal life, such as insulin, insulin-like growth factors, glucocorticoids, as well as some specific molecules such as taurine [43].

In several studies, maternal protein restriction has been shown to program an insulin-resistant phenotype in rodents, especially in consequence of catch-up growth following intrauterine growth restriction. Such mode of malnutrition resulted in expression of early markers of insulin resistance and metabolic disease risk, including alterations in adipocyte cell size and expression levels of several insulin-signalling proteins through post-transcriptional mechanisms [44]. Catch-up growth following maternal protein restriction also favoured the development of obesity in adult male rat offspring [45]. In a mice model, a protein restriction during foetal life followed by catch-up growth led to obesity in adult male mice [46]. These changes were associated with increased relative fat mass, hypercholesterolemia, hyperglycaemia and hyperleptinemia, and also with altered expression profile of several gene-encoding enzymes involved in lipid metabolism.

4. Quasi-Experimental Design in Studying the Developmental Origin of T2D

The experimental research of developmental programming in human populations is not applicable, either for ethical reasons and because the long-term follow-up is required to observe life-long outcomes of early-life experiences. In this regard, an important point is that observational studies in appropriate populations may be realized. The consistent evidence linking the early-life conditions with adult health status has been accumulated from studies conducted with a quasi-experimental design ('natural experiments'), defined as "naturally occurring circumstances in which subsets of the population have different levels of exposure to a supposed causal factor, in a situation resembling an actual experiment where human subjects would be randomly allocated to groups" [47]. Both natural and man-made disasters such as famine obviously provide a lot of advantages to their use in quasi-experimental studies. In the sections below, empirical findings from such a line of research across countries are reviewed.

4.1. Dutch Famine of 1944–1945

The long-term health consequences of the Dutch famine ('Hunger Winter') are the most comprehensively studied up to now. This famine, caused by the Nazi food embargo, affected the western Netherlands from November 1944 to May 1945. Many features of the Dutch famine can be used in a quasi-experimental design. It was a severe famine, distinctly defined in time and place and occurred in a society with a well-developed structure of administrative control. Therefore, exposure to this famine may be accurately defined by region and date of birth in relation to distribution of the food rations and the level of calories consumed. Such circumstances of the Hunger Winter famine provide the opportunity to thoroughly examine the link between inadequate maternal nutrition during particular trimesters of pregnancy and the offspring's adult health status. While a normal daily ration is 2000 kcal and 2500 kcal for women and men, respectively, the average daily rations during the famine were less than 700 kcal [48]. The population that suffered from severe food shortage throughout the famine was generally well fed before and after this period. These features of the Dutch famine provide the researchers with a near-ideal quasi-experimental research design to examine how maternal malnutrition throughout the critical early-life time windows can affect the life-course offspring health status. The prenatal exposure to the Dutch famine has been repeatedly shown to be related to the impaired metabolic phenotypes such as elevated levels of plasma lipids and body mass index (BMI), as well as enhanced risks of obesity and cardiovascular disease (CVD) later in life (for reviews, see refs. [48–50]). Most of these associations have been critically dependent on the timing of exposure. In the majority of the studies, early gestation was found to be the most vulnerable period [48–51]. Childhood and puberty are other sensitive periods with high potential to trigger programming effects. The link between exposure to the Dutch famine between age 0 and 21 years and T2D in adulthood was clearly evident, e.g., from the study by van Abeelen et al. [52]. This relationship was found to be dose-dependent: in those women who self-reported moderate famine exposure during their childhood and young adulthood, the age-adjusted hazard ratio for T2D was 1.36, and in those who reported severe famine exposure, the hazard ratio was 1.64 compared to unexposed women. The exposure to severe malnutrition during the Dutch famine at ages 11−14 was found to be considerably associated with enhanced probability of developing T2D and/or peripheral arterial diseases at ages 60−76 in women, but not in men [53].

In the Dutch famine study, compelling evidence has been obtained that exposure to famine during prenatal development may result in persistent epigenetic changes. Although no relationship between the prenatal exposure to the Dutch famine and overall global DNA methylation in adulthood was observed [54], levels of methylation of particular genes were clearly associated with prenatal famine exposure. The methylation levels of the imprinted gene encoding an insulin-like growth factor 2 (IGF2), known to play a crucial role in human growth and development, have been estimated by Heijmans et al. [51]. This gene was selected for analysis because its methylation marks are stable up to adult age, making *IGF2* gene a good candidate for such a study. In this research, those subjects exposed to the Dutch famine during their early gestation period had much lower *IGF2* methylation levels compared to control unexposed individuals six decades after the hunger exposure. Subsequently, this observation has been extended by examination of a set of 15 additional candidate loci responsible for development of metabolic and cardiovascular phenotypes [55]. Levels of methylation of six of these loci (*GNASAS, IL10, LEP, ABCA1, INSIGF* and *MEG3*) have been found to be associated with prenatal exposure to famine.

4.2. Famines in 20th-Century Austria

Findings from the Dutch Hunger Winter Study on the developmental origin of T2D were also confirmed in populations of other countries such as Austria, which has been subjected to three massive famine episodes during the 20th century. These famines occurred in 1918–19 during the collapse of the Austro-Hungarian Empire; in 1938, following the economic crisis, harvest failure, and food embargo from Nazi Germany; and in 1946–1947 in the period following the Second World War. Based on the data set including 325,000 Austrian diabetic patients, Thurner et al. [56] observed an excess risk of T2D in those persons who were born during or immediately after the periods of these famine episodes. For instance, up to 40% higher chances of having T2D in those individuals who were born in 1919–1921 compared to those who were born in 1918 or 1922, have been revealed in different Austrian regions. Noteworthy, the excess risk of T2D was practically absent in those Austrian provinces that were less affected by hunger. Furthermore, T2D rates have been correlated with the economic wealth of particular regions. The authors concluded that the revealed peaks of T2D in subjects born during and after the periods of severe starvation obviously demonstrate importance of environmental determinants in the period from conception to early childhood, in addition to genetic predisposition and shared life-course factors. These determinants clearly include nutritional triggers, although contribution of other triggering factors such as the famine-related stress and infectious factors, including rodent-borne viral infections, cannot be excluded [57]. The data obtained from this research, however, collectively favoured the hunger hypothesis as the leading explanation for the effects observed [56,58].

4.3. Ukrainian Famine of 1932–1933

The association between prenatal exposure to the famine and adult risk of T2D has been recently examined in large birth cohorts (total n = 43,150) born before, during and after the Great Ukrainian Famine of 1932–1933 ('Holodomor') [59]. This famine was caused by the Soviet Union government's forced agriculture collectivization throughout the early 1930s and led to the deaths from starvation of several million people with a ten-fold increase of mortality rate in April−July 1933 compared to the pre- and post-famine times. The cohorts born during the famine can be well defined with respect to the timing of the famine exposure in relation to the stage of pregnancy and the severity of the famine around the birth date. The odds ratios (ORs) for developing T2D were 1.47 in those individuals born in the first half of 1934 in regions affected by extreme famine, 1.26 in those born in regions with severe famine, and there was no increase (OR = 1.0) in those born in regions with no famine, compared to the births in other examined time periods. The associations observed between T2D and famine exposure around the time of birth have been found to be similar in men and women. The data obtained showed a dose-response relationship between the famine severity during the prenatal development and the risk of T2D later in life, and assumed that early gestational stage is a critical time window for modulating the prenatal environment to affect the adult T2D risk.

4.4. Leningrad Siege of 1941–1944

The Nazi Siege of the Russian city of Leningrad (the modern-day St. Petersburg) in 1941–1944 resulted in extreme hunger and death of about a million city residents. The siege-induced starvation caused an average fall in birth weight of 500–600 g [60]. Follow-up of 549 subjects born in Leningrad before or during the siege, however, demonstrated no effect of intrauterine undernutrition during the siege on dyslipidaemia, glucose intolerance, hypertension and the risk of CVD in adulthood [61,62]. Starvation-exposed individuals demonstrated only evidence for endothelial dysfunction and for a stronger influence of obesity on blood pressure. These results seem to contradict the thrifty phenotype concept since in utero undernutrition was not related to glucose intolerance in adult persons, although prenatal malnutrition influenced their blood pressure and differ from those obtained in the Dutch Hunger Winter study. One possible explanation for such a contradiction suggested by some authors in discussing these data is that the Leningrad siege research was complicated by the fact that malnutrition extended into the postnatal period. Thus, the conflict between prenatal and postnatal environments did not occur [63]. Indeed, in the Netherlands, the food supplies become fully adequate after the war ended, while those babies who were born throughout the Leningrad siege remained malnourished during all their childhood, since this famine lasted for years rather than months and nutrition was poor in subsequent years as well. The association between starvation during the Leningrad siege in early life and the risk of T2D development in adulthood was, however, observed in several more recent studies. Both the increasing incidence and decreasing age of onset of T2D without obesity have been found in women exposed to starvation throughout the Siege of Leningrad during their childhood [64]. This cohort was characterized by higher incidence of conditions associated with metabolic dysregulation such as severe arterial hypertension, and also atherosclerosis of coronary, brain and carotid arteries [65]. Similar health problems were also demonstrated in cohorts exposed to starvation during the Leningrad Siege in their childhood and puberty. Women who were 6−8 years old and men who were 9−15 years old throughout the peak of the famine demonstrated higher systolic blood pressure in their adulthood as compared with unexposed individuals who were born during the same period. Moreover, men exposed to hunger at age 6−8 and 9−15 were characterized by increased mortality from ischaemic heart disease and cerebrovascular disease, respectively [66].

4.5. Chinese Famine of 1959–1961

The long-term health consequences of the Chinese Famine of 1959–1961 ('Great Leap Forward Famine') are extensively studied now. This massive famine occurred in China in the late 1950s following the disastrous social agricultural reform commonly referred to as 'Great Leap Forward.' Over the years of the famine, 25 to 30 million more deaths and 30 to 35 million fewer births were registered in China than would have been expected under normal conditions [67]. In recent years, the Great Leap Forward Famine is the most actively studied famine episode across the globe. It should be noted, however, that one methodological limitation of the Chinese Famine study is that famine exposure data are not available by month; therefore, the periods of the famine exposure cannot be as precisely defined as in the Dutch famine study or in the Ukrainian study.

In most of the studies of long-term impacts of the Chinese Famine, the evidence was obtained that T2D as well as associated metabolic abnormalities were more common among adult Chinese residents born during the famine than among control individuals born after the famine (for a systematic review, see [68]). More specifically, in areas which were severely affected by famine, those subjects who were exposed to famine prenatally had a 3.9-fold enhanced risk of hyperglycaemia in comparison with non-exposed individuals; this difference was not seen in less severely affected regions. Remarkably, the hyperglycaemia risk was 7.6-fold higher in those prenatally exposed subjects who followed an affluent/Western dietary pattern and 6.2-fold higher in those who had a higher economic status in later life compared to non-exposed controls [69]. In a more recent study by Wang et al. [70], both prenatal and childhood exposures to famine were shown to result in higher risk of being diagnosed with T2D in adulthood (1.5-times and 1.8-times, respectively), compared with non-exposed subjects. Individuals residing in Chinese regions with high economic status had a greater T2D risk (OR = 1.46). Interestingly, the timing of association between the famine exposure in early life and adult T2D was gender-specific: an elevated risk of T2D development was evident in the foetal-exposed men (OR = 1.64) and childhood-exposed women (OR = 2.81). These findings were further confirmed in subsequent research by the same authors, where a significant association between the famine severity in the areas of exposure and the risk of T2D was found [71]. Those subjects who were exposed to severe famine during the foetal and childhood periods had substantially higher odds estimates (1.90 and 1.44, respectively). A significant interaction between the level of famine severity in the areas of exposure throughout the prenatal and childhood periods and the risk of T2D in adulthood has been observed. In another Chinese population, 1.44-fold higher risk of T2D development in the middle-childhood-exposed group, and 1.5-fold higher risks of hyperglycaemia in both the middle- and late-childhood-exposed groups were demonstrated compared to the unexposed group [72]. Remarkably, those individuals who experienced more severe famine in childhood had a 38% higher risk of T2D development than those exposed to less severe famine. The revealed association was, however, sex-specific and has been found in women, but not in men. Similar associations have been observed for the hyperglycaemia risk as well.

In a recent study conducted in Suihua, China, the evidence was obtained that programming effects can be manifested not only in those prenatally exposed to famine population (F1 generation), but also in the F2 progeny [73]. In this research, prenatal exposure to the Chinese Famine has been linked to a 1.75-fold enhanced risk of T2D and 1.93-fold enhanced risk of hyperglycaemia in F1 adult offspring in comparison with unexposed individuals. Furthermore, F2 offspring of exposed ancestors had a 2.02-fold elevated risk of adult hyperglycaemia compared to the offspring of non-exposed ancestors. These findings suggest that famine-induced effects can be transmitted via the germ line across generations and translated into increased T2D susceptibility in the descendants of the famine-exposed individuals.

4.6. Nigerian Famine of 1967–1970

The Nigerian Famine (commonly referred to as 'Biafran Famine') occurred during the Nigerian Civil War from 1967–1970. Of the one to three million Nigerians that died during this civil war, only a relatively small fraction (about 10%) had lost their lives from military action as such; the majority died from war-associated starvation [74]. The risks of glucose intolerance, hypertension and being overweight 40 years after prenatal exposure to the Biafran Famine have been assessed in the Hult et al. study [75]. The studied cohorts (total n = 1339) included those adults born before (1965–1967), during (1968–1970), or after (1971–1973) the years of famine. The exposure to famine during both foetal and infant periods has been found to be associated with significantly increased systolic and diastolic blood pressure, higher levels of p-glucose and waist circumference, as well as with substantially elevated risks of systolic hypertension (OR = 2.87), impaired glucose regulation (OR = 1.65) and overweight (OR = 1.41) in adulthood compared with persons who were born after the famine. As in the case of the Chinese Famine study, the lack of birth weight data and the resulting impossibility to separate effects of prenatal and infant famine exposure is the main methodological weakness of Biafran Famine research.

4.7. Holocaust (1939–1945)

The Holocaust was a genocide in which Nazi Germany and its collaborators killed about six million Jews. It was obviously associated with severe starvation and stress in affected populations. The long-term health outcomes of exposure to the Holocaust in the period from preconception to early infancy were determined in recent studies conducted in Israel. The pilot study involved 70 European

Jews born in countries under Nazi rule during the period 1940–1945 (exposed group) and 230 age- and sex-matched Israeli-born individuals (non-exposed group) who self-reported the presence of chronic diseases [76]. The exposed individuals have been shown to be at a higher risk of adult metabolic disturbances, including enhanced BMI, as well as 1.46-fold increased risk of hypertension, 1.58-fold increased risk for dyslipidaemia, and 1.89-fold increased risk of T2D compared to the Holocaust-unexposed group. The associations observed were further confirmed on larger groups of participants (exposed group, n = 653; non-exposed group, n = 433) [77]. The higher risks of hypertension (OR = 1.52), T2D (OR = 1.60), metabolic syndrome (OR = 2.14) and vascular disease (OR = 1.99) were found in exposed individuals.

In general, findings from quasi-experimental studies suggest that exposure to famine in early life may result in serious metabolic disturbances in later life including high risk of development of T2D and associated conditions. The main findings from these studies are summarized in Table 1.

Table 1. Summary of main findings from research on long-term metabolic health consequences of early-life undernutrition exposure

Country	Cause of Starvation	Period	Adult consequence	Ref.
Netherlands ('Dutch Hunger Winter')	Nazi food embargo	1944–1945	Impaired glucose regulation Atherogenic lipid profiles Obesity, CVD T2D Lower *IGF2* methylation Changed methylation of *ABCA1, GNASAS, IL10, LEP, INSIGF* and *MEG3* genes	[78] [79–81] [49,81] [49] [51] [55]
Austria	Empire's collapse Nazi food embargo Post-war period	1918–1919 1938 1946–1947	High risk of T2D	[56]
Ukraine ('Holodomor')	Agriculture collectivization	1932–1933	High risk of T2D	[59]
Russia	Leningrad Siege	1941–1944	Endothelial dysfunction, stronger influence of obesity on blood pressure Increasing incidence of T2D Atherosclerosis, arterial hypertension	[61,62] [64] [65,66]
China ('Great Leap Forward Famine')	Disastrous social agricultural reform	1959–1961	Hyperglycemia High risk of T2D	[69,73] [70–73]
Nigeria ('Biafran Famine')	Civil war	1967–1970	Increased blood pressure, higher levels of p-glucose, increased waist circumference, overweight, high risks of impaired glucose regulation and systolic hypertension	[75]
Europe ('Holocaust')	Nazi genocide	1939–1945	Enhanced BMI, hypertension, dyslipidemia, high risk of T2D and CVD	[76,77]
Spain	Seasonal malnutrition	1935–1954	High systolic blood pressure	[82]
United Kingdom	Seasonal malnutrition	1920–1930	Obesity	[83]
Canada	Seasonal malnutrition	1943–1995	Obesity	[84]
United Kingdom	Seasonal malnutrition	1924–1943	Dyslipidaemia, insulin resistance and CVD	[85]
USA	Seasonal malnutrition	1968–1995	High risk of T2D	[86]
Netherlands	Seasonal malnutrition	1920–1948	High risk of T2D	[87]
Ukraine	Seasonal malnutrition	1930–1938	High risk of T2D	[88]

5. Seasonality of Birth

Season of birth also can be used in quasi-experimental design to examine associations between early-life exposures, including nutritional ones, and later-life health outcomes. In this regard, month of birth presents a good instrument which may help to examine later-life outcomes of early-life exposures independently of life-course factors. This is true since decades ago there were strong seasonal variations in nutrition, especially in developing countries. Availability of cereals, vegetables, fruits and animal proteins varied significantly according to the season. Such differences in the supply of high-quality food might potentially affect the foetal and neonatal development depending on the month of gestation [89]. Other potentially confounding factors for early-life disease programming, including temperature [90], infections [91], sunlight/photoperiod and, correspondingly, production of melatonin and vitamin D [92], as well as maternal lifestyle factors such as physical activity [93] and alcohol intake [94], also tend to vary seasonally.

Seasonal conditions around the period of birth were demonstrated to significantly determine birth weight: lower birth weights were observed in the winter-born newborns and higher birth weights in summer-born newborns in the high- and low-latitude areas, while the summer birth was associated with relatively lower birth weight in the mid-latitude areas [95]. Seasonality of birth has been demonstrated for many aspects of metabolic syndrome, including high systolic blood pressure [82], obesity [83,84] and also dyslipidaemia, insulin resistance and CVD [85]. The seasonal pattern of birth for childhood autoimmune (type 1) diabetic patients was reported repeatedly (see, e.g., [96]), while the seasonality of birth for T2D adult persons was observed only in a few studies. Seasonal patterns of birth were reported, e.g., in small-sample studies conducted in 155 adolescent African-Americans [86] and in 282 T2D patients in the Netherlands [87].

By now, the most obvious evidence for the seasonality of birth in T2D patients is provided in research conducted in a Ukrainian population [88]. In this study, those persons who were born in April−May had increased risk of T2D development. In the climatic conditions characteristic of the Ukraine, these subjects ordinarily experienced their foetal life in the nutritionally marginal period from late autumn to early spring and passed the first neonatal months during the relatively plentiful season. In contrast, a decreased risk of T2D was observed in those born in November–December. In these individuals, prenatal development in a nutritionally abundant season would have been followed by early infancy in the season of relative scarcity (winter−spring). The first scenario is apparently more high-risk for developing T2D than the second one. These results are highly consistent with the thrifty phenotype hypothesis [8]. Interestingly, the seasonal pattern of birth was found to be very similar in type 1 and type 2 diabetic patients, suggesting shared early-life etiological causation for both disorders [97]. In more recent research by Jensen et al. [98], no evidence for seasonality of birth in Danish patients with T2D was found. The authors assumed that difference in effects obtained in Denmark and the Ukraine may be explained by standards of living or by differences in latitude between the countries. Indeed, as the seasonal variations in both weather and nutrition were much more pronounced in the Ukraine than in Denmark throughout the study periods, and since the Ukraine belonged to low-income countries for much of that time, its residents experienced more pronounced seasonal extremes than those experienced by people in a more prosperous country like Denmark.

In discussing the mechanistic basis for seasonal programming of adult-life diseases, one possible explanation is that seasonal factors operating around the time of birth may trigger persistent epigenetic changes that have adaptive significance in postnatal development but can predispose to chronic disorders, including the metabolic ones, at the late stages of life. The evidence for the link between season of birth and long-term changes in DNA methylation has been recently obtained in the epigenome-wide association study (EWAS) by Lockett et al. [99], where methylation at 92 CpG dinucleotides was significantly associated with season of birth. The networks related to the cell cycle, development and apoptosis have been found to be enriched among these differentially methylated CpG sites. Interestingly, the season-associated methylation patterns have been mainly absent in newborns, suggesting they arise postnatally. Although these findings were not confirmed in a more recent study by Dugué et al. [100], they, however, suggest that changes in DNA methylation might mechanistically underlie the season-of-birth effects on the risk of later-life disease.

6. Conclusions and Future Perspectives

A trend to a dramatic enhancing incidence of type 2 diabetes (T2D) has become a serious problem across the globe over the past years. Metabolic syndrome and associated risk factors including dyslipidaemia, high blood pressure, impaired glucose metabolism and T2D, are among the main causes of death in both developed and developing countries. It is widely believed that risk of T2D is mostly dependent on genetic and lifestyle factors. However, while genetic factors undoubtedly contribute to an individual susceptibility to development of obesity and T2D, the identified genetic variants can explain only part of the variation [22,101]. Recent research has demonstrated that exposure to unfavourable environmental stimuli early in life is another important determinant of the risk of T2D and associated conditions during adulthood. Findings from several of these studies suggest that epigenetic regulation can be largely contributed to development of these pathological states. Since epigenetic marks may persist long term, epigenetic modifications triggered by environmental cues throughout early sensitive stages may lead to lasting effects on the metabolic functioning, thereby affecting the risk of metabolic disorders, including T2D, later in life [102]. Prenatal and early postnatal nutrition is likely the most important factor affecting the adult risk of T2D. For instance, in studying the long-term health consequences of prenatal exposure to the Dutch famine, a link between poor nutritional intake in utero and impaired glucose regulation, atherogenic lipid profiles and obesity later in life, all known to be risk factors for development of T2D, has been demonstrated [99–102]. Therefore, it is not surprising that cohorts exposed to starvation in early life are at higher risk of T2D development. In a very recent meta-analysis of 11 published articles, a strong association between exposure to famine in early life and increased risk of T2D in adulthood has been observed (the pooled relative risk (RR) = 1.38, 95% CI 1.17−1.63) [103]. RRs for T2D development were 1.36 (95% CI 1.12−1.65) for cohorts exposed prenatally or during the early postnatal period and 1.40 (95% CI 0.98−1.99) for those cohorts who were exposed in their childhood compared to the unexposed cohorts.

In offspring born to mothers experiencing famine during pregnancy, differential methylation of genes, including those associated with pathogenesis of T2D, has been observed [51,55], indicating the importance of epigenetic processes in mediating early-life starvation exposure to the risk of later-life disease. Data from reviewed studies suggest that a focus on very early periods of gestation, and perhaps even on the periconceptional period, should constitute the next frontier for prevention of T2D over the human life course [104]. Some studies have indicated that epigenetic effects contributing to development of T2D could be transmitted across several generations. In research conducted in the Överkalix, an isolated community in northern Sweden, the possibility of transgenerational effects on T2D mortality was observed. The transgenerational consequences of the ancestors' nutrition throughout their slow growth period (SGP, aged 9 to 12 years), the period of higher susceptibility of organism to environmental influences, were investigated in cohorts born in this region in 1890, 1905 and 1920 [105,106]. In case of limited food availability in the father's SGP, then the descendant cardiovascular mortality was low, while the overeating of paternal grandfathers led to a four-fold increase in diabetes mortality in the offspring [105,106]. Such transgenerational effects were shown to be gender-specific: the paternal grandmother's nutrient supply affected granddaughters' mortality risk, while the paternal grandfather's nutrient supply was shown to be associated with the mortality risk in grandsons [106]. Since epigenetic alterations unlike genetic mutations are potentially reversible [107], pharmacological modification of epigenetic marks contributing to T2D development can provide a novel approach to prevention and treatment of T2D and associated disorders.

Acknowledgments: The author would like to thank Oksana Zabuga for the technical assistance in preparing this manuscript.

Conflicts of Interest: The authors declare no conflict of interest.

References

1. Wilmot, E.; Idris, I. Early onset type 2 diabetes: Risk factors, clinical impact and management. *Ther. Adv. Chronic. Dis.* **2014**, *5*, 234–244. [CrossRef] [PubMed]
2. Jaacks, L.M.; Siegel, K.R.; Gujral, U.P.; Narayan, K.M. Type 2 diabetes: A 21st century epidemic. *Best Pract. Res. Clin. Endocrinol. Metab.* **2016**, *30*, 331–343. [CrossRef] [PubMed]
3. Nielsen, J.H.; Haase, T.N.; Jaksch, C.; Nalla, A.; Søstrup, B.; Nalla, A.A.; Larsen, L.; Rasmussen, M.; Dalgaard, L.T.; Gaarn, L.W. Impact of fetal and neonatal environment on beta cell function and development of diabetes. *Acta Obstet. Gynecol. Scand.* **2014**, *93*, 1109–1122. [CrossRef] [PubMed]

4. Dabelea, D.; Hanson, R.L.; Lindsay, R.S.; Pettitt, D.J.; Imperatore, G.; Gabir, M.M.; Roumain, J.; Bennett, P.H.; Knowler, W.C. Intrauterine exposure to diabetes conveys risks for type 2 diabetes and obesity: A study of discordant sibships. *Diabetes* **2000**, *49*, 2208–2211. [CrossRef] [PubMed]

5. Eriksson, J.G. Developmental Origins of Health and Disease—From a small body size at birth to epigenetics. *Ann. Med.* **2016**, *48*, 456–467. [CrossRef] [PubMed]

6. Kim, J.B. Dynamic cross talk between metabolic organs in obesity and metabolic diseases. *Exp. Mol. Med.* **2016**, *48*, e214. [CrossRef] [PubMed]

7. Nettle, D.; Bateson, M. Adaptive developmental plasticity: What is it, how can we recognize it and when can it evolve? *Proc. Biol. Sci.* **2015**, *282*, 20151005. [CrossRef] [PubMed]

8. Hales, C.N.; Barker, D.J. Type 2 (non-insulin-dependent) diabetes mellitus: The thrifty phenotype hypothesis. 1992. *Int. J. Epidemiol.* **2013**, *42*, 1215–1222. [CrossRef] [PubMed]

9. Thorn, S.R.; Rozance, P.J.; Brown, L.D.; Hay, W.W., Jr. The intrauterine growth restriction phenotype: Fetal adaptations and potential implications for later life insulin resistance and diabetes. *Semin. Reprod. Med.* **2011**, *29*, 225–236. [CrossRef] [PubMed]

10. Carolan-Olah, M.; Duarte-Gardea, M.; Lechuga, J. A critical review: Early life nutrition and prenatal programming for adult disease. *J. Clin. Nurs.* **2015**, *24*, 3716–3729. [CrossRef] [PubMed]

11. Tarry-Adkins, J.L.; Ozanne, S.E. Nutrition in early life and age-associated diseases. *Ageing Res. Rev.* **2016**. [CrossRef] [PubMed]

12. Whincup, P.H.; Kaye, S.J.; Owen, C.G.; Huxley, R.; Cook, D.G.; Anazawa, S.; Barrett-Connor, E.; Bhargava, S.K.; Birgisdottir, B.E.; Carlsson, S.; et al. Birth weight and risk of type 2 diabetes: A systematic review. *J. Am. Med. Assoc.* **2008**, *300*, 2886–2897. [PubMed]

13. Kensara, O.A.; Wootton, S.A.; Phillips, D.I.; Patel, M.; Jackson, A.A.; Elia, M.; Hertfordshire Study Group. Fetal programming of body composition: Relation between birth weight and body composition measured with dual-energy X-ray absorptiometry and anthropometric methods in older Englishmen. *Am. J. Clin. Nutr.* **2005**, *82*, 980–987. [PubMed]

14. Morrison, K.M.; Ramsingh, L.; Gunn, E.; Streiner, D.; van Lieshout, R.; Boyle, M.; Gerstein, H.; Schmidt, L.; Saigal, S. Cardiometabolic health in adults born premature with extremely low birth weight. *Pediatrics* **2016**, *138*. [CrossRef] [PubMed]

15. Stirrat, L.I.; Reynolds, R.M. The effect of fetal growth and nutrient stresses on steroid pathways. *J. Steroid. Biochem. Mol. Biol.* **2016**, *160*, 214–220. [CrossRef] [PubMed]

16. Frankel, S.; Elwood, P.; Sweetnam, P.; Yarnell, J.; Smith, G.D. Birthweight, body-mass index in middle age and incident coronary heart disease. *Lancet* **1996**, *348*, 1478–1480. [CrossRef]

17. Harder, T.; Rodekamp, E.; Schellong, K.; Dudenhausen, J.W.; Plagemann, A. Birth weight and subsequent risk of type 2 diabetes: A meta-analysis. *Am. J. Epidemiol.* **2007**, *165*, 849–857. [CrossRef] [PubMed]

18. Dulloo, A.G. Thrifty energy metabolism in catch-up growth trajectories to insulin and leptin resistance. *Best Pract. Res. Clin. Endocrinol. Metab.* **2008**, *22*, 155–171. [CrossRef] [PubMed]

19. Cho, W.K.; Suh, B.K. Catch-up growth and catch-up fat in children born small for gestational age. *Korean J. Pediatr.* **2016**, *59*, 1–7. [CrossRef] [PubMed]

20. Ong, T.P.; Ozanne, S.E. Developmental programming of type 2 diabetes: Early nutrition and epigenetic mechanisms. *Curr. Opin. Clin. Nutr. Metab. Care* **2015**, *18*, 354–360. [CrossRef] [PubMed]

21. Paluch, B.E.; Naqash, A.R.; Brumberger, Z.; Nemeth, M.J.; Griffiths, E.A. Epigenetics: A primer for clinicians. *Blood Rev.* **2016**, *30*, 285–295. [CrossRef] [PubMed]

22. Van Dijk, S.J.; Tellam, R.L.; Morrison, J.L.; Muhlhausler, B.S.; Molloy, P.L. Recent developments on the role of epigenetics in obesity and metabolic disease. *Clin. Epigenet.* **2015**, *7*, 66. [CrossRef] [PubMed]

23. Vaiserman, A. Epidemiologic evidence for association between adverse environmental exposures in early life and epigenetic variation: A potential link to disease susceptibility? *Clin. Epigenet.* **2015**, *7*, 9. [CrossRef] [PubMed]

24. Geraghty, A.A.; Lindsay, K.L.; Alberdi, G.; McAuliffe, F.M.; Gibney, E.R. Nutrition during pregnancy impacts offspring's epigenetic status—Evidence from human and animal studies. *Nutr. Metab. Insights* **2016**, *8*, 41–47. [CrossRef] [PubMed]

25. Alam, F.; Islam, M.A.; Gan, S.H.; Mohamed, M.; Sasongko, T.H. DNA methylation: An epigenetic insight into Type 2 diabetes mellitus. *Curr. Pharm. Des.* **2016**, *22*, 4398–4419. [CrossRef] [PubMed]

26. Kwak, S.H.; Park, K.S. Recent progress in genetic and epigenetic research on type 2 diabetes. *Exp. Mol. Med.* **2016**, *48*, e220. [CrossRef] [PubMed]

27. Green, A.S.; Rozance, P.J.; Limesand, S.W. Consequences of a compromised intrauterine environment on islet function. *J. Endocrinol.* **2010**, *205*, 211–224. [CrossRef] [PubMed]

28. Portha, B.; Chavey, A.; Movassat, J. Early-life origins of type 2 diabetes: Fetal programming of the beta-cell mass. *Exp. Diabetes Res.* **2011**. [CrossRef] [PubMed]

29. Pinney, S.E. Intrauterine growth retardation–A developmental model of type 2 diabetes. *Drug Discov Today Dis. Models.* **2013**, *10*, e71–e77. [CrossRef] [PubMed]

30. Dumortier, O.; Blondeau, B.; Duvillie, B.; Reusens, B.; Breant, B.; Remacle, C. Different mechanisms operating during different critical time-windows reduce rat fetal beta cell mass due to a maternal low-protein or low-energy diet. *Diabetologia* **2007**, *50*, 2495–2503. [CrossRef] [PubMed]

31. Garofano, A.; Czernichow, P.; Breant, B. In utero undernutrition impairs rat beta-cell development. *Diabetologia* **1997**, *40*, 1231–1234. [CrossRef] [PubMed]

32. Garofano, A.; Czernichow, P.; Breant, B. Beta-cell mass and proliferation following late fetal and early postnatal malnutrition in the rat. *Diabetologia* **1998**, *41*, 1114–1120. [CrossRef] [PubMed]

33. Petrik, J.; Reusens, B.; Arany, E.; Remacle, C.; Coelho, C.; Hoet, J.J.; Hill, D.J. A low protein diet alters the balance of islet cell replication and apoptosis in the fetal and neonatal rat and is associated with a reduced pancreatic expression of insulin-like growth factor-II. *Endocrinology* **1999**, *140*, 4861–4873. [CrossRef] [PubMed]

34. Garofano, A.; Czernichow, P.; Breant, B. Effect of ageing on beta-cell mass and function in rats malnourished during the perinatal period. *Diabetologia* **1999**, *42*, 711–718. [CrossRef] [PubMed]

35. Blondeau, B.; Garofano, A.; Czernichow, P.; Breant, B. Age-dependent inability of the endocrine pancreas to adapt to pregnancy: A long-term consequence of perinatal malnutrition in the rat. *Endocrinology* **1999**, *140*, 4208–4213. [CrossRef] [PubMed]

36. Thamotharan, M.; Shin, B.C.; Suddirikku, D.T.; Thamotharan, S.; Garg, M.; Devaskar, S.U. GLUT4 expression and subcellular localization in the intrauterine growth-restricted adult rat female offspring. *Am. J. Physiol. Endocrinol. Metab.* **2005**, *288*, E935–E947. [CrossRef] [PubMed]

37. Matveyenko, A.V.; Singh, I.; Shin, B.C.; Georgia, S.; Devaskar, S.U. Differential effects of prenatal and postnatal nutritional environment on ss-cell mass development and turnover in male and female rats. *Endocrinology* **2010**, *151*, 5647–5656. [CrossRef] [PubMed]

38. Ong, T.P.; Ozanne, S.E. Developmental programming of type 2 diabetes: Early nutrition and epigenetic mechanisms. *Curr. Opin. Clin. Nutr. Metab Care* **2015**, *18*, 354–360. [CrossRef] [PubMed]

39. Simmons, R.A. Developmental origins of diabetes: The role of epigenetic mechanisms. *Curr Opin. Endocrinol. Diabetes Obes.* **2007**, *14*, 13–16. [CrossRef] [PubMed]

40. Simmons, R.A. Developmental origins of adult disease. *Pediatr. Clin. N. Am.* **2009**, *56*, 449–466. [CrossRef] [PubMed]

41. Blondeau, B.; Avril, I.; Duchene, B.; Breant, B. Endocrine pancreas development is altered in foetuses from rats previously showing intra-uterine growth retardation in response to malnutrition. *Diabetologia* **2002**, *45*, 394–401. [CrossRef] [PubMed]

42. Park, J.H.; Stoffers, D.A.; Nicholls, R.D.; Simmons, R.A. Development of type 2 diabetes following intrauterine growth retardation in rats is associated with progressive epigenetic silencing of Pdx1. *J. Clin. Investig.* **2008**, *118*, 2316–2324. [CrossRef] [PubMed]

43. Reusens, B.; Theys, N.; Dumortier, O.; Goosse, K.; Remacle, C. Maternal malnutrition programs the endocrine pancreas in progeny. *Am. J. Clin. Nutr.* **2011**, *94*, 1824S–1829S. [CrossRef] [PubMed]

44. Berends, L.M.; Fernandez-Twinn, D.S.; Martin-Gronert, M.S.; Cripps, R.L.; Ozanne, S.E. Catch-up growth following intra-uterine growth-restriction programmes an insulin-resistant phenotype in adipose tissue. *Int. J. Obes. (Lond.)* **2013**, *37*, 1051–1057. [CrossRef] [PubMed]

45. Bieswal, F.; Ahn, M.T.; Reusens, B.; Holvoet, P.; Raes, M.; Rees, W.D.; Remacle, C. The importance of catch-up growth after early malnutrition for the programming of obesity in male rat. *Obesity (Silver Spring)* **2006**, *14*, 1330–1343. [CrossRef] [PubMed]

46. Bol, V.V.; Delattre, A.I.; Reusens, B.; Raes, M.; Remacle, C. Forced catch-up growth after fetal protein restriction alters the adipose tissue gene expression program leading to obesity in adult mice. *Am. J. Physiol. Regul. Integr. Comp. Physiol.* **2009**, *297*, R291–R299. [CrossRef] [PubMed]

47. Last, J.M. *A Dictionary of Epidemiology*, 3rd ed.; Oxford University Press: New York, NY, USA, 1995.
48. Heijmans, B.T.; Tobi, E.W.; Lumey, L.H.; Slagboom, P.E. The epigenome: Archive of the prenatal environment. *Epigenetics* **2009**, *4*, 526–531. [CrossRef] [PubMed]
49. Lumey, L.H.; Stein, A.D.; Susser, E. Prenatal famine and adult health. *Annu. Rev. Public Health* **2011**, *32*, 237–262. [CrossRef] [PubMed]
50. Roseboom, T.J.; Painter, R.C.; van Abeelen, A.F.; Veenendaal, M.V.; de Rooij, S.R. Hungry in the womb: What are the consequences? Lessons from the Dutch famine. *Maturitas* **2011**, *70*, 141–145. [CrossRef] [PubMed]
51. Heijmans, B.T.; Tobi, E.W.; Stein, A.D.; Putter, H.; Blauw, G.J.; Susser, E.S.; Slagboom, P.E.; Lumey, L.H. Persistent epigenetic differences associated with prenatal exposure to famine in humans. *Proc. Natl Acad. Sci. USA* **2008**, *105*, 17046–17049. [CrossRef] [PubMed]
52. Van Abeelen, A.F.; Elias, S.G.; Bossuyt, P.M.; Grobbee, D.E.; van der Schouw, Y.T.; Roseboom, T.J.; Uiterwaal, C.S. Famine exposure in the young and the risk of type 2 diabetes in adulthood. *Diabetes* **2012**, *61*, 2255–2260. [CrossRef] [PubMed]
53. Portrait, F.; Teeuwiszen, E.; Deeg, D. Early life undernutrition and chronic diseases at older ages: The effects of the Dutch famine on cardiovascular diseases and diabetes. *Soc. Sci. Med.* **2011**, *73*, 711–718. [CrossRef] [PubMed]
54. Lumey, L.H.; Terry, M.B.; Delgado-Cruzata, L.; Liao, Y.; Wang, Q.; Susser, E.; McKeague, I.; Santella, R.M. Adult global DNA methylation in relation to pre-natal nutrition. *Int. J. Epidemiol.* **2012**, *41*, 116–123. [CrossRef] [PubMed]
55. Tobi, E.W.; Lumey, L.H.; Talens, R.P.; Kremer, D.; Putter, H.; Stein, A.D.; Slagboom, P.E.; Heijmans, B.T. DNA methylation differences after exposure to prenatal famine are common and timing- and sex-specific. *Hum. Mol. Genet.* **2009**, *18*, 4046–4053. [CrossRef] [PubMed]
56. Thurner, S.; Klimek, P.; Szell, M.; Duftschmid, G.; Endel, G.; Kautzky-Willer, A.; Kasper, D.C. Quantification of excess risk for diabetes for those born in times of hunger, in an entire population of a nation, across a century. *Proc. Natl. Acad. Sci. USA* **2013**, *110*, 4703–4707. [CrossRef] [PubMed]
57. Klitz, W.; Niklasson, B. Viral underpinning to the Austrian record of type 2 diabetes? *Proc. Natl. Acad. Sci. USA* **2013**, *110*, E2750. [CrossRef] [PubMed]
58. Thurner, S.; Klimek, P.; Szell, M.; Duftschmid, G.; Endel, G.; Kautzky-Willer, A.; Kasper, D.C. Reply to Klitz and Niklasson: Can viral infections explain the cross-sectional Austrian diabetes data? *Proc. Natl. Acad. Sci. USA* **2013**, *110*, E2751. [CrossRef]
59. Lumey, L.H.; Khalangot, M.D.; Vaiserman, A.M. Association between type 2 diabetes and prenatal exposure to the Ukraine famine of 1932–33: A retrospective cohort study. *Lancet Diabetes Endocrinol.* **2015**, *3*, 787–794. [CrossRef]
60. Sparén, P.; Vågerö, D.; Shestov, D.B.; Plavinskaja, S.; Parfenova, N.; Hoptiar, V.; Paturot, D.; Galanti, M.R. Long term mortality after severe starvation during the siege of Leningrad: Prospective cohort study. *Br. Med. J.* **2004**, *328*, 11. [CrossRef] [PubMed]
61. Stanner, S.A.; Bulmer, K.; Andrès, C.; Lantseva, O.E.; Borodina, V.; Poteen, V.V.; Yudkin, J.S. Does malnutrition in utero determine diabetes and coronary heart disease in adulthood? Results from the Leningrad siege study: A cross sectional study. *Br. Med. J.* **1997**, *315*, 1342–1348. [CrossRef] [PubMed]
62. Stanner, S.A.; Yudkin, J.S. Fetal programming and the Leningrad Siege study. *Twin Res.* **2001**, *4*, 287–292. [CrossRef] [PubMed]
63. Bateson, P. Fetal experience and good adult design. *Int. J. Epidemiol.* **2001**, *30*, 928–934. [CrossRef] [PubMed]
64. Khoroshinina, L.P.; Zhavoronkova, N.V. Starving in childhood and diabetes mellitus in elderly age. *Adv. Gerontol.* **2008**, *21*, 684–687.
65. Khoroshinina, L.P. Peculiarities of somatic diseases in people of middle and old age survived Leningrad siege at childhood. *Adv. Gerontol.* **2004**, *14*, 55–65. (In Russian)
66. Koupil, I.; Shestov, D.B.; Sparén, P.; Plavinskaja, S.; Parfenova, N.; Vågerö, D. Blood pressure, hypertension and mortality from circulatory disease in men and women who survived the siege of Leningrad. *Eur. J. Epidemiol.* **2007**, *22*, 223–234. [CrossRef] [PubMed]
67. Jowett, A.J. The demographic responses to famine: The case of China 1958-61. *GeoJournal* **1991**, *23*, 135–146. [CrossRef] [PubMed]
68. Li, C.; Lumey, L.H. Exposure to the Chinese famine of 1959–61 in early life and current health conditions: A systematic review and meta-analysis. *Lancet* **2016**, *388*, S63. [CrossRef]

69. Li, Y.; He, Y.; Qi, L.; Jaddoe, V.W.; Feskens, E.J.; Yang, X.; Ma, G.; Hu, F.B. Exposure to the Chinese famine in early life and the risk of hyperglycemia and type 2 diabetes in adulthood. *Diabetes* **2010**, *59*, 2400–2406. [CrossRef] [PubMed]

70. Wang, N.; Wang, X.; Han, B.; Li, Q.; Chen, Y.; Zhu, C.; Chen, Y.; Xia, F.; Cang, Z.; Zhu, C.; et al. Is exposure to famine in childhood and economic development in adulthood associated with diabetes? *J. Clin. Endocrinol. Metab.* **2015**, *100*, 4514–4523. [CrossRef] [PubMed]

71. Wang, N.; Cheng, J.; Han, B.; Li, Q.; Chen, Y.; Xia, F.; Jiang, B.; Jensen, M.D.; Lu, Y. Exposure to severe famine in the prenatal or postnatal period and the development of diabetes in adulthood: An observational study. *Diabetologia* **2017**, *60*, 262–269. [CrossRef] [PubMed]

72. Wang, J.; Li, Y.; Han, X.; Liu, B.; Hu, H.; Wang, F.; Li, X.; Yang, K.; Yuan, J.; Yao, P.; et al. Exposure to the Chinese Famine in childhood increases type 2 diabetes risk in adults. *J. Nutr.* **2016**, *146*, 2289–2295. [CrossRef] [PubMed]

73. Li, J.; Liu, S.; Li, S.; Feng, R.; Na, L.; Chu, X.; Wu, X.; Niu, Y.; Sun, Z.; Han, T.; et al. Prenatal exposure to famine and the development of hyperglycemia and type 2 diabetes in adulthood across consecutive generations: A population-based cohort study of families in Suihua, China. *Am. J. Clin. Nutr.* **2016**, *105*, 221–227. [CrossRef] [PubMed]

74. Miller, J.P. Medical relief in the Nigerian civil war. *Lancet* **1970**, *760*, 1330–1334. [CrossRef]

75. Hult, M.; Tornhammar, P.; Ueda, P.; Chima, C.; Bonamy, A.K.; Ozumba, B.; Norman, M. Hypertension, diabetes and overweight: Looming legacies of the Biafran famine. *PLoS ONE* **2010**, *5*, e13582. [CrossRef] [PubMed]

76. Bercovich, E.; Keinan-Boker, L.; Shasha, S.M. Long-term health effects in adults born during the Holocaust. *Isr. Med. Assoc. J.* **2014**, *16*, 203–207. [PubMed]

77. Keinan-Boker, L.; Shasha-Lavsky, H.; Eilat-Zanani, S.; Edri-Shur, A.; Shasha, S.M. Chronic health conditions in Jewish Holocaust survivors born during World War II. *Isr. Med. Assoc. J.* **2015**, *17*, 206–212. [PubMed]

78. Watson, P.E.; McDonald, B.W. Seasonal variation of nutrient intake in pregnancy: Effects on infant measures and possible influence on diseases related to season of birth. *Eur. J. Clin. Nutr.* **2007**, *61*, 1271–1280. [CrossRef] [PubMed]

79. Flouris, A.D.; Spiropoulos, Y.; Sakellariou, G.J.; Koutedakis, Y. Effect of seasonal programming on fetal development and longevity: Links with environmental temperature. *Am. J. Hum. Biol.* **2009**, *21*, 214–216. [CrossRef] [PubMed]

80. Finch, C.E.; Crimmins, E.M. Inflammatory exposure and historical changes in human life-spans. *Science* **2004**, *305*, 1736–1739. [CrossRef] [PubMed]

81. Lowell, W.E.; Davis, G.E., Jr. The light of life: Evidence that the sun modulates human lifespan. *Med. Hypotheses.* **2008**, *70*, 501–507. [CrossRef] [PubMed]

82. Smith, A.D.; Crippa, A.; Woodcock, J.; Brage, S. Physical activity and incident type 2 diabetes mellitus: A systematic review and dose-response meta-analysis of prospective cohort studies. *Diabetologia* **2016**, *59*, 2527–2545. [CrossRef] [PubMed]

83. Vaiserman, A.M. Early-life exposure to substance abuse and risk of type 2 diabetes in adulthood. *Curr. Diabetes Rep.* **2015**, *15*, 48. [CrossRef] [PubMed]

84. Chodick, G.; Flash, S.; Deoitch, Y.; Shalev, V. Seasonality in birth weight: Review of global patterns and potential causes. *Hum. Biol.* **2009**, *81*, 463–477. [CrossRef] [PubMed]

85. Banegas, J.R.; Rodríguez-Artalejo, F.; de la Cruz, J.J.; Graciani, A.; Villar, F.; del Rey-Calero, J. Adult men born in spring have lower blood pressure. *J. Hypertens.* **2000**, *18*, 1763–1766. [CrossRef] [PubMed]

86. Phillips, D.I.; Young, J.B. Birth weight: Climate at birth and the risk of obesity in adult life. *Int. J. Obes. Relat. Metab. Disord.* **2000**, *24*, 281–287. [CrossRef] [PubMed]

87. Wattie, N.; Ardern, C.I.; Baker, J. Season of birth and prevalence of overweight and obesity in Canada. *Early Hum. Dev.* **2008**, *84*, 539–547. [CrossRef] [PubMed]

88. Lawlor, D.A.; Davey-Smith, G.; Mitchell, R.; Ebrahim, S. Temperature at birth, coronary heart disease, and insulin resistance: Cross sectional analyses of the British women's heart and health study. *Heart* **2004**, *90*, 381–388. [CrossRef] [PubMed]

89. Laron, Z.; Lewy, H.; Wilderman, I.; Casu, A.; Willis, J.; Redondo, M.J.; Libman, I.; White, N.; Craig, M. Seasonality of month of birth of children and adolescents with type 1 diabetes mellitus in homogenous and heterogeneous populations. *Isr. Med. Assoc. J.* **2005**, *7*, 381–384. [PubMed]

90. Grover, V.; Lipton, R.B.; Sclove, S.L. Seasonality of month of birth among African American children with diabetes mellitus in the City of Chicago. *J. Pediatr. Endocrinol. Metab.* **2004**, *17*, 289–296. [CrossRef] [PubMed]

91. Jongbloet, P.H.; van Soestbergen, M.; van der Veen, E.A. Month-of-birth distribution of diabetics and ovopathy: A new aetiological view. *Diabetes Res.* **1988**, *9*, 51–58. [PubMed]

92. Vaiserman, A.M.; Khalangot, M.D.; Carstensen, B.; Tronko, M.D.; Kravchenko, V.I.; Voitenko, V.P.; Mechova, L.V.; Koshel, N.M.; Grigoriev, P.E. Seasonality of birth in adult type 2 diabetic patients in three Ukrainian regions. *Diabetologia* **2009**, *52*, 2665–2667. [CrossRef] [PubMed]

93. Vaiserman, A.M.; Khalangot, M.D. Similar seasonality of birth in type 1 and type 2 diabetes patients: A sign for common etiology? *Med. Hypotheses* **2008**, *71*, 604–605. [CrossRef] [PubMed]

94. Jensen, C.B.; Zimmermann, E.; Gamborg, M.; Heitmann, B.L.; Baker, J.L.; Vaag, A.; Sørensen, T.I. No evidence of seasonality of birth in adult type 2 diabetes in Denmark. *Diabetologia* **2015**, *58*, 2045–2050.

95. Lockett, G.A.; Soto-Ramírez, N.; Ray, M.A.; Everson, T.M.; Xu, C.J.; Patil, V.K.; Terry, W.; Kaushal, A.; Rezwan, F.I.; Ewart, S.L.; et al. Association of season of birth with DNA methylation and allergic disease. *Allergy* **2016**, *71*, 1314–1324. [CrossRef] [PubMed]

96. Dugué, P.A.; Geurts, Y.M.; Milne, R.L.; Lockett, G.A.; Zhang, H.; Karmaus, W.; Holloway, J.W. Is there an association between season of birth and blood DNA methylation in adulthood? *Allergy* **2016**, *71*, 1501–1504. [CrossRef] [PubMed]

97. Desiderio, A.; Spinelli, R.; Ciccarelli, M.; Nigro, C.; Miele, C.; Beguinot, F.; Raciti, G.A. Epigenetics: Spotlight on type 2 diabetes and obesity. *J. Endocrinol. Investig.* **2016**, *39*, 1095–1103. [CrossRef] [PubMed]

98. Sterns, J.D.; Smith, C.B.; Steele, J.R.; Stevenson, K.L.; Gallicano, G.I. Epigenetics and type II diabetes mellitus: Underlying mechanisms of prenatal predisposition. *Front. Cell Dev. Biol.* **2014**, *2*, 15. [CrossRef] [PubMed]

99. Ravelli, A.C.; van der Meulen, J.H.; Michels, R.P.; Osmond, C.; Barker, D.J.; Hales, C.N.; Bleker, O.P. Glucose tolerance in adults after prenatal exposure to famine. *Lancet* **1998**, *351*, 173–177. [CrossRef]

100. Lussana, F.; Painter, R.C.; Ocke, M.C.; Buller, H.R.; Bossuyt, P.M.; Roseboom, T.J. Prenatal exposure to the Dutch famine is associated with a preference for fatty foods and a more atherogenic lipid profile. *Am. J. Clin. Nutr.* **2008**, *88*, 1648–1652. [CrossRef] [PubMed]

101. Lumey, L.H.; Stein, A.D.; Kahn, H.S.; Romijn, J.A. Lipid profiles in middle-aged men and women after famine exposure during gestation: The dutch hunger winter families study. *Am. J. Clin. Nutr.* **2009**, *89*, 1737–1743. [CrossRef] [PubMed]

102. Roseboom, T.; de Rooij, S.; Painter, R. The Dutch famine and its long-term consequences for adult health. *Early Hum. Dev.* **2006**, *82*, 485–491. [CrossRef] [PubMed]

103. Liu, L.; Wang, W.; Sun, J.; Pang, Z. Association of famine exposure during early life with the risk of type 2 diabetes in adulthood: A meta-analysis. *Eur. J. Nutr.* **2016**. [CrossRef] [PubMed]

104. Gillman, M.W. Prenatal famine and developmental origins of type 2 diabetes. *Lancet Diabetes Endocrinol.* **2015**, *3*, 751–752. [CrossRef]

105. Kaati, G.; Bygren, L.O.; Edvinsson, S. Cardiovascular and diabetes mortality determined by nutrition during parents' and grandparents' slow growth period. *Eur. J. Hum. Genet.* **2002**, *10*, 682–688. [CrossRef] [PubMed]

106. Pembrey, M.E. Male-line transgenerational responses in humans. *Hum. Fertil. (Camb.)* **2010**, *13*, 268–271. [CrossRef] [PubMed]

107. Vaiserman, A.M.; Pasyukova, E.G. Epigenetic drugs: A novel anti-aging strategy? *Front. Genet.* **2012**, *3*, 224. [CrossRef] [PubMed]

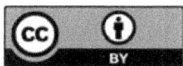

nutrients

MDPI

Article

Serum Magnesium Concentrations in the Canadian Population and Associations with Diabetes, Glycemic Regulation, and Insulin Resistance

Jesse Bertinato [1,2,*], Kuan Chiao Wang [3] and Stephen Hayward [3]

1   Nutrition Research Division, Food Directorate, Health Products and Food Branch, Health Canada,
     Sir Frederick G. Banting Research Centre, 251 Sir Frederick Banting Driveway, Ottawa,
     ON K1A 0K9, Canada
2   Department of Biochemistry, Microbiology and Immunology, University of Ottawa, Ottawa,
     ON K1H 8M5, Canada
3   Bureau of Food Surveillance and Science Integration, Food Directorate, Health Products and Food Branch,
     Health Canada, Ottawa, ON K1A 0K9, Canada;
     kuan.chiao.wang@hc-sc.gc.ca (K.C.W.); stephen.hayward@hc-sc.gc.ca (S.H.)
*   Correspondence: jesse.bertinato@hc-sc.gc.ca; Tel.: +1-613-957-0924; Fax: +1-613-946-6212

Received: 26 January 2017; Accepted: 14 March 2017; Published: 17 March 2017

Abstract: Total serum magnesium (Mg) concentration (SMC) is commonly used to assess Mg status. This study reports current SMCs of Canadians and their associations with demographic factors, diabetes, and measures of glycemic control and insulin resistance using results from the Canadian Health Measures Survey cycle 3 (2012–2013). Associations were examined in adults aged 20–79 years using linear mixed models. Mean SMCs and percentile distributions for 11 sex-age groups between 3 and 79 years (n = 5561) are reported. SMCs were normally distributed and differences ($p < 0.05$) among sex and age groups were small. Between 9.5% and 16.6% of adult sex-age groups had a SMC below the lower cut-off of a population-based reference interval (0.75–0.955 mmol·L^{-1}) established in the United States population as part of the NHANES I conducted in 1971–1974. Having diabetes was associated with 0.04 to 0.07 mmol·L^{-1} lower SMC compared to not having diabetes in the various models. Body mass index, glycated hemoglobin, serum glucose and insulin concentrations, and homeostatic model assessment of insulin resistance were negatively associated with SMC. This is the first study to report SMCs in a nationally representative sample of the Canadian population. A substantial proportion of Canadians are hypomagnesaemic in relation to a population-based reference interval, and SMC was negatively associated with diabetes and indices of glycemic control and insulin resistance.

Keywords: Canada; diabetes; glycemic regulation; homeostatic model assessment of insulin resistance; serum magnesium concentration

---

1. Introduction

Magnesium (Mg) is a mineral nutrient that functions as a catalytic co-factor and structural component of enzymes and plays an important role as a calcium antagonist [1]. Mg is essential for many biological processes including the synthesis of organic molecules, cell proliferation, energy production, muscle contraction and relaxation, bone development, mineral metabolism, and glucose homeostasis [1–4]. In North America, Mg intakes fall short of dietary recommendations for a large segment of the population [5–7]. However, the extent of Mg deficiency in the general population and related health risks are unclear because of the uncertainty regarding Mg intakes needed for optimal health. This is underscored by the large differences in recommended intakes for

Mg established by different scientific bodies [8–10]. In addition, current information on Mg status of the North American population is lacking.

Total serum Mg concentration is the most widely used nutritional biomarker for assessing Mg status [1,11,12]. A recent meta-analysis of randomized controlled trials showed that serum (or plasma) Mg concentrations were significantly increased by oral Mg supplementation in a dose- and time-dependent manner [13]. Notably, little or no change in serum Mg was observed with higher baseline circulating Mg concentrations. Together, these results suggest that serum Mg concentrations can provide meaningful information on Mg status.

Information on serum Mg concentrations in the Canadian or United States populations from nationally-representative health surveys is limited. The last national estimates were based on data collected over 40 years ago in the first National Health and Nutrition Examination Survey (NHANES I) conducted in the United States between 1971 and 1974 [14]. These estimates were used to establish a population-based reference interval for adults of 0.75–0.955 $mmol \cdot L^{-1}$. Based on this reference interval, a serum Mg concentration below 0.75 $mmol \cdot L^{-1}$ is usually defined as hypomagnesaemia (low serum Mg concentration).

Low Mg intakes and/or serum Mg concentrations have been associated with a number of diseases and health conditions including hypertension [15,16], sudden cardiac death [17,18], reduced bone mineral density [19], cardiovascular disease events [20,21], and colorectal cancer [22,23]. Poor Mg status may also impair growth of lean body mass [24] and decrease physical performance [25]. Diabetes (both type 1 and type 2) is the most common metabolic disorder associated with Mg deficiency [26–30], with reported incidence rates of hypomagnesaemia in diabetics as high as 13.5%–47.7% [27]. Multiple factors likely contribute to the hypomagnesaemia, including increased Mg loss through excretion by the kidneys. The higher renal Mg excretion is caused by reduced tubular Mg reabsorption resulting from glucose-induced osmotic diuresis and possibly insulin resistance [27,31]. Serum Mg has been negatively associated with fasting glucose and insulin concentrations and glycated hemoglobin (HbA_{1c}), a measure of long-term glycemic control [32–34]. Negative associations have also been reported with indirect indices of insulin resistance including quantitative insulin sensitivity check index (QUICKI), homeostatic model assessment of insulin resistance (HOMA-IR), and McAuley's index [32,35].

Nationally-representative data are preferred over non-national data for the development of nutrition policies and regulations. National estimates of serum Mg concentrations have never been reported for Canadians. The primary objective of this study was to report current national estimates of serum Mg concentrations for the Canadian population for ages 3–79 years using results from the Canadian Health Measures Survey (CHMS) cycle 3 conducted between 2012 and 2013. In Canada, the high prevalence of obesity [36] and co-morbidities such as insulin resistance and diabetes [37] may have a negative effect on the Mg status of the population. Thus, secondary analyses were performed to examine population-level associations between serum Mg concentrations and demographic factors, diabetes, and measures of glycemic regulation and insulin resistance in adults in order to add to our understanding of subpopulations at increased risk for Mg deficiency.

2. Materials and Methods

2.1. Survey Design

The CHMS is a cross-sectional, population-based survey that collects health information through a household interview and direct physical measures. The CHMS used a multi-stage sampling design. For cycle 3 of the survey, anthropometric measurements and biological samples were collected in a mobile examination centre (MEC) over 2 years from January 2012 to December 2013. Samples were collected from ~5700 volunteers aged 3 to 79 years from 16 collection sites stratified in five regions across Canada: Atlantic, Quebec, Ontario, Prairies, and British Columbia. The survey was designed to provide national estimates for children 3–5 years and for ages 6–11, 12–19, 20–39, 40–59, and 60–79 years for both sexes. Cycle 3 included members of the populations of the 10 provinces. Persons living in the territories, living on reserves and other aboriginal settlements in the provinces, full-time members of the Canadian Forces, the institutionalized, and persons living in certain remote areas were excluded from the survey. Altogether, these exclusions represent ~4% of the target population. The CHMS cycle 3 was approved by the Health Canada and Public Health Agency of Canada Research Ethics Board. Informed written consent was obtained from all participants older than 14 years of age. Parents or legal guardians provided written consent for younger children and the child gave assent. More detailed information on the aims of the CHMS, target population, and methodologies can be found elsewhere [38].

2.2. Biochemical Measurements

Fasted ($\geq$12 h) and nonfasted blood samples were collected and processed in a MEC. Whole blood was collected in 10 mL K_2EDTA tubes (CABD366643L, VWR International, Mississauga, ON, Canada). Serum was isolated from blood collected in 4 mL serum tubes (CABD367812L, VWR International). Whole blood and serum samples were shipped to the Nutrition Laboratory, Health Canada for measurement of HbA_{1c} (whole blood) and serum Mg, albumin, triglyceride, and glucose concentrations using the Vitros 5.1 FS clinical chemistry analyzer (Ortho Clinical Diagnostics, Mississauga, ON, Canada). Serum insulin concentration was measured using the Advia Centaur XP immunoassay analyzer (Siemens Healthcare Diagnostics, Mississauga, ON, Canada). The inter-assay (within lab precision) coefficients of variability (low–high concentration range) for HbA_{1c}, Mg, albumin, triglycerides, glucose and insulin were 1.9%–3.1%, 1.7%–0.9%, 1.7%–0.9%, 1.4%–0.9%, 1.5%–1.2%, and 5.9%–4.8%, respectively. Triglycerides and insulin were only measured in fasted participants. Results from samples with degree of hemolysis exceeding the threshold value for the assay were excluded from the analyses.

2.3. Collection of Demographic Information

Information on age, sex, race (i.e., white, South Asian, Chinese, black, Filipino, Latin American, Arab, Southeast Asian, West Asian, Korean, Japanese, other), diabetes, and yearly household income was collected at a household interview with the participants. The interview was conducted by trained interviewers using a computer-assisted interviewing method [38].

2.4. Calculations

QUICKI, HOMA-IR, and McAuley's index were calculated using the following equations: QUICKI, (log insulin ($\mu IU \cdot mL^{-1}$) + log glucose ($mg \cdot dL^{-1}$))$^{-1}$; HOMA-IR, (glucose ($mmol \cdot L^{-1}$) $\times$ insulin ($\mu IU \cdot mL^{-1}$)) 22.5^{-1}; and McAuley's index, exp(2.63 − 0.28 ln insulin ($\mu IU\ mL^{-1}$) − 0.31 ln triglycerides ($mmol \cdot L^{-1}$)). BMI was calculated from weight and height measurements.

2.5. Statistical Analyses

The CHMS cycle 3 sampling design yields national estimates when survey weights are applied. Bootstrap weights were used for all variance estimations to account for the complex sampling design [39]. The 16 collection sites from five regional strata restricted the statistical analyses to 11 degrees of freedom. Descriptive statistics are presented as arithmetic means and percentiles with 95% confidence intervals. A *t*-test or ANOVA followed by Tukey's test was used for pairwise comparison of means. Association of serum Mg concentration with demographic and biochemical characteristics were assessed via linear mixed models. Age, sex, race (white or non-white), diabetes (type 1 and type 2 combined), BMI, and yearly household income were designated as fixed effects. HbA_{1c}, QUICKI, HOMA-IR, McAuley's index, and serum albumin, glucose, insulin, and triglyceride concentrations were modeled as random effects to account for the inherent variability associated with these measurements during sampling. Model 1 included the full adult sample set (fasted and nonfasted participants), and associations between Mg concentrations and age, sex, race, diabetes, BMI, household income, albumin, and HbA_{1c} were examined. Two additional models were developed using the fasted subsample. In model 2, associations with glucose, insulin, and triglycerides were investigated in addition to the variables examined in Model 1. In Model 3, associations with the indirect indices of insulin resistance QUICKI, HOMA-IR, and McAuley's index were examined instead of the direct measures glucose, insulin, and triglycerides. The SURVEYREG procedure with backwards elimination was used to develop the final models. For the purpose of interpretation, estimates for the continuous variables were also determined after a transformation using the 5th and 95th percentiles:

$$Y \ = \ (X - \text{5th percentile of } X) \ \div \ (\text{95th percentile of } X \ - \ \text{5th percentile of } X) \quad (1)$$

Pregnant women (n = 19) and participants with a missing or invalid value were excluded from the analyses. The coefficients of variation for all estimates were <16.6% and considered acceptable for unrestricted release based on the CHMS sampling variability guidelines [40]. Statistical significance was set a $p < 0.05$. Statistical analyses were performed using SAS/STAT® 9.3 software (SAS Institute Inc., Cary, NC, USA).

3. Results

Means and percentile distributions for total serum Mg concentration for 11 sex-age groups between 3 and 79 years are presented in Table 1. Distributions were symmetrical and thus arithmetic means were reported. In general, differences ($p < 0.05$) among sex and age groups were small. For ages 6–11 years, 20–39 years and 40–59 years females had lower means compared to males. Estimations for adolescents and adults at the 10th percentile were below a population-based reference interval for adults of 0.75–0.955 mmol·L^{-1} [14]. Between 9.5% and 16.6% of the adult sex-age groups had a serum Mg concentration below 0.75 mmol·L^{-1} (Figure 1). Estimates for the 25th and 95th percentiles for all sex-age groups were within the reference interval (Table 1). Boxplots show a greater number of older adults of both sexes with serum Mg concentration below the lower fence (i.e., 1.5 × interquartile range) (Figure S1).

Mean serum Mg concentration between fasted and nonfasted participants were similar ($p \geq 0.05$) for most sex-age groups (Table S1). However, fasted males and females 6–11 years had lower means than corresponding nonfasted participants. Conversely, fasted females aged 60–79 years had a higher mean compared to non-fasting females of the same age range.

Association of serum Mg concentration with demographic factors, diabetes and measures of glycemic control and insulin resistance were examined in adults aged 20–79 years using mixed models (data for children and adolescents aged 3–19 years were excluded from these analyses). Serum albumin concentration was included in the models because of a linear relationship with serum Mg at high and low concentrations [41]. For continuous variables associations were estimated for a defined unit change and after transformation using the 5th and 95th percentiles. After transformation the estimated change in serum Mg corresponds to the change in the continuous variable from the 5th to the 95th percentile in the population. This is a better indication of the relative strengths of the associations among variables since the magnitudes of associations are compared without confounding by their scales. Estimates of the 5th and 95th percentiles for each continuous variable are presented for each model.

In Model 1, associations were estimated in fasted and nonfasted adults (Table 2). Being male was associated with higher serum Mg, whereas white race (compared to non-white) or having diabetes (type 1 or type 2) was associated with lower Mg concentrations. Age, household income, and serum albumin concentration were positively associated with serum Mg, while BMI and HbA_{1c} showed a negative association.

In Models 2 and 3, associations were examined in fasted adults. In Model 2, serum Mg was positively associated with age and household income and negatively associated with diabetes and serum glucose and insulin concentrations (Table 3). In Model 3, age and household income showed positive associations, whereas diabetes and HOMA-IR showed negative associations (Table 4).

Table 1. Means and distributions of serum magnesium concentrations by sex and age in the Canadian population.

Sex and Age	n	Serum Magnesium		Distribution of Serum Magnesium Concentrations													
		Arithmetic Mean [1]	95% CI	5th		10th		25th		50th		75th		90th		95th	
				Estimate	95% CI	Estimate	95% CI	Estimate	95% CI	Estimate	95% CI	Estimate	95% CI	Estimate	95% CI	Estimate	95% CI
										mmol·L^{-1}							
All [2]																	
3–5 years	505	0.83	0.82, 0.84	0.74	0.72, 0.76	0.76	0.74, 0.77	0.78	0.77, 0.80	0.82	0.80, 0.84	0.86	0.84, 0.88	0.90	0.87, 0.93	0.92	0.90, 0.95
Male [3]																	
6–11 years	493	0.83 [a],*	0.82, 0.84	0.73	0.71, 0.76	0.76	0.73, 0.78	0.79	0.78, 0.81	0.83	0.82, 0.84	0.86	0.85, 0.88	0.88	0.86, 0.91	0.91	0.88, 0.94
12–19 years	490	0.80 [c]	0.78, 0.81	0.71	0.68, 0.74	0.73	0.70, 0.75	0.76	0.72, 0.79	0.79	0.77, 0.81	0.83	0.80, 0.85	0.87	0.84, 0.89	0.88	0.87, 0.90
20–39 years	510	0.81 [b,c],*	0.80, 0.82	0.69	0.64, 0.74	0.73	0.70, 0.76	0.77	0.74, 0.79	0.80	0.79, 0.82	0.84	0.83, 0.86	0.87	0.86, 0.89	0.90	0.87, 0.92
40–59 years	538	0.82 [a,b],*	0.81, 0.83	0.71	0.68, 0.73	0.74	0.71, 0.77	0.78	0.76, 0.80	0.82	0.80, 0.84	0.86	0.84, 0.88	0.90	0.88, 0.92	0.91	0.88, 0.94
60–79 years	509	0.81 [b]	0.81, 0.82	0.69	0.67, 0.71	0.72	0.71, 0.74	0.77	0.75, 0.79	0.82	0.80, 0.84	0.86	0.84, 0.87	0.89	0.88, 0.91	0.91	0.89, 0.93
Female [3]																	
6–11 years	455	0.82 [a]	0.81, 0.83	0.74	0.72, 0.76	0.75	0.73, 0.78	0.78	0.77, 0.80	0.82	0.80, 0.84	0.85	0.83, 0.86	0.88	0.86, 0.89	0.89	0.88, 0.90
12–19 years	486	0.79 [d]	0.78, 0.80	0.70	0.68, 0.72	0.72	0.70, 0.73	0.75	0.73, 0.77	0.78	0.77, 0.80	0.82	0.80, 0.83	0.86	0.84, 0.87	0.88	0.86, 0.90
20–39 years	511	0.80 [c,d]	0.79, 0.80	0.71	0.70, 0.72	0.73	0.71, 0.75	0.76	0.74, 0.78	0.79	0.77, 0.80	0.82	0.80, 0.84	0.85	0.82, 0.88	0.87	0.85, 0.89
40–59 years	532	0.81 [b,c]	0.80, 0.82	0.69	0.64, 0.74	0.72	0.69, 0.76	0.76	0.74, 0.78	0.81	0.79, 0.82	0.85	0.83, 0.87	0.88	0.86, 0.89	0.89	0.87, 0.92
60–79 years	532	0.82 [a,b]	0.81, 0.83	0.67	0.65, 0.69	0.71	0.69, 0.73	0.77	0.75, 0.79	0.82	0.80, 0.83	0.86	0.84, 0.88	0.90	0.88, 0.92	0.93	0.90, 0.97

[1] Values in a column and within a sex group without a common superscript letter differ, $p < 0.05$. * Different compared to females in the same age group, $p < 0.05$; [2] Includes nonfasted males and females; [3] Includes fasted and nonfasted participants.

Table 2. Association of serum Mg with demographic factors, diabetes and biochemical measures [1].

IV	Estimate (95% CI) [2,3]	Estimate (95% CI) [3,4]	p	Distribution of Continuous IV	
				5th (95% CI)	95th (95% CI)
	mmol·L^{-1}				
Male [5]	0.01 (0.00, 0.01)	-	<0.01	-	-
White race [6]	−0.01 (−0.02, −0.00)	-	<0.001	-	-
Diabetes [7]	−0.04 (−0.05, −0.02)	-	<0.001	-	-
Age, year	0.01 (0.01, 0.01)	0.05 (0.04, 0.05)	<0.001	21.1 (18.3, 23.9)	71.7 (70.1, 73.3)
BMI, kg·m^{-2}	−0.002 (−0.002, −0.001)	−0.03 (−0.03, −0.02)	<0.001	19.7 (19.1, 20.3)	36.3 (34.7, 38.0)
Household income, K	0.0005 (0.0001, 0.0008)	0.01 (0.00, 0.01)	<0.01	15.0 (11.5, 18.5)	196.7 (166.2, 227.2)
Serum albumin, g·L^{-1}	0.002 (0.001, 0.003)	0.02 (0.01, 0.03)	<0.001	37.8 (36.3, 39.3)	48.9 (47.4, 50.5)
HbA$_{1c}$, %	−0.01 (−0.02, −0.01)	−0.02 (−0.03, −0.02)	<0.001	4.8 (4.6, 5.0)	6.5 (6.1, 6.9)

[1] Results from fasted and nonfasted adults aged 20–79 years, $n = 2838$ (Model 1). Sex, race, diabetes, age, BMI, household income, serum albumin concentration and HbA$_{1c}$ were tested in the model. All variables were statistically significant ($p < 0.05$) and retained in the final model. HbA$_{1c}$: glycated hemoglobin; IV, independent variables; Mg, magnesium; [2] Changes in serum Mg concentrations associated with being male (compared to female), white race (compared to non-white race), diabetes, a 10 years increment in age, a 1 kg·m^{-2} increment in BMI, a \$10 K increment in yearly household income, a 1 g·L^{-1} increment in serum albumin concentration and a 1% increment in HbA$_{1c}$; [3] Estimates are adjusted for all IV in the model; [4] Continuous variables were transformed using the 5th and 95th percentiles prior to analysis; [5] Males, $n = 1438$; [6] Whites, $n = 2331$; [7] Diabetics, $n = 217$.

Table 3. Association of serum Mg with demographic factors, diabetes and serum glucose and insulin concentrations [1].

IV	Estimate (95% CI) [2,3] mmol·L[-1]	Estimate (95% CI) [3,4]	p	Distribution of Continuous IV	
				5th (95% CI)	95th (95% CI)
Diabetes [5]	−0.06 (−0.07, −0.04)	-	<0.001	-	-
Age, year	0.01 (0.01, 0.01)	0.04 (0.03, 0.05)	<0.001	20.6 (17.9, 23.3)	70.8 (69.1, 72.4)
Household income, K	0.0008 (0.0004, 0.0012)	0.02 (0.01, 0.02)	<0.001	14.5 (10.3, 18.7)	199.0 (162.5, 235.6)
Serum glucose, mmol·L[-1]	−0.01 (−0.01, −0.00)	−0.01 (−0.02, −0.01)	<0.001	4.3 (4.1, 4.4)	6.6 (5.9, 7.4)
Serum insulin, pmol·L[-1]	−0.00008 (−0.00013, −0.00004)	−0.01 (−0.02, −0.00)	<0.001	25.1 (21.9, 28.2)	180.1 (156.7, 203.4)

[1] Results from fasted adults aged 20–79 years, $n = 1621$ (Model 2). Sex, race, diabetes, age, BMI, household income, serum albumin concentration, HbA$_{1c}$, serum glucose concentration, serum insulin concentration and serum triglyceride concentration were tested in the model. Statistically significant ($p < 0.05$) variables were selected by backwards elimination and retained in the final model. IV, independent variables; Mg, magnesium; [2] Changes in serum Mg concentrations associated with diabetes, a 10 years increment in age, a \$10 K increment in yearly household income, a 1 mmol·L[-1] increment in serum glucose concentration and a 1 pmol·L[-1] increment in serum insulin concentration; [3] Estimates are adjusted for all IV in the model; [4] Continuous variables were transformed using the 5th and 95th percentiles prior to analysis; [5] Diabetics, $n = 99$.

Table 4. Association of serum Mg with demographic factors, diabetes and HOMA-IR [1].

IV	Estimate (95% CI) [2,3] mmol·L[-1]	Estimate (95% CI) [3,4]	p	Distribution of Continuous IV	
				5th (95% CI)	95th (95% CI)
Diabetes [5]	−0.07 (−0.08, −0.06)	-	<0.001	-	-
Age, year	0.01 (0.01, 0.01)	0.04 (0.03, 0.05)	<0.001	20.6 (18.0, 23.3)	70.8 (69.1, 72.5)
Household income, K	0.0008 (0.0004, 0.0012)	0.02 (0.01, 0.02)	<0.001	14.5 (10.3, 18.7)	199.0 (162.0, 236.0)
HOMA-IR	−0.003 (−0.004, −0.002)	−0.02 (−0.02, −0.01)	<0.001	0.80 (0.67, 0.93)	6.99 (6.34, 7.65)

[1] Results from fasted adults aged 20–79 years, $n = 1621$ (Model 3). Sex, race, diabetes, age, BMI, household income, serum albumin concentration, HbA$_{1c}$, serum triglyceride concentration and HOMA-IR were tested in the model. Statistically significant ($p < 0.05$) variables were selected by backwards elimination and retained in the final model. HOMA-IR, homeostatic model assessment of insulin resistance; IV, independent variables; Mg, magnesium; [2] Changes in serum Mg concentrations associated with diabetes, a 10 years increment in age, a \$10 K increment in yearly household income and an increment of 1 for HOMA-IR; [3] Estimates are adjusted for all IV in the model; [4] Continuous variables were transformed using the 5th and 95th percentiles prior to analysis; [5] Diabetics, $n = 99$.

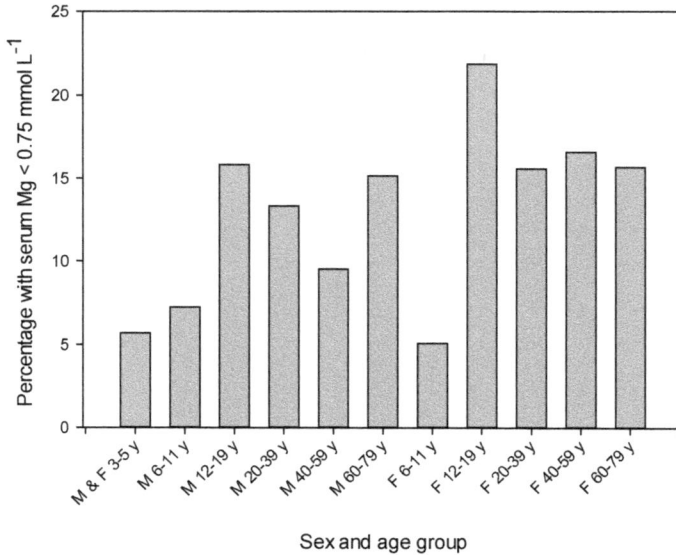

Figure 1. Percentage of each sex and age group with a serum Mg concentration below $0.75 \text{ mmol} \cdot \text{L}^{-1}$. The total number of participants (*n*) examined for each sex-age group is shown in Table 1. F, females; M, males; y, years.

4. Discussion

This study describes current (2012–2013) estimates of serum Mg concentrations in a nationally representative sample of the Canadian population for ages 3–79 years. These results are the first national estimates in Canada or the United States since the NHANES I conducted between 1971 and 1973 [14]. Results from that study showed a normal distribution for serum Mg concentration, with 95% of adults aged 18–74 years having a value between 0.75 and $0.955 \text{ mmol} \cdot \text{L}^{-1}$. Those estimates were considered as normative for the United States population and were used to establish a population-based reference interval. Serum Mg concentrations in the present study were also normally distributed. Substantial proportions of the adult sex-age groups (9.5%–16.6%) and adolescents aged 12–19 years (15.8%–21.8%) had a serum Mg concentration below $0.75 \text{ mmol} \cdot \text{L}^{-1}$, the lower cut-off of the reference interval. All estimates at the 10th percentile for adolescents and adults were also below $0.75 \text{ mmol} \cdot \text{L}^{-1}$. In addition, means in this study were lower than means reported in the NHANES I for comparable sex-age groups [14]. Collectively, these results suggest that present-day serum Mg concentrations in Canada are lower compared to concentrations in the United States population in the early 1970s. Since it has been suggested that a serum Mg concentration below $0.75 \text{ mmol} \cdot \text{L}^{-1}$ represents relatively severe Mg deficiency [11], these results raise suspicions of Mg deficiency in the Canadian population. Estimates at the 95th percentile for all sex-age groups were within the reference interval indicating the rarity of hypermagnesaemia in the population.

Similar to results from the NHANES I, only small differences in serum Mg concentrations were found among sex and age groups. Serum Mg concentrations were highest for children and showed a small increase with age from adolescents 12–19 years to older adults 60–79 years. Among demographic factors, age was the strongest predictor of serum Mg concentration in adults. The magnitudes of associations with sex, race, and household income were considerably smaller. A major finding from the NHANES I was the lower serum Mg in black Americans compared to white Americans [14]. In the present study, being white was associated with a lower serum Mg concentration than being non-white. It should be mentioned that because of the small sample sizes for all racial groups other than whites (including blacks), comparison among races in this study was restricted to the general groups of whites and non-whites.

Boxplot analyses revealed a greater number of older adults with serum Mg values below the lower fence (outliers) indicating that older adults are more prone to marked hypomagnesaemia. Possible explanations include lower dietary Mg intakes, reduced gastrointestinal Mg absorption, and increased renal Mg excretion in the elderly [42]. The higher occurrence of health conditions (e.g., diabetes) and other factors (e.g., use of hypermagnesuric diuretics) that alter Mg metabolism may also contribute [43].

Serum Mg concentrations were compared between fasted and nonfasted participants. Mean serum Mg concentrations were found to be lower for fasted children aged 6–11 years, but higher for fasted females aged 60–79 years. It is presently unclear what accounts for these differences. While the differences could be considered modest, these data offer a caution when interpreting results from a routine serum Mg test for these sex-age groups.

Inverse associations between serum Mg and diabetes and comorbidities such as poor glycemic control and insulin resistance have been well established. However, it is likely that these relationships are affected by factors that can differ among countries or change in populations over time (e.g., dietary Mg intakes, supplement and medication use). Thus, in this study associations of serum Mg concentration with diabetes and measures of glycemic regulation and insulin resistance were investigated in adults to determine the magnitude of these associations in a relatively current nationally-representative dataset. Diabetes was a strong predictor of serum Mg concentration. The estimated lower serum Mg in diabetics (ranging from -0.04 to -0.07 mmol·L^{-1} in the various models) accounts for ~20% to 34% of the spread between the lower and upper limits of the normal reference interval. These estimates are substantial and likely have clinical relevance. Serum Mg was also negatively associated with HbA$_{1c}$ and fasting serum glucose concentration. A negative effect of diabetes on Mg status is noteworthy given the high prevalence of diabetes in Canada which is expected to rise to over 10% by the year 2020 [37].

The hyperinsulinemic euglycemic clamp is considered the "gold standard" for assessment of insulin sensitivity, but the complexity of the method limits its use in large studies [44]. In this study, associations between serum Mg and more practical surrogate indices of insulin resistance [45] were examined. Fasting insulin concentration correlates strongly with insulin resistance [46] and HOMA-IR is considered a robust tool for the evaluation of insulin resistance in large epidemiological studies [47,48]. Serum Mg showed a negative association with both fasting insulin and HOMA-IR, indicating a positive relationship between serum Mg and insulin sensitivity. Notably, these relationships were observed in models controlling for diabetes. It should be mentioned that HOMA-IR was determined to be a better predictor of serum Mg concentration compared to other proxy measures of insulin resistance such as QUICKI or McAuley's index that were insignificant ($p \geq 0.05$) in our selection process.

There is evidence indicating that the relationship between Mg deficiency and type 2 diabetes is bidirectional. Mg deficiency is a common manifestation in type 1 and type 2 diabetics [26,27] and may also increase the risk of diabetes and its complications [29–31]. The negative associations between serum Mg and measures of glycemic regulation observed in this study are in agreement with studies indicating that poor glycemic control lowers serum Mg concentrations [33,34]. However, lower serum Mg may also contribute to poorer glycemic regulation and insulin sensitivity. Studies indicate that Mg supplementation improves glucose and insulin sensitivity parameters [49,50]. A meta-analysis of randomized controlled trials showed that Mg supplementation for over four months improved fasting glucose and HOMA-IR in diabetic and non-diabetic subjects [49]. In another meta-analysis, Mg supplementation was shown to reduce fasting plasma glucose in diabetics and improve HOMA-IR and plasma glucose (in a 2 h oral glucose tolerance test) in persons at high risk of diabetes [50]. The mechanisms by which Mg deficiency may increase diabetes risk are poorly understood but may involve increased oxidative stress and inflammation [35,51,52]. It is important to mention that this study does not provide any information on the temporality of the reported associations with serum Mg given the cross-sectional design.

The main strength of this study is the CHMS cycle 3 study design, including the large sample size that is representative of the Canadian population that is ideal for estimating national serum Mg concentrations and population distributions. The use of mixed models and continuous variables (rather than dichotomizing continuous variables) is also a strength. Limitations include the absence of Mg intake data (including supplement use) for comparison with serum Mg concentrations. The different methodologies used to measure serum Mg in this study and the NHANES I (colorimetric vs. atomic absorption spectroscopy) limits, to some extent, the comparison of results between studies; however, serum Mg measurements by the colorimetric method (the most commonly used method) or atomic absorption show excellent agreement ($R > 0.99$) [53]. Also, based on the responses to the household questionnaire, many diabetics in this study could not be categorized as having type 1 or type 2 diabetes. Thus, in our analyses, diabetics included participants with type 1 or type 2 diabetes or both.

The limitations of total serum Mg concentration as a biomarker of Mg status also merit discussion. Only a small fraction (~0.3%) of total body Mg is present in the serum and fluctuations in serum proteins such as albumin can alter Mg concentrations [41]. Furthermore, serum Mg may not always accurately reflect intracellular Mg deficiency. Serum Mg concentration is tightly regulated primarily at the level of renal excretion. Bone also maintains circulating concentrations by acting as a store for Mg and supplementing the serum under conditions of deficiency. This homeostatic regulation is likely a major factor accounting for the poor association observed between serum Mg concentrations and dietary Mg intakes, particularly when intakes meet nutrient requirements [54,55]. Despite these limitations, low serum Mg is usually indicative of Mg deficiency. Serum Mg is decreased in a dose-dependent manner in animal models of dietary Mg deficiency, demonstrating that low Mg intakes (Mg deficiency) reduce serum Mg concentration [56,57]. Human studies have shown that serum Mg is responsive to long-term changes in dietary Mg intakes [58] and increases with Mg supplementation [13,59,60]. A meta-analysis of randomized controlled trials showed that serum Mg concentrations increase in a dose- and time-dependent manner with oral Mg supplementation, and the response is greater when baseline circulating Mg concentrations are lower, suggesting that serum Mg provides useful information about underlying Mg status [13]. It has been suggested that a serum Mg value below $0.75 \text{ mmol} \cdot \text{L}^{-1}$ is a useful measure of relatively severe Mg deficiency, but Mg deficiency cannot be excluded for persons with a value between 0.75 and $0.85 \text{ mmol} \cdot \text{L}^{-1}$ [11,12].

5. Conclusions

This study reports serum Mg concentrations for 11 sex-age groups between 3 and 79 years in the Canadian population. Between 9.5% and 16.6% of the adult sex-age groups were hypomagnesaemic (serum Mg $< 0.75 \text{ mmol} \cdot \text{L}^{-1}$) in relation to a population-based reference interval [14]. There is a need to establish an evidence-based reference interval (or at minimum a lower cut-off value) for health that will allow more accurate assessment of the prevalence of Mg deficiency in Canada and related health risk based on results from this study [61]. Among demographic factors, age was the strongest predictor of serum Mg concentration. Serum Mg concentration was negatively associated with diabetes, BMI, serum glucose, serum insulin, HbA_{1c}, and HOMA-IR. These results are consistent with a growing body of evidence indicating a negative effect of diabetes, poor glycemic control, and insulin resistance on Mg status.

Supplementary Materials: The following are available online at http://www.mdpi.com/2072-6643/9/3/296/s1, Figure S1: Boxplots of serum Mg concentrations by sex-age group, Table S1: Means and distributions of serum magnesium concentrations by sex and age in fasted and nonfasted Canadians.

Acknowledgments: This research was funded by the Bureau of Nutritional Sciences and the Bureau of Food Surveillance and Science Integration, Health Canada.

Author Contributions: J.B. conceived the study; J.B., K.C.W. and S.H. analyzed the data; J.B. wrote the paper.

Conflicts of Interest: The authors declare no conflict of interest.

References

1. Swaminathan, R. Magnesium metabolism and its disorders. *Clin. Biochem. Rev.* **2003**, *24*, 47–66. [PubMed]
2. Volpe, S.L. Magnesium in disease prevention and overall health. *Adv. Nutr.* **2013**, *4*, 378S–383S. [CrossRef] [PubMed]
3. Elin, R.J. Magnesium: The fifth but forgotten electrolyte. *Am. J. Clin. Pathol.* **1994**, *102*, 616–622. [CrossRef] [PubMed]
4. Wolf, F.I.; Cittadini, A. Magnesium in cell proliferation and differentiation. *Front. Biosci.* **1999**, *4*, D607–D617. [CrossRef] [PubMed]
5. Moshfegh, A.; Goldman, J.D.; Ahuja, J.; Rhodes, D.; LaComb, R. *What We Eat in America, NHANES 2005–2006: Usual Nutrient Intakes from Food and Water Compared to 1997 Dietary Reference Intakes for Vitamin D, Calcium, Phosphorus, and Magnesium*; U.S. Department of Agriculture, Agriculture Research Service: Washington, DC, USA, 2009.
6. Health Canada. Do Canadian Adults Meet Their Nutrient Requirements through Food Intake Alone? Available online: http://www.hc-sc.gc.ca/fn-an/surveill/nutrition/commun/art-nutr-adult-eng.php (accessed on 23 February 2017).
7. Ford, E.S.; Mokdad, A.H. Dietary magnesium intake in a national sample of US adults. *J. Nutr.* **2003**, *133*, 2879–2882. [PubMed]
8. Food and Nutrition Board, Institute of Medicine. *Dietary Reference Intakes for Calcium, Phosphorus, Magnesium, Vitamin D, and Fluoride*; National Academy Press: Washington, DC, USA, 1997; pp. 190–249.
9. EFSA Panel on Dietetic Products, Nutrition and Allergies (NDA). Scientific opinion on dietary reference values for magnesium. *EFSA J.* **2015**, *13*, 4186.
10. Joint FAO/WHO Expert Consultation. *Vitamin and Mineral Requirements in Human Nutrition: Report of a Joint FAO/WHO Expert Consultation*, 2nd ed.; World Health Organization: Geneva, Switzerland, 2004.
11. Arnaud, M.J. Update on the assessment of magnesium status. *Br. J. Nutr.* **2008**, *99*, S24–S36. [CrossRef] [PubMed]
12. Elin, R.J. Assessment of magnesium status for diagnosis and therapy. *Magnes. Res.* **2010**, *23*, S194–S198. [PubMed]
13. Zhang, X.; Del Gobbo, L.C.; Hruby, A.; Rosanoff, A.; He, K.; Dai, Q.; Costello, R.B.; Zhang, W.; Song, Y. The circulating concentration and 24-h urine excretion of magnesium dose- and time-dependently respond to oral magnesium supplementation in a meta-analysis of randomized controlled trials. *J. Nutr.* **2016**, *146*, 595–602. [CrossRef] [PubMed]
14. Lowenstein, F.W.; Stanton, M.F. Serum magnesium levels in the United States, 1971–1974. *J. Am. Coll. Nutr.* **1986**, *5*, 399–414. [CrossRef] [PubMed]
15. Ma, J.; Folsom, A.R.; Melnick, S.L.; Eckfeldt, J.H.; Sharrett, A.R.; Nabulsi, A.A.; Hutchinson, R.G.; Metcalf, P.A. Associations of serum and dietary magnesium with cardiovascular disease, hypertension, diabetes, insulin, and carotid arterial wall thickness: The ARIC study. Atherosclerosis Risk in Communities Study. *J. Clin. Epidemiol.* **1995**, *48*, 927–940. [CrossRef]
16. Zhang, X.; Li, Y.; Del Gobbo, L.C.; Rosanoff, A.; Wang, J.; Zhang, W.; Song, Y. Effects of magnesium supplementation on blood pressure: A meta-analysis of randomized double-blind placebo-controlled trials. *Hypertension* **2016**, *68*, 324–333. [CrossRef] [PubMed]
17. Kieboom, B.C.; Niemeijer, M.N.; Leening, M.J.; van den Berg, M.E.; Franco, O.H.; Deckers, J.W.; Hofman, A.; Zietse, R.; Stricker, B.H.; Hoorn, E.J. Serum magnesium and the risk of death from coronary heart disease and sudden cardiac death. *J. Am. Heart Assoc.* **2016**, *5*, e002707. [CrossRef] [PubMed]
18. Peacock, J.M.; Ohira, T.; Post, W.; Sotoodehnia, N.; Rosamond, W.; Folsom, A.R. Serum magnesium and risk of sudden cardiac death in the Atherosclerosis Risk in Communities (ARIC) Study. *Am. Heart J.* **2010**, *160*, 464–470. [CrossRef] [PubMed]
19. Orchard, T.S.; Larson, J.C.; Alghothani, N.; Bout-Tabaku, S.; Cauley, J.A.; Chen, Z.; LaCroix, A.Z.; Wactawski-Wende, J.; Jackson, R.D. Magnesium intake, bone mineral density, and fractures: Results from the Women's Health Initiative Observational study. *Am. J. Clin. Nutr.* **2014**, *99*, 926–933. [CrossRef] [PubMed]

20. Del Gobbo, L.C.; Imamura, F.; Wu, J.H.; de Oliveira Otto, M.C.; Chiuve, S.E.; Mozaffarian, D. Circulating and dietary magnesium and risk of cardiovascular disease: A systematic review and meta-analysis of prospective studies. *Am. J. Clin. Nutr.* **2013**, *98*, 160–173. [CrossRef] [PubMed]

21. Qu, X.; Jin, F.; Hao, Y.; Li, H.; Tang, T.; Wang, H.; Yan, W.; Dai, K. Magnesium and the risk of cardiovascular events: A meta-analysis of prospective cohort studies. *PLoS ONE* **2013**, *8*, e57720. [CrossRef] [PubMed]

22. Chen, G.C.; Pang, Z.; Liu, Q.F. Magnesium intake and risk of colorectal cancer: A meta-analysis of prospective studies. *Eur. J. Clin. Nutr.* **2012**, *66*, 1182–1186. [CrossRef] [PubMed]

23. Qu, X.; Jin, F.; Hao, Y.; Zhu, Z.; Li, H.; Tang, T.; Dai, K. Nonlinear association between magnesium intake and the risk of colorectal cancer. *Eur. J. Gastroenterol. Hepatol.* **2013**, *25*, 309–318. [CrossRef] [PubMed]

24. Bertinato, J.; Lavergne, C.; Rahimi, S.; Rachid, H.; Vu, N.A.; Plouffe, L.J.; Swist, E. Moderately low magnesium intake impairs growth of lean body mass in obese-prone and obese-resistant rats fed a high-energy diet. *Nutrients* **2016**, *8*, 253. [CrossRef] [PubMed]

25. Veronese, N.; Berton, L.; Carraro, S.; Bolzetta, F.; De Rui, M.; Perissinotto, E.; Toffanello, E.D.; Bano, G.; Pizzato, S.; Miotto, F.; et al. Effect of oral magnesium supplementation on physical performance in healthy elderly women involved in a weekly exercise program: A randomized controlled trial. *Am. J. Clin. Nutr.* **2014**, *100*, 974–981. [CrossRef] [PubMed]

26. De Valk, H.W. Magnesium in diabetes mellitus. *Neth. J. Med.* **1999**, *54*, 139–146. [CrossRef]

27. Pham, P.C.; Pham, P.M.; Pham, S.V.; Miller, J.M.; Pham, P.T. Hypomagnesemia in patients with type 2 diabetes. *Clin. J. Am. Soc. Nephrol.* **2007**, *2*, 366–373. [CrossRef] [PubMed]

28. Kao, W.H.; Folsom, A.R.; Nieto, F.J.; Mo, J.P.; Watson, R.L.; Brancati, F.L. Serum and dietary magnesium and the risk for type 2 diabetes mellitus: The Atherosclerosis Risk in Communities Study. *Arch. Intern. Med.* **1999**, *159*, 2151–2159. [CrossRef] [PubMed]

29. Larsson, S.C.; Wolk, A. Magnesium intake and risk of type 2 diabetes: A meta-analysis. *J. Intern. Med.* **2007**, *262*, 208–214. [CrossRef] [PubMed]

30. Weng, L.C.; Lee, N.J.; Yeh, W.T.; Ho, L.T.; Pan, W.H. Lower intake of magnesium and dietary fiber increases the incidence of type 2 diabetes in Taiwanese. *J. Formos. Med. Assoc.* **2012**, *111*, 651–659. [CrossRef] [PubMed]

31. Gommers, L.M.; Hoenderop, J.G.; Bindels, R.J.; de Baaij, J.H. Hypomagnesemia in type 2 diabetes: A vicious circle? *Diabetes* **2016**, *65*, 3–13. [CrossRef] [PubMed]

32. Bertinato, J.; Xiao, C.W.; Ratnayake, W.M.; Fernandez, L.; Lavergne, C.; Wood, C.; Swist, E. Lower serum magnesium concentration is associated with diabetes, insulin resistance, and obesity in South Asian and white Canadian women but not men. *Food Nutr. Res.* **2015**, *59*, 25974. [CrossRef] [PubMed]

33. Arpaci, D.; Tocoglu, A.G.; Ergenc, H.; Korkmaz, S.; Ucar, A.; Tamer, A. Associations of serum magnesium levels with diabetes mellitus and diabetic complications. *Hippokratia* **2015**, *19*, 153–157. [PubMed]

34. Sinha, S.; Sen, S. Status of zinc and magnesium levels in type 2 diabetes mellitus and its relationship with glycemic status. *Int. J. Diabetes Dev. Ctries.* **2014**, *34*, 220–223. [CrossRef]

35. Kim, D.J.; Xun, P.; Liu, K.; Loria, C.; Yokota, K.; Jacobs, D.R., Jr.; He, K. Magnesium intake in relation to systemic inflammation, insulin resistance, and the incidence of diabetes. *Diabetes Care* **2010**, *33*, 2604–2610. [CrossRef] [PubMed]

36. Shields, M.; Carroll, M.D.; Ogden, C.L. Adult obesity prevalence in Canada and the United States. *NCHS Data Brief* **2011**, *56*, 1–8.

37. Public Health Agency of Canada. Diabetes in Canada: Facts and Figures from a Public Health Perspective. Available online: http://www.phac-aspc.gc.ca/cd-mc/publications/diabetes-diabete/facts-figures-faits-chiffres-2011/index-eng.php (accessed on 23 February 2017).

38. Statistics Canada. Canadian Health Measures Survey (CHMS). Available online: http://www23.statcan.gc.ca/imdb/p2SV.pl?Function=getSurvey&Id=136652 (accessed on 23 February 2017).

39. Giroux, S. Canadian Health Measures Survey: Sampling strategy overview. *Health Rep.* **2007**, *18*, S31–S36.

40. Statistics Canada. Canadian Health Measures Survey (CHMS) Data User Guide: Cycle 1. Available online: http://www23.statcan.gc.ca/imdb-bmdi/document/5071_D2_T1_V1-eng.htm (accessed on 23 February 2017).

41. Kroll, M.H.; Elin, R.J. Relationships between magnesium and protein concentrations in serum. *Clin. Chem.* **1985**, *31*, 244–246. [PubMed]

42. Seelig, M.S.; Preuss, H.G. Magnesium metabolism and perturbations in the elderly. *Geriatr. Nephrol. Urol.* **1994**, *4*, 101–111. [CrossRef]

43. Barbagallo, M.; Belvedere, M.; Dominguez, L.J. Magnesium homeostasis and aging. *Magnes. Res.* **2009**, *22*, 235–246. [PubMed]

44. DeFronzo, R.A.; Tobin, J.D.; Andres, R. Glucose clamp technique: A method for quantifying insulin secretion and resistance. *Am. J. Physiol.* **1979**, *237*, E214–E223. [PubMed]

45. Singh, B.; Saxena, A. Surrogate markers of insulin resistance: A review. *World J. Diabetes* **2010**, *1*, 36–47. [CrossRef] [PubMed]

46. Olefsky, J.; Farquhar, J.W.; Reaven, G. Relationship between fasting plasma insulin level and resistance to insulin-mediated glucose uptake in normal and diabetic subjects. *Diabetes* **1973**, *22*, 507–513. [CrossRef] [PubMed]

47. Matthews, D.R.; Hosker, J.P.; Rudenski, A.S.; Naylor, B.A.; Treacher, D.F.; Turner, R.C. Homeostasis model assessment: Insulin resistance and beta-cell function from fasting plasma glucose and insulin concentrations in man. *Diabetologia* **1985**, *28*, 412–419. [CrossRef] [PubMed]

48. Gutch, M.; Kumar, S.; Razi, S.M.; Gupta, K.K.; Gupta, A. Assessment of insulin sensitivity/resistance. *Indian J. Endocrinol. Metab.* **2015**, *19*, 160–164. [CrossRef] [PubMed]

49. Simental-Mendia, L.E.; Sahebkar, A.; Rodriguez-Moran, M.; Guerrero-Romero, F. A systematic review and meta-analysis of randomized controlled trials on the effects of magnesium supplementation on insulin sensitivity and glucose control. *Pharmacol. Res.* **2016**, *111*, 272–282. [CrossRef] [PubMed]

50. Veronese, N.; Watutantrige-Fernando, S.; Luchini, C.; Solmi, M.; Sartore, G.; Sergi, G.; Manzato, E.; Barbagallo, M.; Maggi, S.; Stubbs, B. Effect of magnesium supplementation on glucose metabolism in people with or at risk of diabetes: A systematic review and meta-analysis of double-blind randomized controlled trials. *Eur. J. Clin. Nutr.* **2016**, *70*, 1354–1359. [CrossRef] [PubMed]

51. Zheltova, A.A.; Kharitonova, M.V.; Iezhitsa, I.N.; Spasov, A.A. Magnesium deficiency and oxidative stress: an update. *BioMedicine* **2016**, *6*, 8–14. [CrossRef] [PubMed]

52. Barbagallo, M.; Dominguez, L.J. Magnesium and type 2 diabetes. *World J. Diabetes* **2015**, *6*, 1152–1157. [CrossRef] [PubMed]

53. Instructions for Use. VITROS Chemistry Products Mg Slides. Available online: https://www.cmmc.org/cmmclab/IFU/Mg_MP2-47_EN_I.pdf (accessed on 23 February 2017).

54. Lakshmanan, F.L.; Rao, R.B.; Kim, W.W.; Kelsay, J.L. Magnesium intakes, balances, and blood levels of adults consuming self-selected diets. *Am. J. Clin. Nutr.* **1984**, *40*, 1380–1389. [PubMed]

55. Misialek, J.R.; Lopez, F.L.; Lutsey, P.L.; Huxley, R.R.; Peacock, J.M.; Chen, L.Y.; Soliman, E.Z.; Agarwal, S.K.; Alonso, A. Serum and dietary magnesium and incidence of atrial fibrillation in whites and in African Americans: Atherosclerosis Risk in Communities (ARIC) Study. *Circ. J.* **2013**, *77*, 323–329. [CrossRef] [PubMed]

56. Bertinato, J.; Lavergne, C.; Plouffe, L.J.; El Niaj, H.A. Small increases in dietary calcium above normal requirements exacerbate magnesium deficiency in rats fed a low magnesium diet. *Magnes. Res.* **2014**, *27*, 35–47. [PubMed]

57. Bertinato, J.; Plouffe, L.J.; Lavergne, C.; Ly, C. Bioavailability of magnesium from inorganic and organic compounds is similar in rats fed a high phytic acid diet. *Magnes. Res.* **2014**, *27*, 175–185. [PubMed]

58. Klevay, L.M.; Milne, D.B. Low dietary magnesium increases supraventricular ectopy. *Am. J. Clin. Nutr.* **2002**, *75*, 550–554. [PubMed]

59. Witkowski, M.; Hubert, J.; Mazur, A. Methods of assessment of magnesium status in humans: A systematic review. *Magnes. Res.* **2011**, *24*, 163–180. [PubMed]

60. Song, Y.; He, K.; Levitan, E.B.; Manson, J.E.; Liu, S. Effects of oral magnesium supplementation on glycaemic control in type 2 diabetes: A meta-analysis of randomized double-blind controlled trials. *Diabet. Med.* **2006**, *23*, 1050–1056. [CrossRef] [PubMed]

61. Costello, R.B.; Elin, R.J.; Rosanoff, A.; Wallace, T.C.; Guerrero-Romero, F.; Hruby, A.; Lutsey, P.L.; Nielsen, F.H.; Rodriguez-Moran, M.; Song, Y.; et al. Perspective: The case for an evidence-based reference interval for serum magnesium: the time has come. *Adv. Nutr.* **2016**, *7*, 977–993. [CrossRef] [PubMed]

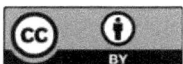

nutrients

MDPI

Article

A Multifunctional Bread Rich in Beta Glucans and Low in Starch Improves Metabolic Control in Type 2 Diabetes: A Controlled Trial

Paolo Tessari [1,*] and Anna Lante [2]

[1] Department of Medicine (DIMED), University of Padova, 35128 Padova PD, Italy
[2] Department of Agronomy, Food, Natural Resources, Animals & Environment (DAFNAE),
     University of Padova, 35123 Padova PD, Italy; anna.lante@unipd.it
*   Correspondence: paolo.tessari@unipd.it; Tel.: +39-049-821-1748; Fax: +39-049-821-7878

Received: 28 December 2016; Accepted: 9 March 2017; Published: 17 March 2017

Abstract: Design: Functional foods may be useful for people with diabetes. The soluble fibers beta glucans can modify starch digestion and improve postprandial glucose response. We analyzed the metabolic effects of a specifically designed 'functional' bread, low in starch, rich in fibers (7 g/100 g), with a beta glucan/starch ratio of (7.6:100, g/g), in people with type 2 diabetes mellitus. Methods: Clinical and metabolic data from two groups of age-, sex- and glycated hemoglobin-matched diabetic subjects, taking either the functional bread or regular white bread, over a roughly six-month observation period, were retrieved. Results: Bread intake did not change during the trial. The functional bread reduced glycated hemoglobin by ~0.5% (absolute units) vs. pre-treatment values ($p = 0.028$), and by ~0.6% vs. the control group ($p = 0.027$). Post-prandial and mean plasma glucose was decreased in the treatment group too. Body weight, blood pressure and plasma lipids did not change. The acceptance of the functional bread was good in the majority of subjects, except for taste. Conclusions: A starch-restricted, fiber-rich functional bread, with an increased beta glucan/starch ratio, improved long term metabolic control, and may be indicated in the dietary treatment of type 2 diabetes.

Keywords: plasma glucose; beta glucan; starch; metabolic control; fibers

1. Introduction

Background and Aims

Type 2 diabetes mellitus (T2DM) is a disease with high prevalence and increasing incidence. The world population currently affected by T2DM is about 400 million, and it is expected to grow to more than 600 million by 2040 [1]. The increase of T2DM is largely due to changes of lifestyle [2], i.e., excess dietary intake combined to low physical activity. Therefore, diet represents a cornerstone for both prevention and therapy of T2DM, and a tool to maintain plasma glucose values close to normal.

Carbohydrates (CHO) are the key nutritional factors conditioning circulating glucose levels, particularly in the post-prandial state. In order to prevent excessive post-prandial glycemicexcursions, dietary CHO should be predominantly represented by starch (>90% of total CHO), with less than 10% by either mono- or di-saccharides [3]. Furthermore, since T2DM is associated with a constellation of conditions (obesity, dyslipidemia, hypertension) and risk factors (e.g., for cardiovascular disease) recognized in the concept of the 'metabolic syndrome' [4–6], food capable of addressing most, if not all these abnormalities, can be recommended. Thus, current understanding is that foods and diets for T2DM patients are considered, for the present, to be energy controlled, with a low glycemic index (GI), and with favorable effects on blood pressure and dyslipidemia. A reduction of cardiovascular (CV) risk and the prevention of long term diabetic complications are also expected to result from long-term use of such 'ideal' foods.

Post-prandial glucose increments in diabetes may be blunted by foods containing starch and/or simple CHO with a slow absorption rate, thus resulting in a low GI. Besides by the CHO type itself, CHO absorption may be modulated by a variety of additional factors, such as starch characteristics (i.e., resistance to digestion), fiber type and content, and by the presence of other compounds that can decrease carbohydrate intestinal digestion and absorption. Conversely, the guidelines for dietary treatment of hypertension, obesity and dyslipidemia include a reduction of sodium and energy intakes, and a control of intestinal lipid absorption. Thus, targeting some, if not all, these risk factors, by means of functional foods seems to be both recommended and promising in the dietary management of both diabetes and the metabolic syndrome, through health-beneficial properties conveyed by natural components and/or by added ingredients [7].

Functional foods rich in natural fibers, such as beta glucans, are among those most-widely studied and employed. Beta glucans are naturally-occurring soluble fibers of some cereals (oats and barley), composed of mixed-linkage (1,3)(1,4)-β-D-glucose units, mainly consisting of the linear polysaccharide (1→3), (1→4)-β-D-glucan. Beta glucans increase viscosity in the upper digestive tract, thus reducing postprandial glucose and insulin responses [8]. An optimal beta glucan/starch ratio has been proposed as a method to decrease starch digestion in functional breads [9].

Bread is a staple food and a fundamental source of CHO worldwide in everyday diet. Therefore, the design of a bread with targeted functional properties could retain a major impact on nutrition and on metabolic parameters.

In this study, we examined the metabolic effects of long-term (roughly six months) substitution of regular white bread with a functional bread, starch-restricted and rich in fiber (mostly beta glucans), in the everyday diet of persons with type 2 diabetes.

2. Methods

2.1. Study Design and Participants

In the context of a comprehensive analysis of clinical and biochemical parameters of people with type 2 diabetes mellitus, data from T2DM subjects of both sexes, collected at their regularly-scheduled outpatient visits at the Diabetes Center of the Padova University Hospital, Italy, were retrieved. This was an observational, controlled study with parallel groups, performed following recently published guidelines and format (http://www.consort-statement.org/). The subjects' inclusion criteria were: a diabetes duration longer than 2 years; an unsatisfactory diabetes control (HbA$_1$c values greater than 7%); age between 50 and 80 years; treatment with diet only, or diet plus oral hypoglycemic agents (OHA) and/or basal insulin; and a reported daily intake of at least 50 g CHO as either white bread, breadsticks or other bread substitutes. The patients were visited at 3–6 months intervals.

2.2. Interventions

The patients had routinely been recommended to consume foods considered to be beneficial to peoples with diabetes, such as low calorie items, with CHO predominantly represented by starch, with a high fiber content and/or a low glycemic index, and low amounts of fats of animal origin. Furthermore, the patients had been informed about the availability in supermarkets, of flour products enriched with fibers and/or other compounds that could be beneficial to control glucose levels. They were encouraged to prepare homemade bread using any of these flour products, as a substitute of their usually consumed white bread made of refined flour.

At subsequent examinations, the type of bread used by every subjects was recorded. Therefore, two groups of subjects could be selected over time: those who had shifted to the use of one of the functional bread types ('functional bread' group), and those who had been still using their regular white bread ('control' group). Among the former, the starting time of consumption of either the functional flour and/or bread, and its type, were retrieved and recorded. For the sake of homogeneity, we report here data of those subjects consuming only one type of these fiber-enriched products, i.e., a flour labelled Salus® (produced by Ruggeri srl, Padova, Italy), that was the most largely used. These subjects were included into the 'functional bread' group. The data of the case-control group, i.e., that of patients who were consuming their regular bread, were collected in a similar fashion. The matching criteria with the 'functional bread' group were age, sex, absolute HbA$_1$c values as well as absence of HbA$_1$c changes between the two selected time intervals (i.e., approximately ~6–7 months. apart), greater than ±1% (absolute value). For both groups, other inclusion criteria were: no variation in both hypoglycemic and other drug therapy, and no major intercurrent diseases over the chosen observation periods. A total of eleven subjects in each group were selected.

The target observations interval after the 'start' time point was set between 3 and 12 months. Each patient had been advised to maintain his/her usual dietary habits and nutrient intake, except for the type of bread used. The 24-h recall method was used to assess dietary intake of the day before each visit. The data of each patients were handled rigorously in anonymous fashion. Of the 20 subjects originally enrolled into the 'functional bread group', only eleven completed the intended observational time period. The causes for drop-out were: insufficient bread intake (less than 40 g of starch equivalents per day, possibly preventing the detection of a significant effect by substitution with the functional bread); intercurrent diseases and/or changes of therapy; major dietary changes and/or failure to observe the standard recommendations for people with T2DM.

As controls, two sets of data were used. First, each patient's own HbA$_1$c value(s) in the 3–12 month period antecedent either the start of consumption of the functional bread/flour, or a comparable period of use of the regular bread in the 'control' group, were recorded. These data are referred to as the 'previous' time points. Each patient was thus the control of him/herself. Second, data collected after use of either the 'functional bread' and of the 'control bread', as described above, recorded over the subsequent 3–12 months from the 'start' time point, were retrieved.

The subjects were either in the fasting state or had consumed their breakfast at home before coming to the Diabetes Centre. Breakfast composition was pretty reproducible in the same subject on the two/three visits, but different from patient to patient. In general, the patients consumed a medium-to-low-calorie Italian breakfast, consisting of milk, coffee (or tea), cereals (or bread slices), dressed with a thin layer of jam with a low sugar content, and/or one fruit, and/or one portion of yoghurt.

On the occasion of each visit, the patients' glucose value (either in the fasting state or 2-h post-breakfast, the latter labeled as 'post-prandial' value), were determined by a reflectometer. These directly determined values were averaged with those retrieved from the home glucose monitoring of each patients, in the two–three days preceding the visit. Thus, both the fasting and post-breakfast data were the mean of these values.

The local Ethics Committee of Padova University Hospital had approved, as part of broader clinical data investigations in diabetes, the retrieval in anonymous form, of clinical and biochemical data from medical records of the diabetic patients (Approval N. 14809, released on 11 March 2016).

2.3. Bread Preparation

The functional bread was prepared at home by every subject using the instructions of the producer(s). Typically, a Moulinex bread machine (model. OW 3101, Moulinex, Groupe Seb Italia Spa, Milan, Italy) was employed. The composition of the functional bread (Salus®) flour and that of the refined flour used for the preparation of the control white bread, are reported on Table 1. The botanical source of the Beta-glucans was oat, as reported by the producers on the label of flour Salus (see Reg. (CE) n. 1924/2006 and Reg. (CE) n. 1160/2011). The mix of ingredients to prepare the functional bread was contained in packs of 500 g containing about 20 g of β-glucan and 200 g of starch.

Table 1. Flour composition of the 'functional' and the 'control' (made with refined wheat white flour) breads.

Expressed per 100 g	Functional Bread	Control Bread
Edible part (%)	100	100
Water (g)	43	29
Protein (g)	12	8.6
Lipid (g)	1.2	0.4
Cholesterol (mg)	n.d.	0
Available carbohydrates (g)	31	66.9
Starch (g)	30.2	59.1
Soluble sugars (g)	0.8	1.9
Solubile fiber (g)	2.3	1.46
as beta-glucan	2.3	0
Insolubile fiber (g)	4.7	1.72
Total fiber (g)	7	3.2
Beta-glucan/starch	7.62	0
Energy (kJ)	827	1209
Energy (kcal)	197	289
Salt (mg)	885	1465
Sodium (mg)	354	586

The carbohydrates unit is expressed as g/100 g of the sum of glucose and starch. In this value, fiber is not included.

Bread baking was carried out using standard conditions for a white bread, as indicated by the manufacturer, as follows. Five hundred grams of the ingredient's mixture and 430 mL of water were added into the bread machine's pan. The bread maker took three hours to bake a loaf of bread. From about 450 g dough, 320–360 g cooked bread are obtained with a moisture percent ranging between 42%–43%. A bread loaf of 100 g contained about 2.3 g of β-glucans.

In order to determine consumer acceptability, a simple 5-point hedonic scale (questionnaire) for each sensorial attribute, was used, where 5 was the highest (i.e., extremely positive) score ('like very much') and 1 the lowest (i.e., extremely negative) ('dislike very much'). Participants were asked to rate odor, taste (salty and sweet), texture (soft and crisp) and general acceptance on the five-point Likert scale [10].

2.4. Outcome

The data of plasma glucose, HbA_1c, lipids, blood pressure, and weight were retrieved from each subject's medical records on the regularly scheduled visits. The methods of analyses were those standardized in the central analysis laboratory of the Padova University Hospital [11]. The post-prandial glucose values refer to measurements taken ~2 h after the meal (breakfast). The mean glucose concentrations resulting from the fasting and the post-prandial values was also calculated.

2.5. Sample Size and Statistical Analysis

By considering the primary end-point, i.e., a relative change of HbA_1c of 0.6% (as absolute units) between the treated vs. the control group, and assuming a population mean of HbA_1c of 8%, and an SD of 10% of the mean, a significant effect ($\alpha = 0.05$, $1 - \beta = 0.80$), would be attained by the sample size here studied.

All data were expressed as means ± standard error (SE). The two-way analysis of variance (ANOVA) for repeated measurements, followed by post-hoc test, was employed, to compare the data of the test group with those of the case-control group. The two tailed Student's *t* test for either paired or unpaired data was employed as appropriate. A *p* value < 0.05 was taken as statistically significant.

3. Results

The basal, pre-treatment clinical data of the patients are reported on Table 2. There was no statistical difference between the treatment and the control groups in any clinical or biochemical parameter. Although there were some differences between the two groups in drug consumption, no subject modified his/her current therapy (including both hypoglycemic agents and other drugs) during the test period, both in the test and in the control group. The subjects allocated to the 'functional bread' group had reported a daily intake of CHO (as bread, breadsticks, cereals or other bread substitutes) of approximately 70 ± 10 g. In the control group, the estimated intake of CHO (starch)-equivalents was similar. From medical records there were no evidence of changes in everyday diet in any of the selected subjects.

Table 2. Clinical characteristics of the type 2 diabetic subjects, included in either the functional bread or the control group. Data are expressed as means $\pm$ SE.

Parameter	Functional Bread Group	Control Bread Group
Number	11	11
Sex (M/F)	4/7	4/7
Age (years)	68.6 ± 1.9	68.0 ± 2.3
Body weight (kg)	72.9 ± 3.6	76.2 ± 4.0
BMI (kg/m^2)	27.8 ± 1.2	27.9 ± 1.3
Months between measurements	6.0 ± 0.5	6.9 ± 0.8
range	4–9	3–11
Therapy:		
Metformin	8	10
Sulphonylureas/Glinides	3	2
Insulin	1	2
Incretins	5	7
Statins	2	8
ACE-I/ARB	2	7
Beta-blockers/Antiadrenergics	4	1
Diuretics	2	4
Aspirin	2	1
Other	7	4

Abbreviations: BMI: Body Mass Index; ACE-I: angiotensin-conversion-enzyme inhibitors; ARB: angiotensin-receptor-blockers.

Following the time point defined as 'start', clinical and biochemical data were retrieved, after 6.0 ± 0.5 months in the 'treatment' group, and after 6.9 ± 0.8 months in the control group (p = NS between the two groups).

In the treatment group, the use of the functional bread resulted in (insignificantly) lower fasting glucose concentrations (by -20.4 ± 16.7 mg/dL, i.e., -1.15 ± 0.92 mmol/L, $p > 0.05$ by paired t test), but in significantly lower postprandial glucose concentrations (by -16.4 ± 6.3 mg/dL, i.e., -0.91 ± 0.35 mmol/L, $p = 0.045$ by paired t test). The resulting average glucose concentrations were reduced by -17.4 ± 8.0 mg/dL (i.e., by -0.97 ± 0.44 mmol/L, $p = 0.08$ by paired t test) (Table 3).

In contrast, in the control group, modest though insignificantly greater fasting (by $+2.8 \pm 9.9$ mg/dL, i.e., $+0.15 \pm 0.55$ mmol/L), post-prandial (by $+29.0 \pm 10.6$ mg/dL, i.e., $+1.6 \pm 0.6$ mmol/L) and mean (by $+12.7 \pm 6.6$ mg/dL, i.e., $+0.71 \pm 0.34$ mmol/L) plasma glucose concentrations were observed. As a result, a significant difference between the two groups was observed (by ANOVA, as interaction effect), as regards both the post-prandial ($p = 0.011$) and the mean ($p = 0.02$) glucose concentrations (Table 3).

Table 3. Hemoglobin A_1c (HbA_1c) (as percent, %), fasting plasma glucose (FPG), post-prandial plasma glucose (PPG) and mean plasma glucose (MPG), in the 'functional bread' and in the 'control' treatment groups, before ('start') and after ('end') the observation periods. Data are expressed as means ± SE.

| | Functional Bread Group | | Control Group | | |
	Start	End	Start	End	*p* Value
HbA_1c (%)	7.97 ± 0.36	7.45 ± 0.31 *	8.03 ± 0.34	8.10 ± 0.31	0.0265
FPG (mmol/L)	9.1 ± 0.8	8.0 ± 0.5	8.7 ± 0.7	8.8 ± 0.5	0.29
PPG (mmol/L)	9.2 ± 0.5	8.4 ± 0.6 *	8.7 ± 0.4	9.9 ± 0.6	0.0113
MPG (mmol/L)	9.2 ± 0.6	8.2 ± 0.4 *	8.5 ± 0.6	9.0 ± 0.5	0.02

* Significant difference between the 'functional bread' and the 'control' groups. The reported *p* values are those resulting from the two-way analysis of variance for repeated measurements, interaction effect.

The HbA_1c values are shown in Figure 1. Between the 'previous' and the 'start' observation time points, no difference between the functional and the control bread groups were observed, both groups showing a slight trend (albeit insignificant) towards worsening of HbA_1c. The observation periods between these two time points were not different between the two groups (treatment group: 6.6 ± 0.6 months; control group: 7.7 ± 1.0 months, $p = 0.34$ between the two).

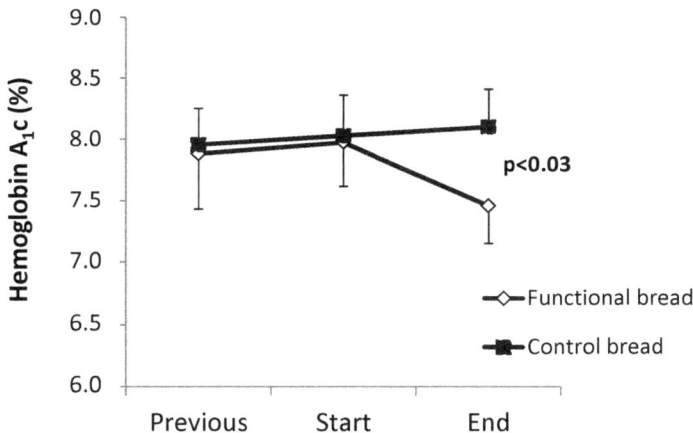

Figure 1. The effect of the functional bread on roughly six-month metabolic control as reflected by HbA_1c. Hemoglobin A_1C values (expressed as percent, mean ± SE) in the seven to eight months before ('previous'), at the beginning ('start') and after six to seven months ('end') of intake of either the functional bread (open symbols) or the control white bread (filled symbols). The data are expressed as mean ± SE. The *p* value in the figure indicates the significant difference in the changes of HbA_1c % values, before and following the intake of between either the functional bread or the control bread (by ANOVA).

Following the 'start' time point, in the group treated with the functional bread, a −0.52% decrease (as absolute value) of HbA_1c levels ($p < 0.028$ by the pair *t* test, Figure 1) was observed. In contrast, in the control group HbA_1c did not change (+0.21% ± 0.13%). As a result, there was a significant difference between the two groups in the post-treatment HbA_1c values ($p = 0.027$ by ANOVA, interaction effect). Again, there was no difference in the duration of the observation periods between the 'start' and the 'end' time points, between the treatments and the control group (Table 2). No significant differences between the two groups were however observed in the other clinical and metabolic parameters (Table 4), such a systolic and diastolic blood pressure, total, low-density lipoprotein (LDL) and high-density lipoprotein (HDL) cholesterol.

Table 4. Body weight, systolic and diastolic blood pressure, and fasting lipid concentrations, in the groups treated with either the 'functional' or the 'control' bread, before ('start') and after ('end') the observation periods. Data are expressed as means ± SE.

Parameter	Functional Bread		Control Bread	
	Start	End	Start	End
Weight (kg)	72.9 ± 3.4	73.9 ± 3.5	77.6 ± 3.3	76.9 ± 3.2
Systolic pressure (mm·Hg)	139.7 ± 5.4	138.6 ± 4.2	137.3 ± 4.9	136.4 ± 6.1
Diastolic pressure (mm·Hg)	75.0 ± 3.4	77.3 ± 3.1	78.6 ± 1.7	79.6 ± 1.9
Total cholesterol (mmol/L)	4.60 ± 0.33	4.55 ± 0.48	4.26 ± 0.16	4.32 ± 0.26
HDL cholesterol (mmol/L)	1.50 ± 0.10	1.46 ± 0.12	1.67 ± 0.08	1.57 ± 0.12
LDL cholesterol (mmol/L)	2.23 ± 0.25	2.36 ± 0.48	2.08 ± 0.15	2.26 ± 0.18
Triglycerides (mmol/L)	1.90 ± 0.29 *	1.60 ± 0.16 *	1.11 ± 0.06	1.08 ± 0.12

* $p < 0.05$ between the 'functional' and the 'control' bread groups (by ANOVA, group effect). Abbreviations: HDL: high-density lipoprotein; LDL: low-density lipoprotein.

Although plasma triglyceride concentrations were greater ($p < 0.015$) in the functional than in the control group at the 'start' time point, they did not significantly change in either group between the start and the end periods. Body weight increased by roughly one kilogram in the treatment group ($p = 0.05$ by paired t test vs. baseline), but it did not significantly change in the controls (though without significance differences between the groups by ANOVA).

The data on consumer acceptability are reported in Supplementary material. The overall response was satisfactory, and positive judgments on texture, odor and general acceptance, were delivered, with ranges between 60% and 80%. In contrast, the responses regarding taste were on the whole 'neutral', as they did not elicit any prevalence between sweet and salty taste. As a matter of fact, the functional bread was well accepted by the subjects who completed the study. The relatively large drop-out rate (9 out of originally enrolled 20 subjects) was due to reasons other than bread acceptability (see Methods). Most subjects really appreciated the functional bread and are still continuing to use it regularly.

4. Discussion

Bread is a staple food, and one of the main sources of carbohydrates and energy worldwide. The diet recommended for a person with diabetes should contain 40%–50% energy as carbohydrates, 15% to 20% as proteins and ~30% as fat. A fiber daily intake of 20–40 g is also suggested [3,12]. Foods with a low glycemic index and/or a low glycemic load would be preferred in diabetes, since they blunt post-prandial hyperglycemia [13,14]. Absolute fiber content [15], type (soluble/insoluble), as well as the presence of active compounds interacting with starch, are important modifiers of carbohydrate digestion and absorption particularly in diabetes. Therefore, the design of a flour containing active ingredients, to be employed for bread preparations, is a 'hot' issue today.

In this study, we report the results of roughly six months' administration of a home-prepared 'functional' bread, made up with a flour enriched with fiber (mainly beta glucan), low in starch and salt, as a substitute for common bread, in subjects with type 2 diabetes in everyday life conditions.

We report that this 'functional bread' significantly improved the metabolic control in the T2DM subjects, as shown by significant reductions of glycated hemoglobin, of post-prandial and mean glucose concentrations. In contrast, both HbA_1c and glucose concentrations did not change in the 'control' bread group (Figure 1 and Table 3). Furthermore, in the six to seven months preceding the observation periods, HbA_1c was nearly stable in both groups (Figure 1). Therefore, these data indicate that the intake of the functional bread was effective in the improvement of metabolic control in type 2 diabetes.

This study was conducted on everyday life conditions, and based on data retrieval of a limited number of patients regularly visited at the diabetes Centre. Although larger prospective, controlled studies would be required to confirm these findings, our data nevertheless suggest that daily intake of a functional bread could be useful in subjects with T2DM. Notably, in this group the percent reduction of HbA_1c (-0.52%, as absolute values) was consistent with the concurrent reduction of mean plasma glucose (-17 mg/dL). Indeed, it is well established that a 'one-point' reduction of % HbA_1c is associated with a reduction of 30–40 mg/dL of mean plasma glucose [16]. In addition, the decrease of HbA_1c values here observed is within the range of changes previously observed after high fiber diets in type 2 diabetes [15].

The efficacy of the functional bread here tested could be due to several, concurring factors. First, as reported in Table 1, the starch content was about half that of the reference, regular bread prepared with refined white wheat flour, on a bread-weight basis. However, no patient reported a *decrease* in bread intake (as grams) with the use of the functional bread. Rather, some of them informed the investigators about a (small) increase in the intake of the functional bread, once they realized that the post-prandial glucose values were improved. Thus, a decrease in the intake (as grams) of the functional bread is very unlikely. Second, the functional bread contained beta glucans, that were absent in the reference bread. Third, the beta glucan/starch ratio in the functional bread was 7.6/100. Such a ratio, although lower than that previously reported to be the optimal value to reduce starch digestion/absorption, could have nevertheless produced a favorable effect [9]. On the other hand, greater ratios than those here tested could further improve post-prandial glucose excursions and the metabolic control in T2DM, should bread palatability be preserved. Fourth, the beta-glucans contained in the functional bread, due to their hydrophilic effect, were probably responsible for its greater water content that, on turn, contributed to bread weight despite the lower starch content. Finally, the total fiber content of the functional bread was nearly double that of the reference bread (Table 1). Therefore, several concurrent variables in the composition of the functional bread could have contributed to its beneficial effects. However, the aim of this study was not to analyze separately the impact of each variable on glucose control in type 2 diabetes. We rather tested the effects of the chosen flour product, available in the supermarket, on glucose control and on sensorial aspects in everyday life conditions.

A high (>40 g/day) dietary fiber intake is usually recommended to subjects with type 2 diabetes [3–12]. However, the fiber effect on medium- as well as on long-term metabolic control in T2DM remains controversial [17,18]. A fiber effect had usually been demonstrated when associated to intake of foods with low glycemic index. On the other hand, a high fiber diet may be difficult to be maintained in the long term, because of its poor palatability [19]. In addition, the large gel volume associated to the intake of fibers such as guar gum, despite their efficacy, is often a hurdle in food consumption. In contrast, using beta glucans, the amount of fiber per serving may be increased without either expanding the volume to be ingested or reducing palatability [20]. In this respect, the peculiar composition of the 'functional flour' here reported may represent an optimal balance between fiber intake, starch reduction, bread 'mass' (i.e., weight), and, last but not least, palatability.

Beta glucans have been reported to improve satiety and to decrease caloric intake and appetite [21]. These effects are likely driven by an increased viscosity [22], a delay in CHO absorption [23], and a 'bulking action' [24]. Beta glucans have also been reported to improve glucose and insulin responses [20]. In addition, the consumption of three grams per day of oat or barley beta-glucans daily was sufficient to decrease blood cholesterol levels [25]. Since beta-glucans reduce the rapidly-digestible starch (RDS) fraction, while increasing that of slowly digestibly starch (SDS) [8], these combined effects would result in a relative increase of resistant starch (RS). However, the beta-glucan-associated reduction of starch digestion rate may also be product- and process-dependent [26]. As a matter of fact, the relationships among beta glucan to starch ratio, starch gelatinization and solubility, and RS formation, are quite complex. At beta glucan to starch ratios below 2 [9], starch solubility was lower at the 1.6/10 than at the 1.1/10 ratio, leading to higher RS and lower SDS values. Our beta-glucan to starch ratio of 0.76/10 probably lead to some increase, although not maximal, of the SDS fraction.

Conversely, others reported that a beta glucan to starch ratio of 0.5/10 ratio nevertheless resulted in a significant reduction in starch gelatinization and in its breakdown rate evaluated in vitro [27]. Further research need to be carried out to elucidate these difficult issues.

An association between beta glucan-induced decrease of post-prandial insulin levels, increase satiety and decrease caloric intake, with increase of cholecystokinin, has also been suggested [28]. In our study, neither cholecystokinin nor insulin were measured. Therefore, no conclusions on possible relationships between changes in these two hormones and the observed effects, can be drawn.

Body weight was not significantly different between the two groups (an analyzed by ANOVA). However, a one kilogram positive change in the treatment group was observed ($p = 0.05$ vs. basal value), whereas weight did not change at all in the control groups. As an explanation of such an unexpected finding, as reported above, some subjects of the treatment group admittedly reported that they had increased the bread intake because they realized that their plasma glucose values were improving, as well as because an increased sense of hunger. Nevertheless, the functional bread was capable to improve the metabolic control, thus independently from any major body weight change. It should also be considered that the raw amount and the energy intake of the diet was generally reported to be unchanged in either group.

At variance with the improvement of the glycemic control, other clinical and biochemical parameters, such systolic and diastolic blood pressure, total, LDL, and HDL cholesterol, were unchanged by the functional bread intake, being rather stable in both groups. Lack of any effect of blood pressure might be due to the hypotensive treatment of most of our subjects (Table 2). Conversely, despite the reported hypocholesterolemic effects of beta glucan [25,29], in our study lack of any change in cholesterol could be due to the already near-normal values of our subjects, of total as well as LDL cholesterol, (also in respect to target values) (Table 2). Nevertheless, the hypolipidemic effects of beta glucans t in medium-term studies (four weeks) are controversial [29].

Since high-fiber products may decrease palatability [19], our subjects were accurately tested for sensorial responses. The overall response to the functional bread was however satisfactory, with positive judgments on texture, odor and general acceptance recorded in >50% of the subjects, and a virtually neutral response regarding taste (see Table S1 in the Supplementary material). In this regard, other authors [30,31] reported that beta-glucan inclusion improves both the rheological and the sensory properties of bread.

Although there were some differences in the pharmacological therapy (other than the hypoglycemic agents) between the two groups, with a lower use of statins and ACE-I/ARB, and increased consumption of beta-blockers, in the functional bread group, these differences likely did not affect the results, since no subject modified drug therapy throughout the study. Although statins have been reported to exhibit deleterious effects on plasma glucose [32], plasma glucose was actually unchanged in the control group. Furthermore, the control subjects as well as those of the functional group were on long term therapy with statins. Therefore, statins use per se should not represent a bias in this study.

5. Conclusions

In conclusion, regular intake of a low-starch functional bread, enriched with beta glucan fibers, could improve the medium- to long-term glycemic control in type 2 diabetes mellitus in addition to the drugs used to control of blood glucose.

Supplementary Materials: The following are available online at http://www.mdpi.com/2072-6643/9/3/297/s1.

Acknowledgments: This study was supported by Institutional Grants of the University of Padova (DOR grants) and by a non conditioned grant from the 'Granaio delle Idee'-Maserà di Padova, Italy.

Author Contributions: P.T. designed the study along with A.L., searched for the clinical and biochemical data in the databases, analyzed the results and wrote the paper. A.L. addressed the technological issues of the functional bread, cooperated in the calculation of the results and co-wrote and reviewed the paper.

Conflicts of Interest: The authors declare no conflict of interest.

Abbreviations

The following abbreviations are used in this manuscript:

CHO   carbohydrates
BMI   Body Mass Index
T2DM   Type 2 Diabetes Mellitus
HbA$_1$c   glycated hemoglobin
CV   cardiovascular
GI   Glycemic Index
ACE-I   angiotensin converting enzyme inhibitors
ARB   angiotensin receptors blockers

References

1. International Diabetes Federation. *IDF Diabetes Atlas*, 7th ed.; International Diabetes Federation: Brussels, Belgium, 2015.
2. Pereira, M.A.; Kartashov, A.I.; Ebbeling, C.B.; van Horn, L.; Slattery, M.L.; Jacobs, D.R., Jr.; Ludwig, D.S.; Jacobs, D.R. Fast-food habits, weight gain, and insulin resistance (the CARDIA study): 15-year prospective analysis. *Lancet* **2005**, *365*, 36–42. [CrossRef]
3. AMD-SID. Standard Italiani per la Cura del Diabete Mellito 2014. Available online: http://www.standarditaliani.it (accessed on 11 November 2016).
4. Reaven, G.M. Insulin resistance, the insulin resistance syndrome, and cardiovascular disease. *Panminerva Med.* **2005**, *47*, 201–210. [PubMed]
5. Pawar, K.; Thompkinson, D.K. Multiple functional ingredient approach in formulating dietary supplement for management of diabetes: A review. *Crit. Rev. Food Sci. Nutr.* **2014**, *54*, 957–973. [CrossRef] [PubMed]
6. Zarich, S.W. Cardiovascular risk factors in the metabolic syndrome: Impact of insulin resistance on lipids, hypertension, and the development of diabetes and cardiac events. *Rev. Cardiovasc. Med.* **2005**, *6*, 194–205. [PubMed]
7. Grajek, W.; Olejnik, A.; Sip, A. Probiotics, prebiotics and antioxidants as functional foods. *Acta Biochim. Pol.* **2005**, *52*, 665–671. [PubMed]
8. Regand, A.; Tosh, S.M.; Wolever, T.M.; Wood, P.J. Physicochemical properties of beta-glucan in differently processed oat foods influence glycemic response. *J. Agric. Food Chem.* **2009**, *57*, 8831–8838. [CrossRef] [PubMed]
9. Regand, A.; Chowdhury, Z.; Tosh, S.M.; Wolever, T.M.S.; Wood, P. The molecular weight solubility and viscosity of oat beta-glucan affect human glycemic response by modifying starch digestibility. *Food Chem.* **2011**, *129*, 297–304. [CrossRef]
10. Lawless, H.T.; Heymann, H. *Sensory Evaluation of Food: Principles and Practices*; Chapman & Hall: New York, NY, USA, 1998; pp. 341–372.
11. Graziani, M.S.; Ceriotti, F.; Zaninotto, M.; Catapano, A.L.; Medea, G.; Parretti, D.; Gulizia, M.; Averna, M.; Ciaccio, M. La diagnostica di laboratorio delle dislipidemie. Documento di consenso SIBIoC, SISA, SIMG, ANMCO. *Biochim. Clin.* **2014**, *40*, 338–346.
12. Evert, A.B.; Boucher, J.L.; Cypress, M.; Dunbar, S.A.; Franz, M.J.; Mayer-Davis, E.J.; Neumiller, J.J.; Urbanski, P.; Verdi, C.L.; Nwankwo, R. American Diabetes Association. Nutrition therapy recommendations for the management of adults with diabetes. *Diabetes Care* **2013**, *36*, 3821–3842. [CrossRef] [PubMed]
13. Augustin, L.S.; Kendall, C.W.; Jenkins, D.J.; Willett, W.C.; Astrup, A.; Barclay, A.W.; Björck, I.; Brand-Miller, J.C.; Brighenti, F.; Buyken, A.E.; et al. Glycemic index, glycemic load and glycemic response: An International Scientific Consensus Summit from the International Carbohydrate Quality Consortium (ICQC). *Nutr. Metab. Cardiovasc.* **2015**, *25*, 795–815. [CrossRef] [PubMed]
14. Riccardi, G.; Rivellese, A.A.; Giacco, R. Role of glycemic index and glycemic load in the healthy state, in prediabetes, and in diabetes. *Am. J. Clin. Nutr.* **2008**, *87*, 269S–274S. [PubMed]
15. Silva, F.M.; Kramer, C.K.; de Almeida, J.C.; Steemburgo, T.; Gross, J.L.; Azevedo, M.J. Fiber intake and glycemic control in patients with type 2 diabetes mellitus: A systematic review with meta-analysis of randomized controlled trials. *Nutr. Rev.* **2013**, *71*, 790–801. [CrossRef] [PubMed]

16. Rohlfing, C.L.; Wiedmeyer, H.M.; Little, R.R.; England, J.D.; Tennill, A.; Goldstein, D.E. Defining the relationship between plasma glucose and HbA(1c): Analysis of glucose profiles and HbA(1c) in the Diabetes Control and Complications Trial. *Diabetes Care* **2002**, *25*, 275–278. [CrossRef] [PubMed]

17. Beattie, V.A.; Edwards, C.A.; Hosker, J.P.; Cullen, D.R.; Ward, J.D.; Read, N.W. Does adding fiber to a low energy, high carbohydrate, low fat diet confer any benefit to the management of newly diagnosed overweight type II diabetics? *Br. Med. J. (Clin. Res. Ed.)* **1988**, *296*, 1147–1149. [CrossRef]

18. Scott, A.R.; Attenborough, Y.; Peacock, I.; Fletcher, E.; Jeffcoate, W.J.; Tattersall, R.B. Comparison of high fibre diets, basal insulin supplements, and flexible insulin treatment for non-insulin dependent (type II) diabetics poorly controlled with sulphonylureas. *BMJ* **1988**, *297*, 707–710. [CrossRef] [PubMed]

19. Wood, P.J. Cereal beta-glucans in diet and health. *J. Cereal Sci.* **2007**, *46*, 230–238. [CrossRef]

20. Jenkins, A.L.; Jenkins, D.J.; Zdravkovic, U.; Würsch, P.; Vuksan, V. Depression of the glycemic index by high levels of beta-glucan fiber in two functional foods tested in type 2 diabetes. *Eur. J. Clin. Nutr.* **2002**, *56*, 622–628. [CrossRef] [PubMed]

21. Rebello, C.J.; O'Neil, C.E.; Greenway, F.L. Dietary fiber and satiety: The effects of oats on satiety. *Nutr. Rev.* **2016**, *74*, 131–147. [CrossRef] [PubMed]

22. Dikeman, C.L.; Fahey, G.C. Viscosity as related to dietary fiber: A review. *Crit. Rev. Food Sci. Nutr.* **2006**, *46*, 649–663. [CrossRef] [PubMed]

23. Battilana, P.; Ornstein, K.; Minehira, K.; Schwarz, J.M.; Acheson, K.; Schneiter, P.L.; Burri, J.; Jequier, E.; Tappy, L. Mechanism of action of beta-glucan in postprandial glucose metabolism in healthy men. *Eur. J. Clin. Nutr.* **2001**, *55*, 327–333. [CrossRef] [PubMed]

24. Burton-Freeman, B. Dietary fibre and energy regulation. *J. Nutr.* **2000**, *130*, 272S–275S. [PubMed]

25. Tiwari, U.; Cummins, E. Meta-analysis of the effect of beta-glucan intake on blood cholesterol and glucose levels. *Nutrition* **2011**, *27*, 1008–1016. [CrossRef] [PubMed]

26. Brennan, C.S. Dietary fibre, glycaemic response, and diabetes. *Mol. Nutr. Food Res.* **2005**, *49*, 560–570. [CrossRef] [PubMed]

27. Symons, L.J.; Brennan, C.S. The effect of barley beta-glucan fiber fractions on starch gelatinization and pasting characteristics. *J. Food Sci.* **2004**, *69*, FCT257–FCT261.

28. Beck, E.J.; Tosh, S.M.; Batterham, M.J.; Tapsell, L.C.; Huang, X.F. Oat beta-glucan increases postprandial cholecystokinin levels, decreases insulin response and extends subjective satiety in overweight subjects. *Mol. Nutr. Food Res.* **2009**, *53*, 1343–1351. [CrossRef] [PubMed]

29. Zhou, X.; Lin, W.; Tong, L.; Liu, X.; Zhong, K.; Wang, L.; Zhou, S. Hypolipidaemic effects of oat flakes and β-glucans derived from four Chinese naked oat (*Avena nuda*) cultivars in Wistar-Lewis rats. *J. Sci. Food Agric.* **2016**, *96*, 644–649. [CrossRef] [PubMed]

30. Flander, L.; Salmenkallio-Marttila, M.; Suortti, T.; Autio, K. Optimization of ingredients and baking process for improved wholemeal oatbread quality. *LWT* **2007**, *40*, 860–870. [CrossRef]

31. Skendi, A.; Biliaderis, C.G.; Papageorgiou, M.; Izydorczyk, M.S. Effects of two barley beta-glucan isolates on wheat flour dough and bread properties. *Food Chem.* **2010**, *119*, 1159–1167. [CrossRef]

32. Erqou, S.; Lee, C.C.; Adler, A.I. Statins and glycaemic control in individuals with diabetes: A systematic review and meta-analysis. *Diabetologia* **2014**, *57*, 2444–2452. [CrossRef] [PubMed]

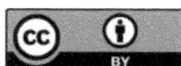

nutrients

MDPI

Article

The Association between Vitamin D Deficiency and Diabetic Retinopathy in Type 2 Diabetes: A Meta-Analysis of Observational Studies

Bang-An Luo [1], Fan Gao [2] and Lu-Lu Qin [2,3,*]

[1] Department of Mental Health, Brain Hospital of Hunan Province, Changsha 410007, Hunan, China; luo276@126.com
[2] Department of Social Medicine and Health Management, Xiangya School of Public Health, Central South University, Changsha 410078, Hunan, China; gfydsl@163.com
[3] Department of Prevention Medicine, Medical School, Hunan University of Chinese Medicine, Changsha 410208, Hunan, China
* Correspondence: powerestlulu@163.com; Tel.: +86-731-8845-9423

Received: 22 January 2017; Accepted: 15 March 2017; Published: 20 March 2017

Abstract: Emerging evidence from in vivo and in vitro studies have shown that vitamin D may play an important role in the development of diabetic retinopathy (DR), but individually published studies showed inconclusive results. The aim of this study was to quantitatively summarize the association between vitamin D and the risk of diabetic retinopathy. We conducted a systematic literature search of Pubmed, Medline, and EMBASE updated in September 2016 with the following keywords: "vitamin D" or "cholecalciferol" or "25-hydroxyvitamin D" or "25(OH)D" in combination with "diabetic retinopathy" or "DR". Fifteen observational studies involving 17,664 subjects were included. In this meta-analysis, type 2 diabetes patients with vitamin D deficiency (serum 25(OH)D levels <20 ng/mL) experienced a significantly increased risk of DR (odds ratio (OR) = 2.03, 95% confidence intervals (CI): 1.07, 3.86), and an obvious decrease of 1.7 ng/mL (95% CI: −2.72, −0.66) in serum vitamin D was demonstrated in the patients with diabetic retinopathy. Sensitivity analysis showed that exclusion of any single study did not materially alter the overall combined effect. In conclusion, the evidence from this meta-analysis indicates an association between vitamin D deficiency and an increased risk of diabetic retinopathy in type 2 diabetes patients.

Keywords: vitamin D; diabetic retinopathy; type 2 diabetes; meta-analysis

1. Introduction

Diabetes mellitus (DM) is a large public health problem which affects more than 300 million individuals in the world, with significant morbidity and mortality worldwide [1]. In addition to the deleterious effects of the disease itself, its long-term complications can conspicuously decrease the quality of life of diabetes patients. Diabetes patients with uncontrolled or poorly-controlled blood glucose are at high risk of microvascular complications. Diabetic retinopathy (DR) is among the most common diabetic complications, and is the leading cause of blindness among working-aged individuals worldwide [2]. The prevalence of DR varies from 20% to 80% in different studies. Recent estimates suggest that the number of people with diabetic retinopathy will increase to 191 million by 2030 [3]. Diabetic retinopathy has a complex process. Many risk factors for DR have been established, such as poor glycemic control, long duration of diabetes, smoking, inflammation, obesity, and hypertension. Stratton et al. have given evidence that poor glycemic control and long duration of diabetes are independent risk factors of DR [4]. Praidou et al. found that increased physical activity is associated with less severe levels of DR, independent of the effects of HbA1c and body mass index (BMI) [5]. However, detailed pathophysiological mechanisms and other DR risk factors are not fully clarified.

Vitamin D is a multi-functional fat-solute metabolite required for humans' growth and development. Vitamin D deficiency (VDD) is seen across all ages, races, and geographic regions. Due to the wide functionality of vitamin D and because vitamin D deficiency is epidemic, vitamin D's non-classical functions are gaining more attention for the close association between vitamin D deficiency and cancers, infectious diseases, autoimmune diseases, diabetes, and diabetic complications [6–8]. The prevalence of vitamin D deficiency is high in type 2 diabetes mellitus (T2DM) patients [9–11]. Vitamin D receptors are expressed extensively in the retina [12], and an animal study showed that calcitriol was a potent inhibitor of retinal neovascularization in an oxygen-induced ischemic retinopathy mouse model [13]. This evidence indicated that vitamin D may play a role in the pathogensis of diabetic retinopathy.

While there are accumulating studies on the effect of vitamin D on diabetic retinopathy, the association between vitamin D and diabetic retinopathy are conflicting. According to some studies, vitamin D deficiency is associated with an increasing risk of diabetic retinopathy. Patrick et al. found an association between serum 25-hydroxyvitamin D concentration and diabetic retinopathy in a cohort of 1790 type 2 diabetes patients [14]. Inukai et al. reported that serum 25-hydroxyvitamin D (25(OH)D) levels were decreased in type 2 patients with retinopathy when compared with type 2 patients who had no microangiopathy [15]. However, others suggested that no significant differences in vitamin D status were found between type 2 diabetes with or without diabetic retinopathy. Alam et al. found no association between serum 25(OH)D levels and the presence and the severity of diabetic retinopathy [16].

Currently, there is insufficient evidence showing whether serum vitamin D deficiency is related to diabetic retinopathy, and the determination of this relationship has rarely been conducted. To address these issues, we carried out this meta-analysis by pooling the results from observation studies to examine the potential association between vitamin D and diabetic retinopathy.

2. Methods

2.1. Data Sources

Relevant articles were identified by a systematic literature search of Pubmed, Medline, and EMBASE through September 2016, using the following keywords: "vitamin D" or "cholecalciferol" or "25-hydroxyvitamin D" or "25(OH)D" in combination with "diabetic retinopathy" or "retinopathy" or "DR". Additionally, we manually searched all eligible original articles, reviews, and other relevant articles. This meta-analysis was performed following the guidelines for observation study protocols (Meta-analysis Of Observational Studies in Epidemiology (MOOSE) guidelines) [17].

2.2. Study Selection

Original articles evaluating the relationship between serum vitamin D status and diabetic retinopathy were reviewed and selected if they met the following inclusion criteria: (a) the study population was type 2 diabetes patients; (b) DR was the outcome, and the control group consisted of type 2 diabetes patients without DR; (c) the study presented sample sizes and odds ratios (OR) with 95% confidence intervals (CI) or information that could be used to infer these results; (d) vitamin D deficiency was defined as a 25(OH)D level below 20 ng/mL, and vitamin D insufficiency was defined as 25(OH)D levels of 21–29 ng/mL; (e) the study was published in English; and (f) the study met the predefined methodological quality assessment criteria for observational studies (Supplementary Data Box 1). Animal experiments, chemistry, or cell-line studies and editorials, commentaries, review articles, and case reports were excluded. Other exclusion criteria consisted of studies with a score of 0 for any item or a total score <7 out of 10 maximal points [18].

Two independent reviewers (Bang-An Luo and Fan Gao) reviewed all the literature searches and acquired full-length articles for all citations meeting the predefined selection criteria. Final inclusion or exclusion decisions were made after reading the full text. We resolved any disagreements through consensus or arbitration by a third reviewer (Lu-Lu Qin).

The following information was extracted from each article: the last name of first author, publication year, location of study, study design, sample size, 25(OH)D assay methods, 25(OH)D concentration, and the prevalence of vitamin D deficiency. In the case of relevant missing data, contacts were made to the main authors for more information.

2.3. Statistical Analysis

We performed this meta-analysis with RevMan Software (Version 5.2, Cochrane Collaboration, London, UK). The odds ratio (OR) and weight mean difference (WMD) were used as measures of associations between vitamin D status and risk for DR. If the OR and 95% CI were not available for the meta-analysis, these data were extracted from the selected articles to construct 2 × 2 tables of serum low vitamin D status versus the presence or absence of diabetic retinopathy.

We used forest plots to visually assess pooled estimates and corresponding 95% CIs for each study. The heterogeneity among the results of the included studies was evaluated with I^2 statistical tests. The percentage of $I^2 < 25$, near 50, and >75 indicated low, moderate, and high heterogeneity, respectively. A fixed-effects model or a random-effects model was used to combine the study results according to the heterogeneity. Once the effects were found to be heterogeneous ($I^2 > 50\%$), a random effects model was used. Otherwise, a fixed effect model was used.

Potential publication bias was assessed using the funnel plots. A sensitivity analysis was conducted to test the robustness of results, as well as to investigate the effect of a single article on the overall risk estimated by removing one article in each turn. Additionally, a subgroup analysis was performed to explore the possible explanations for heterogeneity. All the *p*-values were for a two-tailed and $p < 0.05$ was considered as statistically significant.

3. Results

3.1. Search Results

Of the 238 articles identified from our initial search, a total of 15 studies were finally identified as eligible for inclusion in this meta-analysis through a strict screening process (Figure 1). The quality assessment showed that the quality scores of these studies ranged from 8.5 to 10 according to the MOOSE guidelines, which indicates that all of the selected studies were of high quality (Supplementary Table S1).

3.2. Characteristics of the Included Studies

The characteristics of these articles in this meta-analysis are summarized in Table 1. These studies were published from 2000 to 2016. Among these studies, nine were conducted in Asia, two each in North America and Europe, one in Africa, and one each in three countries (Australia, New Zealand, and Finland). Seven studies had cross-sectional design, five were case–control, two were prospective cohort, and one had a retrospective cohort design. Four different assay techniques were used to measure the serum 25(OH)D levels, and four different ways were used to diagnose DR. Eight of the included studies explored the association between vitamin D deficiency and diabetic retinopathy, four explored the association between vitamin D insufficiency and diabetic retinopathy, and ten explored the mean difference in vitamin D status among diabetic retinopathy and non-diabetic retinopathy.

The diversity of participant characteristics was considerable in these studies. Out of 17,664 participants, 3455 (19.6%) were diagnosed with diabetic retinopathy, consisting of different ages and races. In addition, the age of type 2 diabetes participants were older than 18 years and the mean BMI—if provided by articles—varied from 13.9 to 42.0 kg/m². The vitamin D status of diabetic retinopathy ranged from 9.2 to 32.6 ng/mL.

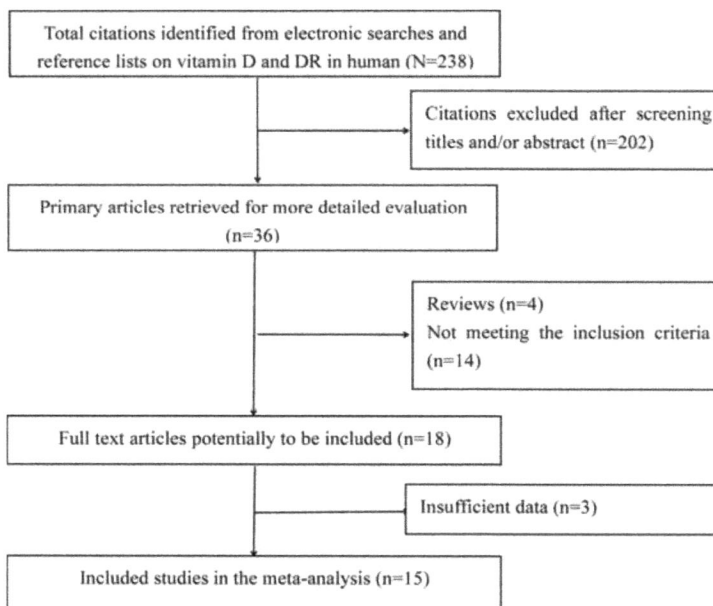

Figure 1. Flow chart of literature search and study selection.

3.3. Main Analysis

The relationship between serum vitamin D deficiency (VDD) and the risk of diabetic retinopathy is shown in Figure 2 and Supplementary Table S2. Eight studies involving 13,435 participants were included. As the results of this meta-analysis show, type 2 diabetes with vitamin D deficiency (serum 25(OH)D levels <20 ng/mL) had an increased risk of developing diabetic retinopathy (OR = 2.03, 95% CI: 1.07, 3.86) in the random-effects model.

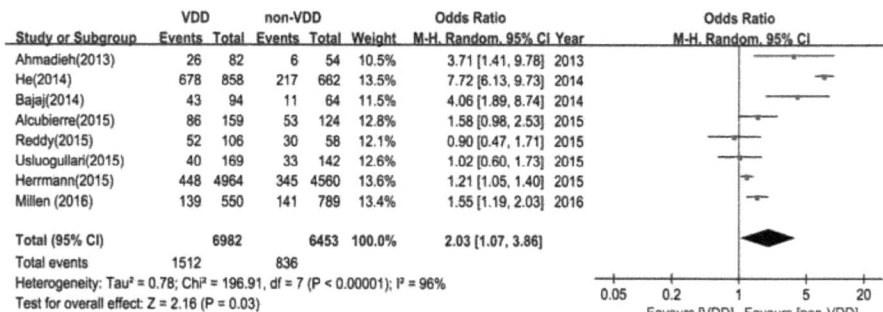

Figure 2. The meta-analysis of the association between vitamin D deficiency (VDD) and diabetic retinopathy (DR).

Based on four studies, the pooled OR for vitamin D insufficiency (VDI, serum 25(OH)D levels <30 ng/mL) was calculated as (OR = 0.89, 95% CI: 0.20, 4.02) (Supplementary Table S2 and Supplementary Figure S1). Only the result of vitamin D deficiency showed that low serum vitamin D status increased the risk of diabetic retinopathy.

The comparison of the mean difference between the DR group and the control group (non-DR group) is shown in Figure 3. From the results of the random-effects model, the pooled effect was -1.7 ng/mL (95% CI: -2.75, -0.66) and significant heterogeneity was observed ($I^2 = 80\%$, $p < 0.001$). It showed that serum 25(OH)D levels were significantly lower in diabetic retinopathy patients than the control in type 2 diabetes. This result demonstrated that vitamin D deficiency is significantly related with an increased risk of DR.

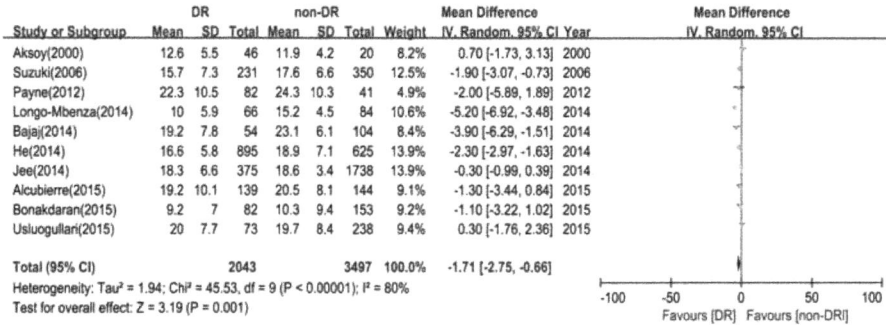

Study or Subgroup	DR Mean	SD	Total	non-DR Mean	SD	Total	Weight	Mean Difference IV, Random, 95% CI	Year
Aksoy(2000)	12.6	5.5	46	11.9	4.2	20	8.2%	0.70 [-1.73, 3.13]	2000
Suzuki(2006)	15.7	7.3	231	17.6	6.6	350	12.5%	-1.90 [-3.07, -0.73]	2006
Payne(2012)	22.3	10.5	82	24.3	10.3	41	4.9%	-2.00 [-5.89, 1.89]	2012
Longo-Mbenza(2014)	10	5.9	66	15.2	4.5	84	10.6%	-5.20 [-6.92, -3.48]	2014
Bajaj(2014)	19.2	7.8	54	23.1	6.1	104	8.4%	-3.90 [-6.29, -1.51]	2014
He(2014)	16.6	5.8	895	18.9	7.1	625	13.9%	-2.30 [-2.97, -1.63]	2014
Jee(2014)	18.3	6.6	375	18.6	3.4	1738	13.9%	-0.30 [-0.99, 0.39]	2014
Alcubierre(2015)	19.2	10.1	139	20.5	8.1	144	9.1%	-1.30 [-3.44, 0.84]	2015
Bonakdaran(2015)	9.2	7	82	10.3	9.4	153	9.2%	-1.10 [-3.22, 1.02]	2015
Usluogullari(2015)	20	7.7	73	19.7	8.4	238	9.4%	0.30 [-1.76, 2.36]	2015
Total (95% CI)			**2043**			**3497**	**100.0%**	**-1.71 [-2.75, -0.66]**	

Heterogeneity: Tau² = 1.94; Chi² = 45.53, df = 9 (P < 0.00001); I² = 80%
Test for overall effect: Z = 3.19 (P = 0.001)

Favours [DR]   Favours [non-DR]

Figure 3. Meta-analysis of the association between 25-hydroxyvitamin D (25(OH)D) levels and DR.

Table 1. Characteristics of observational studies included in this meta-analysis.

Author and Year	Country	Study Design	Sample Size (n)	VD Assay Method	DR Diagnosis	VDD Prevalence (%) DR	VDD Prevalence (%) NDR	Mean 25(OH)D ng/mL (SD) DR	Mean 25(OH)D ng/mL (SD) NDR	Significant	Adjustment
Aksoy (2000) [19]	Turkey	Cross-sectional	66	RIA	Ophthalmologists	NA	NA	12.6 ± 5.5	11.9 ± 4.2	Yes	No
Suzuki (2006) [20]	Japan	Case-control	581	RIA	Ophthalmologists	NA	NA	15.7 ± 7.3	17.6 ± 6.6	Yes	Age, BMI, duration, HbA1c, treatment
Payne (2012) [21]	US	Cross-sectional	123	CL	Ophthalmologists	NA	NA	22.3 ± 10.5	24.3 ± 10.3	Yes	Multivitamin use
Ahmadieh (2013) [22]	Lebanon	Cross-sectional	136	RIA	Ophthalmologists	78.8	53.8	NA	NA	Yes	BMI, duration, smoking
Bajaj (2014) [23]	Indian	Case-control	158	NA	Ophthalmologists	79.6	49.0	NA	NA	Yes	No
He (2014) [24]	China	Cross-sectional	1520	CL	The International Clinical DR Severity Scale	75.7	63.6	16.6 ± 5.8	18.9 ± 7.1	Yes	Age, sex, duration
Jee (2014) [25]	Korea	Cross-sectional	2113	RIA	The Early Treatment Diabetic Retinopathy Study severity scale	NA	NA	18.3 ± 6.6	18.7 ± 3.4	Yes	Sex
Longo-Mbenza (2014) [26]	Congo	Case-control	150	HPLC	The modified Airlie House classification system	NA	NA	10 ± 5.9	15.2 ± 4.5	Yes	No
Alcubierre (2015) [27]	Spain	Case-control	283	CL	Ophthalmologists	61.9	50.7	19.2 ± 10.1	20.5 ± 8.1	Yes	Race, season, physical activity
Bonakdaran (2015) [10]	Iran	Cross-sectional	235	RIA	Ophthalmologists	NA	NA	9.2 ± 7.0	10.3 ± 9.4	No	Age, sex, duration, BMI, HbA1c, BMI, sex, HbA1c
Herrmann (2015) [28]	Australia, New Zealand, and Finland	Prospective	9524	CL	Ophthalmologists	56.5	51.7	NA	NA	Yes	Age, sex, et al. *
Reddy (2015) [29]	Indian	Case-control	164	HPLC	The modified Airlie House classification system	27.0	23.0	NA	NA	No	Duration
Ustuogullari (2015) [30]	Turkey	Retrospective	557	HPLC	Ophthalmologists	45.2	54.2	20.0 ± 7.7	19.7 ± 8.4	No	Age, BMI, sex, HbA1c
Zoppini (2015) [31]	Italy	Cross-sectional	715	CL	Ophthalmologists	NA	NA	NA	NA	Yes	Age
Millen (2016) [32]	US	Prospective	1339	LC-MS	The modified Airlie House classification system	49.6	38.8	NA	NA	Yes	Race, duration, HbA1c, hypertension

DR: diabetic retinopathy; VD: vitamin D; VDD: vitamin D deficiency; NDR: no diabetic retinopathy; NA: not available. CL: chemiluminescence; HPLC: high performance liquid chromatography; RIA: radioimmunoassay; LC-MS: high-sensitivity mass spectrometry; SD: standard deviation; et al. *: diabetes duration, HbA 1c; systolic blood pressure, BMI, lipids (triglycerides and high-density lipoprotein (HDL) and low-density lipoprotein (LDL) cholesterol), smoking, baseline use of oral hypoglycemic agents, and baseline use of insulin.

3.4. Sensitivity and Subgroup Analysis

To explore the impact of various exclusion criteria on the overall risk estimate, we conducted sensitivity and subgroup analyses to examine the potential sources of heterogeneity in this meta-analysis. In the result of the pooled ORs, the study conducted in China [24] was responsible for most of the heterogeneity in this meta-analysis. After excluding this study, the heterogeneity was down to 67% and the pooled OR was 1.50 (95% CI: 1.41, 1.98). Besides, there were no obvious changes in the pooled ORs as a result of the exclusion of any other single study. In the comparison of the mean difference between the DR group and the control group, moderate heterogeneity ($I^2 = 70\%$, $p < 0.001$) was observed among the remaining studies after the exclusion Jee's study [25]. Jee's study was responsible for most of the heterogeneity. Further exclusion of any single study did not alter the overall combined relative risk, with a range from −2.2 ng/mL (−3.28, −1.17) to −1.6 ng/mL (−2.43, −0.69), and each outcome had statistical significance.

In the subgroup with study design, there were moderate heterogeneities in cross-sectional and prospective cohort studies for the pooled OR ($I^2 = 52\%$, $p = 0.15$ for cross-sectional studies; $I^2 = 61\%$, $p = 0.11$ for prospective cohort studies) (Supplementary Materials Figure S2). We found that there were obvious heterogeneities in the cross-sectional and the case–control studies for the pooled WMD ($I^2 = 79\%$, $p = 0.0007$ for cross-sectional studies; $I^2 = 76\%$, $p = 0.006$ for case–control studies) (Supplementary Materials Figure S3). In the subgroup with VD assay methods, there were high heterogeneities in the chemiluminescence (CL) vitamin D assay method for the pooled OR ($I^2 = 99\%$, $p < 0.0001$), and the study conducted in China [24] was responsible for the heterogeneities. After excluding this study, the heterogeneity in the CL subgroup was down to 8% and the pooled OR was 1.25 (95% CI: 1.06, 1.48) (Supplementary Materials Figure S4). In the subgroup with DR diagnosis, there were modern heterogeneities in the ophthalmologists group (OR = 1.71, 95% CI: 1.11, 2.62, $I^2 = 74\%$, $p = 0.0004$) (Supplementary Materials Figure S5). Subgroup analyses of BMI, season, duration of diabetes, race, and age were not conducted due to insufficient data in some studies.

3.5. Publication Bias

No obvious publication bias was observed in the funnel plots of this meta-analysis (Supplementary Materials Figure S6).

4. Discussion

Vitamin D's non-classical functions have attracted much public health attention for its closer association with some diseases. This is the first meta-analysis of the relationship between serum vitamin D status and DR in type 2 diabetes. In this meta-analysis, the results of 15 observational studies provided strong evidence that serum 25(OH)D levels were associated with an increased risk of DR in type 2 diabetes patients. Both the results of the pooled OR for vitamin D deficiency (serum 25(OH)D levels <20 ng/mL) and the pooled effect of WMD showed that the serum 25(OH)D levels in type 2 diabetes had a relationship with DR, while the pooled OR for vitamin D insufficiency (serum 25(OH)D levels <30 ng/mL) did not. Considering the results of vitamin D deficiency and that serum 25(OH)D levels were more reliable and accurate than the result of vitamin D insufficiency (only four studies), we concluded that low 25(OH)D levels were associated with an increased risk of DR.

The quality of the studies included in this meta-analysis was high. From the funnel plots, we concluded that there was no obvious publication bias in this meta-analysis. We further conducted sensitivity and subgroup analyses to explore potential sources of heterogeneity. From the forest plots, we observed high heterogeneity among the pooled OR and WMD as the association of DR (Figures 2 and 3), which was not surprising given the different characteristics of participants and adjustments for confounding factors. Regarding the results of sensitivity analyses, two studies probably contributed to the heterogeneity [24,25]. After excluding the two studies, there was moderate heterogeneity, and there may be other factors contributing to the heterogeneity in this study. Firstly, there was no consensus on the levels of vitamin D denoting deficiency and insufficiency, and the diagnosis standards of DR might not be uniform among different ophthalmologists in these studies. Secondly, there were four methods for measuring vitamin D, such as HPLC (high performance liquid chromatography) and RIA (radioimmunoassay). Thirdly, the time of collecting blood sample were different. Fourthly, the heterogeneity might be a result of differences in the study populations—there were several races included in this meta-analysis. Fifthly, the duration of diabetes, the age of patients, the diet, the treatment of diabetes, and the sunlight exposure are confounding factors in this meta-analysis. Hence, more studies are needed to give full proof.

There is an epidemic of vitamin D deficiency around the world [6]. From this meta-analysis, the prevalence of vitamin D deficiency was high among type 2 diabetes patients, although it may vary from different latitude, ethnicity, body mass index, season, and supplementation of vitamin D. VDD was consistent with previous studies [9–11]. For patients with diabetes, the association with vitamin D deficiency and risk of developing diabetes has been acknowledged. Vitamin D deficiency is associated with an increased risk for diabetes [9,22,29].

In patients with diabetic retinopathy, the level of serum 25(OH)D was lower than patients without diabetic retinopathy. The characteristic feature of diabetic retinopathy is the appearance of vascular lesions of increasing severity, ending up in the growth of new vessels (neovascularization). Vitamin D has anti-inflammation properties and inhibits vascular smooth muscle cell growth and effects on the expression of transforming growth factor $\beta1$ [13,33–35]. Vitamin D is an important regulator of hundreds of genes regulating key biological processes from cell division to apoptosis [36]. It is well known that poor glycemic control is a risk factor for the development and progression of DR, and vitamin D deficiency has been shown to impair insulin synthesis and secretion in animal models of diabetes [37]. On the other hand, an optimal concentration of vitamin D is strongly proven to be necessary for efficient insulin secretion and function [38–40], and vitamin D receptors (VDR) are ubiquitously expressed in every human tissue, including retina. Active vitamin D mediates its biological function by binding to vitamin D receptors. Vitamin D receptors have been found to be associated with insulin secretion and sensitivity, and have been identified in pancreatic beta cells [41]. Additionally, some genes associated with the development of diabetic retinopathy have been found, such as *Bsm1*, *rs2228570*, and *TT*. So, vitamin D status is related with the development and progression of diabetic retinopathy among type 2 diabetes patients.

Increasing studies have given more evidence of this. Annwelier et al. found that the serum 25(OH)D levels were associated with optic chiasm volume [42], and in a vitro experiment, vitamin D was found to inhibit neovascularization in retinal tissue in a model of ischemic retinopathy [13]. What is more, proof of the VDR polymorphisms related with diabetic retinopathy was found. Hong et al. showed that patients with the B allele (BB or Bb) of Bsm1 polymorphism in VDR were associated with lower risk of diabetic retinopathy compared to patients without the B allele (bb) in Korean type 2 diabetic patients [41]. Bucan et al. showed that the bb genotype in VDR has a higher risk of developing diabetic retinopathy [43]. Zhong et al. found that rs2228570 was associated with increased risk of diabetic retinopathy in Han Chinese type 2 diabetes patients [44]. Benjamin et al. reported that the anticipation of retinopathy onset is significantly associated with the exaggeration of oxidative stress biomarkers or decrease of antioxidants in African type 2 diabetics, and supplementation with vitamin D should be recommended as complement therapies of T2DM [26]. Therefore, low serum 25(OH)D levels are association with an increased risk of diabetic retinopathy, but more studies are required to identify the mechanism of the relationship between vitamin D and diabetic retinopathy fully.

It is well known that one of the two major sources of vitamin D is cutaneous synthesis by solar ultraviolet B radiation and the other is dietary intake. The cutaneous synthesis of vitamin D is affected by many factors, such as season, latitude, time of day, skin pigmentation, the amount of skin exposed, and whether makeup with sunscreen is used, so serum 25-hydroxyvitamin D levels vary between areas and persons. Hence, dietary vitamin D supplementation and physical activity might be a feasible way for patients with diabetes to maintain sufficient 25-hydroxyvitamin D levels. Physical activity may increase blood 25-hydroxyvitamin D concentrations as a consequence of an associated increase in sunlight exposure. Praidou et al. reported that increased physical activity is associated with less severe levels of diabetic retinopathy, independent of the effects of HbA1c and BMI [5]. Lee et al. showed that 3 months of vitamin D supplementation improved neuropathic symptoms by 50% in diabetic patients whose 25-hydroxyvitamin D status was deficient at baseline [45]. However, there has yet to be a dietary vitamin D supplementation trial on diabetic retinopathy. Thus, large randomized controlled trials researching on reducing diabetic retinopathy in type 2 diabetes are needed to accurately evaluate the potential benefits of these low-cost interventions in the future.

Diabetic retinopathy may develop and progress to advanced stages without producing any immediate symptoms to the patient. Screening for DR is essential in order to establish early treatment of sight-threatening retinopathy and has been demonstrated to be successful at achieving vision loss [46]. Considering the heavy burden of DR and the association between serum 25(OH)D level and diabetic retinopathy, low 25(OH)D levels may help us to find more early stage diabetic retinopathy patients. Therefore, screening low 25(OH)D levels may be a potential simple way for screening diabetic retinopathy among type 2 diabetes in primary hospitals—especially where there is a shortage of ophthalmic equipment or ophthalmologists.

The main strength of this study is giving strong evidence of the association of serum vitamin D and diabetic retinopathy. However, there were several limitations in this study. Firstly, different diagnostic criteria of diabetic retinopathy and different measured assays could have influenced the pooled effect. Secondly, there were some confounding factors in this meta-analysis, such as age, race, diet, the treatment of diabetes, sun exposure, physical activity, and so on. Some, but not all, of the studies generated adjusted OR, so we could not pool the findings by adjusting for confounding factors. Thirdly, there was a lack of access to complete data of all related published papers, despite correspondence with the authors. Fourthly, the association between vitamin D and the severity of diabetic retinopathy was not analyzed in this meta-analysis because of a lack of enough data and information. Finally, only published articles in English were included.

5. Conclusions

In conclusion, this meta-analysis indicates an association between vitamin D deficient type 2 diabetes mellitus patients and an increased risk of diabetic retinopathy. Type 2 diabetes patients with vitamin D deficiency experienced an increased risk of diabetic retinopathy. However, further studies are required to better understand the relationship between vitamin D deficient type 2 diabetes patients and diabetic retinopathy, and well-designed randomized controlled trials are needed to determine the explicit effect of vitamin D supplementation on the prevention of diabetic retinopathy. Considering the high prevalence of vitamin D deficiency and the burden of the diabetic retinopathy, screening type 2 diabetes patients who are at risk of vitamin D deficiency should be considered.

Supplementary Materials: The following are available online at http://www.mdpi.com/2072-6643/9/3/307/s1, Table S1. Quality scores of included studies on vitamin D status and pregnancy outcomes. Table S2. Results of meta-analysis according to 25-hydroxyvitamin D (25(OH)D) level. DR: diabetic retinopathy; NDR: no diabetic retinopathy. Figure S1. Meta-analysis of the association between vitamin D insufficiency (<30 ng/mL) and DR. Figure S2. Subgroup analysis of pooled ORs according to study design. Figure S3. Subgroup analysis of weight mean difference (WMD) according to study design. Figure S4. Subgroup analysis of pooled ORs according to vitamin D assay method. Figure S5. Subgroup analysis of pooled ORs according to different DR diagnosis. Figure S6. Result of funnel plots.

Author Contributions: All authors participated in the process of this meta-analysis.

Conflicts of Interest: The authors declare no conflict of interest.

References

1. Sherwin, R.; Jastreboff, A.M. Year in diabetes 2012: the diabetes tsunami. *J. Clin. Endocrinol. Metab.* **2012**, *97*, 4293–4301. [CrossRef] [PubMed]
2. Klein, B.E. Overview of epidemiologic studies of diabetic retinopathy. *Ophthalmic Epidemiol.* **2007**, *14*, 179–183. [CrossRef] [PubMed]

3.   Zheng, Y.; He, M.; Congdon, N. The worldwide epidemic of diabetic retinopathy. *Indian J. Ophthalmol.* **2012**, *60*, 428–431. [PubMed]

4.   Stratton, I.M.; Kohner, E.M.; Aldington, S.J.; Turner, R.C.; Holman, R.R.; Manley, S.E.; Matthews, D.R. UKPDS50: Risk factors for incidence and progression of retinopathy in Type II diabetes over 6 years from diagnosis. *Diabetologia* **2001**, *44*, 156–163. [CrossRef] [PubMed]

5.   Praidou, A.; Harris, M.; Niakas, D.; Labiris, G. Physical activity and its correlation to diabetic retinopathy. *J. Diabetes Complicat.* **2017**, *31*, 456–461. [CrossRef] [PubMed]

6.   Holick, M.F. Vitamin D deficiency. *N. Engl. J. Med.* **2007**, *357*, 266–281. [CrossRef] [PubMed]

7.   Holick, M.F.; Chen, T.C. Vitamin D deficiency: A worldwide problem with health consequences. *Am. J. Clin. Nutr.* **2008**, *87*, 1080s–1086s. [CrossRef] [PubMed]

8.   Mitri, J.; Muraru, M.D.; Pittas, A.G. Vitamin D and Type 2 diabetes: A systematic review. *Eur. J. Clin. Nutr.* **2011**, *65*, 1005–1015. [CrossRef] [PubMed]

9.   Rhee, S.Y.; Hwang, Y.C.; Chung, H.Y.; Woo, J.T. Vitamin D and diabetes in Koreans: Analyses based on the Fourth Korea National Health and Nutrition Examination Survey (KNHANES), 2008–2009. *Diabet. Med.* **2012**, *29*, 1003–1010. [CrossRef] [PubMed]

10.   Bonakdaran, S.; Shoeibi, N. Is there any correlation between vitamin D insufficiency and diabetic retinopathy? *Int. J. Ophthalmol.* **2015**, *8*, 326–331. [PubMed]

11.   Isaia, G.; Giorgino, R.; Adami, S. High prevalence of hypovitaminosis D in female type diabetic population. *Diabetes Care* **2001**, *24*, 1496. [CrossRef] [PubMed]

12.   Taverna, M.J.; Selam, J.L.; Slama, G. Association between a protein polymorphism in the start codon of the vitamin D receptor gene and severe diabetic retinopathy in C-peptide-negative type 1 diabetes. *J. Clin. Endocrinol. Metab.* **2005**, *90*, 4803–4808. [CrossRef] [PubMed]

13.   Albert, D.M.; Scheef, E.A.; Wang, S.; Mehraein, F.; Darjatmoko, S.R.; Sorenson, C.M.; Sheibani, N. Calcitriol is a potent inhibitor of retinal neovascularization. *Investig. Ophthalmol. Vis. Sci.* **2007**, *48*, 2327–2334. [CrossRef] [PubMed]

14.   Patrick, P.A.; Visintainer, P.F.; Shi, Q.; Weiss, I.A.; Brand, D.A. Vitamin D and Retinopathy in Adults with Diabetes Mellitus. *Arch. Ophthalmol.* **2012**, *130*, 756–760. [CrossRef] [PubMed]

15.   Inukai, T.; Fujiwara, Y.; Tayama, K.; Aso, Y.; Takemura, Y. Alterations in serum levels of 1 alpha, 25(OH)2 D3 and osteocalcin in patients with early diabetic nephropathy. *Diabetes Res. Clin. Pract.* **1997**, *38*, 53–59. [CrossRef]

16.   Alam, U.; Amjad, Y.; Chan, A.W.; Asghar, O.; Petropoulos, I.N.; Malik, R.A. Vitamin D Deficiency Is Not Associated with Diabetic Retinopathy or Maculopathy. *J. Diabetes Res.* **2016**, *2016*, 6156217. [CrossRef] [PubMed]

17.   Stroup, D.F.; Berlin, J.A.; Morton, S.C.; Olkin, I.; Williamson, G.D.; Rennie, D.; Moher, D.; Becker, B.J.; Sipe, T.A.; Thacker, S.B. Meta-analysis of observational studies in epidemiology: A proposal for reporting. Meta-analysis of observational studies in epidemiology (moose) group. *JAMA* **2000**, *283*, 2008–2012. [CrossRef] [PubMed]

18.   Duckitt, K.; Harrington, D. Risk factors for pre-eclampsia at antenatal booking: Systematic review of controlled studies. *BMJ (Clin. Res. Ed.)* **2005**, *330*, 565. [CrossRef] [PubMed]

19.   Aksoy, H.; Akçay, F.; Kurtul, N.; Baykal, O.; Avci, B. Serum 1,25 Dihydroxy Vitamin D (1,25(OH)2D3), 25 Hydroxy Vitamin D (25(OH)D) and Parathormone Levels in Diabetic Retinopathy. *Clin. Biochem.* **2000**, *33*, 47–51. [CrossRef]

20.   Suzuki, A.; Kotake, M.; Ono, Y.; Kato, T.; Oda, N.; Hayakawa, N.; Hashimoto, S.; Itoh, M. Hypovitaminosis D in type 2 diabetes mellitus: Association with microvascular complications and type of treatment. *Endocr. J.* **2006**, *53*, 503–510. [CrossRef] [PubMed]

21.   Payne, J.F.; Ray, R.; Watson, D.G.; Delille, C.; Rimler, E.; Cleveland, J.; Lynn, M.J.; Tangpricha, V.; Srivastava, S.K. Vitamin D Insufficiency in Diabetic Retinopathy. *Endocr. Pract.* **2012**, *18*, 185–193. [CrossRef] [PubMed]

22.   Ahmadieh, H.; Azar, S.T.; Lakkis, N.; Arabi, A. Hypovitaminosis D in Patients with Type 2 Diabetes Mellitus: A Relation to Disease Control and Complications. *ISRN Endocrinol.* **2013**, *2013*, 641098. [CrossRef] [PubMed]

23.   Bajaj, S.; Singh, R.P.; Dwivedi, N.C.; Singh, K.; Gupta, A.; Mathur, M. Vitamin D levels and microvascular complications in type 2 diabetes. *Indian J. Endocrinol. Metab.* **2014**, *18*, 537–541. [CrossRef] [PubMed]

24. He, R.; Shen, J.; Liu, F.; Zeng, H.; Li, L.; Yu, H.; Lu, H.; Lu, F.; Wu, Q.; Jia, W. Vitamin D deficiency increases the risk of retinopathy in Chinese patients with Type 2 diabetes. *Diabet. Med.* **2014**, *31*, 1657–1664. [CrossRef] [PubMed]

25. Jee, D.; Han, K.; Kim, E.C. Inverse Association between High Blood 25 Hydroxyvitamin D Levels and Diabetic Retinopathy in a Representative Korean Population. *PLoS ONE* **2014**, *9*, e115199. [CrossRef] [PubMed]

26. Longo-Mbenza, B.; Mvitu Muaka, M.; Masamba, W.; Muizila Kini, L.; Longo Phemba, I.; Kibokela Ndembe, D.; Tulomba Mona, D. Retinopathy in non diabetics, diabetic retinopathy and oxidative stress: A new phenotype in Central Africa? *Int. J. Ophthalmol.* **2014**, *7*, 293–301. [PubMed]

27. Alcubierre, N.; Valls, J.; Rubinat, E.; Cao, G.; Esquerda, A.; Traveset, A.; Granado-Casas, M.; Jurjo, C.; Mauricio, D. Vitamin D Deficiency Is Associated with the Presence and Severity of Diabetic Retinopathy in Type 2 Diabetes Mellitus. *J. Diabetes Res.* **2015**, *2015*, 374178. [CrossRef] [PubMed]

28. Herrmann, M.; Sullivan, D.R.; Veillard, A.S.; McCorquodale, T.; Straub, I.R.; Scott, R.; Laakso, M.; Topliss, D.; Jenkins, A.J.; Blankenberg, S.; Burton, A.; et al. Serum 25-Hydroxyvitamin D: A Predictor of Macrovascular and Microvascular Complications in Patients With Type 2 Diabetes. *Diabetes Care* **2015**, *38*, 521–528. [CrossRef] [PubMed]

29. Reddy, G.B.; Sivaprasad, M.; Shalini, T.; Satyanarayana, A.; Seshacharyulu, M.; Balakrishna, N.; Viswanath, K.; Sahay, M. Plasma vitamin D status in patients with type 2 diabetes with and without retinopathy. *Nutrition* **2015**, *31*, 959–963. [CrossRef] [PubMed]

30. Usluogullari, C.A.; Balkan, F.; Caner, S.; Ucler, R.; Kaya, C.; Ersoy, R.; Cakir, B. The relationship between microvascular complications and vitamin D deficiency in type 2 diabetes mellitus. *BMC Endocr. Disord.* **2015**, *15*, 33. [CrossRef] [PubMed]

31. Zoppini, G.; Galletti, A.; Targher, G.; Brangani, C.; Pichiri, I.; Trombetta, M.; Negri, C.; de Santi, F.; Stoico, V.; Cacciatori, V.; et al. Lower levels of 25-hydroxyvitamin D3 are associated with a higher prevalence of microvascular complications in patients with type 2 diabetes. *BMJ Open Diabetes Res. Care* **2015**, *3*, e000058. [CrossRef] [PubMed]

32. Millen, A.E.; Sahli, M.W.; Nie, J.; LaMonte, M.J.; Lutsey, P.L.; Klein, B.E.; Mares, J.A.; Meyers, K.J.; Andrews, C.A.; Klein, R. Adequate vitamin D status is associated with the reduced odds of prevalent diabetic retinopathy in African Americans and Caucasians. *Cardiovasc. Diabetol.* **2016**, *15*, 128. [CrossRef] [PubMed]

33. Zittermann, A.; Koerfer, R. Protective and toxic effects of vitamin D on vascular calcification: Clinical implications. *Mol. Asp. Med.* **2008**, *29*, 423–432. [CrossRef] [PubMed]

34. Targher, G.; Bertolini, L.; Padovani, R.; Zenari, L.; Scala, L.; Cigolini, M.; Arcaro, G. Serum 25-hydroxyvitamin D3 concentrations and carotid artery intima–media thickness among Type 2 diabetic patients. *Clin. Endocrinol. (Oxf.)* **2006**, *65*, 593–597. [CrossRef] [PubMed]

35. Ren, Z.; Li, W.; Zhao, Q.; Ma, L.; Zhu, J. The impact of 1,25-dihydroxy vitamin D3 on the expressions of vascular endothelial growth factor and transforming growth factor-b1 in the retinas of rats with diabetes. *Diabetes Res. Clin. Pract.* **2012**, *98*, 474–480. [CrossRef] [PubMed]

36. Temmerman, J.C. Vitamin D and cardiovascular disease. *J. Am. Coll. Nutr.* **2011**, *30*, 167–170. [CrossRef] [PubMed]

37. Mathieu, C.; Gysemans, C.; Giulietti, A.; Bouillon, R. Vitamin D and diabetes. *Diabetologia* **2005**, *48*, 1247–1257. [CrossRef] [PubMed]

38. Michos, E.D. Vitamin D deficiency and the risk of incident Type 2 diabetes. *Future Cardiol.* **2009**, *5*, 15–18. [CrossRef] [PubMed]

39. Danescu, L.G.; Levy, S.; Levy, J. Vitamin D and diabetes mellitus. *Endocrine* **2009**, *35*, 11–17. [CrossRef] [PubMed]

40. Cavalier, E.; Delanaye, P.; Souberbielle, J.C.; Radermecker, R.P. Vitamin D and type 2 diabetes mellitus: where do we stand? *Diabetes Metab.* **2011**, *37*, 265–272. [CrossRef] [PubMed]

41. Hong, Y.J.; Kang, E.S.; Ji, M.J.; Choi, H.J.; Oh, T.; Koong, S.S.; Jeon, H.J. Association between Bsm1 Polymorphism in Vitamin D Receptor Gene and Diabetic Retinopathy of Type 2 Diabetes in Korean Population. *Endocrinol. Metab. (Seoul)* **2015**, *30*, 469–474. [CrossRef] [PubMed]

42. Annweiler, C.; Beauchet, O.; Bartha, R.; Graffe, A.; Milea, D.; Montero-Odasso, M. Association between serum 25-hydroxyvitamin D concentration and optic chiasm volume. *J. Am. Geriatr. Soc.* **2013**, *61*, 1026–1028. [CrossRef] [PubMed]

43. Bućan, K.; Ivanisević, M.; Zemunik, T.; Boraska, V.; Skrabić, V.; Vatavuk, Z.; Galetović, D.; Znaor, L. Retinopathy and nephropathy in type 1 diabetic patients association with polymorphysms of vitamin D-receptor, TNF, Neuro-D and IL-1 receptor 1 genes. *Coll. Antropol.* **2009**, *33*, 99–105. [PubMed]

44. Zhong, X.; Du, Y.; Lei, Y.; Liu, N.; Guo, Y.; Pan, T. Effects of vitamin D receptor gene polymorphism and clinical characteristics on risk of diabetic retinopathy in Han Chinese type 2 diabetes patients. *Gene* **2015**, *566*, 212–216. [CrossRef] [PubMed]

45. Lee, P.; Chen, R. Vitamin D as an analgesic for patients with type 2 diabetes and neuropathic pain. *Arch. Intern. Med.* **2008**, *168*, 771–772. [CrossRef] [PubMed]

46. Stitt, A.W.; Curtis, T.M.; Chen, M.; Medina, R.J.; McKay, G.J.; Jenkins, A.; Gardiner, T.A.; Lyons, T.J.; Hammes, H.P.; Simó, R.; et al. The progress in understanding and treatment of diabetic retinopathy. *Prog. Retin. Eye Res.* **2016**, *51*, 156–186. [CrossRef] [PubMed]

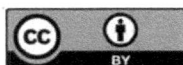

nutrients

MDPI

Article

Daily Intake of Grape Powder Prevents the Progression of Kidney Disease in Obese Type 2 Diabetic ZSF1 Rats

Salwa M. K. Almomen [1], Qiunong Guan [1,2], Peihe Liang [1,3], Kaidi Yang [1], Ahmad M. Sidiqi [1,4], Adeera Levin [4] and Caigan Du [1,2,*]

[1]   Department of Urologic Sciences, University of British Columbia, Vancouver, BC V6H3Z6, Canada; sa.momen@windowslive.com (S.M.K.A.); qiunong@hotmail.com (Q.G.); lph1972@163.com (P.L.); kaidiyang1994@gmail.com (K.Y.); ahmad.sidiqi@alumni.ubc.ca (A.M.S.)
[2]   Immunity and Infection Research Centre, Vancouver Coastal Health Research Institute, Vancouver, BC V6H3Z6, Canada
[3]   Department of Urology, The Second Affiliated Hospital, Chongqing Medical University, Chongqing 400010, China
[4]   Division of Nephrology, Department of Medicine, University of British Columbia, Vancouver, BC V6Z1Y6, Canada; alevin@providencehealth.bc.ca
*   Correspondence: caigan@mail.ubc.ca; Tel.: +1-604-875-4111 (ext. 63793)

Received: 10 March 2017; Accepted: 29 March 2017; Published: 31 March 2017

Abstract: Individuals living with metabolic syndrome (MetS) such as diabetes and obesity are at high risk for developing chronic kidney disease (CKD). This study investigated the beneficial effect of whole grape powder (WGP) diet on MetS-associated CKD. Obese diabetic ZSF1 rats, a kidney disease model with MetS, were fed WGP (5%, w/w) diet for six months. Kidney disease was determined using blood and urine chemical analyses, and histology. When compared to Vehicle controls, WGP intake did not change the rat bodyweight, but lowered their kidney, liver and spleen weight, which were in parallel with the lower serum glucose and the higher albumin or albumin/globin ratio. More importantly, WGP intake improved the renal function as urination and proteinuria decreased, or it prevented kidney tissue damage in these diabetic rats. The renal protection of WGP diet was associated with up-regulation of antioxidants (*Dhcr24, Gstk1, Prdx2, Sod2, Gpx1 and Gpx4*) and downregulation of *Txnip* (for ROS production) in the kidneys. Furthermore, addition of grape extract reduced H_2O_2-induced cell death of cultured podocytes. In conclusion, daily intake of WGP reduces the progression of kidney disease in obese diabetic rats, suggesting a protective function of antioxidant-rich grape diet against CKD in the setting of MetS.

Keywords: metabolic syndrome; chronic kidney disease; grape powder; antioxidants; natural products; dietary supplements

---

1. Introduction

Chronic kidney disease (CKD) is multifactorial, and is defined as abnormalities of kidney structure or function that is present for more than three months. While not progressive in all, it can lead to end-stage renal disease (ESRD)—total and permanent kidney failure [1,2]. CKD places a major public health burden on our community as it affects more than 10% of adults aged 20 years or older, or more than 40% in those aged 65 years or older in the United States (source: Centers for Disease Control and Prevention), and 12.5% of adults, representing approximately three million, in Canada [3,4]. Like other chronic diseases, many cases of CKD are not curable, but there are substantial numbers of people who can benefit from prevention or delay of progression [5], suggesting that an effective and feasible preventive strategy is expected to reduce the burden of CKD in our community. However, there are a limited number of these that are proven or used in our daily practice. Recently, there is an increasing interest in diet, the interaction of gut microbiome and CKD progression. Dietary supplements or natural health products is definitely an attractive and feasible strategy for CKD prevention.

Metabolic syndrome (MetS) is a collective term for several clinical measures, which include insulin resistance, high serum glucose, overweight or obesity, high triglyceride or low high-density lipoprotein cholesterol and hypertension [6]. Literature suggests that MetS may increase the risk of the development of CKD [7–9], mainly seen as hypertensive and diabetic nephropathy (DN). While the etiology for MetS-induced CKD remains unknown [9], oxidative stress is theorized to a play a role [8,10,11]. The oxidative stress is induced by the imbalance between the level of reactive oxygen species (ROS, free radicals) and the capacity of antioxidant defenses, which leads to the generation of excessive ROS and consequently tissue damage [11,12]. One of major antioxidant defense mechanisms in our body is exogenous antioxidants, such as flavonoids, vitamins, resveratrol, anthocyanine, curcumin and phenolic acid that come from our food and other dietary sources [11,13–15]. There are some data that antioxidant rich berry diet has benefit in preventing or mitigating MetS [15,16], suggesting that a dietary strategy of using antioxidant-rich food may be a novel strategy to employ to reduce the incidence of CKD among individuals who are living with MetS.

Grapes are one of the most widely cultivated and popularly consumed fruits in the world, and contain over 1600 phytonutrients including some major antioxidant flavonoids, such as catechins (catechin and epicatechin), anthocyanins (peonidin, cyaniding, and malvidin), flavonols (quercetin, kaempferol, and isorhamnetin) and resveratrol (source: the California Table Grape Commission report, Fresno, CA, USA). The renoprotective activities of these compounds have been demonstrated in various experimental models. For example, epicatechin, quercetin or resveratrol has been shown to lower the oxidative stress in the kidneys and reduce renal damage in animals with cisplatin nephropathy [17–19], and feeding with anthocyanin-rich food reduces diabetes-associated kidney failure in db/db mice [20]. A recent study shows that daily drinking of whole grape powder (WGP) prevents age-related decline of kidney function in rats [21], but its beneficial effect on MetS-associated CKD, a common public health problem in our community [22], has not been investigated. Obese ZSF1 male rats are generated by a cross between a Zucker diabetic fatty (ZDF) female and a spontaneously hypertensive heart failure (SHHF) male rat, which have MetS similar to humans, including hypertension, type 2 diabetes, hyperlipidemia and nephropathy [23–27]. Hence, these rats have been widely used as a disease model for renal failure in the condition of MetS [27–30]. The objective of this study was to examine the effect of daily feeding with the WGP on the progression of kidney disease in obese ZSF1 rats, as compared to control animals.

2. Materials and Methods

2.1. Animals and Cells

Obese ZSF1 male rats (~300 g bodyweight, 8 weeks old) were purchased from Charles River Laboratories International, Inc. (Wilmington, MA, USA). These rats were F1 hybrids from a cross between a female ZDF rat and a male SHHF rat [27], and were maintained in the animal facility of the Jack Bell Research Centre (Vancouver, BC, Canada). All animal experiments were performed in accordance with the Canadian Council on Animal Care guidelines under protocols approved by the Animal Use Subcommittee at the University of British Columbia (Vancouver, BC, Canada).

Heat-sensitive mouse podocyte (HSMP) cell line was a gift from Dr. Stuart Shankland (University of Washington School of Medicine, Seattle, WA, USA). HSMP cells were maintained and grown in RPMI 1640 culture medium supplemented with 10% fetal bovine serum and 0.2 ng·mL^{-1} of IFN-γ in a CO_2 incubator at 33 °C as described previously [31]. To induce quiescence and the differentiated phenotype for experiments, HSMP cells were grown at 37 °C in the same medium but in the absence of IFN-γ (growth restrictive conditions) [31].

2.2. Whole Grape Powder (WGP)

WGP was provided by the California Table Grape Commission (CTGC), and was a freeze-dried grape product developed for the usage of research purposes only. WGP was composed of seeded and seedless varieties of fresh green, red and black California grapes that were initially frozen, and then ground with food-quality dry ice. The processing and storage of the WGP were done properly for preserving the bioactivities of the compounds found in the grapes. Approximately 90% of the WGP by weight was sugars (glucose and fructose found in a 1:1 ratio), and the remainder consisted of organic acids, phenolic compounds, nitrogenous compounds, aroma compounds, and minerals and pectic substances. Antioxidants, such as resveratrol, flavans (including catechin), flavonols (including quercetin), anthocyanins and many simple phenolics (as per the CTGC report) were also found. This product was stored at −80 °C in moisture-proof containers until it was mixed with regular rat chow for the animal experiments.

2.3. Food Supplements

According to the CTGC guideline of the usage of WGP as food supplements for animal studies, WGP supplement food (denoted as WGP here) was prepared for this study by mixing regular chow (95%, *w/w*) with WGP (5%, *w/w*), and its Vehicle control the regular chow (95.5%, *w/w*) with 2.25% (*w/w*) glucose and 2.25% (*w/w*) fructose. Rats were randomly assigned to two groups (WGP and Vehicle), in which they were fed with either WGP or sugar control. The animal experiment was repeated twice with total 15 rats in each group. One rat in WGP group suffered a urinary tract infection diagnosed early during the second month of the feeding experiment, and was consequently excluded from the experiment and data analysis.

2.4. Preparation of WGP Extract

The WGP extract was prepared for both cell culture experiments to determine its antioxidative activity. In brief, WGP (4 g) was dissolved in 200 mL of methanol (anhydrous, 99.8%) and was stirred for 72 h at room temperature, followed by centrifugation at 3000 rpm for 15 min. The resultant supernatant fraction was subsequently dried by lyophilization using a centrifugal evaporator. Around 3.3 g of WGP-methanol extract was produced from 4 g of WGP by this procedure. The stock solution of WGP extract was prepared by dissolving the dried extract pellet in culture medium at the concentration of 5 mg·mL^{-1}.

2.5. Primary Outcomes from This Study

Our primary outcomes were to measure renal function through assessment of urine volume, proteinuria, urine protein to creatinine ratio (uPCR), and estimated glomerular filtration rate (GFR). Renal injury was also measured via the kidney organ index and histological analysis.

2.6. Urine Collection and Determination of Kidney Function

A 24-h urine sample was collected using metabolic caging, in which the rat had unrestricted access to food and drinking water. The collected urine was immediately centrifuged at 3000 rpm for 15 min to remove any food scraps and fecal matters. After its volume was measured, the sample was stored in aliquots at −20 °C until all the samples were collected for the determination of both protein and creatinine levels at the same time.

The levels of urine creatinine (UCr) were measured in the Chemistry Laboratory at the Vancouver Coastal Health Regional Laboratory Medicine (Vancouver, BC, Canada) by using the Dimension Vista® System with CRE2 reagent cartridges (Siemens Healthcare Diagnostics Inc., Newark, DE, USA). The levels of urine protein were determined using Bio-Rad protein assay following manufacturer's instruction (Bio-Rad Laboratories-Canada, Mississauga, ON, Canada). In brief, the protein in the urine was precipitated using 10% trichloroacetic acid, followed by centrifugation at 10,000 rpm for 10 min.

The protein pellet was suspended in 3% sodium hydroxide (NaOH) solution, and 1 μL of this protein solution was added to 200 μL of Bio-Rad dye (10 × dilution). The optical density (OD) of urine protein samples, background control and bovine serum albumin (BSA) standards at 595 nm was measured using an ELx808 Ultra Microplate Reader (BioTek, Winooski, VT, USA), and protein concentration (mg·mL^{-1}) in the urine sample was calculated based on the BSA standard curve.

2.7. Blood Collection and Chemical Analysis

Blood samples were collected from the tail vein using a lithium heparin tube after 1, 3 and 6 months of WGP feeding. A comprehensive metabolic panel of 14 blood substances, including alanine aminotransferase (ALT), albumin (ALB), alkaline phosphatase (ALP), amylase (AMY), total calcium (Ca^{2+}), creatinine (CRE), globulin (GLOB), glucose (GLU), phosphorus (PHOS), potassium (K$^+$), sodium (Na$^+$), total bilirubin (TBIL), total protein (TP), and urea nitrogen (BUN), were determined using the VetScan® Comprehensive Diagnostic Profile reagent rotor with the VetScan Chemistry Analyzer VS2 (Abaxis, Inc., Union City, CA, USA) in the Animal Unit Hematology Diagnostic Laboratory at Jack Bell Research Centre (Vancouver, BC, Canada).

2.8. Glomerular Filtration Rate (GFR)

The renal function was estimated using GFR that was calculated based on the creatinine clearance using the following: GFR = (UCr × V)/SCr, where UCr was creatinine level in urine sample, V the volume of the 24-h urine sample, and SCr the creatinine in serum.

2.9. Renal Histopathology

The kidney tissues (6 rats/group) were randomly selected. The tissues were fixed in 10% neutral buffered formalin, followed by embedding in paraffin wax. Sections were cut at 4-μm thickness, and were stained with hematoxylin and eosin (HE) or periodic acid-Schiff (PAS). The stained tissue sections were scanned with Leica SCN400 Slide scanner (Leica Microsystens Inc., Concord, ON, Canada), and the pathological parameters of renal disease were determined in two separate sections of each kidney using the Digital Image Hub—A slidepath Software Solution (Leica Microsystems Inc.) in a blinded fashion.

The number of intratubular protein cast formation or glomerular atrophy in each microscopic view was counted in HE-stained section, and the average number of at least 20 randomly selected views under 40× magnification represented these two parameters in each kidney.

A semi-quantitative scoring system using a 0 to 4 scale was established to determine the severity of the tubular atrophy (including tubular dilution and/or cellular flatting) in the renal cortex of HE-stained kidney sections. The scale/score was measured based on the percentage of damaged tubules occupying a microscopic view: 1 (0%–24% of the area affected with damaged tubules), 2 (25%–49%), 3 (50%–74%), and 4 (>75%). The average of at least 30 randomly selected views under 200× magnification represented the tubular atrophy in each kidney.

The mesangial expansion was also determined using a 0 to 4 scale based on the percentage of the area stained strongly with PAS, indicating the mesangial expansion in an affected glomerulus: 1 (0%–24% of the area affected with densely stain, minimal), 2 (25%–49%, mild), 3 (50%–74%, moderate), and 4 (>75%, severe). A range of 180 to 250 glomeruli were counted and averaged for each kidney.

2.10. PCR Array Analysis of Oxidative Stress

The expression of 84 oxidative stress-associated genes in kidney tissues was quantitatively examined using PCR Arrays kits (Cat. No.: PARN-065Z, SABiosciences—QIAGEN Inc., Valencia, CA, USA) following manufacturer's instruction. Four samples/rats (one from each rat) were randomly selected from each group. In brief, one piece of kidney cortex was snap-frozen in liquid nitrogen and stored at −80 °C until all the samples were ready for the experiment. The total RNA from the tissues was extracted and purified using the RNeasy Microarray Tissue Mini kit

(QIAGEN), and converted to cDNA using RT^2 First Strand Kit (QIAGEN). The expression of selected genes was amplified by real-time PCR using RT^2 Profile PCR arrays (QIAGEN). Data were analyzed using Web-based PCR Array Data Analysis Software at the website of the manufacturer (http://www.SABiosciences.com/pcrarraydataanalysis.php).

2.11. Flow Cytometric Analysis

Cell death or viability was quantitatively determined by using fluorescence-activated cell sorter (FACS) analysis following the manufacturer's protocol (BD Biosciences, Mississauga, ON, Canada). Annexin-V conjugated with phycoerythrin (Annexin-V-PE) stained apoptotic cells, and 7-amino-actinomycin D (7-AAD) positivity indicated late apoptotic and necrotic cells. Briefly, cells were stained with both Annexin-V-PE and 7-AAD for 15 min in the dark, and cell apoptosis and necrosis were detected by using a flow cytometry and further quantified using FlowJo software (Tree Star Inc., Ashland, OR, USA). In a FACS graph, the lower right quadrant—only Annexin V positive indicated early apoptosis; the upper right quadrant—Annexin V/7-AAD double positive showed late apoptosis; and the upper left quadrant—7-AAD positive cells were necrosis. Finally, negative staining (the lower left quadrant—Annexin V/7-AAD double negative) showed the population of viable cells.

2.12. Statistical Analysis

Data were presented as mean $\pm$ standard derivation (SD) of each group. Statistical analysis of difference between groups was performed using GraphPad Prism software (GraphPad, San Diego, CA, USA) by *t*-test or analysis of variance (ANOVA) as indicated in the text. A *p* value of ≤ 0.05 was considered statistically significant.

3. Results

3.1. Daily Intake of WGP Is Associated with Lower Organ Index of the Kidney, Liver and Spleen but Does Not Affect Bodyweight in Obese Diabetic Rats

Both bodyweight and diet consumption were monitored once a week. As shown in Figure 1, the weight gain of rats during six months of WGP feeding was the same as sugar-fed Vehicle control group, indicated by a complete overlap of growth curves between these two groups (WGP vs. Vehicle: $p = 0.7701$, two-way ANOVA). This observation was correlated with their diet consumption, which remained the same at 25 ± 2 g·day^{-1}·animal^{-1} between these two groups throughout the experiment. Interestingly, at the end of feeding experiment, significantly lower organ weight index was seen in the kidney (WGP vs. Vehicle: $p = 0.0127$, two-tailed *t*-test), liver (WGP vs. Vehicle: $p < 0.0001$, two-tailed *t*-test) and spleen (WGP vs. Vehicle: $p = 0.0341$, two-tailed *t*-test) of WGP-fed rats compared to Vehicle controls, whereas both the heart and the lung remained the same (Table 1). The data suggested that daily intake of WGP reduced the weight/size of these three organs—the liver, kidney and spleen—as compared to those in control group in these obese diabetic rats.

The bodyweight of rats in both Vehicle ($n = 15$) and WGP ($n = 14$) groups was recorded during a period of six months of dietary supplements. Data were presented as mean $\pm$ SD of each group. Vehicle vs. WGP: $p = 0.7701$ (two-way ANOVA).

Table 1. Organ index (organ weight/bodyweight) after six months of feeding sugar (Vehicle) or whole grape powder (WGP).

	Kidneys	Liver	Spleen	Heart	Lung
Vehicle ($n = 15$)	0.0070 ± 0.00072	0.0627 ± 0.00418	0.00135 ± 0.00010	0.00289 ± 0.00115	0.00356 ± 0.00096
WGP ($n = 14$)	0.0063 ± 0.00069	0.0544 ± 0.00546	0.00129 ± 0.00001	0.00251 ± 0.00022	0.00371 ± 0.00103
p value *	0.0127	<0.0001	0.0341	0.2351	0.6880

* The difference between Vehicle and WGP was compared using two-tailed *t*-test.

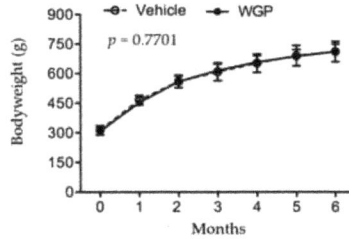

Figure 1. No effect of daily intake of whole grape powder (WGP) on bodyweight gain or obesity in obese diabetic ZSF1 rats.

3.2. Daily Intake of WGP Is Associated with Higher Serum Albumin and Lower Blood Glucose in Obese Diabetic Rats

The overall metabolism status of these rats was determined by using the changes in a comprehensive metabolic panel of 14 blood substances that represent the basic metabolism (GLU), electrolytes (Na^+, K^+, Ca^{2+}, and PHOS) and both kidney and liver functions (BUN, CRE, ALB, GLOB. ALB/GLOB ratio, ALP, ALT, AMY, TP and TBIL). Over six months of feeding experiment, the rats in both groups experienced a significant decline in ALB (including ALB/GLOB ratio), ALP, BUN, K^+ and PHOS, and at the same time an increase in GLU, AMY, TBIL, GLOB, TP, Ca^{2+} and Na^+ (Table S1). Only CRE and ALT remained unchanged (Table S1). The importance for this examination was that as compared to the Vehicle group, WGP-fed rats had significantly higher levels of serum ALB ($p = 0.0013$, two-way ANOVA) or ALB/GLOB ratio ($p = 0.0092$, two-way ANOVA), and lower levels of blood GLU ($p = 0.0276$, two-way ANOVA) (Table S1 and Figure 2), at the end of the six-month period.

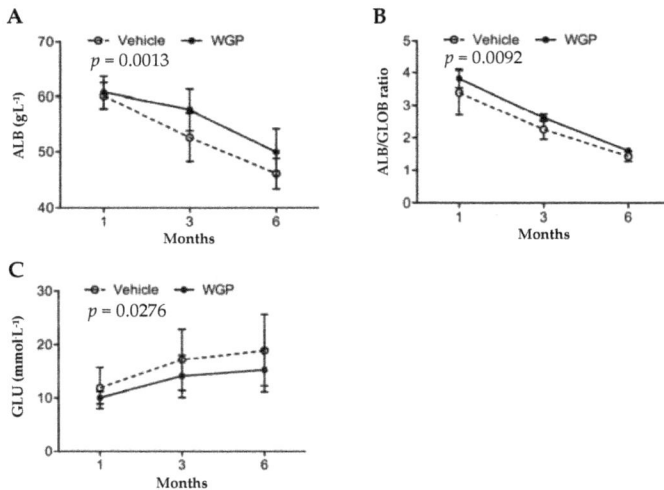

Figure 2. Daily intake of WGP has beneficial effect on the maintenance of blood albumin and the reduction of blood glucose in obese diabetic ZSF1 rats. The blood levels of albumin (ALB), globulin (GLOB) and glucose (GLU) were measured in randomly selected rats in Vehicle ($n = 8$–12) or WGP ($n = 8$–11) group after one, three or six months of dietary supplements. Data were presented as mean ± SD of each group. (**A**) Blood ALB levels. Vehicle vs. WGP: $p = 0.0013$ (two-way ANOVA); (**B**) ALB/GLOB ratio. Vehicle vs. WGP: $p = 0.0092$ (two-way ANOVA); (**C**) Blood GLU levels. Vehicle vs. WGP: $p = 0.0276$ (two-way ANOVA).

3.3. Daily Intake of WGP Significantly Is Associated with Lower Urine Volume and Urine Protein Excretion but Does Not Impact GFR after Six Months in Obese Diabetic Rats

The baseline ranges for renal function in obese ZSF1 rats at the age of eight weeks were 164.8 ± 14.5 mL·kg^{-1}·day^{-1} of urine volume, 307 ± 23 mg·kg^{-1}·day^{-1} of proteinuria or 5.98 ± 0.41 of urine protein to creatinine ratio (uPCR) [28], and the average of bodyweight of the rats at this age was approximately 300 g (Figure 1). After six months of feeding, a 24-h urine sample was collected from each rat. As shown in Figure 3A, WGP-fed rats had lower urine output than Vehicle controls ($p = 0.0092$, one-tailed *t*-test). Similarly, the WGP group had significantly lower proteinuria ($p = 0.0412$, one-tailed *t*-test) (Figure 3B), and uPCR ($p = 0.0084$, one-tailed *t*-test) (Figure 3C), when compared to the Vehicle controls. When GFR (mL·24 h^{-1}) between these two groups was compared, no significant difference was found between the WGP-fed and control groups ($p = 0.3474$, one-tailed *t*-test) (Figure 3D).

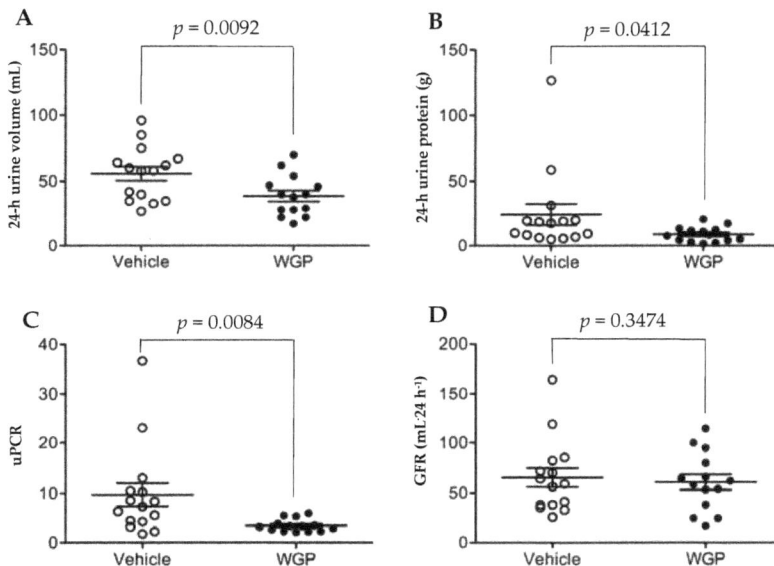

Figure 3. Daily intake of WGP reduces urine production and proteinuria but no effect on GFR in obese diabetic ZSF1 rats. A 24-h urine sample was collected from each rat in both Vehicle ($n = 15$) and WGP ($n = 14$) at the end of six months of dietary supplements. (**A**) Total volume of urine production from each rat during 24 h. Vehicle vs. WGP: $p = 0.0092$ (one-tailed *t*-test); (**B**) Total amount of protein in 24-h urine sample of each rat. Vehicle vs. WGP: $p = 0.0412$ (one-tailed *t*-test); (**C**) Protein to creatinine ratio (uPCR) in the urine sample of each rat. Vehicle vs. WGP: $p = 0.0084$ (one-tailed *t*-test); (**D**) GFR of each rat calculated based on creatinine clearance. Vehicle vs. WGP: $p = 0.3474$ (one-tailed *t*-test). Line: mean with the standard error of the mean (SEM).

3.4. Daily Intake of WGP Partially Prevents Renal Pathological Changes in Obese Diabetic Rats

To further explore the beneficial effect of daily intake of WGP on the prevention of kidney damage in obese diabetic rats, histological analysis of kidney sections was performed and compared between these two groups. The histological score of all four renal pathological parameters in WGP group were significantly lower than that in Vehicle group (Figure 4A–E). The WGP group had lower scores of glomerular atrophy per view ($p = 0.0225$, two-tailed *t*-test, $n = 9$) (Figure 4B), reduced mesangial expansion ($p < 0.0001$, two-tailed *t*-test, $n = 9$) (Figure 4C), fewer tubular protein cast formation per view ($p = 0.0006$, two-tailed *t*-test, $n = 12$) (Figure 4D), and less severe tubular dilation and atrophy ($p = 0.0036$, two-tailed *t*-test, $n = 12$ (Figure 4E), when compared to the Vehicle controls. Together, the histological data indicated less kidney injury in all compartments of the kidneys in WGP-fed rats.

A

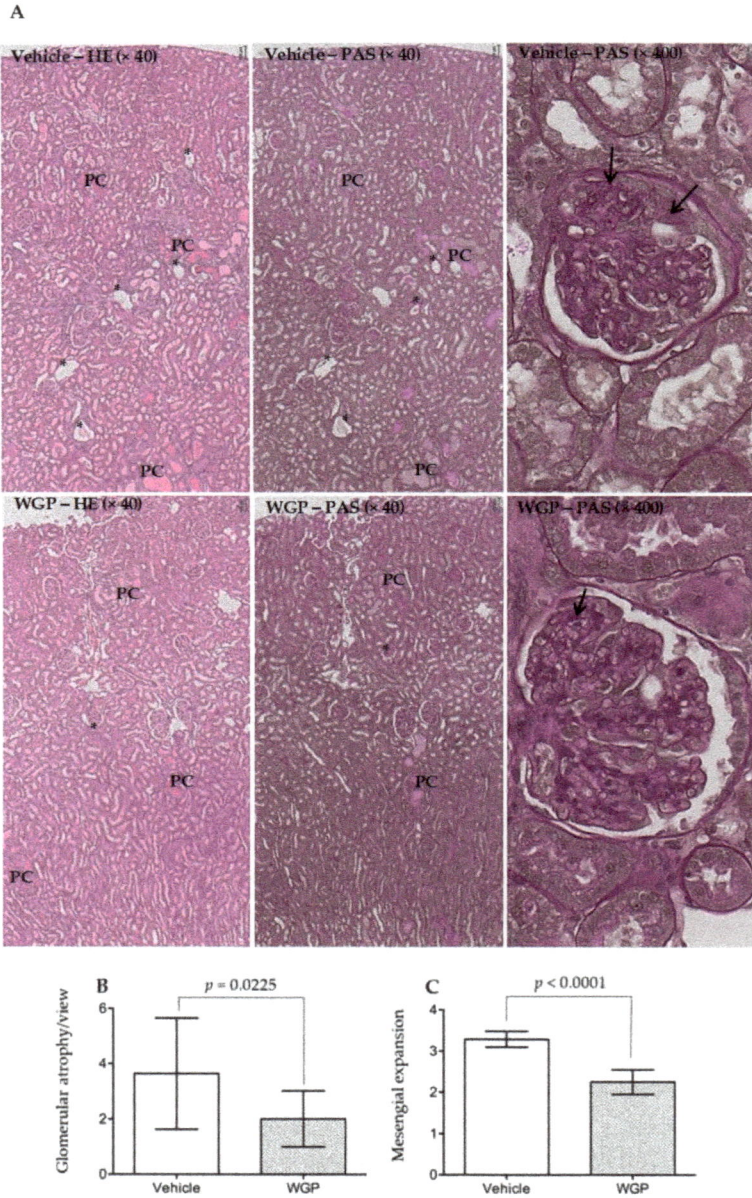

Figure 4. *Cont.*

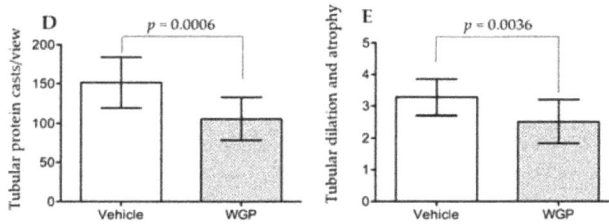

Figure 4. Daily intake of WGP reduces kidney injury in obese diabetic ZSF1 rats. At the end of six months of dietary supplements, six kidneys/rats were randomly selected from each group (Vehicle vs. WGP), and kidney sections were stained with either hematoxylin and eosin (HE) or Periodic acid-Schiff (PAS). (**A**) Typical microscopic images of renal cortex, outer medulla and a glomerulus in each group (Vehicle: top panel; WGP: bottom panel); data showed the same area of renal cortex and outer medulla stained with either HE or PAS. PC: protein cast formation; black stars (*): damaged glomerulus (glomerular atrophy); arrows: PAS-stained mesangial expansion; (**B**) The glomerular atrophy was scored in at least 20 randomly selected views in two separate sections of each kidney, and was presented in average per view; data are presented as mean ± SD of each group ($n = 9$); vehicle vs. WGP: $p = 0.0225$ (two-tailed *t*-test); (**C**) The mesangial expansion was determined using a 0 to 4 scale based on the percentage of the area stained strongly with PAS; a range of 180 to 250 glomeruli were counted and averaged for each kidney. Data are presented as mean ± SD of each group ($n = 9$); vehicle vs. WGP: $p < 0.0001$ (two-tailed *t*-test); (**D**) The number of intratubular protein cast formation in each microscopic view was counted in HE-stained section, and the average number of at least 20 randomly selected views under 40× magnification represented in each kidney; data are presented as mean ± SD of each group ($n = 12$); vehicle vs. WGP: $p = 0.0006$ (two-tailed *t*-test); (**E**) Tubular dilation and atrophy were determined using a 0–4 scale based on the percentage of damaged tubules occupying an area in each microscopic view; the average of at least 30 randomly selected views under 200× magnification represented the tubular atrophy in each kidney; data are presented as mean ± SD of each group ($n = 12$). Vehicle vs. WGP: $p = 0.0036$ (two-tailed *t*-test).

3.5. Daily Intake of WGP Is Associated with Increasing Local Antioxidant Defense in the Kidney of Obese Diabetic Rats

To understand the mechanisms by which the daily intake of WGP reduced the progression of kidney disease in these rats, the transcriptional profile of 84 genes that are involved in oxidative stress and antioxidant defense in the kidney was examined using PCR array. In the kidneys of WGP-fed rats compared to Vehicle controls, the expression levels of antioxidants (*Gpx1, Gpx4, Gstk1 and Prdx2*) and reactive oxygen species (ROS) metabolism (*Sod2, Cyba, Dhcr24 and Park7*) were significantly up-regulated while oxidative stress response genes (*Hmox1, Ercc6, Gstp1 and Txnip*) downregulated (Table S2 and Table 2). These results suggest an increase in antioxidant defense in the kidneys by WGP diet.

Table 2. Significant changes of oxidative stress-related gene expression in renal cortex of WGP-fed rats as compared to Vehicle controls, analyzed using PCR array.

Gene Symbol	Gene Names	Functions	Fold Change *	*p* Value ($n = 4$)
Dhcr24	24-dehydrocholesterol reductase	H_2O_2 scavenger, preventing H_2O_2-induced cell death	4.265	0.00222
Cyba	Cytochrome *b*-245, alpha polypeptide	NADPH oxidase subunit, optimizing immunity	4.215	0.00875
Gstk1	Glutathione S-transferase kappa 1	Cellular detoxification (lipid peroxide detoxification)	1.1475	0.01279
Prdx2	Peroxiredoxin 2	H_2O_2 and Alkyl hydroperoxide antioxidant	1.7625	0.02746
Sod2	Superoxide dismutase, mitochondrial	Limiting ROS detrimental effect, and moderating ROS release	2.3375	0.02983

Table 2. *Cont.*

Gene Symbol	Gene Names	Functions	Fold Change *	*p* Value (*n* = 4)
Park7	Parkinson disease (autosomal recessive, early onset) 7	Redox-sensitive chaperone	1.24	0.03723
Gpx4	Glutathione peroxidase 4	H_2O_2, lipid peroxide and hydroperoxide reduction	1.96	0.03756
Gpx1	Glutathione peroxidase 1	H_2O_2 antioxidant	3.235	0.04614
Hmox1	Heme oxygenase (decycling) 1	Heme degradation to CO	−101.533	0.01283
Ercc6	Excision repair cross-complementing rodent repair deficiency, complementation group 6	Damaged DNA repair	−3.9575	0.02908
Gstp1	Glutathione S-transferase pi 1	Cellular detoxification	−22.4875	0.0405
Txnip	Thioredoxin interacting protein	Increasing ROS production	−37.8825	0.04436

* Minus: decreased.

3.6. Addition of WGP Extract Reduced H_2O_2-Induced Cell Death in Cultured Podocytes

Podocyte injury plays a key role in the initiation and early progression of DN [32]. To investigate if the antioxidant compounds from WGP prevented podocyte injury under oxidative stress, the protective activity of WGP extract was tested in cultured podocytes in the presence of H_2O_2. Methanol extraction of WGP exhibited a high antioxidative activity, indicated by the equivalence of approximately 1.7 mg of the extract to 5 µg of ascorbic acid in all three different assays (Figure S1). H_2O_2 induced significant podocyte cell death through apoptosis (positive stain with Annexin-V) (Figure 5A). However, cells that were co-treated with WGP extract (200 mg·mL^{-1}) and H_2O_2 had significantly more cell viability than cells that were treated with H_2O_2 only (p = 0.037, two-tailed t-test, n = 8). The viability of cells treated with both H_2O_2 and WGP extract was not different from that in cultures treated with the extract only (p = 0.2732, two-tailed t-test. n = 8), suggesting that the extract significantly inhibited H_2O_2-induced cell death under this condition.

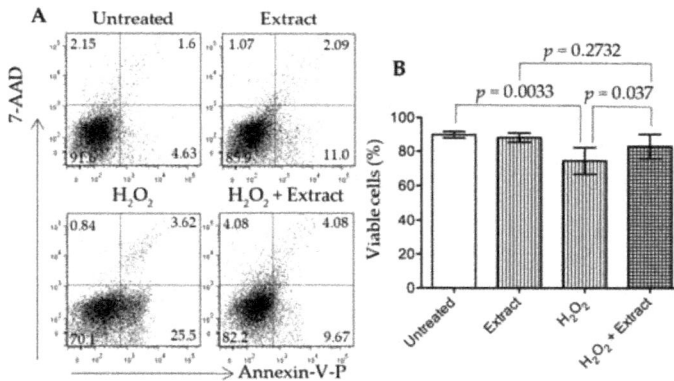

Figure 5. Grape extract protects cultured podocytes from H_2O_2-induced cell death. Grape extract was prepared by using methanol extraction. HSMP cells (0.25 × 10^6 cells/well) were grown in RPMI 1640 culture medium in 24-well plates at 37 °C overnight, followed by grape extract treatment (200 mg·mL^{-1}) in the presence or absence of H_2O_2 (1 µM). (**A**) Cell viability or apoptosis was determined by FACS analysis with Annexin-V-PE and 7-AAD staining after 24-h treatment with the grape extract. Data were represented as a typical FACS graph in each group; (**B**) Cell viability represented the percentage of viable cells (double-Annexin-V-PE/7-AAD negative cells in lower left quadrant). Data were presented as mean ± SD of eight separate experiments in each group. Untreated vs. H_2O_2, p = 0.0033 (two-tailed t-test); H_2O_2 vs. H_2O_2 + Extract, p = 0.037 (two-tailed t-test); or Extract vs. H_2O_2 + Extract, p = 0.2732 (two-tailed t-test).

4. Discussion

CKD is a major health problem in our society. In addition to pharmacological therapy, such as through angiotensin converting enzyme (ACE) inhibitors or angiotensin receptor blockers (ARB) for proteinuria and/or hypertension control, nutritional interventions have been widely recommended in the management of CKD [33]. A low-protein diet is a popular and practical nutritional management of CKD [34–36]. Interestingly, a recent pilot clinical study shows that dietary supplementation with two gram of grape seed extract a day for six months can improve some kidney function parameters of 2–4 stage CKD in patients, in which the grape seed extract likely acts through the strong antioxidative activity and anti-inflammation of phytochemicals [37]. This study may suggest that a diet containing the antioxidative grape extract can potentially become a nutritional management strategy for the prevention of CKD.

In the present study, when the rats started diet supplement at 8 weeks old, compared to the reference range [38] (Table S3), they had significant higher levels of blood GLU, BUN, TBIL, ALT, ALP and AMY, which may represent a sign of mild diabetes (higher GLU), pancreatic (higher AMY) and nonalcoholic fatty liver disease (higher ALT, ALP, TBIL and BUN). During six months of feeding experiments, the serum levels of AMY, Ca^{2+}, GLOB, GLU, Na^+, TBIL and TB were increased and of ALB (including ALB/GLOB ratio), ALP, BUN, K^+ and PHOS decreased in both groups (Table S1). These data may suggest progressively worsening diabetic (high GLU) and pancreatic (high AMY), fatty liver (high GLOB, TB and TBIL, low ALB and BUN), and kidney disease (low ALB or ALB/GLOB ratio for albumin loss, and the imbalance of Na^+, Ca^{2+}, K^+ and PHOS). When compared to the vehicle control group, with no difference in their bodyweight (Figure 1) the lower organ index of WGP-fed rats may indicate the reduced fatty liver, kidney hypertrophy and perhaps low-degree systemic immune response activity (indicated by the smaller size of the spleens) (Table 1). Further chemical tests showed that daily intake of WGP improved blood ALB and ALB/GLOB ratio and decreased GLU levels (Figure 2), and lower proteinuria, uPCR and urination (probably due to higher renal water reabsorption) (Figure 3). Histologically, we found that glomerular atrophy, mesangial expansion, tubular injury and protein cast formation, all of which are elevated in early stages of diabetic related CKD [39,40], were reduced in the WGP-fed rats (Figure 4). In vitro, the grape extract inhibited H_2O_2-induced cell death in cultured podocytes and exhibited a high antioxidative activity (Figure 5). In consistent with our study, a recently study demonstrates similar benefits of the grape powder to age-related kidney functions in Fischer 344 rats [21].

We described higher urine volumes in the vehicle fed rats versus WGP fed rats (Figure 3A), which may be due to either a manifestation of higher glycemic levels (Figure 2C) or worsened MetS, resulting in increasing hyperfiltration and renal injury. Hyperglycemia-induced hyperfiltration is an early manifestation of diabetes that causes polyuria and is an early predictor of glomerular damage in late stages of kidney disease [41–43]. While there was no evidence of better renal function (eGFR levels) in the WGP group (Figure 3D), this may have been due to the short duration of the study, since decline in GFR is a late marker of nephropathy when around 50% of nephrons are already lost [39,44]. The obese ZSF1 rats in this study indeed show the signs of early stages of CKD where an evidence of kidney damage such as proteinuria is present with normal or slightly decreased eGFR.

The renal protective pathway of WGP diet in obese diabetic ZSF1 rats is not fully understood. A previous study has demonstrated that the kidney disease of these rats is mostly independent on hypertension and/or hypertensive nephropathy [45], suggesting the attribution of renal pathophysiology strictly to other components of MetS, such as obesity and/or hyperglycemia. Indeed, many studies in literature use these rats as an appropriate model for the purposes of investigating MetS-related kidney disease or DN [28,46]. Our data show that the daily intake of WGP had no impact on the bodyweight or obesity of these rats (Figure 1). Therefore, the beneficial effect of WGP diet on the diseased kidney may act through direct and/or indirect pathways, which include the improvement of glucose metabolism and/or fatty liver disease (Figure 2), and the probability of suppressing low-degree immune response activity as indicated by the smaller size of the spleens

(Table 1), but not relate to hypertension and obesity. The mechanism by which a WGP diet protects the kidney under the influence of both diabetic mellitus and fatty liver disease remains unknown and requires further investigation.

Oxidative stress is induced by the excess levels of ROS that are generated in many different situations, including the mitochondrial injury [47], the increased activity of oxidases (e.g., cytochrome p450s, xanthine oxidase, 5-lipoxygenase, and NADPH oxidase) in the response to inflammatory stimuli (e.g., hypoxia and immunologic stimuli) [48–50] and the loss of antioxidant defense system that includes enzymes (e.g., SOD, CAT and GSH-Px) and small molecular antioxidant scavengers (e.g., vitamin E, N-acetylcysteine and α-lipoic acid) [51,52]. The oxidative stress or ROS causes cellular damage by reacting with and/or denaturing cellular macromolecules including lipid, protein and nucleic acids, and/or even mediating or activating intracellular death signaling pathways [53], which plays an important role in the pathogenesis and progression of diabetes, fatty liver disease and their associated CKD including DN [52,54–56]. Grape products are rich in antioxidant chemicals, such as phenolic, flavonoid, and anthocyanidin [57–59], and exhibit anti-oxidative activities in both humans and animals [37,60,61]. Our study showed that each gram of WGP extract from methanol extraction contained approximately 21.5 mg of phenolics (reference: tannic acid), 0.25 mg of total flavonoids (reference: quercetin) and 5.2 mg of proanthocyandins (reference: catechine). The antioxidative activity of approximately 1.7 mg of this extract was equivalent to that of 5 μg of ascorbic acid in all three different assays (ABTS, DPPH, and FRAP) (Figure S1), and addition of this extract prevented H_2O_2-induced podocyte injury in cultures (Figure 5). Consist with these data, the anti-oxidative stress system in the kidneys of the rats receiving WGP diet was improved (Table 2). Taken together, these findings from both the literature and our study imply that WGP diet may improve antioxidant capability not only systemically (e.g., in the liver and the immune system/spleen and glucose metabolism) but also locally specific in the kidneys, resulting in less cellular damage in the setting of MetS and CKD.

The US Department of Agriculture considers 1.5 to 2 cups (250 g to 340 g, or 3.125 $g \cdot kg^{-1}$ to 4.25 $g \cdot kg^{-1}$ based on 80 kg, an average bodyweight of an adult) of fresh grapes per day as a standard serving size. In this experimental study, each ZSF1 rat (300 g to 600 g) consumed an average of approximately 25 g of food or 1.25 g of WGP a day that was equal to 2.8 $g \cdot kg^{-1} \cdot day^{-1}$. There are two simple ways to converse this dose between rats and humans [62]; one is based on the equivalent surface area (1 for rats = 1/7 for humans), so that the equivalent dose for humans will be 2.8 $\times$ 1/7 = 0.4 $g \cdot kg^{-1}$; the other is based on the representative surface area to weight ratio (Km), whereas rat Km = 5.9 and human (adult) Km = 37, then the dose for adult humans will be 2.8 $\times$ (5.9/37) = 0.45 $g \cdot kg^{-1}$. The result from both calculations is similar. Given that grapes are approximately 80% water by weight, 0.45 $g \cdot kg^{-1}$ of WGP dose equals to 2.25 $g \cdot kg^{-1}$ of fresh grapes, indicating that the dose we used in this experimental study was less than the standard serving size recommended by the US Department of Agriculture.

There are several limitations of this study. First, this is an experimental study using a relatively small number of animals from one strain, so the results may just limit to this strain and disease type. It is not certain if the same results would be seen in different species, or in different models of kidney disease. Second, a relatively short duration of this study may not represent the most of metabolic conditions and strategies that require life-long exposure and long duration of intervention. Finally, if the findings of the renoprotective effects of WGP diet are possibly attributable to better glycemic control, so there is a need to test the WGP diet in non-diabetic animal models.

5. Conclusions

CKD has been known as an initially silent condition where clinical manifestations are usually underreported at its early stages. By the time SCr reaches abnormally high levels, there already is 50% nephron loss in the kidneys [44]. This highlights the importance of early stage management, such as lifestyle and dietary modifications, which may be able to improve disease prognosis [63]. In this experimental study, we demonstrate that a daily intake of WGP for six months shows renoprotection in a MetS animal model (obese diabetic ZSF1 rats), as evidenced by decreased proteinuria, lower uPCR, improved diabetic uremia and reduced renal injury in DN (early stages of CKD). Our findings suggest that a daily intake of grape product rich in antioxidants may delay the progression of early CKD to late or ESRD in humans, and warrants further investigation.

Supplementary Materials: The following are available online at http://www.mdpi.com/2072-6643/9/4/345/s1, Figure S1: Antioxidant activity of WGP extract, Table S1: The blood chemistry of obese male ZSF1 rats over six months of daily intake of whole grape powder (WGP) compared to sugar (Vehicle) group, Table S2: Oxidative stress-related gene expression in kidney cortex of WGP-fed rats compared to Vehicle controls at the end of six months of feeding experiment, Table S3: Blood chemistry of metabolism of obese male ZSF1 rats (approximately eight weeks old) compared with a reference in the literature [36].

Acknowledgments: This study was supported by a grant from the California Table Grape Commission (CA, USA); S.M.K.A. received the scholarship from King Abdullah Scholarship Program of the Kingdom of Saudi Arabia; P.L. the funding support from the Second Affiliated Hospital of Chongqing Medical University; and K.Y. the Canadian Mitacs Globalink Internship.

Author Contributions: A.L. and C.D. were responsible for the concept and design of the study; S.M.K.A., Q.G., P.L. and K.Y. for the lab work; S.M.K.A., Q.G., A.M.S., A.L. and C.D. for the data analysis and interpretation; S.M.K.A., A.M.S., A.L. and C.D. for drafting the article; and A.M.S., A.L. and C.D. for revising the article critically for intellectual content. All authors gave the approval of the final version to the manuscript.

Conflicts of Interest: The authors declare no potential conflicts of interest.

References

1.   Coresh, J.; Astor, B.C.; Greene, T.; Eknoyan, G.; Levey, A.S. Prevalence of chronic kidney disease and decreased kidney function in the adult us population: Third national health and nutrition examination survey. *Am. J. Kidney Dis.* **2003**, *41*, 1–12. [CrossRef] [PubMed]

2.   Levin, A.; Hemmelgarn, B.; Culleton, B.; Tobe, S.; McFarlane, P.; Ruzicka, M.; Burns, K.; Manns, B.; White, C.; Madore, F.; et al. Guidelines for the management of chronic kidney disease. *CMAJ* **2008**, *179*, 1154–1162. [CrossRef] [PubMed]

3.   Stigant, C.; Stevens, L.; Levin, A. Nephrology: 4. Strategies for the care of adults with chronic kidney disease. *CMAJ* **2003**, *168*, 1553–1560. [PubMed]

4.   Arora, P.; Vasa, P.; Brenner, D.; Iglar, K.; McFarlane, P.; Morrison, H.; Badawi, A. Prevalence estimates of chronic kidney disease in canada: Results of a nationally representative survey. *CMAJ* **2013**, *185*, E417–E423. [CrossRef] [PubMed]

5.   Levey, A.S.; Coresh, J. Chronic kidney disease. *Lancet* **2012**, *379*, 165–180. [CrossRef]

6.   Kaur, J. A comprehensive review on metabolic syndrome. *Cardiol. Res. Pract.* **2014**, *2014*, 943162. [CrossRef] [PubMed]

7.   Singh, A.K.; Kari, J.A. Metabolic syndrome and chronic kidney disease. *Curr. Opin. Nephrol. Hypertens.* **2013**, *22*, 198–203. [CrossRef] [PubMed]

8.   Prasad, G.V. Metabolic syndrome and chronic kidney disease: Current status and future directions. *World J. Nephrol.* **2014**, *3*, 210–219. [CrossRef] [PubMed]

9.   Thomas, G.; Sehgal, A.R.; Kashyap, S.R.; Srinivas, T.R.; Kirwan, J.P.; Navaneethan, S.D. Metabolic syndrome and kidney disease: A systematic review and meta-analysis. *Clin. J. Am. Soc. Nephrol.* **2011**, *6*, 2364–2373. [CrossRef] [PubMed]

10. Nashar, K.; Egan, B.M. Relationship between chronic kidney disease and metabolic syndrome: Current perspectives. *Diabetes Metab. Syndr. Obes.* **2014**, *7*, 421–435. [CrossRef] [PubMed]

11. Asmat, U.; Abad, K.; Ismail, K. Diabetes mellitus and oxidative stress-a concise review. *Saudi Pharm. J.* **2016**, *24*, 547–553. [CrossRef] [PubMed]

12. Betteridge, D.J. What is oxidative stress? *Metabolism* **2000**, *49*, 3–8. [CrossRef]

13. Sadowska-Bartosz, I.; Bartosz, G. Effect of antioxidants supplementation on aging and longevity. *Biomed. Res. Int.* **2014**, *2014*, 404680. [CrossRef] [PubMed]

14. Williamson, G.; Faulkner, K.; Plumb, G.W. Glucosinolates and phenolics as antioxidants from plant foods. *Eur. J. Cancer Prev.* **1998**, *7*, 17–21. [PubMed]

15. Vendrame, S.; Del Bo, C.; Ciappellano, S.; Riso, P.; Klimis-Zacas, D. Berry fruit consumption and metabolic syndrome. *Antioxidants (Basel)* **2016**, *5*, 34. [CrossRef] [PubMed]

16. Kowalska, K.; Olejnik, A. Current evidence on the health-beneficial effects of berry fruits in the prevention and treatment of metabolic syndrome. *Curr. Opin. Clin. Nutr. Metab. Care* **2016**, *19*, 446–452. [CrossRef] [PubMed]

17. El-Mowafy, A.M.; Salem, H.A.; Al-Gayyar, M.M.; El-Mesery, M.E.; El-Azab, M.F. Evaluation of renal protective effects of the green-tea (EGCG) and red grape resveratrol: Role of oxidative stress and inflammatory cytokines. *Nat. Prod. Res.* **2011**, *25*, 850–856. [CrossRef] [PubMed]

18. Sanchez-Gonzalez, P.D.; Lopez-Hernandez, F.J.; Perez-Barriocanal, F.; Morales, A.I.; Lopez-Novoa, J.M. Quercetin reduces cisplatin nephrotoxicity in rats without compromising its anti-tumour activity. *Nephrol. Dial. Transplant.* **2011**, *26*, 3484–3495. [CrossRef] [PubMed]

19. Tanabe, K.; Tamura, Y.; Lanaspa, M.A.; Miyazaki, M.; Suzuki, N.; Sato, W.; Maeshima, Y.; Schreiner, G.F.; Villarreal, F.J.; Johnson, R.J.; et al. Epicatechin limits renal injury by mitochondrial protection in cisplatin nephropathy. *Am. J. Physiol. Ren. Physiol.* **2012**, *303*, F1264–F1274. [CrossRef] [PubMed]

20. Li, J.; Kang, M.K.; Kim, J.K.; Kim, J.L.; Kang, S.W.; Lim, S.S.; Kang, Y.H. Purple corn anthocyanins retard diabetes-associated glomerulosclerosis in mesangial cells and db/db mice. *Eur. J. Nutr.* **2012**, *51*, 961–973. [CrossRef] [PubMed]

21. Pokkunuri, I.; Ali, Q.; Asghar, M. Grape powder improves age-related decline in mitochondrial and kidney functions in fischer 344 rats. *Oxid. Med. Cell. Longev.* **2016**, *2016*, 6135319. [CrossRef] [PubMed]

22. Laguardia, H.A.; Hamm, L.L.; Chen, J. The metabolic syndrome and risk of chronic kidney disease: Pathophysiology and intervention strategies. *J. Nutr. Metab.* **2012**, *2012*, 652608. [CrossRef] [PubMed]

23. Tofovic, S.P.; Kusaka, H.; Kost, C.K., Jr.; Bastacky, S. Renal function and structure in diabetic, hypertensive, obese ZDFxSHHF-hybrid rats. *Ren. Fail.* **2000**, *22*, 387–406. [CrossRef] [PubMed]

24. Baynes, J.; Murray, D.B. Cardiac and renal function are progressively impaired with aging in zucker diabetic fatty type II diabetic rats. *Oxid. Med. Cell. Longev.* **2009**, *2*, 328–334. [CrossRef] [PubMed]

25. Rafikova, O.; Salah, E.M.; Tofovic, S.P. Renal and metabolic effects of tempol in obese ZSF1 rats—Distinct role for superoxide and hydrogen peroxide in diabetic renal injury. *Metab. Clin. Exp.* **2008**, *57*, 1434–1444. [CrossRef] [PubMed]

26. Vora, J.P.; Zimsen, S.M.; Houghton, D.C.; Anderson, S. Evolution of metabolic and renal changes in the ZDF/DRT-fa rat model of type II diabetes. *J. Am. Soc. Nephrol.* **1996**, *7*, 113–117. [PubMed]

27. Tofovic, S.P.; Jackson, E.K. Rat models of the metabolic syndrome. *Methods Mol. Med.* **2003**, *86*, 29–46. [PubMed]

28. Bilan, V.P.; Salah, E.M.; Bastacky, S.; Jones, H.B.; Mayers, R.M.; Zinker, B.; Poucher, S.M.; Tofovic, S.P. Diabetic nephropathy and long-term treatment effects of rosiglitazone and enalapril in obese ZSF1 rats. *J. Endocrinol.* **2011**, *210*, 293–308. [CrossRef] [PubMed]

29. Tofovic, S.P.; Kusaka, H.; Jackson, E.K.; Bastacky, S.I. Renal and metabolic effects of caffeine in obese (fa/fa(cp)), diabetic, hypertensive ZSF1 rats. *Ren. Fail.* **2001**, *23*, 159–173. [CrossRef] [PubMed]

30. Zhang, X.; Jia, Y.; Jackson, E.K.; Tofovic, S.P. 2-methoxyestradiol and 2-ethoxyestradiol retard the progression of renal disease in aged, obese, diabetic ZSF1 rats. *J. Cardiovasc. Pharmacol.* **2007**, *49*, 56–63. [CrossRef] [PubMed]

31. Griffin, S.V.; Hiromura, K.; Pippin, J.; Petermann, A.T.; Blonski, M.J.; Krofft, R.; Takahashi, S.; Kulkarni, A.B.; Shankland, S.J. Cyclin-dependent kinase 5 is a regulator of podocyte differentiation, proliferation, and morphology. *Am. J. Pathol.* **2004**, *165*, 1175–1185. [CrossRef]

32. Brosius, F.C.; Coward, R.J. Podocytes, signaling pathways, and vascular factors in diabetic kidney disease. *Adv. Chronic Kidney Dis.* **2014**, *21*, 304–310. [CrossRef] [PubMed]

33. Anderson, C.A.; Nguyen, H.A.; Rifkin, D.E. Nutrition interventions in chronic kidney disease. *Med. Clin. N. Am.* **2016**, *100*, 1265–1283. [CrossRef] [PubMed]

34. Chan, M. Protein-controlled versus restricted protein versus low protein diets in managing patients with non-dialysis chronic kidney disease: A single centre experience in Australia. *BMC Nephrol.* **2016**, *17*, 129. [CrossRef] [PubMed]

35. Shah, B.V.; Patel, Z.M. Role of low protein diet in management of different stages of chronic kidney disease—Practical aspects. *BMC Nephrol.* **2016**, *17*, 156. [CrossRef] [PubMed]

36. Wang, M.; Chou, J.; Chang, Y.; Lau, W.L.; Reddy, U.; Rhee, C.M.; Chen, J.; Hao, C.; Kalantar-Zadeh, K. The role of low protein diet in ameliorating proteinuria and deferring dialysis initiation: What is old and what is new. *Panminerva Med.* **2017**, *59*, 157–165. [PubMed]

37. Turki, K.; Charradi, K.; Boukhalfa, H.; Belhaj, M.; Limam, F.; Aouani, E. Grape seed powder improves renal failure of chronic kidney disease patients. *EXCLI J.* **2016**, *15*, 424–433. [PubMed]

38. Bernardi, C.; Moneta, D.; Brughera, M.; DiSalvo, M.; Lamparelli, D.; Mazue, G.; Iatropoulos, M.J. Haematology and clinical chemistry in rats: Comparison of different blood collection sites. *Comp. Haematol. Int.* **1996**, *6*, 160–166. [CrossRef]

39. Vassalotti, J.A.; Stevens, L.A.; Levey, A.S. Testing for chronic kidney disease: A position statement from the national kidney foundation. *Am. J. Kidney Dis.* **2007**, *50*, 169–180. [CrossRef] [PubMed]

40. Arici, M. *Management of Chronic Kidney Disease: A Clinician's Guide*; Springer: Berlin/Heidelberg, Germany, 2014.

41. Spira, A.; Gowrishankar, M.; Halperin, M.L. Factors contributing to the degree of polyuria in a patient with poorly controlled diabetes mellitus. *Am. J. Kidney Dis.* **1997**, *30*, 829–835. [CrossRef]

42. Ahloulay, M.; Schmitt, F.; Dechaux, M.; Bankir, L. Vasopressin and urinary concentrating activity in diabetes mellitus. *Diabetes Metab.* **1999**, *25*, 213–222. [PubMed]

43. Mogensen, C.E. Early glomerular hyperfiltration in insulin-dependent diabetics and late nephropathy. *Scand. J. Clin. Lab. Investig.* **1986**, *46*, 201–206. [CrossRef]

44. Ahmed, S.; Lowder, G. Severity and stages of chronic kidney disease. *Age* **2012**, *140*, 13–25.

45. Griffin, K.A.; Abu-Naser, M.; Abu-Amarah, I.; Picken, M.; Williamson, G.A.; Bidani, A.K. Dynamic blood pressure load and nephropathy in the ZSF1 (fa/fa cp) model of type 2 diabetes. *Am. J. Physiol. Renal. Physiol.* **2007**, *293*, F1605–F1613. [CrossRef] [PubMed]

46. Tofovic, S.P.; Salah, E.M.; Jackson, E.K.; Melhem, M. Early renal injury induced by caffeine consumption in obese, diabetic zsf1 rats. *Ren. Fail.* **2007**, *29*, 891–902. [CrossRef] [PubMed]

47. Rocha, M.; Hernandez-Mijares, A.; Garcia-Malpartida, K.; Banuls, C.; Bellod, L.; Victor, V.M. Mitochondria-targeted antioxidant peptides. *Curr. Pharm. Des.* **2010**, *16*, 3124–3131. [CrossRef] [PubMed]

48. Novo, E.; Parola, M. Redox mechanisms in hepatic chronic wound healing and fibrogenesis. *Fibrogenesis Tissue Repair* **2008**, *1*, 5. [CrossRef] [PubMed]

49. Babior, B.M. NADPH oxidase: An update. *Blood* **1999**, *93*, 1464–1476. [PubMed]

50. Forman, H.J.; Torres, M. Redox signaling in macrophages. *Mol. Aspects Med.* **2001**, *22*, 189–216. [CrossRef]

51. Birben, E.; Sahiner, U.M.; Sackesen, C.; Erzurum, S.; Kalayci, O. Oxidative stress and antioxidant defense. *World Allergy Organ. J.* **2012**, *5*, 9–19. [CrossRef] [PubMed]

52. Du, C.; Wang, X.; Chen, H. Oxidative stress to renal tubular epithelial cells—A common pathway in renal pathologies. In *Systems Biology of Free Radicals and Anti-Oxidants*; Laher, I., Ed.; Springer: Berlin/Heidelberg, Germany, 2014; pp. 2606–2624.

53. Rhee, S.G. Redox signaling: Hydrogen peroxide as intracellular messenger. *Exp. Mol. Med.* **1999**, *31*, 53–59. [CrossRef] [PubMed]

54. Turkmen, K. Inflammation, oxidative stress, apoptosis, and autophagy in diabetes mellitus and diabetic kidney disease: The four horsemen of the apocalypse. *Int. Urol. Nephrol.* **2016**. [CrossRef] [PubMed]

55. Sunny, N.E.; Bril, F.; Cusi, K. Mitochondrial adaptation in nonalcoholic fatty liver disease: Novel mechanisms and treatment strategies. *Trends Endocrinol. Metab.* **2017**, *28*, 250–260. [CrossRef] [PubMed]

56. Newsholme, P.; Cruzat, V.F.; Keane, K.N.; Carlessi, R.; de Bittencourt, P.I., Jr. Molecular mechanisms of ROS production and oxidative stress in diabetes. *Biochem. J.* **2016**, *473*, 4527–4550. [CrossRef] [PubMed]

57. Yilmaz, Y.; Toledo, R.T. Major flavonoids in grape seeds and skins: Antioxidant capacity of catechin, epicatechin, and gallic acid. *J. Agric. Food Chem.* **2004**, *52*, 255–260. [CrossRef] [PubMed]

58. Ross, C.F.; Hoye, C., Jr.; Fernandez-Plotka, V.C. Influence of heating on the polyphenolic content and antioxidant activity of grape seed flour. *J. Food Sci.* **2011**, *76*, C884–C890. [CrossRef] [PubMed]

59. Yang, J.; Xiao, Y.Y. Grape phytochemicals and associated health benefits. *Crit. Rev. Food Sci. Nutr.* **2013**, *53*, 1202–1225. [CrossRef] [PubMed]

60. Aloui, F.; Charradi, K.; Hichami, A.; Subramaniam, S.; Khan, N.A.; Limam, F.; Aouani, E. Grape seed and skin extract reduces pancreas lipotoxicity, oxidative stress and inflammation in high fat diet fed rats. *Biomed. Pharmacother.* **2016**, *84*, 2020–2028. [CrossRef] [PubMed]

61. Oueslati, N.; Charradi, K.; Bedhiafi, T.; Limam, F.; Aouani, E. Protective effect of grape seed and skin extract against diabetes-induced oxidative stress and renal dysfunction in virgin and pregnant rat. *Biomed. Pharmacother.* **2016**, *83*, 584–592. [CrossRef] [PubMed]

62. Freireich, E.J.; Gehan, E.A.; Rall, D.P.; Schmidt, L.H.; Skipper, H.E. Quantitative comparison of toxicity of anticancer agents in mouse, rat, hamster, dog, monkey, and man. *Cancer Chemother. Rep.* **1966**, *50*, 219–244. [PubMed]

63. Johnson, D.W. Evidence-based guide to slowing the progression of early renal insufficiency. *Intern. Med. J.* **2004**, *34*, 50–57. [CrossRef] [PubMed]

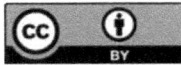

nutrients

MDPI

Review

Effects of Ketogenic Diets on Cardiovascular Risk Factors: Evidence from Animal and Human Studies

Christophe Kosinski [1] **and François R. Jornayvaz** [2,*]

[1] Service of Endocrinology, Diabetes and Metabolism, Lausanne University Hospital (CHUV), Avenue de la Sallaz 8, 1011 Lausanne, Switzerland; christophe.kosinski@chuv.ch

[2] Service of Endocrinology, Diabetes, Hypertension and Nutrition, Geneva University Hospitals, Rue Gabrielle-Perret-Gentil 4, 1205 Geneva, Switzerland

* Correspondence: françois.jornayvaz@hcuge.ch; Tel.: +41-22-372-9302

Received: 7 March 2017; Accepted: 16 May 2017; Published: 19 May 2017

Abstract: The treatment of obesity and cardiovascular diseases is one of the most difficult and important challenges nowadays. Weight loss is frequently offered as a therapy and is aimed at improving some of the components of the metabolic syndrome. Among various diets, ketogenic diets, which are very low in carbohydrates and usually high in fats and/or proteins, have gained in popularity. Results regarding the impact of such diets on cardiovascular risk factors are controversial, both in animals and humans, but some improvements notably in obesity and type 2 diabetes have been described. Unfortunately, these effects seem to be limited in time. Moreover, these diets are not totally safe and can be associated with some adverse events. Notably, in rodents, development of nonalcoholic fatty liver disease (NAFLD) and insulin resistance have been described. The aim of this review is to discuss the role of ketogenic diets on different cardiovascular risk factors in both animals and humans based on available evidence.

Keywords: ketogenic diets; obesity; NAFLD; fibroblast growth factor (FGF21); insulin resistance; type 2 diabetes; cardiovascular risk factors

1. Introduction

As a consequence of the rising obesity prevalence in industrialized countries, the incidence of cardiovascular diseases also increases [1]. Obesity is also a major risk factor for insulin resistance and type 2 diabetes [2]. This state of insulin resistance is frequently associated with ectopic lipid accumulation, notably in the liver and skeletal muscle. This can lead to the development of nonalcoholic fatty liver disease (NAFLD), which is an independent predictor of cardiovascular disease [3,4]. NAFLD is defined as steatosis which is not due to excess consumption of alcohol, viral or autoimmune causes, and iron overload [5,6]. No evidence-based pharmacological treatment for NAFLD exists so far. NAFLD is an important risk factor for the development of insulin resistance and type 2 diabetes, which may be associated with other cardiovascular risk factors such as dyslipidemia and high blood pressure. As NAFLD is present in almost 90% of obese patients [7], weight loss represents one of the pillars of the treatments among others, such as physical activity.

In the literature, diets rich in carbohydrates, and notably rich in refined sugars and fructose, are associated with the metabolic syndrome [8,9]. Therefore, to lose weight, different diets have been suggested. Among them, carbohydrate restriction has been proposed to be the single most effective intervention for reducing all features of the metabolic syndrome [10–12]. Since the publication of Atkins's book in the early 1970s [13], low-carbohydrate diets have become increasingly popular, particularly ketogenic diets (KD). These diets are known for being very low in carbohydrates, but usually high in fats and/or proteins. In practice, KD are characterized by a reduction in carbohydrates (usually less than 50 g/day) and a relative increase in the proportions of proteins and fats [14]. Some variations exist, like very-low-carbohydrate KD, which are even more restrictive, with less than 30 g/day (Table 1).

Table 1. Standard composition of ketogenic diets in adults * (calculated for a 2000 kcal diet/day).

Classical KD	Defined as <130 g carbohydrate per day or <26% of caloric intake by the American Diabetes Association
Modified Atkins Diet	65% caloric intake from fat, 30% protein, 6% carbohydrates
Very low-carbohydrate KD	Carbohydrates < 30 g/day

KD, Ketogenic Diet. * Adapted from Kossoff et al. [15], Feinman et al. [16], Accurso et al. [17].

After a few days of such diets, glucose reserves (i.e., glycogen stored in liver and skeletal muscle) become insufficient to provide body energy needs. This leads to the production of ketone bodies by the liver, which will be used as an alternative energy source notably by the central nervous system [18].

KD are known to be efficient in the treatment of seizures and can be used as an alternative treatment [19], but this aspect will not be discussed in this review. Nevertheless, for about forty years, the potential use of KD has also been investigated in the prevention and treatment of cardiovascular risk factors. The aim of this review is to discuss the available evidence in animal and human studies, and the role of KD on different cardiovascular risk factors, namely obesity, NAFLD, insulin resistance and type 2 diabetes, dyslipidemia and high blood pressure. To our knowledge, this is the first review comparing the effects of KD on cardiovascular risk factors in animals and humans.

2. Method

This article is neither a systematic review nor a meta-analysis. We searched Medline (PubMed) for trials in animals and humans, reviews or meta-analyses, using the query "ketogenic diet" + "weight loss", "obesity", "fibroblast growth factor (FGF21)", "NAFLD", "diabetes", "insulin resistance", "dyslipidemia" or "blood pressure". Then, we selected the most recent papers (less than 15 years) and publications with potential practical usefulness. Finally, we only kept studies of adults, not children.

3. Results

3.1. KD and Obesity

Studies in rodents (obese or non obese) show that KD are efficient for weight loss [20,21]. Nevertheless, it is important to assess body composition changes, as it is always better to lose fat mass than lean mass. Indeed, in a study by Garbow et al., after 12 weeks KD led to a significantly lower weight gain compared to chow-fed and high-simple-carbohydrate high-fat Western diet fed mice, but lean mass was significantly reduced in KD-fed mice compared to chow-fed mice [22]. In another study, accumulation of visceral fat mass was significantly higher (at least 30%) in rats fed a KD (two compositions of KD were tested: a high-protein "Atkins-style" or a low-protein diet, both with a low-carbohydrate and high-fat content), compared with chow-fed controls, after 4 weeks of diet [23]. Finally, Jornayvaz et al. showed that KD-fed mice during 5 weeks gained significantly less weight than regular-chow fed mice. Nevertheless, KD-fed mice had an increased fat mass percentage than regular-chow fed mice, without differences in the percentage of lean body mass between diets [24].

It is also important to assess whether weight loss can be maintained. Long-term studies reveal an absence of weight loss after 22 weeks of KD in mice, despite an initial weight loss during the first week of diet [25]. Moreover, another study showed that mice fed a KD for 80 weeks initially lost weight, but after 18 weeks, their weight returned to baseline and then increased gradually [26]. Nevertheless, they gained less weight than chow-fed mice, and, with body composition analysis, the authors showed that this difference resulted from both a lower lean mass and a lower fat mass. Moreover, the survival curves were the same between the two diets. Finally, KD-fed mice also had an increased energy expenditure and a loss of the diurnal pattern of the respiratory exchange ratio, which indicated continuous use of fatty acids as an energy substrate [26]. This rise in energy expenditure was analyzed in another study which showed that KD promotes weight loss (20% of total body weight) through an increased energy expenditure and this correlated with a rise in plasma fibroblast growth factor 21 (FGF21) levels [27]. The role of FGF21 in KD will be further discussed later. In another study, compared to non-KD, rats fed a low protein (10% of total content) KD had a waste of energy in urine. [28]. Indeed, KD-fed rats had a lower urine nitrogen excretion due to a lower protein intake and a urine energy-to-nitrogen ratio almost twice as high as the other diets.

Overall, an increase in energy expenditure in mice fed a KD compared to mice fed a chow diet could be the mechanism responsible for decreased weight gain or weight loss seen in rodents, despite a similar caloric intake [24]. As a potential component of the increased energy expenditure, other authors performed microarrays in the liver of KD-fed mice and described an increased expression of genes involved in fatty acid oxidation and a reduced expression in genes involved in lipid synthesis [20].

A recent study analyzed the effects of KD on exercising rats and sedentary rats [29]. Compared to other diets (Western diet, standard chow), after 6 weeks, sedentary KD-fed rats had an approximately 25% lower body mass, a lower size of adipocytes from omental adipose tissue, 80% lower levels of serum insulin, 50% lower levels of glucose, 55% lower levels of triglycerides and 20% lower levels of total cholesterol. Activity did not confer a benefit, as KD-fed exercising rats did not show better results than the sedentary rats. Nevertheless, exercising rats had 40% lower serum β-hydroxybutyrate levels than sedentary rats, independent of diet, while they had more favorable adipose tissue characteristics. These results suggest that body fat regulation (e.g., reduced adipose tissue mass and cell size) under a KD (with or without exercise) could rather be due to lower insulin levels. Therefore, increased serum ketones may have a smaller role.

In humans, KD are known to be an effective weight-loss therapy [30–33] (in average up to 5% of body weight at 6 months), but the mechanisms are not clearly established. Some authors suggest that it results simply from reduced caloric intake and an increased satiety effect of proteins [34]. Other studies suggest a metabolic effect of KD: possibly, the use of energy from proteins in KD is an expensive process and therefore increases weight loss [35–37]. Also, there is the suggestion that gluconeogenesis, which is increased with carbohydrate restriction, is energy demanding [35,38]. Another hypothesis of KD-induced weight loss is decreased appetite induced by ketosis [39]. Some authors also suggest digestive metabolic changes: with ketogenic very-low energy diets, ghrelin levels and subjective appetite (usually increased in a hypocaloric diet) were reduced when patients were in a ketotic state [39]. Surprisingly, leptin levels were lower under ketosis. A study in 132 severely obese patients (mean body mass index (BMI) 43 kg/m^2) with a high prevalence of type 2 diabetes or metabolic syndrome showed that participants using a low-carbohydrate diet lost more weight than those using other diets, suggesting a greater reduction in overall caloric intake, rather than a direct effect of macronutrient composition [32].

As discussed in rodents, the problem is that a lot of studies are of short duration. For example, a small study [40] of 17 obese men, randomized to two different high-protein diets (one low-carbohydrate, "ketogenic"; one medium-carbohydrate, "non-ketogenic") with a cross-over design, eating ad libitum during 4 weeks each, revealed that KD reduced hunger and was associated with a lower food intake. Weight loss was also significantly greater with the ketogenic diet than with the non-ketogenic diet, and weight loss was equally comprised of fat mass and fat-free mass. Only 35% of the difference in total weight loss between the two diets was due to water depletion; the remainder was attributed to fat mass and lean mass loss [40]. In a bigger study of 311 participants [41], a very low-carbohydrate KD followed by a period of slow re-insertion of a Mediterranean diet and alimentary education was associated with an overall improvement (mean total body weight loss of 14 ± 10 kg, BMI 5 ± 3 kg/m^2, waist circumference 13 ± 7 cm) at 1–4 months, which remained stable after 1 year [41]. The limitations were the composition of the diet (low-carbohydrate, but also low-fat) and the fact that it was an observational study. Other authors [42] compared different diets in the same group of patients eating alternatively a KD (two different periods of 20 days), a low-carbohydrate non-KD (two different periods of 20 days), and a normal Mediterranean diet (4 months during the rotation of the two other diets, then 6 months) during 1 year. Significant weight loss and reduction of body fat percentages were observed only during ketogenic periods compared to the two other diets. Moreover, if the patients were compliant to the prescribed Mediterranean diet (which was relatively strict: 1800 kcal/day) during the maintenance period, no weight regain was observed at 12 months [42]. In an older study in obese non-diabetic participants, a low-carbohydrate diet led to a greater weight loss after 6 months, but no significant difference at 1 year [33]. The authors suggested that weight loss was probably due to a greater energy deficit, but the mechanisms remain unknown, and no relation between weight loss and ketosis was found at any time during the study. Finally, in a study with obese type 2 diabetes patients [43], the authors compared a low-carbohydrate high unsaturated fat diet to a high-carbohydrate low-fat diet, in adjunction with structured exercise: weight loss was similar in both groups (−9.1%), but a trend toward regaining more weight was observed in the low-carbohydrate diet group at 52 weeks. Weight loss is usually related to a high intensity of lifestyle interventions. Thus, it would be interesting to know the evolution on the next months/years of follow-up, and if the weight loss would be maintained without structured exercise. Exercise has an impact on body weight, but also on body composition as described in a study that analyzed the association of KD or regular diet in combination with exercise (resistance training) in overweight women [44]. The KD group lost fat mass without experiencing a significant alteration in lean mass, while the other group gained lean mass without a significant change in fat mass [44].

To summarize, in rodents and humans, KD seem to have a benefit on weight loss, notably by increased energy expenditure in animals and decreasing food intake in humans. In humans, weight loss affects both fat mass and lean mass. Greater weight loss is also associated with structured professional support, which may be difficult and expensive to maintain over time. Long-term studies are nevertheless needed to assess the evolution of weight loss.

3.2. KD and NAFLD

In mice, KD induce hepatic inflammation and lipid accumulation [22], while inflammation is reduced in white adipose tissue [27]. KD also lead to hepatic steatosis in both short-term [24,25] and long-term feeding in mice [26]. Biological markers such as aspartate aminotransferase (AST) and alanine aminotransferase (ALT) are increased at least twofold in parallel with increased intrahepatic triglyceride content [24,25]. On the contrary, a study described that compared to other diets (Western diet, standard chow), KD-fed mice display reduced ALT levels, hepatic triglyceride accumulation and markers of liver inflammation [29]. The authors explained that these results, different from previous studies, could be due to the protein content of the diet (they used a KD with 20% protein, versus <10% in other studies) and differences in animal models (rat in this study, versus mice in others). Thus, this shows the importance of the diet's composition. Another study reported an increase in hepatic triglyceride content in KD-fed mice after 12 weeks, and this correlated with an elevation in ALT levels, suggesting that chronic KD feeding causes an injury pattern similar to a NAFLD phenotype [22]. Another interesting marker of NAFLD is FGF21. In humans, FGF21 levels are increased in NAFLD and correlate with hepatic triglyceride content [45–47]. Nevertheless, the role of FGF21 in NAFLD induced by a KD has mostly been studied in rodents [26,27,48,49]. Notably, a study in mice showed that FGF21 plasma levels and liver expression are increased by 5 weeks of KD feeding, and this was accompanied by an increased hepatic fat content as revealed by increased hepatic triglycerides, diacylglycerols and ceramides levels [24]. Moreover, KD-fed mice developed hepatic insulin resistance and this was due to increased hepatic diacylglycerol content, as diacylglycerols are known to activate protein kinase Cε [50]. In this study [24], the authors suggested that increased plasma FGF21 levels and hepatic expression in KD-fed mice was probably secondary to hepatic fat accumulation and may represent a compensatory mechanism to counteract hepatic insulin resistance, suggesting that FGF21 may be beneficial in reversing hepatic insulin resistance. This has been further verified in high-fat diet fed mice treated with exogenous FGF21. In a study in wild-type mice, FGF21 decreased hepatic fat content, notably hepatic diacylglycerol content, and improved hepatic insulin sensitivity [51]. The beneficial role of FGF21 on hepatic insulin sensitivity was also shown by other authors [52]. Moreover, mice lacking FGF21 gain weight, have an increased fat mass and develop glucose intolerance. Moreover, when the chow diet was changed for a KD, these mice not only gained weight and developed glucose intolerance, but also developed NAFLD [53]. Finally, another study revealed that FGF21 knock-out mice fed a KD develop NAFLD and severe hepatic insulin resistance as assessed by the gold-standard technique, the hyperinsulinemic-euglycemic clamp [54]. Finally, FGF21 has been shown to act as an endocrine signal of protein restriction [55]. In summary, these studies suggest an important role of FGF21 in the pathophysiology of NAFLD.

In humans, liver fat content was shown to be increased during an isocaloric high-fat low-carbohydrate diet [56]. This result should be analyzed with caution, as with 31% of carbohydrates the diet is not a "real" KD. Caloric restriction also had an impact: compared to the high-carbohydrate ("standard") hypocaloric diet, reduction of liver fat content was significantly higher with the hypocaloric low-carbohydrate diet [57,58]. This effect was limited in time, with no significant difference at 11 weeks [57]. KD have also been associated with a higher decrease in liver volume compared with a standard hypocaloric diet, probably due to the depletion of liver glycogen [59]. Finally, the response to KD may be influenced by genetic predisposition to NAFLD, as shown by two studies with a better response to KD for patients with variants of the PNPLA3 gene [60,61]. When fed a KD, subjects with PNPLA3 variants had a lower liver fat content than controls.

To summarize, the effect of KD on the liver was mostly investigated in rodents. The results are rather negative, with induction of hepatic inflammation and NAFLD, but these findings have not been reported in humans. An alteration of FGF21 expression could be a potential cause or consequence. More studies are warranted in humans to assess whether KD could induce or improve NAFLD.

3.3. KD and Insulin Resistance / Type 2 Diabetes

Obesity is often associated with the development of NAFLD, insulin resistance and type 2 diabetes. Notably, as already discussed, KD can lead to decreased weight gain in mice but with concomitant development of NAFLD and associated hepatic insulin resistance [24]. In the latter study, mice fed a KD for 5 weeks developed whole body insulin resistance despite reduced basal plasma glucose and insulin levels. In this case, the use of indices of insulin sensitivity, such as the homeostatic model assessment for insulin resistance (HOMA-IR) and quantitative insulin-sensitivity check index (QUICKI) indices, would lead to the conclusion that insulin sensitivity is improved in KD fed mice [62]. However, using the hyperinsulinemic-euglycemic clamp, glucose infusion rates were 47% lower in KD-fed mice than in chow-fed mice, demonstrating whole body insulin resistance in KD-fed mice [24]. KD-fed mice also had an impaired insulin ability to suppress endogenous glucose production confirming insulin resistance at the level of the liver. In this case, KD induced severe hepatic insulin resistance in mice despite lower body weight gain, and this was attributed to an increased hepatic diacylglycerol content. Finally, insulin resistance was also attributed to a decreased insulin-stimulated whole body glucose disposal, which was notably due to decreased glucose uptake in brown adipose tissue and the heart [24].

In another study, mice fed a KD during 12 weeks remained euglycemic, but had reduced mean serum insulin levels and HOMA-IR indices, and exhibited glucose intolerance as assessed by intra-peritoneal glucose tolerance tests [22]. However, despite mild hepatic steatosis, systemic response to insulin was preserved, unlike in other studies. The authors explained this discrepancy by a relatively reduced lean body mass in KD-fed mice, resulting in higher insulin dose in insulin-tolerance tests. Also, hepatic insulin resistance may confer a smaller contribution to overall glucose homeostasis than peripheral glucose disposal [22]. In studies using rats, KD also induced glucose intolerance and insulin resistance [23,63], despite reduced glucose and insulin levels [23]. In the latter study, the authors showed that these effects were not due to energy overconsumption. Moreover, as KD-fed rats had a significant accumulation of visceral fat, the effects on glucose homeostasis were not dependent upon visceral fat mass. In the same study, short term KD feeding in rats was also associated with decreased β-cell mass, but this effect could be due to a lower lean body mass of KD fed rats [23]. Nevertheless, these findings were corroborated by another study where long term KD feeding in mice led to glucose intolerance that was associated with insufficient insulin secretion from β-cells, potentially due to a decrease in β-cell mass [25]. Interestingly, after only 6 days of KD feeding, mice showed impairments in glucose tolerance and insulin sensitivity, and this was attributed to a possible adaptation to maintain blood glucose levels against insufficient amounts of carbohydrates [48]. In this case, insulin signaling was impaired only in white adipose tissue, but not in liver and muscle. The authors suggested that this impairment in white adipose tissue could not be the only culprit for whole body glucose intolerance in KD fed mice. Indeed, a low-carbohydrate diet might account for an impaired nutritional state compared to a chow diet. These results were explained by a lower lean mass and a proportionally higher insulin dose in insulin tolerance tests. The possible role of KD in inducing insulin resistance is nevertheless controversial. Indeed, several authors reported that long term KD fed mice had normal glucose tolerance, lower baseline insulin levels and improved insulin sensitivity [26,29].

In humans, the effect of KD on glucose homeostasis is more controversial, and notably depends on the presence of type 2 diabetes or not at baseline. A study showed that a high-fat, low-carbohydrate intake reduces the ability of insulin to suppress endogenous glucose production in healthy men, by using the gold standard method, the hyperinsulinemic-euglycemic clamp [64]. The limitation is the small number of participants (only 6). Other studies described the opposite: with a KD, obese non-diabetic participants had a significant lower HOMA-IR and fasting glucose after a KD than at baseline [40], and an improvement in insulin sensitivity using the QUICKI [32]. Finally, another trial also described a better insulin sensitivity by consuming a KD [33], but this improvement does not seem to be permanent. Indeed, Forster et al. found a significant improvement in insulin sensitivity at 6 months, but not at 1 year [33]. This reduction in insulin levels could be explained by the satietogenic effect of this diet [65].

In type 2 diabetic patients, KD could be an interesting approach, as most patients have glycemic variability due to food carbohydrate content. A lot of studies have been designed around this purpose. KD are frequently associated with a diminution of blood glucose levels (up to 0.5 mmol/L) [41,66–68], glycosylated hemoglobin (HbA1c (up to 0.3%) [41,66,68,69], glycemic variability [70] and improvement in insulin sensitivity [32,68], sometimes without weight loss [67]. Low-carbohydrate diets can lead to a reduction in medications in type 2 diabetic patients [69–74]. An important aspect is to assess the long-term effect of a KD on these outcomes. In studies in obese type 2 diabetic patients fed a KD, a significant improvement in fasting glucose levels was seen after 12 weeks and continued after 56 weeks [75]. Nevertheless, in another study, a short-term decrease in HbA1c was observed at 6 months, but was not sustained at 24 months [76]. The latter study is probably more relevant to daily clinical practice because it was a low-intensity intervention. A recent study in obese type 2 diabetic patients compared a hypocaloric high-unsaturated/low-saturated fat very-low-carbohydrate diet to a high-carbohydrate low-fat diet [43]. After 52 weeks, the low-carbohydrate diet group showed a decrease in glycemic variability two times greater that the low-fat diet group, which indicates a greater diurnal blood glucose stability. However, improvement in HbA1c was similar in both diets (−1%). Nevertheless, the low-carbohydrate diet led to a greater reduction in antidiabetic medications, which could overall be helpful to optimize glycemic control [43]. Still, long-term effects of such dietary changes need to be evaluated.

In a prospective cohort of non-diabetic men, health professionals younger than 65 years old followed during 20 years, a low-carbohydrate diet high in animal proteins and fats was associated with a twofold increased risk of type 2 diabetes [77]. On the other hand, a low-carbohydrate diet high in vegetal proteins and fats was associated with a decreased risk of type 2 diabetes [77]. These findings suggest that a low-carbohydrate diet should contain proteins and fats from foods other than red and processed meat. However, these results were found from non-ketogenic diets. Therefore, further studies with "vegetal versus animal protein and fat content" KD are necessary to assess if these assumptions are validated. In another trial [32], a greater decrease of mean fasting glucose levels (−9%) was observed in all subjects of the low-carbohydrate group, but was significant only in diabetic patients (−15%), with more reduction of oral hypoglycemic agents or insulin in the low-carbohydrate group. Interestingly, in a study in obese non diabetic patients, after 8 weeks, a very-low-energy KD led to a rise in postprandial glucose levels, but not in fasting glucose levels [39]. The authors postulated that KD reduces insulin ability to suppress endogenous glucose production and impairs insulin-stimulated glucose oxidation, suggesting that there may be a different effect of ketosis on glucose homeostasis between diabetic and non-diabetic patients. For example, in obese type 2 diabetic patients, a strong inverse correlation between circulating ketones and hepatic glucose output has been described [78], suggesting that higher levels of ketones are associated with more favorable effects on glycemic control in these subjects.

An interesting study using biology systems approaches found a strong relationship between the insulin resistance pathway and the ketosis main pathway, providing a possible explanation for the improvement in glucose homeostasis found in clinical trials using low-carbohydrate diets. Notably, maps analyses suggest a direct implication of glucose transporters and inflammatory processes [79].

In summary, in rodents, KD mostly induces insulin resistance and glucose intolerance, while in type 2 diabetic humans KD is associated with a better control in glucose homeostasis and a reduction in antidiabetic medications. Nevertheless, these improvements seem to be limited in time. Further studies should evaluate if a higher weight loss correlates with a better glucose control or with higher ketones levels.

3.4. KD and Dyslipidemia

Dyslipidemia is a well-known risk factor for cardiovascular diseases. As KD are usually high in fats, it is necessary to assess their potential effect on the lipid profile.

In rodents, short term (14 days) studies showed no change in fatty acids and triglycerides levels in mice fed a KD [48]. The duration and the composition of KD feeding are very important. In a study of 4 weeks, Bielohuby et al. compared the effects on rats of chow diet and two different KD: one with 78.7% fat, 19.1% protein, 2.2% carbohydrates, and the other with 92.8% fat, 5.5% protein, 1.7% carbohydrates. The very high-fat KD-fed group had a reduction in high-density lipoproteins (HDL) cholesterol levels and higher triglycerides levels. No significant difference in total cholesterol levels was found between the three groups [23]. It should be noticed that the authors did not mention the effect on low-density lipoproteins (LDL) cholesterol levels. In another study, Jornayvaz et al. showed that mice fed a KD during 5 weeks had similar levels of LDL cholesterol than mice fed a chow diet [24]. In longer term (28–80 weeks) studies, KD fed mice displayed a twofold increase in plasma total cholesterol and triglyceride levels [25,26]. On the opposite, a recent study reported that mice fed a KD during 6 weeks had lower total cholesterol and triglycerides levels than with other diets [29]. The authors suggested that there was a KD-induced reduction in insulin levels, which further decreased liver fatty acids and cholesterol biosynthesis pathways [20,29]. Overall, most studies in animals used KD rich in saturated fats, which may have detrimental effects on the lipid profile compared to KD rich in unsaturated fats, and therefore limits definitive conclusions on the role of KD on dyslipidemia.

In humans, KD have been associated with significant reductions in total cholesterol [75], increases in HDL cholesterol levels [33,70,75,80–83], decreases in triglycerides levels [32,33,70,75,82,83] and reductions in LDL cholesterol levels [75]. These results were obtained in non epileptic obese participants with [32,70,75,83] or without [33,82] at least one risk factor of the metabolic syndrome, but also in healthy normal weight participants [80]. This is of importance as the effects of KD on the lipid profile may differ in epileptic subjects [84]. KD have also been associated with an increase in size and volume of LDL cholesterol particles, which is considered to reduce cardiovascular risk by decreasing atherogenicity [81]. Nevertheless, several studies showed an increase in LDL cholesterol levels [82,83,85,86], but not significantly in the trial by Westman et al. [85]; in these cases, KD were mostly composed of saturated fats. In other studies, total and LDL cholesterol were significantly more reduced with a high-protein medium-carbohydrate diet than with a KD [40]. Another study [33] reported no significant difference in total and LDL cholesterol levels after 12 months of a KD compared to a conventional diet, except at 3 months, where LDL cholesterol levels were lower in the conventional diet group. The absence of improvement suggests that weight loss with a low-carbohydrate diet is not associated with a decrease in LDL cholesterol usually observed with moderate weight loss [33]. Interestingly, the effect of a KD on lipid profile may be associated with ethnicity: in a study, white subjects lost more weight and had a bigger decrease in triglycerides levels than black subjects [32]. However, in this study, there was no significant change in total cholesterol, HDL cholesterol and LDL cholesterol levels.

As discussed for other cardiovascular risk factors, the composition of the diet used is very important. For example, in a study that reported a benefit of a KD on triglycerides and HDL cholesterol levels [70], the authors decided to use a low-carbohydrate diet rich in unsaturated but low in saturated fatty acids, which may greatly influence the lipid profile, but also the development of other metabolic complications such as NAFLD, insulin resistance and type 2 diabetes, as discussed earlier.

The impact of KD on the lipid profile differs between rodents and humans. In rodents, KD seem to be associated with worsened levels of total, HDL and LDL cholesterol, and triglycerides. In humans, the opposite is reported. These differences are mostly explained by differences in the composition of the diets, which are usually higher in total fat, but also in saturated fat in animal studies. Both in rodents and humans, comparison between saturated fat and unsaturated fat KD in long-term studies would be necessary. Later in this review, we will discuss whether saturated fat diets are as harmful as once thought.

3.5. KD and Blood Pressure

Studies reporting a potential effect of KD on blood pressure are scarce. We could not find studies in animals. In humans, KD are usually associated with a slight but not significant reduction in systolic and/or diastolic blood pressure [32]. Moreover, no change in antihypertensive therapy was observed [32,33]. Nevertheless, a study described an improvement in both systolic and diastolic blood pressure in obese participants when fed a KD during 48 weeks compared to a low-fat diet plus orlistat [69]. Weight loss was not a confounding factor as weight loss was similar in both arms. Finally, a reduction in systolic blood pressure was found in a study using a KD, but only after 3 months, without change after 1 year of observation [41].

Overall, there is a clear lack of conclusive data on the potential beneficial effect of KD on arterial blood pressure and further studies are therefore needed.

4. Discussion

Both in rodents and humans, controversies remain regarding the effect of KD on metabolic risk factors such as NAFLD, insulin resistance, type 2 diabetes and dyslipidemia. The potential beneficial and adverse effects of KD are summarized in Figure 1, and the effects of KD on different biomolecular markers in Figure 2.

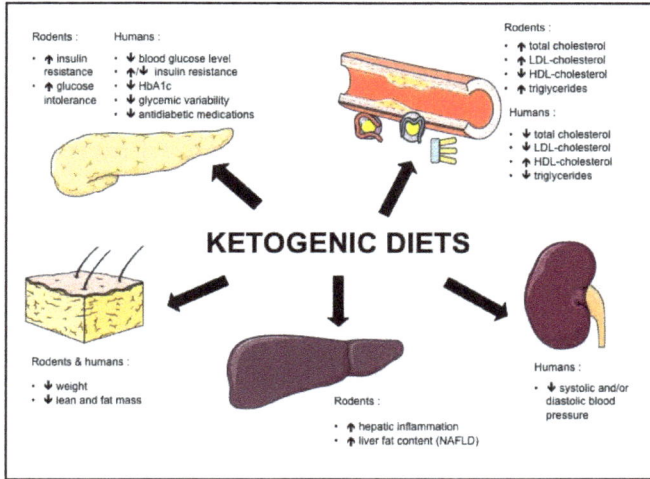

Figure 1. Effects of ketogenic diets in rodents and humans.

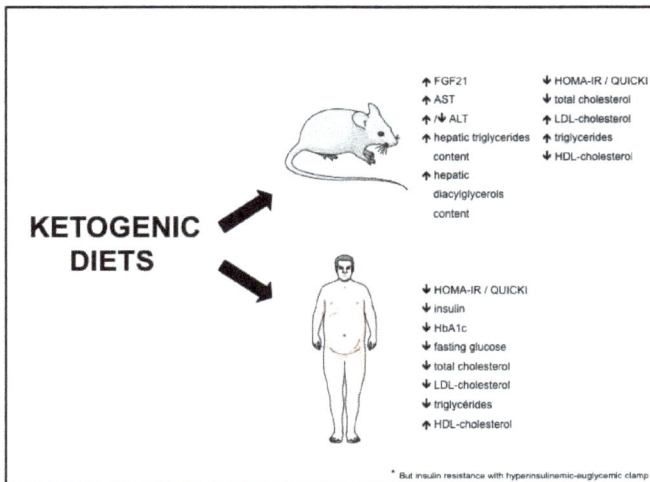

Figure 2. Effects of ketogenic diets on biomolecular markers. FGF21: fibroblast growth factor-21; ALT: alanine aminotransferase; AST: aspartate aminotransferase; QUICKI: quantitative insulin-sensitivity check index; HOMA-IR: homeostasis model assessment of insulin resistance.

Overall, KD composition greatly differs between studies. KD used in rodents are usually not similar to KD used in humans (almost no carbohydrates and low protein content in rodent KD). Moreover, low-carbohydrate diets can be different in macronutrient composition, i.e., high-fat versus high-protein content, which may account for some of the differences between the studies. Moreover, as previously mentioned, fat composition can substantially differ between studies, some using KD rich in unsaturated fatty acids and others rich in saturated fatty acids. Nevertheless, a recent systematic review and meta-analysis revealed that saturated fat intake was not associated with all-cause and cardiovascular mortality, coronary heart disease, ischemic stroke or type 2 diabetes, but with heterogenous evidence [87]. The authors conclude that trans fats were associated with all-cause and cardiovascular mortality and also with coronary heart disease. Moreover, it is well known that different ratios of some unsaturated and saturated fatty acids in diet compositions can alter metabolic parameters such as insulin sensitivity [9]. Therefore, it is a real challenge for physicians to advise patients with different metabolic diseases about the best diet composition to use. If a KD has to be prescribed, maybe it could be better to favor a vegetable-based KD, as vegetable-based low-carbohydrate diets have been correlated with a decrease in all-cause and cardiovascular-related mortality [88]. In the latter study, two US cohorts (121,700 females, 51,529 males) were followed during 26 and 20 years, respectively. Both in men and women, animal-based low-carbohydrate diets were found to be associated with higher all-cause (especially cardiovascular mortality) and cancer mortality, compared to vegetable-based low-carbohydrate diets. Nevertheless, similar studies with "real" KD need to be performed to confirm this assumption, as a low-carbohydrate diet is not necessarily inducing ketosis and is therefore not a ketogenic diet per se. Another problem when using a KD is the long-term effect and sustainability of effects, notably due to a lack of long-term studies in metabolic diseases such as type 2 diabetes. Restrictive diets are often associated with poor long-term adherence [89]. Nevertheless, some evidence suggests that adherence to low-carbohydrate diets is better than to low-fat diets, because of the allowance to unlimited access to food as long as carbohydrates are reduced, given that proteins and fats are known to induce satiety [16].

Three meta-analyses about the effect of KD on cardiovascular risk factors were published recently [90–92]. Their conclusions are unanimous about general positive effects, but not unanimous about each single variable. Santos et al. concluded in 2012 that low-carbohydrate diets lead to a significant decrease in body weight, BMI, abdominal circumference, both systolic and diastolic blood pressure, triglycerides levels, fasting plasma glucose and HbA1c, an increase in HDL cholesterol levels, and no change in LDL cholesterol levels. As we mentioned before, the authors suggested a possible duration effect, specifically for body weight and blood pressure, where benefits seem to decrease over time [90]. Bezerra Bueno et al. compared very-low carbohydrate diets to low-fat diets and their effects after a follow-up of at least 12 months. Very-low carbohydrate diets confer a greater weight loss, reduction in triglycerides and diastolic blood pressure, and increase in HDL and LDL cholesterol levels. There was however no difference in systolic blood pressure. There was no significant difference between diets for fasting blood glucose and insulin levels, and HbA1c. It is interesting to note that in the studies (only 4) with 24 months of follow-up, only the change in HDL cholesterol levels remained significant [91]. The latest meta-analysis on KD by Naude et al. included 19 randomized controlled trials (RCT) and revealed that there is probably little or no difference in changes in weight or cardiovascular risk factors when comparing low-carbohydrate diets to isoenergetic diets (both showed weight loss) after two years of follow-up. These results were found in overweight and obese patients, with or without type 2 diabetes. This meta-analysis showed that strict adherence failed and declined with follow-up in most trials [92].

It is also important to keep in mind that KD could have some adverse side effects when chronically used. Indeed, studies in children using KD to treat epilepsy and other neurological disorders show an increase in kidney stones, osteoporosis, hyperlipidemia and impaired growth [93,94]. While several authors found that a low-carbohydrate high-protein diet was not associated with higher mortality after 12 years of follow-up [95], others described a weak statistically significant higher mortality rate after 10 years [96]. However, they did not evaluate sources of proteins and fats.

Finally, it should be mentioned that it is difficult to really know in studies if low-carbohydrate diets were "real" KD. Indeed, most of the time there is no report about a potential induction of ketosis, by for example reporting measurements of plasma ketone bodies.

5. Conclusions

Based on the available literature, KD may be associated with some improvements in some cardiovascular risk factors, such as obesity, type 2 diabetes and HDL cholesterol levels, but these effects are usually limited in time. As KD are often rich in fats, some negative effects could happen. Mainly in rodents, developments of NAFLD and insulin resistance were described. In humans, insulin resistance is also a potential negative effect, but some studies have shown improvements in insulin sensitivity. Nevertheless, many subjects contemplating such diets are overweight or obese at baseline, and even a moderate weight loss could be metabolically beneficial for them. However, it is mandatory to maintain body weight after weight loss, which is usually a major problem. More studies are therefore warranted to better assess the effects of long term use of KD on metabolic diseases and cardiovascular risk factors, but also to better define which dietary macronutrient composition is optimal.

Acknowledgments: F.R.J. is supported by a grant from the Gottfried und Julia Bangerter-Rhyner-Stiftung and from the Fondation de l'Association Suisse du Diabète.

Author Contributions: C.K. and F.R.J. wrote the paper and contributed equally.

Conflicts of Interest: The authors declare no conflict of interest.

References

1. Ng, M.; Fleming, T.; Robinson, M.; Thomson, B.; Graetz, N.; Margono, C.; Mullany, E.C.; Biryukov, S.; Abbafati, C.; Abera, S.F.; et al. Global, regional, and national prevalence of overweight and obesity in children and adults during 1980–2013: A systematic analysis for the Global Burden of Disease Study 2013. *Lancet* **2014**, *384*, 766–781. [CrossRef]

2. Koh-Banerjee, P.; Wang, Y.; Hu, F.B.; Spiegelman, D.; Willett, W.C.; Rimm, E.B. Changes in body weight and body fat distribution as risk factors for clinical diabetes in US men. *Am. J. Epidemiol.* **2004**, *159*, 1150–1159. [CrossRef] [PubMed]

3. Fabbrini, E.; Magkos, F.; Mohammed, B.S.; Pietka, T.; Abumrad, N.A.; Patterson, B.W.; Okunade, A.; Klein, S. Intrahepatic fat, not visceral fat, is linked with metabolic complications of obesity. *Proc. Natl. Acad. Sci. USA* **2009**, *106*, 15430–15435. [CrossRef] [PubMed]

4. Fabbrini, E.; Sullivan, S.; Klein, S. Obesity and nonalcoholic fatty liver disease: Biochemical, metabolic, and clinical implications. *Hepatology* **2010**, *51*, 679–689. [CrossRef] [PubMed]

5. Chalasani, N.; Younossi, Z.; Lavine, J.E.; Diehl, A.M.; Brunt, E.M.; Cusi, K.; Charlton, M.; Sanyal, A.J. The diagnosis and management of non-alcoholic fatty liver disease: Practice guideline by the American Gastroenterological Association, American Association for the Study of Liver Diseases, and American College of Gastroenterology. *Gastroenterology* **2012**, *142*, 1592–1609. [CrossRef] [PubMed]

6. Gariani, K.; Philippe, J.; Jornayvaz, F.R. Non-alcoholic fatty liver disease and insulin resistance: From bench to bedside. *Diabetes Metab.* **2013**, *39*, 16–26. [CrossRef] [PubMed]

7. Machado, M.; Marques-Vidal, P.; Cortez-Pinto, H. Hepatic histology in obese patients undergoing bariatric surgery. *J. Hepatol.* **2006**, *45*, 600–606. [CrossRef] [PubMed]

8. McKeown, N.M.; Meigs, J.B.; Liu, S.; Saltzman, E.; Wilson, P.W.F.; Jacques, P.F. Carbohydrate nutrition, insulin resistance, and the prevalence of the metabolic syndrome in the Framingham Offspring Cohort. *Diabetes Care* **2004**, *27*, 538–546. [CrossRef] [PubMed]

9. Asrih, M.; Jornayvaz, F.R. Diets and nonalcoholic fatty liver disease: The good and the bad. *Clin. Nutr.* **2014**, *33*, 186–190. [CrossRef] [PubMed]

10. Volek, J.S.; Fernandez, M.L.; Feinman, R.D.; Phinney, S.D. Dietary carbohydrate restriction induces a unique metabolic state positively affecting atherogenic dyslipidemia, fatty acid partitioning, and metabolic syndrome. *Prog. Lipid Res.* **2008**, *47*, 307–318. [CrossRef] [PubMed]

11. Volek, J.S.; Phinney, S.D.; Forsythe, C.E.; Quann, E.E.; Wood, R.J.; Puglisi, M.J.; Kraemer, W.J.; Bibus, D.M.; Fernandez, M.L.; Feinman, R.D. Carbohydrate restriction has a more favorable impact on the metabolic syndrome than a low fat diet. *Lipids* **2009**, *44*, 297–309. [CrossRef] [PubMed]

12. Volek, J.S.; Feinman, R.D. Carbohydrate restriction improves the features of Metabolic Syndrome. Metabolic Syndrome may be defined by the response to carbohydrate restriction. *Nutr. Metab.* **2005**, *2*, 31. [CrossRef] [PubMed]

13. Atkins, R.C. *Dr Atkins' Diet Revolution: The High Calorie Way to Stay Thin Forever*; D. McKay Co.: New York, NY, USA, 1972.

14. Veech, R.L. The therapeutic implications of ketone bodies: The effects of ketone bodies in pathological conditions: Ketosis, ketogenic diet, redox states, insulin resistance, and mitochondrial metabolism. *Prostaglandins Leukot. Essent. Fat. Acids* **2004**, *70*, 309–319. [CrossRef] [PubMed]

15. Kossoff, E.H.; Cervenka, M.C.; Henry, B.J.; Haney, C.A.; Turner, Z. A decade of the modified Atkins diet (2003–2013): Results, insights, and future directions. *Epilepsy Behav.* **2013**, *29*, 437–442. [CrossRef] [PubMed]

16. Feinman, R.D.; Pogozelski, W.K.; Astrup, A.; Bernstein, R.K.; Fine, E.J.; Westman, E.C.; Westman, E.C.; Accurso, A.; Frassetto, L.; Gower, B.A.; et al. Dietary carbohydrate restriction as the first approach in diabetes management: Critical review and evidence base. *Nutrition* **2015**, *31*, 1–13. [CrossRef] [PubMed]

17. Accurso, A.; Bernstein, R.K.; Dahlqvist, A.; Draznin, B.; Feinman, R.D.; Fine, E.J.; Gleed, A.; Jacobs, D.B.; Larson, G.; Lustig, R.H.; et al. Dietary carbohydrate restriction in type 2 diabetes mellitus and metabolic syndrome: Time for a critical appraisal. *Nutr. Metab.* **2008**, *5*, 9. [CrossRef] [PubMed]

18. Owen, O.E.; Morgan, A.P.; Kemp, H.G.; Sullivan, J.M.; Herrera, M.G.; Cahill, G.F. Brain metabolism during fasting. *J. Clin. Invest.* **1967**, *46*, 1589–1595. [CrossRef] [PubMed]

19. Kessler, S.K.; Neal, E.G.; Camfield, C.S.; Kossoff, E.H. Dietary therapies for epilepsy: Future research. *Epilepsy Behav.* **2011**, *22*, 17–22. [CrossRef] [PubMed]

20. Kennedy, A.R.; Pissios, P.; Otu, H.; Roberson, R.; Xue, B.; Asakura, K.; Furukawa, N.; Marino, F.E.; Liu, F.F.; Kahn, B.B.; et al. A high-fat, ketogenic diet induces a unique metabolic state in mice. *Am. J. Physiol. Endocrinol. Metab.* **2007**, *292*, E1724–E1739. [CrossRef] [PubMed]

21. Badman, M.K.; Kennedy, A.R.; Adams, A.C.; Pissios, P.; Maratos-Flier, E. A very low carbohydrate ketogenic diet improves glucose tolerance in ob/ob mice independently of weight loss. *Am. J. Physiol. Endocrinol. Metab.* **2009**, *297*, E1197–E1204. [CrossRef] [PubMed]

22. Garbow, J.R.; Doherty, J.M.; Schugar, R.C.; Travers, S.; Weber, M.L.; Wentz, A.E.; Ezenwajiaku, N.; Cotter, D.G.; Brunt, E.M.; Crawford, P.A. Hepatic steatosis, inflammation, and ER stress in mice maintained long term on a very low-carbohydrate ketogenic diet. *Am. J. Physiol. Gastrointest. Liver Physiol.* **2011**, *300*, G956–G967. [CrossRef] [PubMed]

23. Bielohuby, M.; Sisley, S.; Sandoval, D.; Herbach, N.; Zengin, A.; Fischereder, M.; Menhofer, D.; Stoehr, B.J.M.; Stemmer, K.; Wanke, R.; et al. Impaired glucose tolerance in rats fed low-carbohydrate, high-fat diets. *Am. J. Physiol. Endocrinol. Metab.* **2013**, *305*, E1059–E1070. [CrossRef] [PubMed]

24. Jornayvaz, F.R.; Jurczak, M.J.; Lee, H.-Y.; Birkenfeld, A.L.; Frederick, D.W.; Zhang, D.; Zhang, X.M.; Samuel, V.T.; Shulman, G.I. A high-fat, ketogenic diet causes hepatic insulin resistance in mice, despite increasing energy expenditure and preventing weight gain. *Am. J. Physiol. Endocrinol. Metab.* **2010**, *299*, E808–E815. [CrossRef] [PubMed]

25. Ellenbroek, J.H.; van Dijck, L.; Tons, H.A.; Rabelink, T.J.; Carlotti, F.; Ballieux, B.E.; de Koning, E.J.P. Long-term ketogenic diet causes glucose intolerance and reduced B- and a-cell mass but no weight loss in mice. *Am. J. Physiol. Endocrinol. Metab.* **2014**, *306*, E552–E558. [CrossRef] [PubMed]

26. Douris, N.; Melman, T.; Pecherer, J.M.; Pissios, P.; Flier, J.S.; Cantley, L.C.; Locasale, J.W.; Maratos-Flier, E. Adaptive changes in amino acid metabolism permit normal longevity in mice consuming a low-carbohydrate ketogenic diet. *Biochim. Biophys. Acta* **2015**, *1852*, 2056–2065. [CrossRef] [PubMed]

27. Asrih, M.; Altirriba, J.; Rohner-Jeanrenaud, F.; Jornayvaz, F.R. Ketogenic Diet Impairs FGF21 Signaling and Promotes Differential Inflammatory Responses in the Liver and White Adipose Tissue. *PLoS ONE* **2015**, *10*, e0126364. [CrossRef] [PubMed]

28. Frommelt, L.; Bielohuby, M.; Menhofer, D.; Stoehr, B.J.M.; Bidlingmaier, M.; Kienzle, E. Effects of low carbohydrate diets on energy and nitrogen balance and body composition in rats depend on dietary protein-to-energy ratio. *Nutrition* **2014**, *30*, 863–868. [CrossRef] [PubMed]

29. Holland, A.M.; Kephart, W.C.; Mumford, P.W.; Mobley, C.B.; Lowery, R.P.; Shake, J.J.; Patel, R.K.; Healy, J.C.; McCullough, D.J.; Kluess, H.A.; et al. Effects of a ketogenic diet on adipose tissue, liver, and serum biomarkers in sedentary rats and rats that exercised via resisted voluntary wheel running. *Am. J. Physiol. Regul. Integr. Comp. Physiol.* **2016**, *311*, R337–R351. [CrossRef] [PubMed]

30. Partsalaki, I.; Karvela, A.; Spiliotis, B.E. Metabolic impact of a ketogenic diet compared to a hypocaloric diet in obese children and adolescents. *J. Pediatr. Endocrinol. Metab.* **2012**, *25*, 697–704. [CrossRef] [PubMed]

31. Saisho, Y.; Butler, A.E.; Manesso, E.; Elashoff, D.; Rizza, R.A.; Butler, P.C. β-cell mass and turnover in humans: Effects of obesity and aging. *Diabetes Care* **2013**, *36*, 111–117. [CrossRef] [PubMed]

32. Samaha, F.F.; Iqbal, N.; Seshadri, P.; Chicano, K.L.; Daily, D.A.; McGrory, J.; Williams, T.; Williams, M.; Gracely, E.J.; Stem, L. A Low-Carbohydrate as Compared with a Low-Fat Diet in Severe Obesity. *N. Engl. J. Med.* **2003**, *348*, 2074–2081. [CrossRef] [PubMed]
33. Foster, G.D.; Wyatt, H.R.; Hill, J.O.; McGuckin, B.G.; Brill, C.; Mohammed, B.S.; Szapary, P.O.; Rader, D.J.; Edman, J.S.; Klein, S. A Randomized Trial of a Low-Carbohydrate Diet for Obesity. *N. Engl. J. Med.* **2003**, *348*, 2082–2090. [CrossRef] [PubMed]
34. Westerterp-Plantenga, M.S.; Nieuwenhuizen, A.; Tomé, D.; Soenen, S.; Westerterp, K.R. Dietary protein, weight loss, and weight maintenance. *Annu. Rev. Nutr.* **2009**, *29*, 21–41. [CrossRef] [PubMed]
35. Fine, E.J.; Feinman, R.D. Thermodynamics of weight loss diets. *Nutr. Metab.* **2004**, *1*, 15. [CrossRef] [PubMed]
36. Feinman, R.D.; Fine, E.J. Nonequilibrium thermodynamics and energy efficiency in weight loss diets. *Theor. Biol. Med. Model.* **2007**, *4*, 27. [CrossRef] [PubMed]
37. Halton, T.L.; Hu, F.B. The effects of high protein diets on thermogenesis, satiety and weight loss: A critical review. *J. Am. Coll. Nutr.* **2004**, *23*, 373–385. [CrossRef] [PubMed]
38. Veldhorst, M.A.B.; Westerterp-Plantenga, M.S.; Westerterp, K.R. Gluconeogenesis and energy expenditure after a high-protein, carbohydrate-free diet. *Am. J. Clin. Nutr.* **2009**, *90*, 519–526. [CrossRef] [PubMed]
39. Sumithran, P.; Prendergast, L.A.; Delbridge, E.; Purcell, K.; Shulkes, A.; Kriketos, A.; Proietto, J. Ketosis and appetite-mediating nutrients and hormones after weight loss. *Eur. J. Clin. Nutr.* **2013**, *67*, 759–764. [CrossRef] [PubMed]
40. Johnstone, A.M.; Horgan, G.W.; Murison, S.D.; Bremner, D.M.; Lobley, G.E. Effects of a high-protein ketogenic diet on hunger, appetite, and weight loss in obese men feeding ad libitum. *Am. J. Clin. Nutr.* **2008**, *87*, 44–55. [PubMed]
41. Cicero, A.F.G.; Benelli, M.; Brancaleoni, M.; Dainelli, G.; Merlini, D.; Negri, R. Middle and Long-Term Impact of a Very Low-Carbohydrate Ketogenic Diet on Cardiometabolic Factors: A Multi-Center, Cross-Sectional, Clinical Study. *High Blood Press. Cardiovasc. Prev.* **2015**, *22*, 389–394. [CrossRef] [PubMed]
42. Paoli, A.; Bianco, A.; Grimaldi, K.A.; Lodi, A.; Bosco, G. Long term successful weight loss with a combination biphasic ketogenic Mediterranean diet and Mediterranean diet maintenance protocol. *Nutrients* **2013**, *5*, 5205–5217. [CrossRef] [PubMed]
43. Tay, J.; Luscombe-Marsh, N.D.; Thompson, C.H.; Noakes, M.; Buckley, J.D.; Wittert, G.A.; Yancy, W.S.; Brinkworth, G.D. Comparison of low- and high-carbohydrate diets for type 2 diabetes management: A randomized trial. *Am. J. Clin. Nutr.* **2015**, *102*, 780–790. [CrossRef] [PubMed]
44. Jabekk, P.T.; Moe, I.A.; Meen, H.D.; Tomten, S.E.; Høstmark, A.T. Resistance training in overweight women on a ketogenic diet conserved lean body mass while reducing body fat. *Nutr. Metab.* **2010**, *7*, 17. [CrossRef] [PubMed]
45. Morris-Stiff, G.; Feldstein, A.E. Fibroblast growth factor 21 as a biomarker for NAFLD: Integrating pathobiology into clinical practice. *J. Hepatol.* **2010**, *53*, 795–796. [CrossRef] [PubMed]
46. Dushay, J.; Chui, P.C.; Gopalakrishnan, G.S.; Varela-Rey, M.; Crawley, M.; Fisher, F.M.; Badman, M.K.; Martinez-Chantar, M.L.; Maratos-Flier, E. Increased fibroblast growth factor 21 in obesity and nonalcoholic fatty liver disease. *Gastroenterology* **2010**, *139*, 456–463. [CrossRef] [PubMed]
47. Li, H.; Fang, Q.; Gao, F.; Fan, J.; Zhou, J.; Wang, X.; Zhang, H.; Pan, X.; Bao, Y.; Xiang, K.; et al. Fibroblast growth factor 21 levels are increased in nonalcoholic fatty liver disease patients and are correlated with hepatic triglyceride. *J. Hepatol.* **2010**, *53*, 934–940. [CrossRef] [PubMed]
48. Murata, Y.; Nishio, K.; Mochiyama, T.; Konishi, M.; Shimada, M.; Ohta, H.; Itoh, N. Fgf21 Impairs Adipocyte Insulin Sensitivity in Mice Fed a Low-Carbohydrate, High-Fat Ketogenic Diet. *PLoS ONE* **2013**, *8*, e69330. [CrossRef] [PubMed]
49. Badman, M.K.; Pissios, P.; Kennedy, A.R.; Koukos, G.; Flier, J.S.; Maratos-Flier, E. Hepatic fibroblast growth factor 21 is regulated by PPARalpha and is a key mediator of hepatic lipid metabolism in ketotic states. *Cell Metab.* **2007**, *5*, 426–437. [CrossRef] [PubMed]
50. Jornayvaz, F.R.; Shulman, G.I. Diacylglycerol activation of protein kinase Cε and hepatic insulin resistance. *Cell Metab.* **2012**, *15*, 574–584. [CrossRef] [PubMed]
51. Camporez, J.P.G.; Jornayvaz, F.R.; Petersen, M.C.; Pesta, D.; Guigni, B.A.; Serr, J.; Zhang, D.; Kahn, M.; Samuel, V.T.; Jurczak, M.J.; et al. Cellular mechanisms by which FGF21 improves insulin sensitivity in male mice. *Endocrinology* **2013**, *154*, 3099–3109. [CrossRef] [PubMed]

52. Xu, J.; Lloyd, D.J.; Hale, C.; Stanislaus, S.; Chen, M.; Sivits, G.; Vonderfecht, S.; Hecht, R.; Li, Y.S.; Lindberg, R.A.; et al. Fibroblast growth factor 21 reverses hepatic steatosis, increases energy expenditure, and improves insulin sensitivity in diet-induced obese mice. *Diabetes* **2009**, *58*, 250–259. [CrossRef] [PubMed]

53. Badman, M.K.; Koester, A.; Flier, J.S.; Kharitonenkov, A.; Maratos-Flier, E. Fibroblast growth factor 21-deficient mice demonstrate impaired adaptation to ketosis. *Endocrinology* **2009**, *150*, 4931–4940. [CrossRef] [PubMed]

54. Camporez, J.P.G.; Asrih, M.; Zhang, D.; Kahn, M.; Samuel, V.T.; Jurczak, M.J.; Jornayvaz, F.R. Hepatic insulin resistance and increased hepatic glucose production in mice lacking Fgf21. *J. Endocrinol.* **2015**, *226*, 207–217. [CrossRef] [PubMed]

55. Laeger, T.; Henagan, T.M.; Albarado, D.C.; Redman, L.M.; Bray, G.A.; Noland, R.C.; Münzberg, H.; Hutson, S.M.; Gettys, T.W.; Schwartz, M.W.; et al. FGF21 is an endocrine signal of protein restriction. *J. Clin. Investig.* **2014**, *124*, 3913–3922. [CrossRef] [PubMed]

56. Westerbacka, J.; Lammi, K.; Häkkinen, A.-M.; Rissanen, A.; Salminen, I.; Aro, A.; Yki-Järvinen, H. Dietary fat content modifies liver fat in overweight nondiabetic subjects. *J. Clin. Endocrinol. Metab.* **2005**, *90*, 2804–2809. [CrossRef] [PubMed]

57. Kirk, E.; Reeds, D.N.; Finck, B.N.; Mayurranjan, S.M.; Mayurranjan, M.S.; Patterson, B.W.; Klein, S. Dietary fat and carbohydrates differentially alter insulin sensitivity during caloric restriction. *Gastroenterology* **2009**, *136*, 1552–1560. [CrossRef] [PubMed]

58. Browning, J.D.; Baker, J.A.; Rogers, T.; Davis, J.; Satapati, S.; Burgess, S.C. Short-term weight loss and hepatic triglyceride reduction: Evidence of a metabolic advantage with dietary carbohydrate restriction. *Am. J. Clin. Nutr.* **2011**, *93*, 1048–1052. [CrossRef] [PubMed]

59. Bian, H.; Hakkarainen, A.; Lundbom, N.; Yki-Järvinen, H. Effects of dietary interventions on liver volume in humans. *Obesity* **2014**, *22*, 989–995. [CrossRef] [PubMed]

60. Sevastianova, K.; Kotronen, A.; Gastaldelli, A.; Perttilä, J.; Hakkarainen, A.; Lundbom, J.; Orho-Melander, M.; Lundbom, N.; Ferrannini, E.; Rissanen, A.; et al. Genetic variation in PNPLA3 (adiponutrin) confers sensitivity to weight loss-induced decrease in liver fat in humans. *Am. J. Clin. Nutr.* **2011**, *94*, 104–111. [CrossRef] [PubMed]

61. Shen, J.; Wong, G.L.-H.; Chan, H.L.-Y.; Chan, R.S.-M.; Chan, H.-Y.; Chu, W.C.-W.; Cheung, B.H.-K.; Yeung, D.K.-W.; Li, L.S.; Sea, M.M.-M.; et al. PNPLA3 gene polymorphism and response to lifestyle modification in patients with nonalcoholic fatty liver disease. *J. Gastroenterol. Hepatol.* **2015**, *30*, 139–146. [CrossRef] [PubMed]

62. Jornayvaz, F.R. Fibroblast growth factor 21, ketogenic diets, and insulin resistance. *Am. J. Clin. Nutr.* **2011**, *94*, 955. [CrossRef] [PubMed]

63. Kinzig, K.P.; Honors, M.A.; Hargrave, S.L. Insulin sensitivity and glucose tolerance are altered by maintenance on a ketogenic diet. *Endocrinology* **2010**, *151*, 3105–3114. [CrossRef] [PubMed]

64. Bisschop, P.H.; de Metz, J.; Ackermans, M.T.; Endert, E.; Pijl, H.; Kuipers, F.; Meijer, A.J.; Sauerwein, H.P.; Romijn, J.A. Dietary fat content alters insulin-mediated glucose metabolism in healthy men. *Am. J. Clin. Nutr.* **2001**, *73*, 554–559. [PubMed]

65. Westman, E.C.; Feinman, R.D.; Mavropoulos, J.C.; Vernon, M.C.; Volek, J.S.; Wortman, J.A.; Yancy, W.S.; Phinney, S.D. Low-carbohydrate nutrition and metabolism. *Am. J. Clin. Nutr.* **2007**, *86*, 276–284. [PubMed]

66. Hussain, T.A.; Mathew, T.C.; Dashti, A.A.; Asfar, S.; Al-Zaid, N.; Dashti, H.M. Effect of low-calorie versus low-carbohydrate ketogenic diet in type 2 diabetes. *Nutrition* **2012**, *28*, 1016–1021. [CrossRef] [PubMed]

67. Gannon, M.C.; Nuttall, F.Q. Control of blood glucose in type 2 diabetes without weight loss by modification of diet composition. *Nutr. Metab.* **2006**, *3*, 16. [CrossRef] [PubMed]

68. Boden, G.; Sargrad, K.; Homko, C.; Mozzoli, M.; Stein, T.P. Effect of a low-carbohydrate diet on appetite, blood glucose levels, and insulin resistance in obese patients with type 2 diabetes. *Ann. Intern. Med.* **2005**, *142*, 403–411. [CrossRef] [PubMed]

69. Mayer, S.B.; Jeffreys, A.S.; Olsen, M.K.; McDuffie, J.R.; Feinglos, M.N.; Yancy, W.S. Two diets with different haemoglobin A1c and antiglycaemic medication effects despite similar weight loss in type 2 diabetes. *Diabetes Obes. Metab.* **2014**, *16*, 90–93. [CrossRef] [PubMed]

70. Tay, J.; Luscombe-Marsh, N.D.; Thompson, C.H.; Noakes, M.; Buckley, J.D.; Wittert, G.A.; Yancy, W.S.; Brinkworth, G.D. A Very Low-Carbohydrate, Low–Saturated Fat Diet for Type 2 Diabetes Management: A Randomized Trial. *Diabetes Care* **2014**, *37*, 2909–2918. [CrossRef] [PubMed]

71. Gannon, M.C.; Nuttall, F.Q. Effect of a high-protein, low-carbohydrate diet on blood glucose control in people with type 2 diabetes. *Diabetes* **2004**, *53*, 2375–2382. [CrossRef] [PubMed]

72. Halton, T.L.; Liu, S.; Manson, J.E.; Hu, F.B. Low-carbohydrate-diet score and risk of type 2 diabetes in women. *Am. J. Clin. Nutr.* **2008**, *87*, 339–346. [PubMed]

73. Yancy, W.S.; Foy, M.; Chalecki, A.M.; Vernon, M.C.; Westman, E.C. A low-carbohydrate, ketogenic diet to treat type 2 diabetes. *Nutr. Metab.* **2005**, *2*, 34. [CrossRef] [PubMed]

74. Saslow, L.R.; Kim, S.; Daubenmier, J.J.; Moskowitz, J.T.; Phinney, S.D.; Goldman, V.; Murphy, E.J.; Cox, R.M.; Moran, P.; Hecht, F.M. A randomized pilot trial of a moderate carbohydrate diet compared to a very low carbohydrate diet in overweight or obese individuals with type 2 diabetes mellitus or prediabetes. *PLoS ONE* **2014**, *9*, e91027. [CrossRef] [PubMed]

75. Dashti, H.M.; Al-Zaid, N.S.; Mathew, T.C.; Al-Mousawi, M.; Talib, H.; Asfar, S.K.; Behbahani, A.I. Long term effects of ketogenic diet in obese subjects with high cholesterol level. *Mol. Cell. Biochem.* **2006**, *286*, 1–9. [CrossRef] [PubMed]

76. Iqbal, N.; Vetter, M.L.; Moore, R.H.; Chittams, J.L.; Dalton-Bakes, C.V.; Dowd, M.; Williams-Smith, C.; Cardillo, S.; Wadden, T.A. Effects of a low-intensity intervention that prescribed a low-carbohydrate vs. a low-fat diet in obese, diabetic participants. *Obesity* **2010**, *18*, 1733–1738. [CrossRef] [PubMed]

77. De Koning, L.; Fung, T.T.; Liao, X.; Chiuve, S.E.; Rimm, E.B.; Willett, W.C.; Spiegelman, D.; Hu, F.B. Low-carbohydrate diet scores and risk of type 2 diabetes in men. *Am. J. Clin. Nutr.* **2011**, *93*, 844–850. [CrossRef] [PubMed]

78. Gumbiner, B.; Wendel, J.A.; McDermott, M.P. Effects of diet composition and ketosis on glycemia during very-low-energy-diet therapy in obese patients with non-insulin-dependent diabetes mellitus. *Am. J. Clin. Nutr.* **1996**, *63*, 110–115. [PubMed]

79. Farrés, J.; Pujol, A.; Coma, M.; Ruiz, J.; Naval, J.; Mas, J.; Molins, A.; Fondevila, J.; Aloy, P. Revealing the molecular relationship between type 2 diabetes and the metabolic changes induced by a very-low-carbohydrate low-fat ketogenic diet. *Nutr. Metab.* **2010**, *7*, 88. [CrossRef] [PubMed]

80. Sharman, M.J.; Kraemer, W.J.; Love, D.M.; Avery, N.G.; Gómez, A.L.; Scheett, T.P.; Volek, J.S. A ketogenic diet favorably affects serum biomarkers for cardiovascular disease in normal-weight men. *J. Nutr.* **2002**, *132*, 1879–1885. [PubMed]

81. Volek, J.S.; Sharman, M.J.; Forsythe, C.E. Modification of lipoproteins by very low-carbohydrate diets. *J. Nutr.* **2005**, *135*, 1339–1342. [PubMed]

82. Foster, G.D.; Wyatt, H.R.; Hill, J.O.; Makris, A.P.; Rosenbaum, D.L.; Brill, C.; Stein, R.I.; Mohammed, B.S.; Miller, B.; Rader, D.J.; et al. Weight and metabolic outcomes after 2 years on a low-carbohydrate versus low-fat diet: A randomized trial. *Ann. Intern. Med.* **2010**, *153*, 147–157. [CrossRef] [PubMed]

83. Brinkworth, G.D.; Noakes, M.; Buckley, J.D.; Keogh, J.B.; Clifton, P.M. Long-term effects of a very-low-carbohydrate weight loss diet compared with an isocaloric low-fat diet after 12 mo. *Am. J. Clin. Nutr.* **2009**, *90*, 23–32. [CrossRef] [PubMed]

84. Lima, P.A.; de Brito Sampaio, L.P.; Damasceno, N.R.T. Ketogenic diet in epileptic children: Impact on lipoproteins and oxidative stress. *Nutr. Neurosci.* **2015**, *18*, 337–344. [CrossRef] [PubMed]

85. Westman, E.C.; Yancy, W.S.; Mavropoulos, J.C.; Marquart, M.; McDuffie, J.R. The effect of a low-carbohydrate, ketogenic diet versus a low-glycemic index diet on glycemic control in type 2 diabetes mellitus. *Nutr. Metab.* **2008**, *5*, 36. [CrossRef] [PubMed]

86. Stern, L.; Iqbal, N.; Seshadri, P.; Chicano, K.L.; Daily, D.A.; McGrory, J.; Williams, M.; Gracely, E.J.; Samaha, F.F. The effects of low-carbohydrate versus conventional weight loss diets in severely obese adults: One-year follow-up of a randomized trial. *Ann. Intern. Med.* **2004**, *140*, 778–785. [CrossRef] [PubMed]

87. De Souza, R.J.; Mente, A.; Maroleanu, A.; Cozma, A.I.; Ha, V.; Kishibe, T.; Uleryk, E.; Budylowski, P.; Schünemann, H.; Beyene, J.; et al. Intake of saturated and trans unsaturated fatty acids and risk of all cause mortality, cardiovascular disease, and type 2 diabetes: Systematic review and meta-analysis of observational studies. *BMJ* **2015**, *351*, h3978. [CrossRef] [PubMed]

88. Fung, T.T.; van Dam, R.M.; Hankinson, S.E.; Stampfer, M.; Willett, W.C.; Hu, F.B. Low-carbohydrate diets and all-cause and cause-specific mortality: Two cohort studies. *Ann. Intern. Med.* **2010**, *153*, 289–298. [CrossRef] [PubMed]

89. Ye, F.; Li, X.-J.; Jiang, W.-L.; Sun, H.-B.; Liu, J. Efficacy of and Patient Compliance with a Ketogenic Diet in Adults with Intractable Epilepsy: A Meta-Analysis. *J. Clin. Neurol.* **2015**, *11*, 26. [CrossRef] [PubMed]

90. Santos, F.L.; Esteves, S.S.; da Costa Pereira, A.; Yancy, W.S., Jr.; Nunes, J.P. Systematic review and meta-analysis of clinical trials of the effects of low carbohydrate diets on cardiovascular risk factors: Low carbohydrate diets and cardiovascular risk factors. *Obes. Rev.* **2012**, *13*, 1048–1066. [CrossRef] [PubMed]

91. Bueno, N.B.; de Melo, I.S.; de Oliveira, S.L.; da Rocha Ataide, T. Very-low-carbohydrate ketogenic diet v. low-fat diet for long-term weight loss: A meta-analysis of randomised controlled trials. *Br. J. Nutr.* **2013**, *110*, 1178–1187. [CrossRef] [PubMed]

92. Naude, C.E.; Schoonees, A.; Senekal, M.; Young, T.; Garner, P.; Volmink, J. Low carbohydrate versus isoenergetic balanced diets for reducing weight and cardiovascular risk: A systematic review and meta-analysis. *PLoS ONE* **2014**, *9*, e100652. [CrossRef] [PubMed]

93. Bergqvist, A.G.C. Long-term monitoring of the ketogenic diet: Do's and Don'ts. *Epilepsy Res.* **2012**, *100*, 261–266. [CrossRef] [PubMed]

94. Kossoff, E.; Wang, H.-S. Dietary Therapies for Epilepsy. *Biomed. J.* **2013**, *36*, 2. [CrossRef] [PubMed]

95. Lagiou, P.; Sandin, S.; Weiderpass, E.; Lagiou, A.; Mucci, L.; Trichopoulos, D.; Adami, H.-O. Low carbohydrate-high protein diet and mortality in a cohort of Swedish women. *J. Intern. Med.* **2007**, *261*, 366–374. [CrossRef] [PubMed]

96. Trichopoulou, A.; Psaltopoulou, T.; Orfanos, P.; Hsieh, C.-C.; Trichopoulos, D. Low-carbohydrate-high-protein diet and long-term survival in a general population cohort. *Eur. J. Clin. Nutr.* **2007**, *61*, 575–581. [CrossRef] [PubMed]

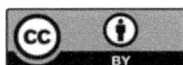

nutrients

MDPI

Article

Leucine Supplementation Differently Modulates Branched-Chain Amino Acid Catabolism, Mitochondrial Function and Metabolic Profiles at the Different Stage of Insulin Resistance in Rats on High-Fat Diet

Rui Liu, Hui Li, Wenjuan Fan, Qiu Jin, Tingting Chao, Yuanjue Wu, Junmei Huang, Liping Hao and Xuefeng Yang *

Department of Nutrition and Food Hygiene, Hubei Key Laboratory of Food Nutrition and Safety, MOE Key Laboratory of Environment and Health, School of Public Health, Tongji Medical College, Huazhong University of Science and Technology, Wuhan 430030, Hubei, China; amicable123lr@163.com (R.L.); 15032280368@163.com (H.L.); fanwenjuan0706@163.com (W.F.); 15927486696@163.com (Q.J.); weikeccs@sina.com (T.C.); wuyuanjue@hust.edu.cn (Y.W.); huangjunmeihust@163.com (J.H.); haolp@mails.tjmu.edu.cn (L.H.)
* Correspondence: xxyxf@mails.tjmu.edu.cn; Tel.: +86-(0)27-8365-0522

Received: 3 April 2017; Accepted: 26 May 2017; Published: 2 June 2017

Abstract: The available findings concerning the association between branched-chain amino acids (BCAAs)—particularly leucine—and insulin resistance are conflicting. BCAAs have been proposed to elicit different or even opposite effects, depending on the prevalence of catabolic and anabolic states. We tested the hypothesis that leucine supplementation may exert different effects at different stages of insulin resistance, to provide mechanistic insights into the role of leucine in the progression of insulin resistance. Male Sprague-Dawley rats were fed a normal chow diet, high-fat diet (HFD), HFD supplemented with 1.5% leucine, or HFD with a 20% calorie restriction for 24 or 32 weeks. Leucine supplementation led to abnormal catabolism of BCAA and the incompletely oxidized lipid species that contributed to mitochondrial dysfunction in skeletal muscle in HFD-fed rats in the early stage of insulin resistance (24 weeks). However, leucine supplementation induced no remarkable alternations in BCAA catabolism, but did enhance mitochondrial biogenesis with a concomitant improvement in lipid oxidation and mitochondrial function during the hyperglycaemia stage (32 weeks). These findings suggest that leucine trigger different effects on metabolic signatures at different stages of insulin resistance, and the overall metabolic status of the organisms should be carefully considered to potentiate the benefits of leucine.

Keywords: leucine; BCAAs; BCAA catabolism; insulin resistance; metabolomic; mitochondria

1. Introduction

Branched-chain amino acids (BCAAs), comprising leucine, isoleucine and valine, are essential amino acids and important nutrient signals that have direct and indirect effects on metabolism. Substantial evidence indicates that increased dietary intake of BCAAs, particularly leucine, has positive effects on the regulation of body weight, muscle protein synthesis, glucose homeostasis, lipid metabolism, and the ageing process [1–4]. Nevertheless, the idea that BCAAs or their supplementation might have a positive role in glucose metabolism and insulin resistance remains controversial. In other studies, leucine supplementation has no effect, or leads to deterioration in insulin sensitivity [5,6]. Along with these effects on metabolic health, it has long been recognized that elevated levels of circulating BCAAs and related metabolites are strongly associated with obesity and insulin resistance and are predictive of future type 2 diabetes mellitus (T2DM) in humans and in some rodent models [7–10]. The mechanisms underlying these paradoxical findings are not completely understood.

BCAAs modulate insulin resistance via multiple mechanisms. Generally, BCAAs have been shown to induce insulin resistance by phosphorylation of serine IRS-1 via activating mammalian targets of the rapamycin complex 1 (mTORC1) signaling pathway, and lead to a negative feedback loop of insulin signaling [11]. However, several previous studies, including a study conducted in our laboratory, have indicated that BCAA–associated mTORC1 activation is not required or sufficient to elicit insulin resistance [12,13]. Alternatively, the Lynch group have observed that abnormal tissue-specific BCAA metabolism in obesity results in the accumulation of BCAAs and related toxic metabolites, thereby triggering "anaplerotic stress" and mitochondrial dysfunction associated with insulin resistance and type 2 diabetes mellitus (T2DM) [14,15]. In contrast, BCAAs supplementation has been shown to promote mitochondrial biogenesis and extend the lifespan of yeast and middle-aged mice [16]. Recently, BCAAs and leucine have been hypothesised to elicit different or even opposing effects, depending on the catabolic and anabolic states of the organism [17]. Development of T2DM is a time-dependent process accompanied with different metabolic characteristics [18]. Notably, during the progression of insulin resistance to T2DM, the predominantly anabolic processes transition to predominantly catabolic processes, with the loss of insulin activity. This complexity introduces interpretive limitations, when using data derived from a static time point, on understanding how BCAAs affect the progression of insulin resistance [19].

In the present study, we performed comprehensive metabolic and physiological profiling to investigate dynamic alterations in BCAA catabolism, mitochondrial function, and metabolic responses to long-term leucine supplementation in rats with hyperinsulinaemia or hyperglycaemia induced by a high-fat diet (HFD). We aimed to provide mechanistic insights into the role of leucine in insulin resistance progression. Furthermore, we compared the effects of leucine with those of calorie restriction (CR), a well-known approach for improving insulin sensitivity.

2. Materials and Methods

2.1. Animals, Diets and Treatments

Male Sprague-Dawley rats at six weeks of age (160–180 g) were obtained from Sino-British Sipper/BK Lab Animal Co., Ltd. (Shanghai, China) and housed in a temperature- and humidity-controlled environment on a 12 h light/dark cycle with free access to food and water. After acclimation, the rats were randomly divided into four groups (n = 20 per group) based on body weight and fed a normal chow diet (ND; D12450B, Research Diet Inc., New Brunswick, NJ, USA), HFD (D12451, Research Diet Inc., New Brunswick, NJ, USA), HFD supplemented with 1.5% leucine (HFD + Leu) or HFD with 20% CR (HFD + CR). The administered leucine dose was determined in our preliminary experiments [12] and nearly doubled the total daily leucine intake from food. The diet of the HFD + Leu group was also supplemented with small amounts of valine and isoleucine to prevent valine and isoleucine deficiencies. The HFD was rendered isonitrogenous and isocalorie to the HFD + Leu diet by the addition of a mixture of non-essential amino acids (alanine, glycine, proline, aspartate and serine in isomolar amounts) (Table 1). Food intake was monitored daily, and that of HFD controls was used as a reference to calculate the amount of food provided to the rats subjected to CR (80% of food consumption of controls). Half of the rats in each group were killed at week 24, and the other half were killed at week 32 after overnight fasting. Blood samples were obtained and centrifuged at $4000\times g$ for 20 min. The serum was then collected and stored in a freezer at −80 °C until further analysis. Tissues were rapidly excised, weighed, flash-frozen in liquid nitrogen and then stored at −80 °C until use. All animal studies were conducted in accordance with the National Institutes of Health guide for the Care and Use of Laboratory Animals and approved by the Institutional Animal

Care and Use Committee of Tongji Medical College, Huazhong University of Science and Technology (IACUC No. 417, Date: 2015.3.28).

Table 1. Composition of the experimental diets (/100g).

	ND	HFD	HFD + Leu
Macronutrients (g)			
Protein	20.3	20.3	20.3
Carbohydrate	64.5	44.6	44.6
Fat	4.5	24.4	24.4
Fiber	5.0	5.0	5.0
Minerals	3.0	3.0	3.0
Calories (kcal)	379.7	479.2	479.2
Fat (energy %)	10.7	45.8	45.8
Protein (energy %)	21.3	17.0	17.0
Carbohydrate (energy %)	68.0	37.2	37.2
Amino acids (g)			
Leucine	1.3	1.5	2.9
Isoleucine	0.6	0.7	1.0
Valine	0.7	0.9	1.1
Alanine	0.8	0.8	0.5
Aspartic acid	1.5	1.6	1.2
Glycine	0.7	0.5	0.3
Threonine	0.7	0.7	0.7
Serine	0.8	1.0	0.8
Glutamic acid	3.4	3.2	3.2
Tyrosine	0.5	0.7	0.6
Phenylalanine	0.7	0.8	0.8
Lysine	1.1	1.2	1.2
Histidine	0.5	0.5	0.4
Proline	1.2	1.7	1.6
Arginine	1.0	0.5	0.6
Methionine	0.4	0.3	0.4
Serine	0.8	1.0	0.8

ND: Normal chow diet; HFD: High fat diet.

2.2. Insulin Sensitivity Analysis

After 24 or 32 weeks on the respective diets, the fasting serum glucose levels were determined by colorimetric assay (Nanjing Jiancheng Bioengineering Institute, Nanjing, China), and insulin levels were assessed using a commercial ELISA kit (Mercodia AB, Uppsala, Sweden), according to the manufacturer's instructions. The HOMA-IR index was calculated using the following formula: HOMA-IR = [fasting glucose levels (mmol/L)] × [fasting serum insulin (mU/L)]/22.5. The glucose tolerance test (GTT) and insulin tolerance test (ITT) were performed following intragastric glucose administration and intraperitoneal insulin injection, respectively, after overnight starvation of the rats. Blood samples were collected from the tail vein at 0, 15, 30, 60 and 120 min, and the glucose levels were measured with a Glucose Meter (Roche Diagnostics, Shanghai, China).

2.3. Western Blot Analysis

Frozen gastrocnemius muscle, liver and adipose tissues were lysed in RIPA buffer (Beyotime Biotechnology, Shanghai, China) supplemented with phosphatase inhibitors and PMSF (Roche, Ltd., Basel, Switzerland) before use. For the total MitoProfile Oxidative phosphorylation complexes (OXPHOS) analysis, mitochondrial proteins were extracted from the gastrocnemius muscle according to the manufacturer's instructions (Nanjing Jiancheng Bioengineering Institute, Nanjing, China). Protein concentrations were assayed using a bicinchoninic acid (BCA) kit (Beyotime Biotechnology, Shanghai, China). A total of 20–50 µg of protein were resolved on SDS-PAGE gels and then transferred to polyvinylidene difluoride (PVDF) membranes. Information regarding the primary antibodies used in this study is provided in Table S1. Protein bands were visualized with Molecular Imager VersaDoc MP 4000 System (Bio-Rad, Berkeley, CA, USA).

2.4. Transmission Electron Microscopy

The mitochondrial morphology was investigated using electron microscopy. Briefly, gastrocnemius muscles were isolated and fixed with 2.5% glutaraldehyde for 1 day. The muscles were washed and cut longitudinally into 0.5 mm thick strips. Following osmification with 2% osmium tetroxide and 1% uranyl acetate en bloc, the stained tissue was routinely dehydrated in a methanol gradient and embedded in Eponate-12. After polymerization, the ultrastructural features of the mitochondria were observed and photographed using a Tecnai G2 12 transmission electron microscope (FEI Company, Holland, The Netherlands).

2.5. Quantitative Real-Time PCR Analysis

Total RNA was extracted from gastrocnemius muscles with Trizol reagent (Invitrogen, New York, NY, USA) and reverse transcribed into cDNA using a high-capacity cDNA archive kit (Takara, Dalian, China). Real-time PCR was performed using the StepOnePlus^{TM} Real-Time PCR System (Applied Biosystems, Grand Island, NY, USA) with the cDNA templates, gene-specific primers and the SYBR Green qPCR Master mix (Takara, Dalian, China). Calculations were performed using a comparative method ($2^{-\Delta\Delta Ct}$), with GAPDH as the internal control. Total DNA was extracted from the gastrocnemius muscles using acommercial kit (Tiangen Biotech Co., Ltd., Beijing, China), according to the manufacturer's instructions. The mitochondrial DNA (mtDNA) content was assessed using RT-PCR by measuring the threshold cycle ratio of a mitochondria-encoded gene (COXII) to a nucleus-encoded gene (β-globin). All RT-PCR experiments were performed in triplicate using the same sample. The primer pairs for each gene are shown in Table S2.

2.6. Statistical Analysis

Unless otherwise stated, data are presented as means $\pm$ SD. Statistical analyses were performed using the SPSS 15.0 software package (SPSS, Inc., Chicago, IL, USA). Significant differences were assessed by student t test or one-way ANOVA followed by the Student-Newman-Keuls test. $p < 0.05$ were considered statistically significant.

2.7. Serum Preparation and Metabolite Profiling

A targetedLC-MS/MSbased analysis was performed in the State Key Laboratory of Quality Research in Chinese Medicine at Macau University of Science and Technology and Beijing Mass Spectrometry Medical Research Co., Ltd. Broad metabolite profiling of serum was performed using LC-MS/MS (ACQUITYTM ultra-Performance LC (Waters, Milford, MA, USA) equipped with an AB 4000 Q-TRAP mass spectrometer (Applied Biosystems, Grand Island, NY, USA). Serum (200 µL) was mixed with 200 µL of n-Ethylmaleimide (10 mol/L) in PBS buffer and 1000 µL of methanol containing the internal standard L-phenylalanine-d5 (Phe-d5) at a concentration of 10 ng/mL. The mixture was incubated at -20 °C for 20 min and centrifuged at 12,000 rpm for 10 min at 4 °C. The supernatant was evaporated under a vacuum, and the dry residue was reconstituted with distilled water in preparation for analysis.

In addition to the internal standards used for quality control, a quality control (QC) sample was prepared and analyzed after every 10 serum samples. The blank serum used for QC was prepared from serum that had been stripped of endogenous materials by adding 6 g of charcoal activated powder (Sigma-Aldrich, St. Louis, MO, USA) to 100 mL of serum. This suspension was stirred at room temperature for 2 h and centrifuged at 13,500 rpm for 20 min at 4 °C. Then, the supernatant was filtered using a Millipore Express PES Membrane (Merck Millipore, Ltd., Hesse, Germany). The obtained blank serumwas confirmed to be free of biomarkers using LC-MS/MS.

For quantitative amino acid profiling, the LC-MS/MS analysis was performed on an UltiMate3000 (Dionex, Sunnyvale, CA, USA) equipped with an API 3200 Q TRAP MS System (Applied Biosystems, Grand Island, NY, USA). The samples were thawed, extracted and derivatized before analysis. In detail, after dilution with 80 μL of water, the sample was extracted with 500 μL of a mixture of methanol and acetonitrile (1:9, *v*/*v*). The extraction procedure was performed at −20 °C for 10 min after 2 min of vortexing and 1 min of ultrasonication. Then, the residue was re-dissolved in 100 μL of a mixture of methanol and water (1:1, *v*/*v*) with 1 μg/mL of L-2-chlorophenylalanine, and the same steps were repeated (vortexing, ultrasonication and centrifugation). The supernatant (80 μL) was transferred into the sample vial for the analysis.

2.8. Metabolomics Data Processing and Multivariate Analysis

The pre-processed LC-MS/MS data were log-transformed, and the resulting data were analyzed by orthogonal partial least squares projection to latent structure-discriminant analysis (OPLS-DA) using SIMCA-P version 14.0 (Umetrics, Umea, Sweden). OPLS-DA was also used to identify and rank signature metabolites that discriminated the different groups. Qualities of the OPLS-DA models were assessed by R2 indicative of variation described by all components in the model and by Q2, measuring the model ability to predict class membership.

Variables with a variable importance in the projection (VIP) score >1 were considered relevant for group discrimination. Serum metabolite concentrations in HFD + Leu and HFD + CR rats at different time points were compared with their age-matched HFD controls and significantly changed metabolites were analyzed by One-way ANOVA. *p* value < 0.05 was considered statistically significant. In addition, metabolic pathway interpretation of differential metabolites were performed using the MetaboAnalyst 3.0 and KEGG database.

3. Results

3.1. Body Weight and Calorie Intake

As expected, HFD-fed rats exhibited a higher body weight than controls. However, HFD-induced weight gain was significantly attenuated by CR or leucine supplementation from 3 or 13 weeks, respectively. The rats supplemented with leucine had significantly higher body weight when compared to CR rat from 7 weeks (Figure S1A). Consistent with our experimental design, the total calorie intake of CR rats was reduced by 20% over the 32-week feeding period compared with that of HFD-fed rats. Leucine addition to the high fat diet did not significantly alter calorie intake across all time points, with the exception of a slight decrease during week 3 (Figure S1B). The average daily leucine intake in ND, HFD, HFD + CR and HFD + Leu-fed rats were 0.68 g, 0.69 g, 0.54 g and 1.28 g, respectively.

3.2. Insulin Sensitivity

As shown in Figure 1A,B, the 24-week HFD did not alter fasting blood glucose but significantly increased fasting serum insulin. Leucine addition to the HFD for 24 weeks had no obvious effects on fasting serum glucose or insulin, but CR prevented the HFD-induced increase in fasting insulin. Accordingly, the HOMA-IR index was unchanged in leucine-supplemented rats, but was decreased in CR rats (Figure 1C). CR rats had lower insulin level and HOMA-IR than HFD + Leu rats at 24 weeks (Figure 1B,C). After 32 weeks, both fasting blood glucose and insulin were elevated in HFD-fed rats compared with ND-fed rats. HFD + Leu diet induced no significant effect on fast serum glucose and insulin levels. CR largely prevented HFD-induced hyperglycaemia and hyperinsulinaemia (Figure 1A,B). The HOMA-IR index was lower in rats treated with either leucine or CR than that in the corresponding HFD-fed controls (Figure 1C), while the CR rats had lower glucose than HFD + Leu rats at 32 weeks (Figure 1A). The results of the OGTT and ITT confirmed that CR or leucine-supplemented rats were significantly more glucose-tolerant and insulin-sensitive than HFD-fed rats (Figure 1D–I) at the two time points. As expected, insulin-stimulated Protein kinase B (PKB/AKT) phosphorylation in the skeletal muscle was increased in CR rats compared with the HFD-fed controls at both time points (Figure 1J). However, leucine-induced AKT phosphorylation was only observed at 32 weeks. The insulin-stimulated AKT phosphorylation protein expression in CR rats was higher than HFD + Leu rats at week 24 (Figure 1J).

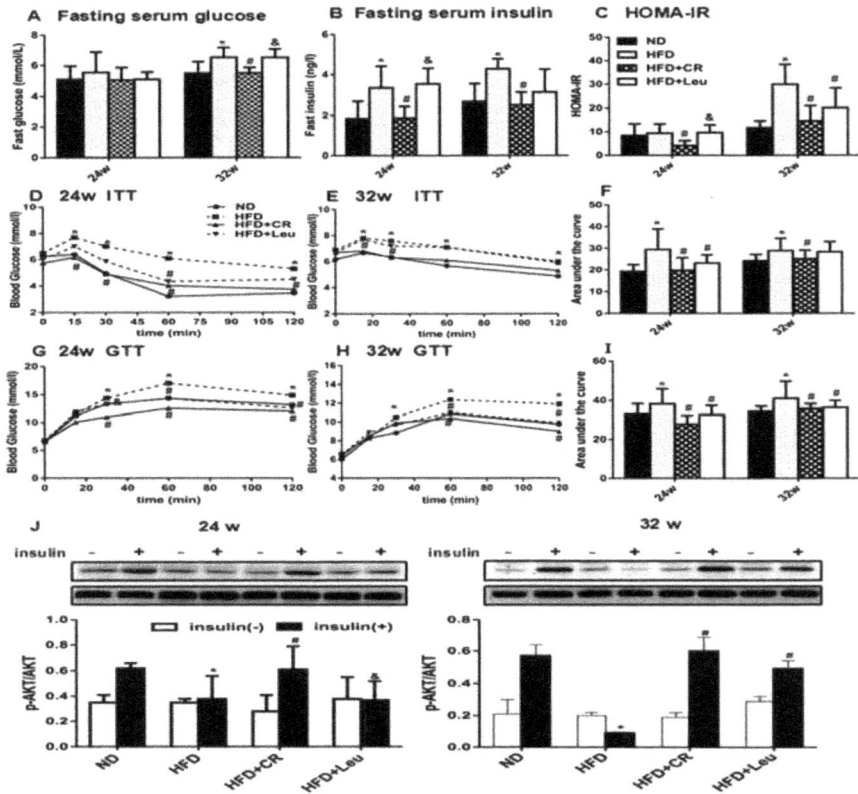

Figure 1. Leucine supplementation improved insulin sensitivity in HFD-fed rats. (**A**) Serum glucose and (**B**) insulin levels were measured after overnight fasting. (**C**) HOMA-IR indices were calculated from fasting glucose and insulin levels. (**D,E**) The intraperitoneal ITT (0.8 IU/kg.bw) and (**G,H**) OGTT (2 g/kg.bw) were performed after overnight fasting at the end of 24 and 32 weeks, respectively. (**F,I**) The area under the curve was calculated ($n = 8$). The results are presented as the mean ± SD. (**J**) AKT and phospho-AKT (Ser473) protein levels in skeletal muscle before (insulin−) and after (insulin+) 2 IU/kg insulin stimulation for 15 min were determined by immunoblotting ($n = 3$–6). * $p < 0.05$ versus ND-fed rats, # $p < 0.05$ versus HFD-fed rats, & $p < 0.05$ versus HFD + CR rats. HFD: High fat diet; ND: Normal chow diet; CR: Calorie restriction; ITT: Insulin tolerance test; OGTT: Oral glucose tolerance test; AKT: Protein kinase B.

3.3. Serum Amino Acid Profiles

Over 24 weeks of feeding, serum concentrations of BCAAs (valine and leucine), glucogenic amino acids (alanine, asparagine and glutamate), and gluconeogenic and ketogenic amino acids (phenylalanine and tryptophan) were significantly lower in HFD-fed rats relative to ND control, While the ketogenic amino acids (lysine) was significantly increased (Table 2). However, BCAA (except for isoleucine) concentrations were significantly elevated after leucine supplementation for 24 weeks compared with those in HFD-fed rats. The concentrations of other amino acids, such as aromatic amino acids (phenylalanine and tryptophan) and several gluconeogenic amino acids (asparagine, proline and alanine), were also significantly elevated (Table 3).

Table 2. Amino acids profile in HFD rats.

Parameter	24 weeks	32 weeks
BCAAs		
isoleucine	1.01 (0.93, 1.09)	0.97 (0.89, 1.06)
valine	0.62 (0.55, 0.70) *	1.04 (0.96, 1,11)
leucine	0.70 (0.56, 0.84) *	0.92 (0.84, 1.01)
Glucogenogenic amino acids		
alanine	0.48 (0.37, 0.59) *	1.02 (0.89, 1.16)
asparagine	0.72 (0.65, 0.80) *	1.36 (1.14, 1.59) *
aspartic acid	1.01 (0.60, 1.43)	1.01 (0.83, 1.20)
cysteine	1.06 (0.92, 1.20)	1.33 (1.24, 1.42) *
glutamate	0.79 (0.69, 0.90) *	1.65 (1.38, 1.92) *
glutamine	1.04 (0.98, 1.10)	1.08 (1.02, 1.14)
glycine	1.46 (1.24, 1.68)	0.94 (0.83, 1.05)
histidine	1.02 (0.95, 1.09)	0.83 (0.77, 0.88) *
methionine	1.01 (0.93, 1.08)	1.09 (0.94, 1.24)
proline	0.91 (0.84, 0.99)	1.23 (1.06, 1.41) *
serine	1.23 (1.04, 1.42)	1.08 (1.02, 1.15)
arginine	1.19 (1.06, 1.32)	0.95 (0.83, 1.08)
Gluconeogenic and ketogenic amino acids		
phenylalanine	0.54 (0.48, 0.59) *	1.10 (0.94, 1.25)
threonine	1.05 (0.95, 1.15)	1.34 (1.25, 1.42) *
tryptophan	0.76 (0.68, 0.85) *	0.90 (0.83, 0.98)
tyrosine	1.12 (0.95, 1.29)	0.89 (0.82, 0.96)
Ketogenic amino acids		
lysine	1.37 (1.20, 1.54) *	1.46 (1.21, 1.71) *

Data were expressed as mean fold difference (95% CI) of HFD-fed rats relative to their corresponding ND-fed controls at week 24 and 32, respectively ($n = 8$). * $p < 0.05$ versus age-matched ND controls. HFD: High-fat diet; ND: Normal chow diet; CR: Calorie restriction; BCAAs, branched-chain amino acids.

At week 32, serum BCAA levels were not significantly changed in HFD rats compared to corresponding controls, but glucogenogenic amino acids (asparagine, cysteine, glutamate and proline), gluconeogenic and ketogenic amino acids (threonine) and ketogenic amino acid lysine were significantly increased (Table 2). However, after 32 weeks of leucine treatment, serum BCAA and aromatic amino acid levels did not significantly differ, whereas asparagine and glycine were significantly reduced and proline was increased. The concentrations of most amino acids in CR rats were reduced at week 24 compared with those in HFD controls, but the observed differences were not statistically significant (except for leucine, isoleucine, alanine, phenylalanine and lysine). However, CR-induced alterations in serum amino acid concentrations were not remarkable at 32 weeks, but alanine and proline were significantly increased (Table 3).

Table 3. Amino acids profile.

Parameter	24 weeks		32 weeks	
	CR	HFD + Leu	CR	HFD + Leu
BCAAs				
isoleucine	0.82 (0.76, 0.88) *	0.91 (0.84, 0.98)	0.88 (0.79, 0.96)	0.94 (0.77, 1.11)
valine	0.91 (0.86, 0.96)	1.38 (1.18, 1.58) *	0.94 (0.85, 1.03)	0.95 (0.74, 1.15)
leucine	0.85 (0.79, 0.91) *	1.43 (1.02, 1.84) *	0.91 (0.84, 0.98)	0.98 (0.69, 1.27)
Glucogenogenic amino acids				
alanine	0.79 (0.71, 0.87) *	1.49 (1.34, 1.65) *	1.29 (1.02, 1.56) *	0.92 (0.71, 1.12)
asparagine	0.91 (0.76, 1.06)	1.49 (1.25, 1.72) *	0.90 (0.73, 1.06)	0.79 (0.60, 0.98) *
aspartic acid	0.93 (0.82, 1.03)	0.91 (0.74, 1.08)	1.08 (0.96, 1.20)	1.14 (0.97, 1.31)
cysteine	1.19 (1.08, 1.30) *	0.96 (0.85, 1.08)	1.09 (0.93, 1.25)	0.93 (0.77, 1.08)
glutamate	0.93 (0.80, 1.07)	1.07 (0.92, 1.23)	1.08 (0.86, 1.31)	1.00 (0.83, 1.17)
glutamine	0.93 (0.85, 1.01)	0.92 (0.84, 1.00)	1.03 (0.88, 1.18)	1.06 (0.91, 1.21)
glycine	0.96 (0.90, 1.03)	0.95 (0.91, 0.99)	0.89 (0.81, 0.98)	0.82 (0.71, 0.93) *
histidine	0.98 (0.90, 1.05)	0.97 (0.83, 1.11)	1.09 (0.98, 1.20)	1.05 (0.92, 1.18)
methionine	0.94 (0.86, 1.03)	1.01 (0.94, 1.08)	0.94 (0.86, 1.02)	0.97 (0.89, 1.04)
proline	1.04 (0.80, 1.29)	1.28 (1.00, 1.57) *	1.24 (1.00, 1.49) *	1.27 (1.02, 1.52) *
serine	0.98 (0.91, 1.04)	0.92 (0.85, 0.98)	1.08 (0.98, 1.18)	0.95 (0.84, 1.05)
arginine	0.86 (0.82, 0.91)	0.98 (0.84, 1.12)	1.08 (1.00, 1.15)	1.16 (0.96, 1.36)
Gluconeogenic and ketogenic amino acids				
phenylalanine	0.89 (0.83, 0.95) *	1.35 (1.20, 1.50) *	0.94 (0.90, 0.97)	1.07 (0.91, 1.21)
threonine	1.17 (1.05, 1.29)	0.92 (0.81, 1.02)	1.08 (0.92, 1.25)	1.09 (0.97, 1.21)
tryptophan	1.00 (0.69, 1.31)	1.43 (1.17, 1.69) *	1.22 (0.94, 1.50)	0.97 (0.77, 1.16)
tyrosine	0.87 (0.71, 1.04)	1.00 (0.87, 1.14)	1.08 (0.92, 1.25)	1.09 (0.97, 1.21)
Ketogenic amino acids				
lysine	0.82 (0.74, 0.90) *	0.65 (0.55, 0.74) *	0.90 (0.75, 1.06)	0.99 (0.79, 1.19)

Data were expressed as mean fold difference (95% CI) of HFD + Leu and HFD + CR rats relative to their corresponding HFD control at week 24 and 32, respectively ($n = 8$). * $p < 0.05$ versus age-matched HFD controls. HFD: High-fat diet; CR: Calorie restriction.

3.4. Serum Metabolic Profiles

An LC-MS/MS-based metabolic approach was used to obtain more insights into the mechanisms underlying the different effects of leucine supplementation on insulin resistance. OPLS-DA model was carried out for ND, HFD, HFD + Leu and HFD + CR groups at week 24 and 32, respectively, and the R2 and Q2 values confirmed good qualities for all models (Figure 2A,B). The score plots for each model showed clear separation among the different groups suggesting they had different metabolic features at different pathological stages of HFD induced insulin resistance.

The metabolites detected in the serum were almost decreased in HFD-fed rats compared to the ND controls at week 24. Prominent decreases were observed for metabolites from amino acids including aromatic amino acid catabolites (5-hydroxytryptophan, 4,6-dihydroxyquinoline, and L-kynurenine), methionine catabolites (spermidine and S-adenosylhomocysteine) and nitrogenous compounds derived from amino acid catabolism (creatinine, Creatine, and uridine), fatty acid metabolites (3-hydroxybutyric, Acetylcarnitine and Carnitine), tricarboxylic acid (TCA) cycle intermediates (Fumaric acid and a-Ketoglutaric acid), bile acid metabolites (Ursodeoxycholic acid, Glycochenodeoxycholic acid) and some lysophosphatidylcholines (LPCs). However, fatty acid metabolism (palmitic acid) and TCA intermediate (malic acid) were marked elevated (Table 4). The serum metabolites that discriminated between leucine-supplemented and HFD-fed rats were primarily involved in the TCA cycle, fatty acid, bile acid and amino acid metabolism (Table 5). Specifically, the serum levels ofTCA intermediates (fumaric acid, malic acid and α-ketoglutarate) and metabolites related to lipid metabolism (acylcarnitine, palmitoyl-L-carnitine, carnitine, palmitic acid and 3-hydroxybutyrate) were markedly higher in leucine-treated rats than in HFD-fed controls at week 24.

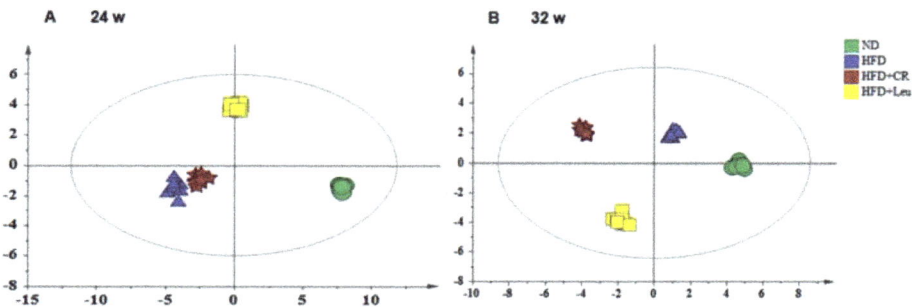

Figure 2. Orthogonal partial least squares projection to latent structure-discriminant analysis (OPLS-DA) score plots displaying the separation of the ND-fed, HFD-fed, Calorie-restricted and HFD + leurats after (**A**) 24 and (**B**) 32 weeks of treatment. Model parameters: (**A**) R2X = 0.944, Q2 = 0.424; (**B**) R2X = 0.938, Q2 = 0.652.HFD: High-fat diet; ND: Normal chow diet.

Table 4. Fold difference of serum metabolites significantly changed in HFD rats relative to the corresponding ND controls.

Metabolites	24 weeks	32 weeks
Amino acids derivatives		
L-Kynurenine	0.72 (0.64, 0.79) *	1.09 (0.87, 1.31)
5-hydroxytryptophan	0.55 (0.44, 0.66) *	1.11 (0.93, 1.29) *
Spermidine	0.52 (0.48, 0.57) *	1.26 (1.10, 1.42)
2-hydroxyisobutyrate	0.86 (0.77, 0.95)	2.23 (1.87, 2.59) *
2-hydroxyglutarate	0.55 (0.47, 0.62) *	1.37 (1.20, 1.54) *
S-(adenosyl)-L-homocysteine	0.49 (0.41, 0.58) *	1.28 (0.96, 1.60)
4,6-dihydroxyquinoline	0.55 (0.49, 0.62) *	1.20 (0.93, 1.46)
Creatinine	0.43 (0.33, 0.54) *	1.19 (0.98, 1.40)
Creatine	0.41 (0.31, 0.52) *	1.34 (1.04, 1.64) *
Uridine	0.39 (0.25, 0.52) *	1.36 (1.17, 1.54) *
Fatty acid metabolism		
3-hydroxybutyric	0.77 (0.70, 0.85) *	1.92 (1.56, 2.27) *
Palmitic acid	3.92 (3.25, 4.59) *	1.53 (0.93, 2.12)
Acetylcarnitine	0.70 (0.64, 0.77) *	1.02 (0.84, 1.19)
Palmitoyl-L-carnitine	0.91 (0.75, 1.08)	1.48 (1.11, 1.86)
Carnitine	0.46 (0.38, 0.54) *	1.04 (0.68, 1.41)
Phospholipids		
Lysophosphatidylcholine (C18:1)	0.50 (0.43, 0.57) *	1.18 (0.99, 1.37)
Lysophosphatidylcholine (C16:1)	0.38 (0.34, 0.41) *	0.99 (0.82, 1.16)
Lysophosphatidylcholine (C16:0)	0.65 (0.58, 0.72) *	0.97 (0.83, 1.12)
Lysophosphatidylcholine (C20:4)	0.16 (0.12, 0.20) *	1.21 (0.94, 1.48)
TCA cycle intermediates		
Fumaric acid	0.82 (0.74, 0.89) *	1.12 (0.93, 1.31)
Malic acid	3.54 (2.81, 4.27) *	1.23 (1.07, 1.39) *
Citric acid	0.91 (0.80, 1.03)	1.22 (1.10, 1.34) *
a-Ketoglutaric acid	0.52 (0.45, 0.59) *	1.13 (0.98, 1.29)

Table 4. *Cont.*

Metabolites	24 weeks	32 weeks
Bile acid metabolism		
Ursodeoxycholic acid	0.28 (0.19, 0.38) *	1.15 (0.73, 1.56)
Glycochenodeoxycholic acid	0.32 (0.28, 0.35) *	0.73 (0.60, 0.86)
Glycocholic acid	0.71 (0.13, 1.28)	0.65 (0.22, 1.08)
Purine metabolism		
Xanthosine	0.71 (0.46, 0.96)	0.93 (0.71, 1.16)
Allantoin	0.42 (0.33, 0.50) *	1.00 (0.85, 1.14)
Uric acid	0.88 (0.77, 0.98)	1.10 (0.95, 1.25)
Xanthine	0.83 (0.56, 1.09)	1.00 (0.71, 1.29)

Data were expressed as mean fold difference (95% Confidence Interval) of HFD-fed rats relative to their corresponding ND controls at week 24 and 32, respectively ($n = 8$). * $p < 0.05$ versus age-matched ND controls. HFD: High fat diet; ND: Normal chow diet; TCA, tricarboxylic acid.

Table 5. Fold difference of serum metabolites significantly changed in HFD + CR or HFD + Leu rats relative to the corresponding HFD-fed controls.

Metabolites	24 weeks		32 weeks	
	HFD + CR	HFD + Leu	HFD + CR	HFD + Leu
Amino acids derivatives				
L-Kynurenine	1.30 (0.66, 1.95)	1.70 (1.23, 2.19) *	1.10 (0.43, 1.78)	1.10 (0.81, 1.39)
5-hydroxytryptophan	1.10 (0.96, 1.25)	1.58 (1.16, 1.92) *	1.29 (0.82, 1.76)	1.43 (1.07, 1.79) *
Spermidine	1.17 (1.02, 1.33) *	1.43 (1.26, 1.60) *	1.18 (1.04, 1.32) *	1.05 (0.89, 1.21)
2-hydroxyisobutyrate	0.90 (0.70, 1.10)	1.54 (1.26, 1.81) *	0.82 (0.56, 1.09)	0.67 (0.38, 0.95) *
2-hydroxyglutarate	0.88 (0.73, 1.03)	1.71 (1.50, 1.92) *	1.07 (0.86, 1.28)	1.01 (0.86, 1.16)
S-(adenosyl)-L-homocysteine	1.24 (0.87, 1.60)	1.57 (1.28, 1.86) *	1.51 (1.20, 1.83) *	1.34 (1.03, 1.66) *
4,6-dihydroxyquinoline	1.54 (1.21, 1.87) *	1.81 (1.56, 2.06) *	1.50 (1.17, 1.82) *	0.90(0.75, 1.05)
Creatinine	1.31 (1.19, 1.43) *	1.50 (1.36, 1.64) *	1.14 (0.91, 1.37)	1.16 (0.91, 1.40)
Creatine	0.91 (0.76, 1.06)	1.33 (0.99, 1.68)	1.04 (0.70, 1.37)	1.71 (1.34, 2.08) *
Uridine	1.32 (0.93, 1.72)	1.61 (1.37, 1.85*	1.02 (0.88, 1.17)	0.92 (0.68, 1.17)
Fatty acid metabolism				
3-hydroxybutyric	0.92 (0.71, 1.13)	1.36 (1.13, 1.59) *	0.92 (0.60, 1.24)	0.91 (0.48, 1.33)
Palmitic acid	1.28 (1.03, 1.53) *	1.81 (1.47, 2.15) *	1.55 (1.17, 1.94) *	0.54 (0.38, 0.70) *
Acetylcarnitine	1.12 (0.96, 1.30)	1.34 (1.21, 1.48) *	1.15 (0.92, 1.39)	0.87 (0.67, 1.07)
Palmitoyl-L-carnitine	1.17 (0.97, 1.37)	1.90 (1.54, 2.26) *	0.99 (0.59, 1.40)	0.49 (0.39, 0.58) *
Carnitine	1.29 (1.09, 1.48) *	1.86 (1.46, 2.26) *	1.28 (1.09, 1.47)	1.04 (0.93, 1.15)
Phospholipids				
Lysophosphatidylcholine (C18:1)	1.35 (1.13, 1.56) *	1.42 (1.19, 1.65) *	1.55 (1.19, 1.90) *	1.49 (1.14, 1.83) *
Lysophosphatidylcholine (C16:1)	1.40 (1.15, 1.64) *	1.42 (1.23, 1.60) *	1.41 (1.00, 1.83) *	0.91 (0.71, 1.10)
Lysophosphatidylcholine(C16:0)	1.20 (1.05, 1.36) *	1.34 (1.18, 1.49) *	1.31 (1.13, 1.48) *	1.21 (1.03, 1.40) *
Lysophosphatidylcholine (C20:4)	1.06 (0.87, 1.25)	1.04 (0.77, 1.30)	0.87 (0.50, 1.24)	3.82 (3.23, 4.41) *
TCA cycle intermediates				
Fumaric acid	1.09 (0.93, 1.24)	1.23 (1.08, 1.38) *	1.09 (0.96, 1.22)	0.82 (0.72, 0.93) *
Malic acid	0.87 (0.74, 1.00)	1.33 (1.11, 1.55) *	0.97 (0.48, 1.47)	0.15 (0.09, 0.22) *
Citric acid	1.02 (0.90, 1.15)	1.18 (0.97, 1.39)	0.94 (0.77, 1.11)	0.86 (0.74, 0.97) *
a-Ketoglutaric acid	0.95 (0.80, 1.09)	1.32 (1.13, 1.50) *	1.23 (1.00, 1.47)	1.05 (0.85, 1.25)
Bile acid metabolism				
Ursodeoxycholic acid	1.57 (0.96, 2.19)	2.58 (1.91, 3.24) *	1.37 (1.06, 1.68) *	1.35 (1.08, 1.61) *
Glycochenodeoxycholic acid	1.45 (1.19, 1.71) *	1.26 (0.92, 1.60)	1.63 (1.13, 2.13) *	1.43 (1.19, 1.66) *
Glycocholic acid	2.20 (1.04, 3.36) *	4.17 (0.60, 7.74)	3.17 (1.08, 5.27) *	3.76 (1.45, 6.07) *
Purine metabolism				
Xanthosine	0.90 (0.63, 1.18)	1.20 (0.77, 1.62)	1.49 (1.13, 1.85) *	1.05 (0.90, 1.19)
Allantoin	1.05 (0.86, 1.24)	1.33 (1.00, 1.66) *	1.27 (1.04, 1.50) *	1.41 (1.23, 1.59) *
Uric acid	0.91 (0.77, 1.05)	1.24 (1.07, 1.41) *	1.08 (0.93, 1.23)	0.90 (0.83, 0.96)
Xanthine	1.05 (0.55, 1.55)	1.26 (0.76, 1.76)	1.71(1.38, 2.02) *	1.12 (0.96, 1.27)

Data were expressed as mean fold difference (95% Confidence Interval) of HFD + Leu and HFD + CR rats relative to their corresponding HFD controls at week 24 and 32, respectively ($n = 8$). * $p < 0.05$ versus age-matched HFD controls. HFD: High fat diet; CR: Calorie restriction.

The amino acid derivatives (5-hydroxytryptophan, 2-hydroxyisobutyrate, 2-hydroxyglutarate, Creatine and Uridine), fatty acid metabolites (3-hydroxybutyric), TCA cycle intermediates (Malic acid, Citric acid) were significantly elevated after 32 weeks of HFD feeding relative to the age-matched ND control (Table 4). Notably, we observed sharp decreases in the levels of TCA intermediates (fumaric acid, malic acid and citric acid) and lipid-related metabolites (palmitoyl-L-carnitine and palmitic acid) at week 32 relative to HFD-fed controls (Table 5).

In addition, leucine supplementation for 24 weeks contributed to the accumulation of metabolites associated with amino acid catabolism, including aromatic amino acid catabolites (5-hydroxytryptophan, 4,6-dihydroxyquinoline, and L-kynurenine), methionine catabolites (spermidine and S-adenosylhomocysteine) and nitrogenous compounds derived from amino acid catabolism (creatinine, uric acid, and uridine).In contrast, at week 32, the levels of amino acid catabolites that discriminated the leucine group from the HFD-fed controls were reduced. Moreover, prominentincreases in bile acid metabolites and some lysophosphatidylcholines (LPCs) were detected at both 24 and 32 weeks (Table 5).

Metabolites related to lipid metabolism (palmitic acid and LPCs), bile acid metabolism (glycochenodeoxycholic acid and glycocholic acid) and some amino acid catabolites were significantly elevated at week 24 and 32 in CR rats compared with the corresponding HFD-fed controls (Table 5).

3.5. BCAA Catabolizing Enzymes and Metabolites

HFD feeding for 24 weeks, the levels of transamination products of BCAAs— branched-chain α-keto acids (BCKAs)—did not change significantly compared with ND-fed control at 24 weeks (Figure 3B). Mitochondrial branched-chain aminotransferase (BCATm) protein expression in skeletal muscle and adipose tissue were both significantly increased. Branched-chain α-keto acid dehydrogenase kinase (BCKDK) protein expression in HFD rats was lower in skeletal muscle, while higher in adipose tissue than ND controls (Figure 4A–C). BCATm protein expression was significantly increased in skeletal muscle and adipose tissue, concurrent with a significant increase in BCKDKandno change in branched-chain α-keto acid dehydrogenase E1 α (BCKDHE1α) in skeletal muscles, livers and adipose tissues of leucine-supplemented rats, compared with those of HFD-fed controls at week 24 (Figure 4A–C). Furthermore, the levels of transamination products of leucine (α-Ketoisocaproate, KIC) were also increased (Figure 3B).

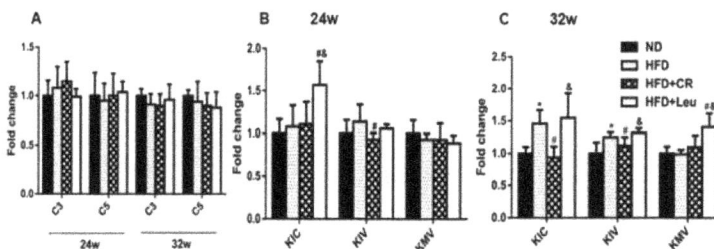

Figure 3. Leucine supplementation-induced alterations in the levels of BCAA derivatives. (**A**) Serum levels of short-chain acylcarnitines (C3 and C5) and (**B**,**C**) Branched-chain α-keto acids (BCKAs) ($n = 8$). The results are presented as means $\pm$ SD. * $p < 0.05$ versus ND-fed rats, # $p < 0.05$ versus HFD-fed rats, & $p < 0.05$ versus HFD + CR rats. HFD: High fat diet; ND: Normal chow diet; CR: Calorie restriction.

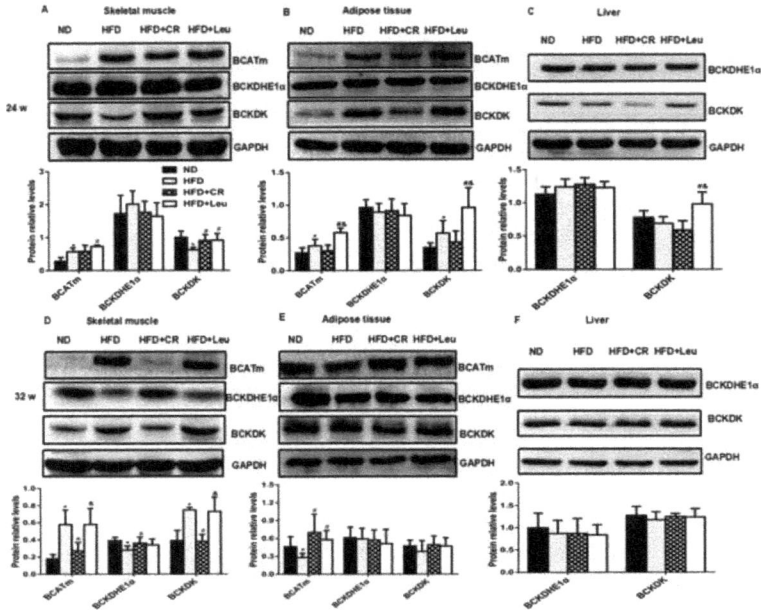

Figure 4. Leucine supplementation-induced alterations in BCAA catabolic enzyme protein expression. Representative immunoblots of total mBCAT, BCKDHE1α and BCKDK protein levels in skeletal muscle (**A,D**), adipose tissue (**B,E**) and liver (**C,F**); $n = 6$. The results are presented as the mean ± SD. * $p < 0.05$ versus ND-fed rats, # $p < 0.05$ versus HFD-fed rats, & $p < 0.05$ versus HFD + CR rats. mBCAT: Mitochondrial branched-chain aminotransferase; BCKDHE1α: Branched-chain α-keto acid dehydrogenase E1 α; BCKDK: Branched-chain α-keto acid dehydrogenase kinase, HFD: High fat diet; ND: Normal chow diet; CR: Calorie restriction.

However, HFD feeding for 32 weeks led to significantly increase in the levels of transamination products of leucine (α-Ketoisocaproate, KIC) and transamination products of valine (α-Ketoisovalerate, KIV) compared to corresponding ND control (Figure 3C). BCATm and BCKDK protein expression were significantly elevated, but BCKDHE1αprotein expression was significantly decreased in skeletal muscle. In addition, BCATm protein expression in adipose tissue was significantly decreased compared with ND-fed control at 32 weeks (Figure 4D–F). In contrast, the only changes observed in the levels of BCAA catabolizing enzymes and metabolites were an increased expression of BCATm in adipose tissue (Figure 4D–F) and increased isoleucine-derived KMV (α-Keto-β-methylvalerate, KMV) levels compared to the HFD-fed controls after 32 weeks of leucine supplementation (Figure 3C). BCAA-catabolizing enzyme protein expression did not significantly differ between CR rats and HFD-fed controls at week 24 (Figure 4A–C). However, BCATm and BCKDK protein expression was significantly decreased, whereas BCKDHE1α expression was significantly increased in skeletal muscle in CR rats at week 32 compared to the HFD-fed controls (Figure 4D–F). Notably, neither leucine supplementation nor CR had a significant impact on serum BCAA-derived short-chain acylcarnitine (C3 and C5) levels throughout the experiment (Figure 3A).

3.6. Mitochondrial Properties

Long-term HFD feeding-induced mitochondrial structural damage was exacerbated by leucine supplementation at 24 weeks (Figure 5A). Mitochondrial function was also impaired, as indicated by the reduced expression of enzymes involved in OXPHOSand serum ATP production (Figure 5B,D).

The expression of genes controlling mitochondrial biogenesis, including mitochondrial transcription factor A (TFAM), peroxisome proliferator-activated receptor γ coactivator-1-α (PGC-1α) and sirtuin 1 (SIRT1), were greatly decreased (Figure 5F) in HFD + Leurats at this time point. In contrast, HFD-induced mitochondrial damage was partially restored by leucine supplementation at 32 weeks (Figure 5A), accompanied by increases in the mtDNA content (Figure 5E), the expression of genes involved in mitochondrial biogenesis (TFAM) (Figure 5G) and ATP production (Figure 5D). As expected, CR ameliorated HFD-induced mitochondrial damage at both time points. At week 24, CR enhanced expression of enzymes involved in OXPHOS, and the gene expression related to mitochondrial biogenesis (TFAM, NRF-1, PGC-1α and SIRT1) (Figure 5B,F). At week 32, CR-induced mitochondrial biogenesis was not greatly changed, but ATP production was significantly increasedcompared to HFD controls (Figure 5D,E,G). CR exhibited better effects on improving HFD-induced mitochondrial damage at week 24 as demonstrated by increases in OXPHOS protein levels (Figure 5B), ATP production (Figure 5D), and mitochondrial biogenesis compared to leucine supplementation (Figure 5F).

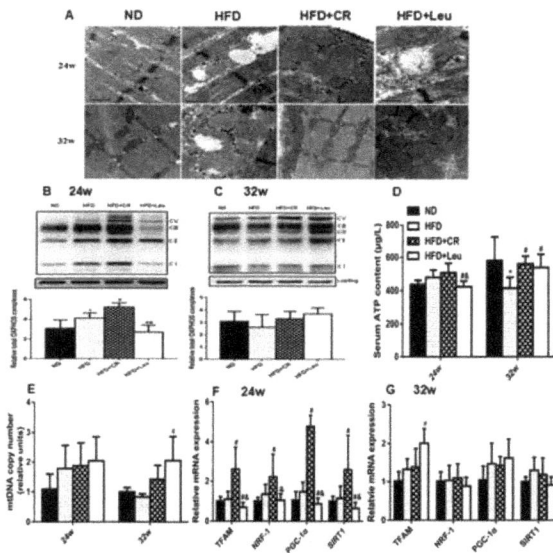

Figure 5. Leucine supplementation-induced alterations in mitochondrial properties. (**A**) Transmission electronic microscopy ($\times 20,000$) of the mitochondrial ultrastructure in skeletal muscle ($n = 4$). (**B**,**C**) Protein expression of Oxidative phosphorylation complexes (OXPHOS) complexes I to V in the electron transport chain in skeletal muscle were analyzed by western blotting ($n = 6$). (**D**) Serum ATP levels ($n = 8$). (**E**) Mitochondrial DNA (mtDNA) copy number ($n = 6$). (**F**,**G**) Expression of mitochondrial biogenesis-related genes ($n = 6$). The results are presented as the mean $\pm$ SD. * $p < 0.05$ versus ND-fed rats, # $p < 0.05$ versus HFD-fed rats, & $p < 0.05$ versus HFD + CR rats. ND: Normal chow diet; HFD: High fat diet; CR: Calorie restriction.

4. Discussion and Conclusions

The effects of BCAA (especially leucine) supplementation on insulin resistance remains elusive. Numerous studies have shown that leucine supplementation may prevent HFD-induced obesity [1,2,20], modulate glucose metabolism [21,22] and improve insulin sensitivity in rodent models. However, Newgard et al. suggested that excess BCAAs could contribute to development of insulin resistance, at least under conditions of high fat feeding or elevated tissue fatty acid availability [7]. The underlying mechanisms contributing to these inconsistent results are incompletely understood.

Exactly how leucine exerts effects on insulin resistance is complex, and may depend on the study design, dietary composition, the animal models typically used and the BCAA concentrations, duration and form of administration. Recently, it has been supposed that BCAAs can trigger different and even opposite effects, depending on the catabolic and anabolic state of the organisms [17]. Given the different metabolic signature in the progression of T2DM, and leucine's ability to stimulate both anabolic and catabolic processes [23], we applied an integrative, time-resolved approach to gain a deeper understanding the effects of leucine supplementation in the complexity of the disease on BCAA metabolism, mitochondrial properties and metabolic profiling. Several interesting and important findings were obtained.

In the present study, HFD feeding induced hyperinsulinaemia at 24 weeks. During this period, the rats became increasingly obese, and exhibited lower concentrations of amino acids and related metabolites, fatty acid metabolites and TCA intermediates compared to corresponding ND controls. Studies have shown that insulin signaling functions at an increased basal level in the presence of insulin resistance and hyperinsulinaemia [24,25]. Compensatory increased insulin secretion response to overnutrition may slow fat oxidation and promote anabolism (syntheses of glycogen, proteins, and fats), leading to body weight gain and glucose homeostasis. In contrast, after HFD feeding for 32 weeks, the rats progressively developed hyperglycaemia. The increased insulin level could not maintain glucose at normal levels, and was accompanied by elevated levels of amino acids and related metabolites, fatty acid metabolites and TCA intermediates relative to corresponding ND-fed rats. These data suggested that at this stage the anabolic response to hyperinsulinaemia was blunted, HFD rats were transition from predominantly anabolic condition to predominantly catabolic condition.

The effect of supplementation of HFD with leucine was examined in these two different metabolic conditions, respectively. Our results indicated that doubling dietary leucine globally improved HFD-induced insulin resistance but caused different changes in BCAA catabolism in rats with hyperinsulinaemia or hyperglycaemia. These results seem inconsistent with the finding that elevated circulation of BCAAs and related metabolites promotes insulin resistance, particularly in response to HFD feeding [5,7]. Leucine supplementation ameliorated HFD-induced insulin resistance to different extents at the two time points, as indicated by the improved HOMA-IR values, insulin tolerance and glucose tolerance. Interestingly, this leucine-induced elevation in insulin sensitivity may not be correlated with changes in serum BCAAs, which were increased in HFD + Leu rats at 24 weeks and unaltered at 32 weeks compared with those in HFD-fed rats.

Recent metabolomic, proteomic and genomic studies have suggested that altered BCAA catabolism contributes to elevated BCAAs [14,26,27]. The enzymes involved in the first two steps of the BCAA catabolic pathway, BCATm and Branched-chain α-keto acid dehydrogenase (BCKDH), were examined in the present study. Leucine supplementation increased BCATm protein expression in adipose tissue and skeletal muscle at 24 weeks, suggesting a substrate-induced effect of increased dietary BCAAs (~70% increase for three BCAAs) compared with that in HFD-fed rats. No differences were observed in protein expression of BCKDHE1α, whereas that of BCKDK, a kinase that inactivates BCKDH by phosphorylating the subunit E1α, was increased in observed tissues, including skeletal muscle, liver and adipose tissues. BCKDK participates in a key mechanism for the nutritional and hormonal regulation of BCAA oxidative flux [28,29], and its expression is increased by insulin [30]. This potentially impaired BCKD activity may contribute to the accumulation of BCKAs, such as KIC, in leucine-supplemented rats during the early stage of insulin resistance, which was characterized by hyperinsulinaemia in the present study. Following the progression of insulin resistance to hyperglycaemia, no significant leucine-induced alterations were observed in serum BCAAs or BCAA-catabolizing enzyme levels, with the exception of increased BCATm in adipose tissue. This tight regulation of BCAA catabolism suggests that an elegant method exists for increasing the degradation of BCAAs when they are present in excess and sparing them [31] when they are needed for anabolic or other necessary processes during the different stages of insulin resistance.

In addition to alterations in BCAA catabolism, we identified several leucine-associated changes in TCA cycle intermediates, lipids and other amino acid metabolites in rats with hyperinsulinaemia or hyperglycaemia. Leucine-induced alterations in serum amino acid concentrations at 24 weeks included increased aromatic amino acid (phenylalanine and tryptophan), alanine and asparagine levels, which may have occurred because BCAAs share a competitive transport system with aromatic amino acids [32]. In addition, BCAA transamination provides a nitrogen source for the synthesis of other dispensable amino acids. The levels of almost all amino acid catabolites investigated in the present study were increased in leucine-supplemented rats at 24 weeks, but were unaltered or decreased at 32 weeks, compared with those in HFD-fed controls. It is noteworthy that various factors affect serum amino acid concentrations, including protein turnover (protein synthesis and degradation), and the metabolism of individual amino acids. The exact mechanisms by which leucine supplementation affect the levels of amino acids and their metabolites at different stage of insulin resistance are still unknown, and warrant further study.

Acylcarnitines are intermediates of fatty acid oxidation, and accumulate as a consequence of the metabolic dysfunction resulting from the insufficient integration between β-oxidation and the TCA cycle [33–35]. Elevated BCAAs in a lipotoxic environment have been proposed to induce the accumulation of BCAA-derived acylcarnitines and incompletely oxidized lipid species [5,7]. In HFD-induced hyperinsulinaemic rats in the present study, leucine supplementation caused increases in acylcarnitine species (carnitine, acylcarnitine and palmitoyl-L-carnitine), but no remarkable changes in BCAA-derived short-chain acylcarnitines (C3 and C5). However, TCA cycle intermediates were significantly elevated, reflecting an early compensatory response to substrate overload. Accumulated by-products of BCAA transamination are catabolized to BCAA-related acetyl-CoAs, ketones and other intermediates, leading to competitive inhibition of lipid-derived acetyl-CoA entry into the TCA cycle [36–38]; in turn, this process may reduce fatty acid oxidation and induce acylcarnitine accumulation and ketogenesis, as indicated by the results (Table 3). Interestingly, as insulin resistance progressed, leucine promoted reductions in the accumulation of serum acylcarnitine species and levels of multiple TCA cycle intermediates at 32 weeks compared with those in age-matched HFD-fed controls.Skeletal muscle serves as a major reservoir of free carnitine and is thought to be a principal contributor to the serum acylcarnitine pool. The accumulation of acylcarnitine species is mitotoxic and promotes mitochondrial dysfunction. The above-mentioned alterations in the metabolic phenotype might be correlated with changes in skeletal muscle mitochondrial properties. Consistent with this hypothesis, the HFD + Leu treatment caused increased mitochondrial damage, accompanied by decreases in mitochondrial biogenesis, ATP production and mitochondrial oxidative enzyme levels in skeletal muscle compared with those in HFD-fed controls.These data were seemingly in conflict with the favorable effects of leucine on overall insulin sensitivity at this stage. It is well-known that insulin resistance is associated with mitochondrial dysfunction, but the causality of this association is controversial. More recent findings suggest that mitochondrial dysfunction is not an early event in the development of insulin resistance [39], but rather an adaptation to excess nutrients [40,41]. Skeletal muscle is the initial site for most BCAA catabolism and major insulin-target tissue. Thus, at this stage, improved insulin sensitivity by leucine supplementation may facilitate both the anabolic effects of insulin and the adaptive catabolic effects of "nutrient overload" in skeletal muscle under the background of a HFD, leading to an impaired mitochondrial function. Notably, the HFD-induced mitochondrial damage was relieved and mitochondrial biogenesis was increased by leucine supplementation after 32 weeks. These results are consistent with previous studies reporting that leucine supplementation increases mitochondrial biogenesis while simultaneously enhancing lipid oxidation [42–44], leading to the reduced accumulation of acylcarnitine species. Therefore, we speculate that BCAAs are primarily used for anabolism at this stage; thus, BCAAs and their derivatives that flow into the mitochondria are decreased. This hypothesis is consistent with our observations of decreased levels of TCA cycle intermediates and no obvious changes in BCAAs and amino acids related catabolites concentrations in circulation. The reduced mitochondrial load occurred simultaneously with improved mitochondrial function, leading to increased ATP production. Thus, altered mitochondrial function may partly account for the improvement in skeletal muscle insulin sensitivity. Moreover, Li et al. observed that in HFD-induced obese mice, leucine supplementation prevented obesity and insulin resistance in association with attenuation of mitochondrial dysfunction [45].

Taken together, these results indicated that abnormal BCAA metabolism induced by dietary supplementation coupled with HFD intake might lead to the accumulation of BCKAs and incompletely oxidized lipid species, which contributed to mitochondrial dysfunction in skeletal muscle during the early stage of insulin resistance (24 weeks). In contrast, during the hyperglycaemic stage (32 weeks), when catabolic processes predominate, leucine supplementation enhanced mitochondrial biogenesis, with concomitantly improved lipid oxidation and mitochondrial function in skeletal muscle (Figure 6).

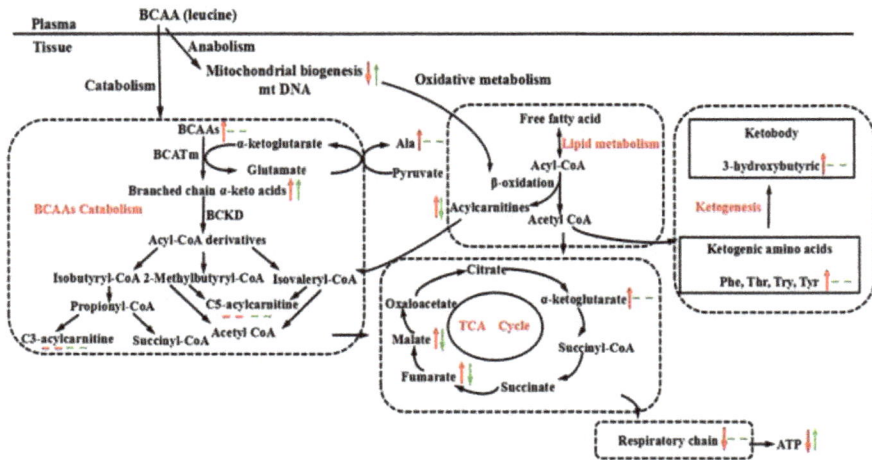

Figure 6. Summary of the possible metabolic alterations induced by leucine supplementation at the different stage of insulin resistance in high-fat diet-fed rats. The red arrows indicate the changes observed at 24 weeks, whereas the blue arrows represent the changes observed at 32 weeks compared with the age-matched high-fat diet-fed controls. The up-arrows indicate an increase in concentration; the down-arrows indicate a decrease in concentration; the dotted lines indicate no significant change in concentration.

CR without malnutrition has long been considered an effective strategy for protecting againstage-associated disorders by modulating mitochondrial biogenesis and activating the reactive oxygen species defense system [46–48]. However, long-term CR is hard for compliance and its possible disadvantages remain to be determined, particularly in the elderly [49]. There has been a growing interest in developing dietary strategies that mimic the beneficial effects of CR. Dietary supplementation with BCAAs has been shown to improve mitochondrial biogenensis and prevent oxidative damage in middle-aged mice [4,16]. In this study, both CR and leucine supplementation improved HFD-induced insulin resistance, but they differently modulated mitochondrial properties at the different stage of insulin resistance. At the hyperinsulinaemia stage, CR improved skeletal muscle mitochondrial biogenesis and function in HFD rats. However, leucine supplementation increased metabolic overload in mitochondria of skeletal muscle accompanied by impaired mitochondrial biogenesis and function. Interestingly, at the hyperglycaemic stage, both CR and leucine supplementationalleviate the HFD-induced mitochondrial damage, whereas HFD + Leu showed a more pronounced effect on mitochondrial biogenesis than CR.

Our study has several limitations. First, T2DM progression and development are long-term processes, with different metabolic characteristics at different stages. Our animal studies only revealed alterations at two time points; thus, they may not reflect the total metabolic changes associated with leucine supplementation. Second, the metabolites detected in our study were limited and we only observed the skeletal muscle's response to leucine supplementation, further investigation should use untargeted metabolomic analysis to capture a large number of differences in metabolite levels and metabolic responses in multiple organs to improve our understanding of the relevant mechanisms. Third, our data demonstrated that the effects of leucine supplementation on insulin resistance were associated with the metabolic condition of the organisms, but the metabolic conditions of HFD rats in the progression of insulin resistance were mainly estimated by the serum metabolites in the present study;this should be further verified by other experiments.

To our knowledge, this study is the first to report that leucine exerts different effects during different stages of insulin resistance in a diet-induced animal model, depending on the prevalence of catabolic and anabolic signals in the organism [17]. During the early stage of insulin resistance, increased insulin levels to maintain normal blood glucose by promoting anabolism (glycogen, protein and fat synthesis) and suppressing fat oxidation [50–52]. Thus, strategies that improve insulin sensitivity may facilitate both the anabolic effects of insulin and the adaptive catabolic effects of "nutrient overload" in the context of a HFD, leading to an adverse metabolic phenotype and mitochondrial dysfunction. Leucine supplementation may not be beneficial if calorie intake is not restricted at this stage. However, as insulin resistance progresses and insulin loses its effectiveness, the condition is characterized by a catabolic state. BCAA or leucine supplementation improves insulin sensitivity, mitochondrial function and other metabolic outcomes, as demonstrated in many conditions, including muscle sarcopaenia, burns, trauma and T2DM in elderly patients [53–55]. The findings of this study help explain the conflicting results reported by different studies and indicate that the patients' overall metabolic status should be carefully considered to potentiate the health benefits of leucine or BCAAs in each clinical setting.

Supplementary Materials: The following are available online at www.mdpi.com/2072-6643/9/6/565/s1.

Acknowledgments: We thank Ying Xie and Zhongwen Yuan at Macau University of Science and Technology and Xude Zhang at Beijing Mass Spectrometry Medical Research Co., Ltd. for expert technical support. This study was supported by The National Natural Science Foundation of China (NSFC) Grant No. 81373006 (to X.Y.).

Author Contributions: R.L. and X.Y. designed the study, analyzed the data and drafted the article. R.L., H.L., W.F., Q.J., T.C., Y.W., J.H. and L.H. contributed to the animal studies and acquisition of data. All authors interpreted the data, revised the manuscript critically for important intellectual content and approved the final version to be published. X.Y. is the guarantor of the article.

Conflicts of Interest: The authors declare no conflict of interest.

References

1. Zhang, Y.; Guo, K.; LeBlanc, R.E.; Loh, D.; Schwartz, G.J.; Yu, Y.H. Increasing dietary leucine intake reduces diet-induced obesity and improves glucose and cholesterol metabolism in mice via multimechanisms. *Diabetes* **2007**, *56*, 1647–1654. [CrossRef] [PubMed]
2. Eller, L.K.; Saha, D.C.; Shearer, J.; Reimer, R.A. Dietary leucine improves whole-body insulin sensitivity independent of body fat in diet-induced obese Sprague-Dawley rats. *J. Nutr. Biochem.* **2013**, *24*, 1285–1294. [CrossRef] [PubMed]
3. Nagata, C.; Nakamura, K.; Wada, K.; Tsuji, M.; Tamai, Y.; Kawachi, T. Branched-chain amino acid intake and the risk of diabetes in a japanese community: The takayama study. *Am. J. Epidemiol.* **2013**, *178*, 1226–1232. [CrossRef] [PubMed]
4. Valerio, A.; D'Antona, G.; Nisoli, E. Branched-chain amino acids, mitochondrial biogenesis, and healthspan: An evolutionary perspective. *Aging (Albany NY)* **2011**, *3*, 464–478. [CrossRef] [PubMed]

5. Newgard, C.B.; An, J.; Bain, J.R.; Muehlbauer, M.J.; Stevens, R.D.; Lien, L.F.; Haqq, A.M.; Shah, S.H.; Arlotto, M.; Slentz, C.A.; et al. A branched-chain amino acid-related metabolic signature that differentiates obese and lean humans and contributes to insulin resistance. *Cell Metab.* **2009**, *9*, 311–326. [CrossRef] [PubMed]

6. Nairizi, A.; She, P.; Vary, T.C.; Lynch, C.J. Leucine supplementation of drinking water does not alter susceptibility to diet-induced obesity in mice. *J. Nutr.* **2009**, *139*, 715–719. [CrossRef] [PubMed]

7. Newgard, C.B. Interplay between lipids and branched-chain amino acids in development of insulin resistance. *Cell Metab.* **2012**, *15*, 606–614. [CrossRef] [PubMed]

8. Wang, T.J.; Larson, M.G.; Vasan, R.S.; Cheng, S.; Rhee, E.P.; McCabe, E.; Lewis, G.D.; Fox, C.S.; Jacques, P.F.; Fernandez, C.; et al. Metabolite profiles and the risk of developing diabetes. *Nat. Med.* **2011**, *17*, 448–453. [CrossRef] [PubMed]

9. Batch, B.C.; Shah, S.H.; Newgard, C.B.; Turer, C.B.; Haynes, C.; Bain, J.R.; Muehlbauer, M.; Patel, M.J.; Stevens, R.D.; Appel, L.J.; et al. Branched chain amino acids are novel biomarkers for discrimination of metabolic wellness. *Metabolism* **2013**, *62*, 961–969. [CrossRef] [PubMed]

10. Shah, S.H.; Crosslin, D.R.; Haynes, C.S.; Nelson, S.; Turer, C.B.; Stevens, R.D.; Muehlbauer, M.J.; Wenner, B.R.; Bain, J.R.; Laferrere, B.; et al. Branched-chain amino acid levels are associated with improvement in insulin resistance with weight loss. *Diabetologia* **2012**, *55*, 321–330. [CrossRef] [PubMed]

11. Sengupta, S.; Peterson, T.R.; Sabatini, D.M. Regulation of the mTOR complex 1 pathway by nutrients, growth factors, and stress. *Mol. Cell* **2010**, *40*, 310–322. [CrossRef] [PubMed]

12. Li, X.; Wang, X.; Liu, R.; Ma, Y.; Guo, H.; Hao, L.; Yao, P.; Liu, L.; Sun, X.; He, K.; et al. Chronic leucine supplementation increases body weight and insulin sensitivity in rats on high-fat diet likely by promoting insulin signaling in insulin-target tissues. *Mol. Nutr. Food Res.* **2013**, *57*, 1067–1079. [CrossRef] [PubMed]

13. Houde, V.P.; Brule, S.; Festuccia, W.T.; Blanchard, P.G.; Bellmann, K.; Deshaies, Y.; Marette, A. Chronic rapamycin treatment causes glucose intolerance and hyperlipidemia by upregulating hepatic gluconeogenesis and impairing lipid deposition in adipose tissue. *Diabetes* **2010**, *59*, 1338–1348. [CrossRef] [PubMed]

14. Herman, M.A.; She, P.; Peroni, O.D.; Lynch, C.J.; Kahn, B.B. Adipose tissue branched chain amino acid (BCAA) metabolism modulates circulating bcaa levels. *J. Biol. Chem.* **2010**, *285*, 11348–11356. [CrossRef] [PubMed]

15. Lynch, C.J.; Adams, S.H. Branched-chain amino acids in metabolic signalling and insulin resistance. *Nat. Rev. Endocrinol.* **2014**, *10*, 723–736. [CrossRef] [PubMed]

16. D'Antona, G.; Ragni, M.; Cardile, A.; Tedesco, L.; Dossena, M.; Bruttini, F.; Caliaro, F.; Corsetti, G.; Bottinelli, R.; Carruba, M.O.; et al. Branched-chain amino acid supplementation promotes survival and supports cardiac and skeletal muscle mitochondrial biogenesis in middle-aged mice. *Cell Metab.* **2010**, *12*, 362–372. [CrossRef] [PubMed]

17. Bifari, F.; Nisoli, E. Branched-chain amino acids differently modulate catabolic and anabolic states in mammals: A pharmacological point of view. *Br. J. Pharmacol.* **2016**. [CrossRef] [PubMed]

18. Kleemann, R.; van Erk, M.; Verschuren, L.; van den Hoek, A.M.; Koek, M.; Wielinga, P.Y.; Jie, A.; Pellis, L.; Bobeldijk-Pastorova, I.; Kelder, T.; et al. Time-resolved and tissue-specific systems analysis of the pathogenesis of insulin resistance. *PLoS ONE* **2010**, *5*, e8817. [CrossRef] [PubMed]

19. Adams, S.H. Emerging perspectives on essential amino acid metabolism in obesity and the insulin-resistant state. *Adv. Nutr.* **2011**, *2*, 445–456. [CrossRef] [PubMed]

20. Macotela, Y.; Emanuelli, B.; Bang, A.M.; Espinoza, D.O.; Boucher, J.; Beebe, K.; Gall, W.; Kahn, C.R. Dietary leucine—An environmental modifier of insulin resistance acting on multiple levels of metabolism. *PLoS ONE* **2011**, *6*, e21187. [CrossRef] [PubMed]

21. Binder, E.; Bermudez-Silva, F.J.; Elie, M.; Leste-Lasserre, T.; Belluomo, I.; Clark, S.; Duchampt, A.; Mithieux, G.; Cota, D. Leucine supplementation modulates fuel substrates utilization and glucose metabolism in previously obese mice. *Obesity (Silver Spring)* **2014**, *22*, 713–720. [CrossRef] [PubMed]

22. Guo, K.; Yu, Y.H.; Hou, J.; Zhang, Y. Chronic leucine supplementation improves glycemic control in etiologically distinct mouse models of obesity and diabetes mellitus. *Nutr. Metab. (Lond.)* **2010**, *7*, 57. [CrossRef] [PubMed]

23. Gannon, N.P.; Vaughan, R.A. Leucineinduced anabolic-catabolism: Two sides of the same coin. *Amino Acids* **2016**, *48*, 321–336. [CrossRef] [PubMed]

24. Kim, B.; McLean, L.L.; Philip, S.S.; Feldman, E.L. Hyperinsulinemia induces insulin resistance in dorsal root ganglion neurons. *Endocrinology* **2011**, *152*, 3638–3647. [CrossRef] [PubMed]

25. Kim, B.; Sullivan, K.A.; Backus, C.; Feldman, E.L. Cortical neurons develop insulin resistance and blunted akt signaling: A potential mechanism contributing to enhanced ischemic injury in diabetes. *Antioxid. Redox Signal.* **2011**, *14*, 1829–1839. [CrossRef] [PubMed]

26. Tai, E.S.; Tan, M.L.; Stevens, R.D.; Low, Y.L.; Muehlbauer, M.J.; Goh, D.L.; Ilkayeva, O.R.; Wenner, B.R.; Bain, J.R.; Lee, J.J.; et al. Insulin resistance is associated with a metabolic profile of altered protein metabolism in Chinese and Asian-Indian men. *Diabetologia* **2010**, *53*, 757–767. [CrossRef] [PubMed]

27. She, P.; Van Horn, C.; Reid, T.; Hutson, S.M.; Cooney, R.N.; Lynch, C.J. Obesity-related elevations in plasma leucine are associated with alterations in enzymes involved in branched-chain amino acid metabolism. *Am. J. Physiol. Endocrinol. Metab.* **2007**, *293*, E1552–E1563. [CrossRef] [PubMed]

28. Harris, R.A.; Joshi, M.; Jeoung, N.H. Mechanisms responsible for regulation of branched-chain amino acid catabolism. *Biochem. Biophys. Res. Commun.* **2004**, *313*, 391–396. [CrossRef] [PubMed]

29. Shimomura, Y.; Obayashi, M.; Murakami, T.; Harris, R.A. Regulation of branched-chain amino acid catabolism: Nutritional and hormonal regulation of activity and expression of the branched-chain alpha-keto acid dehydrogenase kinase. *Curr. Opin. Clin. Nutr. Metab. Care* **2001**, *4*, 419–423. [CrossRef] [PubMed]

30. Nellis, M.M.; Doering, C.B.; Kasinski, A.; Danner, D.J. Insulin increases branched-chain alpha-ketoacid dehydrogenase kinase expression in clone 9 rat cells. *Am. J. Physiol.Endocrinol. Metab.* **2002**, *283*, E853–E860. [CrossRef] [PubMed]

31. Brosnan, J.T.; Brosnan, M.E. Branched-chain amino acids: Enzyme and substrate regulation. *J. Nutr.* **2006**, *136*, 207S–211S. [PubMed]

32. Fernstrom, J.D. Branched-chain amino acids and brain function. *J. Nutr.* **2005**, *135*, 1539S–1546S. [PubMed]

33. Koves, T.R.; Ussher, J.R.; Noland, R.C.; Slentz, D.; Mosedale, M.; Ilkayeva, O.; Bain, J.; Stevens, R.; Dyck, J.R.; Newgard, C.B.; et al. Mitochondrial overload and incomplete fatty acid oxidation contribute to skeletal muscle insulin resistance. *Cell Metab.* **2008**, *7*, 45–56. [CrossRef] [PubMed]

34. Aguer, C.; McCoin, C.S.; Knotts, T.A.; Thrush, A.B.; Ono-Moore, K.; McPherson, R.; Dent, R.; Hwang, D.H.; Adams, S.H.; Harper, M.E. Acylcarnitines: Potential implications for skeletal muscle insulin resistance. *FASEB J.* **2015**, *29*, 336–345. [CrossRef] [PubMed]

35. Adams, S.H.; Hoppel, C.L.; Lok, K.H.; Zhao, L.; Wong, S.W.; Minkler, P.E.; Hwang, D.H.; Newman, J.W.; Garvey, W.T. Plasma acylcarnitine profiles suggest incomplete long-chain fatty acid beta-oxidation and altered tricarboxylic acid cycle activity in type 2 diabetic African-American women. *J. Nutr.* **2009**, *139*, 1073–1081. [CrossRef] [PubMed]

36. Hutson, S.M.; Sweatt, A.J.; Lanoue, K.F. Branched-chain [corrected] amino acid metabolism: Implications for establishing safe intakes. *J. Nutr.* **2005**, *135*, 1557S–1564S. [PubMed]

37. White, P.J.; Lapworth, A.L.; An, J.; Wang, L.; McGarrah, R.W.; Stevens, R.D.; Ilkayeva, O.; George, T.; Muehlbauer, M.J.; Bain, J.R.; et al. Branched-chain amino acid restriction in zucker-fatty rats improves muscle insulin sensitivity by enhancing efficiency of fatty acid oxidation and acyl-glycine export. *Mol. Metab.* **2016**, *5*, 538–551. [CrossRef] [PubMed]

38. Lerin, C.; Goldfine, A.B.; Boes, T.; Liu, M.; Kasif, S.; Dreyfuss, J.M.; De Sousa-Coelho, A.L.; Daher, G.; Manoli, I.; Sysol, J.R.; et al. Defects in muscle branched-chain amino acid oxidation contribute to impaired lipid metabolism. *Mol. Metab.* **2016**, *5*, 926–936. [CrossRef] [PubMed]

39. Di Meo, S.; Iossa, S.; Venditti, P. Skeletal muscle insulin resistance: Role of mitochondria and other ROS sources. *J. Endocrinol.* **2017**, *233*, R15–R42. [CrossRef] [PubMed]

40. Affourtit, C. Mitochondrial involvement in skeletal muscle insulin resistance: A case of imbalanced bioenergetics. *Biochim. Biophys. Acta* **2016**, *1857*, 1678–1693. [CrossRef] [PubMed]

41. Liesa, M.; Shirihai, O.S. Mitochondrial dynamics in the regulation of nutrient utilization and energy expenditure. *Cell Metab.* **2013**, *17*, 491–506. [CrossRef] [PubMed]

42. Vaughan, R.A.; Garcia-Smith, R.; Gannon, N.P.; Bisoffi, M.; Trujillo, K.A.; Conn, C.A. Leucine treatment enhances oxidative capacity through complete carbohydrate oxidation and increased mitochondrial density in skeletal muscle cells. *Amino Acids* **2013**, *45*, 901–911. [CrossRef] [PubMed]

43. Sun, X.; Zemel, M.B. Leucine modulation of mitochondrial mass and oxygen consumption in skeletal muscle cells and adipocytes. *Nutr. Metab. (Lond.)* **2009**, *6*, 26. [CrossRef] [PubMed]

44. Vaughan, R.A.; Mermier, C.M.; Bisoffi, M.; Trujillo, K.A.; Conn, C.A. Dietary stimulators of the PGC-1 superfamily and mitochondrial biosynthesis in skeletal muscle. A mini-review. *J. Physiol. Biochem.* **2014**, *70*, 271–284. [CrossRef] [PubMed]

45. Li, H.; Xu, M.; Lee, J.; He, C.; Xie, Z. Leucine supplementation increases sirt1 expression and prevents mitochondrial dysfunction and metabolic disorders in high-fat diet-induced obese mice. *Am. J. Physiol. Endocrinol. Metab.* **2012**, *303*, E1234–E1244. [CrossRef] [PubMed]

46. Lopez-Lluch, G.; Hunt, N.; Jones, B.; Zhu, M.; Jamieson, H.; Hilmer, S.; Cascajo, M.V.; Allard, J.; Ingram, D.K.; Navas, P.; et al. Calorie restriction induces mitochondrial biogenesis and bioenergetic efficiency. *Proc. Natl. Acad. Sci. USA* **2006**, *103*, 1768–1773. [CrossRef] [PubMed]

47. Guarente, L. Mitochondria—A nexus for aging, calorie restriction, and sirtuins? *Cell* **2008**, *132*, 171–176. [CrossRef] [PubMed]

48. Nisoli, E.; Tonello, C.; Cardile, A.; Cozzi, V.; Bracale, R.; Tedesco, L.; Falcone, S.; Valerio, A.; Cantoni, O.; Clementi, E.; et al. Calorie restriction promotes mitochondrial biogenesis by inducing the expression of enos. *Science* **2005**, *310*, 314–317. [CrossRef] [PubMed]

49. Ingram, D.K.; Roth, G.S. Glycolytic inhibition as a strategy for developing calorie restriction mimetics. *Exp. Gerontol.* **2011**, *46*, 148–154. [CrossRef] [PubMed]

50. Liu, H.Y.; Hong, T.; Wen, G.B.; Han, J.; Zuo, D.; Liu, Z.; Cao, W. Increased basal level of akt-dependent insulin signaling may be responsible for the development of insulin resistance. *Am. J. Physiol. Endocrinol. Metab.* **2009**, *297*, E898–E906. [CrossRef] [PubMed]

51. Cao, W.; Ning, J.; Yang, X.; Liu, Z. Excess exposure to insulin is the primary cause of insulin resistance and its associated atherosclerosis. *Curr. Mol. Pharmacol.* **2011**, *4*, 154–166. [CrossRef] [PubMed]

52. Nolan, C.J.; Ruderman, N.B.; Kahn, S.E.; Pedersen, O.; Prentki, M. Insulin resistance as a physiological defense against metabolic stress: Implications for the management of subsets of type 2 diabetes. *Diabetes* **2015**, *64*, 673–686. [CrossRef] [PubMed]

53. Solerte, S.B.; Fioravanti, M.; Locatelli, E.; Bonacasa, R.; Zamboni, M.; Basso, C.; Mazzoleni, A.; Mansi, V.; Geroutis, N.; Gazzaruso, C. Improvement of blood glucose control and insulin sensitivity during a long-term (60 weeks) randomized study with amino acid dietary supplements in elderly subjects with type 2 diabetes mellitus. *Am. J. Cardiol.* **2008**, *101*, 82E–88E. [CrossRef] [PubMed]

54. Leenders, M.; van Loon, L.J. Leucine as a pharmaconutrient to prevent and treat sarcopenia and type 2 diabetes. *Nutr. Rev.* **2011**, *69*, 675–689. [CrossRef] [PubMed]

55. Kawaguchi, T.; Nagao, Y.; Matsuoka, H.; Ide, T.; Sata, M. Branched-chain amino acid-enriched supplementation improves insulin resistance in patients with chronic liver disease. *Int. J. Mol. Med.* **2008**, *22*, 105–112. [CrossRef] [PubMed]

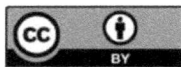

nutrients

MDPI

Article

Effect of *n*-3 Polyunsaturated Fatty Acid Supplementation on Metabolic and Inflammatory Biomarkers in Type 2 Diabetes Mellitus Patients

M. Gorety Jacobo-Cejudo [1], Roxana Valdés-Ramos [1,*], Ana L. Guadarrama-López [1],
Rosa-Virgen Pardo-Morales [2], Beatriz E. Martínez-Carrillo [1] and Laurence S. Harbige [3]

[1]   Faculty of Medicine, Universidad Autónoma del Estado de México, Paseo Tollocan esq. Jesús Carranza,
      Col. Moderna de la Cruz, Toluca 50180, Mexico; ln_gorejace@yahoo.com.mx (M.G.J.-C.);
      anag3075@hotmail.com (A.L.G.-L.); martinez_elina9@hotmail.com (B.E.M.-C.)
[2]   Instlituto Materno-Infantil del Estado de México, Paseo Colón s/n, Col. Villa Hogar, Toluca 50170, Mexico;
      rvpardo@gmail.com
[3]   Faculty of Life Sciences and Computing, London Metropolitan University, 166-220 Holloway Road,
      London N7 8DB, UK; L.Harbige@londonmet.ac.uk
*   Correspondence: rvaldesr@uaemex.mx; Tel.: +52-722-217-4831 (ext. 232)

Received: 25 April 2017; Accepted: 1 June 2017; Published: 3 June 2017

Abstract: Background: Type 2 diabetes mellitus (T2DM) is accompanied by chronic low-grade inflammation, with an imbalance in the secretion of adipokines and, worsening insulin resistance. Supplementation with *n*-3 PUFA in T2DM decreases inflammatory markers, the purpose of the study was to investigate the effect of *n*-3 PUFA supplementation on adipokines, metabolic control, and lipid profile in T2DM Mexican adults. Methods: In a randomized, single-blind, placebo-controlled pilot study, 54 patients with T2DM received 520 mg of DHA + EPA-enriched fish-oil (FOG) or a placebo (PG) daily. Baseline and 24-week anthropometric and biochemical measurements included glucose, insulin, glycosylated hemoglobin (Hb1Ac), leptin, adiponectin, resistin, and lipid profile; *n*-3 PUFA intake was calculated in g/day. Results: Waist circumference and blood glucose showed significant reductions in the FOG group ($p = 0.001$ and $p = 0.011$, respectively). Hb1Ac ($p = 0.009$ and $p = 0.004$), leptin ($p < 0.000$ and $p < 0.000$), and leptin/adiponectin ratio ($p < 0.000$ and $p < 0.000$) decreased significantly in both groups after 24 weeks (FOG and PG respectively). Serum resistin (FOG $p < 0.000$ and PG $p = 0.001$), insulin (FOG $p < 0.000$ and PG $p < 0.000$), and HOMA-IR (FOG $p = 0.000$ and PG $p < 0.000$) increased significantly in both groups. FOG had an overall improvement in the lipid profile with a significant decrease in triacylgycerols ($p = 0.002$) and atherogenic index ($p = 0.031$); in contrast, the PG group had increased total cholesterol ($p < 0.000$), non-HDL cholesterol ($p < 0.000$), and atherogenic index ($p = 0.017$). Conclusions: We found a beneficial effect of *n*-3 PUFA supplementation on waist circumference, glucose, Hb1Ac, leptin, leptin/adiponectin ratio, and lipid profile, without significant changes in adiponectin, and increases in resistin, insulin, and HOMA-IR in both groups.

Keywords: type 2 diabetes mellitus; adipokines; lipid profile; *n*-3 PUFAs

---

1. Introduction

Type 2 diabetes mellitus (T2DM) is one of the most prevalent chronic diseases around the world, with an increase in its prevalence due to the increase in its risk factors such as obesity and physical inactivity [1]. According to the National Health and Nutrition Survey, in 2012, in Mexico there were 6.4 million people with T2DM, which means an increase in prevalence from 7% in 2006 to 9.2% in 2012 [2]. T2DM is characterized by impaired pancreatic β-cell function that causes impaired insulin secretion and insulin resistance (IR) mainly in liver, muscle, and adipose tissue [3].

It is well recognized that the actively secreted products of adipose tissue known as adipokines can modulate different functions [4]; adipokines play a pivotal role in the regulation of whole-body metabolism, as well as in inflammatory and immune responses, and are considered a link between obesity and the development of T2DM [5].

Adiponectin is a collagen-like protein exclusively expressed in adipose tissue [6], which possesses potent antidiabetic and anti-inflammatory properties [7]. In humans, plasma adiponectin levels are closely related to whole-body insulin sensitivity [8] and are correlated negatively with IR and T2DM. Prospective and longitudinal studies have indicated that lower adiponectin levels are associated with a higher incidence of T2DM [4]. Adiponectin regulates glucose and lipid metabolism through the reduction of fat storage (lipogenesis) and the promotion of fat utilization (fatty acid oxidation) [9].

Leptin is a cytokine-like molecule secreted by adipose tissue which regulates adipose tissue mass and body weight by inhibiting food intake and stimulating energy expenditure [6], thus maintaining energy homeostasis. Leptin correlates directly with adipose tissue mass. Obesity and T2DM are associated with increased plasma leptin levels, which fail to correct hyperglycemia in these patients because of the presence of leptin resistance [5], and these elevated plasma leptin levels are associated with IR, independent of obesity and insulin sensitivity [10].

In humans, resistin is mainly secreted by macrophages and monocytes and by organs such as spleen and bone marrow [11]. Since its discovery, resistin has been related to obesity and IR in many animal experiments, but the application of these findings to human studies has been difficult to determine. However, studies in humans have shown that serum resistin levels are higher in obese patients with T2DM compared with non-diabetic obese and that mRNA levels of resistin are higher in female patients with T2DM compared to healthy women [12].

Dyslipidemias are very common in type 2 diabetes mellitus and are the cause of cardiovascular disease in uncontrolled patients. Hypertriacylglyceridemia as well as low HDL-cholesterol concentrations, together with high LDL- and non-HDL-cholesterol is a common lipid profile pattern observed in subjects with diabetes [13–16].

Eicosapentaenoic acid (EPA) and docosahexaenoic acid (DHA) are polyunsaturated fatty acids found at high levels in fish oils [17]. Accumulating evidence suggests that *n*-3 PUFAs from fish oil may counteract the adipokine dysregulation that occurs in obesity and its related diseases like T2DM [9], but it is not well established if the consumption of *n*-3 PUFAs affects circulating adiponectin, resistin, and leptin in humans; the results are inconclusive [18]. Furthermore, research in humans and animal models show a lipid normalizing effect of PUFA supplementation [19,20].

For these reasons, we undertook a pilot study with the aim of investigating the effect of a six-month supplementation trial with *n*-3 PUFAs on adiponectin, resistin, leptin, and the lipid profile in adults with T2DM from Toluca, Mexico.

2. Materials and Methods

2.1. Study Design

This study was a randomized, single-blind and placebo-controlled pilot study conducted in eight Urban Public Health Centers (UPHC) in Toluca, Mexico, from February to September 2015. The inclusion criteria were the following: men and women with T2DM, between 25 and 60 years, without other chronic diseases such as hypertension, arthritis, kidney disease, cancer, and HIV, with a BMI ≤ 29.9, without fish allergies or insulin treatment, and not lactating or pregnant.

2.2. Methods

Sixty-five Mexican subjects with T2DM were enrolled from the eight UPHC in Toluca as follows: Capultitlán (*n* = 1), Emiliano Zapata (*n* = 6), Nueva Oxtototitlán (*n* = 2), Reforma (21), Seminario (3), Tlacotepec (1), San Diego de los Padres (*n* = 16), and Ejido de la Y (*n* = 15). The 65 subjects were randomly and blindly separated into an experimental group (fish oil group: FOG) of 34 patients

(10 males, 24 females) and a control group (placebo group: PG) of 31 patients (5 males, 26 females). The majority of patients were medicated with Glibenclamide plus Metformin or Metformin alone and were controlled by their family practitioner, we did not give them additional dietary or lifestyle advice; we only asked them to continue with their regular medication and diet.

Written informed consent was given to all participants. The study was approved by the Research and Ethics Committee of the Universidad Autónoma del Estado de Mexico and the Institute for Health of the State of Mexico's Research and Education Coordination. The protocol was conducted following the regulations of the Helsinki Declaration of 1975 and its amendment of 2013, as well as the principles for experiments with human beings from the Nüremberg Code for medical ethics. Individual data is being maintained confidential.

Once obtained the sample, the baseline evaluation was performed as follows:

Anthropometric evaluation:

All measurements were recorded with light clothes and height without shoes by a trained nutritionist who was previously standardized. Weight was measured in a TANITA® scale (Mod. 1631) and was registered in kg; height was measured in cm using a portable SECA 206 stadiometer; the percentage of body fat was obtained by electrical bioimpedance with the same TANITA scale; body mass index (BMI) was calculated as body weight in kilograms divided by the square of height in meters. Waist and hip circumferences were measured with a Gülick™ fiberglass tape and the waist/hip ratio was calculated.

Biochemical evaluation:

After an overnight fast ($\geq$12 h), collection of a venous blood sample into an 8.5 mL tiger-top tube containing gel and clotting activator for the subsequent biochemical analysis of glucose, insulin, adipokines, and lipid profile was undertaken. Another venous blood sample in a 3 mL tube with EDTA for the analysis of glycosylated hemoglobin was also obtained.

Serum was obtained after centrifugation at 900 g or 3400 rpm for 10 min at 4 °C, within 30 min after blood sample collection; serum samples for glucose and lipid profile were processed within one hour, and the rest of the samples were aliquoted and stored at −80 °C until assayed.

Serum glucose, triacylglycerols, total cholesterol, HDL-cholesterol, LDL-cholesterol, and glycosylated hemoglobin levels (in total blood) were measured by enzymatic colorimetric assays in the auto-analyzer Selectra II (ROCHE™), using reagents from RANDOX™ (Cat. GL1611, Cat. Tr213, Cat. CHO215, Cat. CH3811A, Cat. CH3811B and Cat. HA3830A). Non-HDL-cholesterol was calculated by difference (total cholesterol − HDL-cholesterol).

Serum levels of insulin were measured with a Human Insulin ELISA kit from EMD Millipore Corporation® (Cat. # EZHI-14K) according to the manufacturer's instructions. We evaluated IR with glucose and insulin concentrations using the Homeostatic model assessment as follows:

HOMA-IR = (fasting insulin (μU/mL)) × (fasting glucose (mg/dL))/405 [21].

Commercially available kits from Merck Millipore® (Cat. # HADK1MAG-61K and HADK2MAG-61K) were used to measure the serum levels of adiponectin, resistin, and leptin in the Luminex® 100™ analyzer by luminometry according to the manufacturer's recommended protocols.

2.3. Supplementation

The supplementation period started after basal evaluation. Patients took two softgels per day of the assigned supplement for 24 weeks. Each 1.4 g *n*-3 PUFAs softgel contained a combination of 160 mg of eicosapentaenoic acid (EPA) with 100 mg of docosahexaenoic acid (DHA) from fish oil, so the total daily oral dose was 520 mg of *n*-3 PUFAs (320 mg of EPA and 200 mg of DHA, 2 g of total fat, 1.2 mg of vitamin E, gelatin and glycerine) during the six months of intervention. PUFA supplements were purchased from General Nutrition Centers™. The placebo softgels were identical to the *n*-3 PUFAs softgels in appearance and contained cornstarch (1 g carbohydrates and 1.7 mg of sodium per softgel).

2.4. Follow-up

After basal evaluation, patients were monitored by 6 monthly visits, in which they received their corresponding supplement and were followed-up every two weeks by telephone to make sure that they were taking their capsules, as well as to remind them not to change their habitual diet, medication, or physical activity regimes.

2.5. Diet Analysis

A trained nutritionist performed 24-h recalls, one at the beginning and one at the end of the study to analyze the diet. The dietary nutrient intake and the consumption of polyunsaturated fatty acids were calculated in grams and percentages using DIAL® (ver 3.3.2., Universidad Complutense, Madrid, Spain) software. In the final 24 h recalls of the FOG, we added the nutritional composition of *n*-3 PUFA softgels.

2.6. Statistical Analysis

Data were expressed as mean $\pm$ SD. To compare differences in the same group after intervention, paired *t*-test was used for parametric variables and Wilcoxon signed rank test for non-parametric variables. In the diet analysis, unpaired two-sample *t*-test was used to compare differences between groups in a parametric way and a Mann–Whitney U-test for non-parametric data. Normality of data was assessed by the Kolmogorov–Smirnoff test. All analyses were performed using the statistical software SPSS (version 19.0; SPSS Inc., Chicago, IL, USA). A *p*-value < 0.05 was considered statistically significant.

3. Results

During the study, 10 subjects, 4 in the omega-3 group and 6 in the placebo group, were eliminated for not completing the six-month supplementation for personal reasons, and the drop-out rate in both groups was less than 20%. When analyzing the causes for drop-out, it is important to note that all patients had low-education and socioeconomic levels, and even though we tried to reach them by phone or house-visits, they were not located either to follow-up or to obtain data at the end of the trial. We analyzed basal data for differences between those who dropped out and those who stayed, and there were no significant differences between groups that indicated that they stopped attending due to the variables we were evaluating.

Age, gender distribution, and diabetes duration were similar between groups without significant differences; in the FOG, 7 subjects were males, and 22 were females; in the PG, 5 subjects were males and 20 were females. The mean age of the FOG was of 50.4 $\pm$ 6.3 years, while in the PG it was 48.1 $\pm$ 6.8 years (*p* = 0.208), and the average time of diabetes duration was of 6.6 $\pm$ 5.0 years in the FOG and of 6.5 $\pm$ 5.8 years in the PG (*p* = 0.954).

In anthropometric measurements, only the FOG showed a significant decrease in waist circumference after supplementation (*p* = 0.001) (Table 1). No significant changes in body weight (*p* = 0.250 and 0.578), BMI (*p* = 0.278 and 0.485), body fat (*p* = 0.889 and 0.614), and waist/hip ratio (*p* = 0.288 and 0.076) were observed in FOG and PG, respectively, after intervention.

At baseline, there was only a significant difference between groups in serum resistin levels (*p* = 0.006). The results of biochemical analysis are summarized in Table 2. Glucose serum levels only showed a significant decrease in FOG (*p* = 0.001), and there were significant reductions in glycosylated hemoglobin (*p* = 0.009 and *p* = 0.004), leptin (*p* = 0.000 and *p* = 0.000), and leptin/adiponectin ratio in both groups (FOG and PG, respectively). Adiponectin did not show significant changes (*p* = 0.177 for FOG and *p* = 0.563 for PG). Contrary to expected, resistin showed a significant increase in both groups (*p* = 0.000 for FOG and *p* = 0.001 for PG). With respect to IR, there were significant increases in insulin serum levels ($p = 0.000$ for FOG and $p = 0.000$ for PG) and in HOMA-IR ($p = 0.000$ for FOG and $p = 0.000$ for PG).

Table 1. Anthropometric measurements.

Variables	Fish Oil Group ($n = 29$)			Placebo Group ($n = 25$)		
	Basal	Final	p	Basal	Final	p
Body weight (kg)	63.0 ± 9.3	62.7 ± 9.4	0.250	60.2 ± 6.4	60.0 ± 7.3	0.578
BMI (kg/m^2)	25.6 ± 2.4	25.4 ± 2.7	0.278	26.0 ± 1.6	25.9 ± 2.0	0.485
Body fat (%)	30.9 ± 9.1	31.1 ± 7.2	0.889	29.9 ± 5.3	30.4 ± 6.1	0.614
Waist circumference (cm)	86.4 ± 7.6	83.1 ± 6.2	**0.001**	83.2 ± 5.3	83.1 ± 6.1	0.893
Waist/hip ratio	0.89 ± 0.05	0.90 ± 0.05	0.288	0.90 ± 0.05	0.92 ± 0.04	0.076

BMI: body mass index. Paired *t*-test was performed to compare differences in time (before and after supplementation). A *p*-value < 0.05 was considered statistically significant, marked in bold numbers.

Table 2. Biochemical measurements.

Variables	Omega-3 ($n = 29$)			Placebo ($n = 25$)		
	Basal	Final	p	Basal	Final	p
Glucose (mg/dL) [‡]	177.2 ± 68.4	156.1 ± 69.4	**0.011**	184.6 ± 71.1	183.3 ± 53.3	0.326
Glycosylated hemoglobin (%) [†]	9.6 ± 3.1	8.2 ± 1.9	**0.009**	10.0 ± 2.1	9.0 ± 1.8	**0.004**
Adiponectin (μg) [‡]	23.6 ± 20.3	24.5 ± 13.0	0.177	22.8 ± 10.5	24.3 ± 13.3	0.563
Leptin (ng) [†]	21.7 ± 15.5	3.9 ± 2.5	**0.000**	18.4 ± 13.2	3.5 ± 2.3	**0.000**
Resistin (ng) [‡]	30.2 ± 14.0	65.9 ± 23.4	**0.000**	39.2 ± 12.5	61.3 ± 20.6	**0.000**
Leptin/adiponectin ratio [†]	1.3 ± 1.2	0.24 ± 0.26	**0.000**	0.88 ± 0.68	0.17 ± 0.12	**0.000**
Insulin μU/mL [‡]	7.6 ± 3.0	14.2 ± 8.2	**0.000**	6.5 ± 1.6	10.2 ± 3.3	**0.000**
HOMA-IR [‡]	3.1 ± 1.3	5.3 ± 3.8	**0.000**	2.9 ± 1.2	4.4 ± 1.6	**0.000**
Total Cholesterol (mg/dL) [†]	203.38 ± 33.72	199.10 ± 47.63	0.542	180.32 ± 30.56	209.75 ± 36.80	**0.000**
Triacylglycerides (mg/dL) [†]	186.24 ± 85.58	137.28 ± 65.39	**0.002**	269.40 ± 169.30	251.20 ± 149.76	0.503
HDL-Cholesterol (mg/dL) [†]	43.52 ± 7.95	48.13 ± 14.59	0.076	38.35 ± 9.51	40.01 ± 9.28	0.384
LDL-Cholesterol (mg/dL) [†]	131.00 ± 34.66	129.82 ± 44.74	0.869	109.40 ± 34.22	127.26 ± 38.80	0.076
Non-HDL-Cholesterol (mg/dL) [†]	159.52 ± 31.28	150.97 ± 44.26	0.152	141.97 ± 24.98	169.74 ± 38.15	**0.000**
Atherogenic Index [†]	5.04 ± 1.77	4.37 ± 1.04	**0.031**	4.86 ± 1.06	5.52 ± 1.63	**0.017**

[†] Paired *t*-test was used for parametric variables and [‡] Wilcoxon signed rank test for non-parametric variables. A *p*-value ≤ 0.05 was considered statistically significant, marked in bold numbers.

Table 2 shows changes in lipid profile indicators, FOG significantly decreased triacylglycerides ($p < 0.01$) and the atherogenic index ($p < 0.05$), whereas the placebo group showed a statistically significant increase in total cholesterol ($p < 0.000$), non-HDL-cholesterol ($p < 0.000$), and the atherogenic index ($p < 0.05$).

The results of diet analysis are shown in Table 3. The FOG showed a significant increase in total omega-3 fatty acids ($p < 0.001$), particularly in EPA and DHA ($p < 0.000$); *n*-6 to *n*-3 ratio decreased from 16:1 to 10:1 ($p < 0.05$). The placebo group showed a statistically significant increase in protein and monounsaturated fatty acid intake ($p < 0.05$). No differences were found in any other nutrient analyzed.

Table 3. Diet analysis.

Variable	Omega-3 ($n = 29$)			Placebo ($n = 25$)		
	Basal	Final	p	Basal	Final	p
Energy (kcal/day)	1562.2 ± 387.4	1672.8 ± 665.2	0.476	1751.4 ± 479.9	1875.9 ± 698.5	0.276
Protein (g/day)	57.3 ± 17.2	59.4 ± 24.3	0.737	50.8 ± 19.4	60.5 ± 27.8	* 0.030
Carbohydrates (g/day)	192.1 ± 60.4	187.8 ± 68.8	0.729	258.2 ± 73.1	255.0 ± 104.7	0.905
Lipids (g/day)	59.5 ± 21.2	72.2 ± 38.4	0.097	54.2 ± 27.7	65.2 ± 31.1	0.092
Saturated fatty acids (g/day)	16.4 ± 7.2	19.3 ± 11.9	0.271	11.4 ± 9.0	14.7 ± 9.7	0.065
Monounsaturated fatty acids (g/day)	20.2 ± 8.2	24.6 ± 15.5	0.160	15.4 ± 10.6	22.6 ± 14.3	* 0.013
Polyunsaturated fatty acids (g/day)	13.2 ± 8.1	16.5 ± 12.7	0.197	13.2 ± 11.9	13.0 ± 6.4	0.367
Omega-3 fatty acids (g/day)	0.89 ± 0.76	1.32 ± 0.34	* 0.001	0.79 ± 1.12	0.75 ± 0.53	0.178
Omega-6 fatty acids (g/day)	10.5 ± 7.7	13.6 ± 12.0	0.221	9.4 ± 11.0	8.8 ± 5.2	0.382
*n*6:*n*3 Ratio	14:1	10:1	* 0.025	16:1	14:1	0.882
EPA (g/day)	0.077 ± 0.317	0.330 ± 0.018	* 0.000	0.016 ± 0.037	0.047 ± 0.177	0.837
DHA (g/day)	0.103 ± 0.236	0.287 ± 0.089	* 0.000	0.086 ± 0.109	0.155 ± 0.187	0.074

Mann–Whitney U test for differences between groups. * A *p*-value < 0.05 was considered significant, marked with bold numbers.

4. Discussion

In this study, we investigated the effect of supplementation with *n*-3 PUFAs on serum levels of adiponectin, resistin, and leptin in an adult Mexican population with T2DM.

The results of the anthropometric analysis (Table 1) are similar to the results observed in previous similar studies such as a study of supplementation with *n*-3 PUFAs in diabetic patients [22]; patients with impaired fasting glucose (IFG) or impaired glucose tolerance (IGT) [23]; and two more in women with polycystic ovarian syndrome [24,25], which regularly present insulin resistance. All of these studies showed no significant change in body weight, BMI, body fat, waist circumference, or waist/hip ratio after the supplementation period, even at higher doses of *n*-3 PUFAs and longer periods of supplementation. However, in a crossover model in which 16 T2DM patients were assigned to one of two consecutive 3.5-week periods of diabetic diets (foods rich in *n*-6 or *n*-3 PUFAs), the authors found a slight but significant reduction in body weight and BMI in both dietary periods [26]. This suggests that *n*-3 PUFAs from food are more effective in controlling body weight than *n*-3 PUFAs from supplements. In our study, supplementation with *n*-3 PUFAs for 24 weeks only helped to significantly reduce waist circumference and did not help control body weight or reduce BMI, body fat percentage, or waist/hip ratio. Furthermore, one of the studies in women with polycystic ovarian syndrome reported that effects of *n*-3 PUFAs on anthropometric measurements might be dependent on gender, age, and BMI of subjects at baseline [25].

The effect of *n*-3 PUFAs on glucose and glycosylated hemoglobin is not clear. A study of supplementation with DHA-rich fish oil in an Iranian diabetic population [27] and reviews of clinical trials of supplementation with *n*-3 PUFAs in different diabetic populations, have not found significant positive effects on glycemic control [17,28]. However, a recent study [23] showed that *n*-3 PUFA supplementation with high doses for 18 months was effective in reducing glycemia and IR in patients affected by IFG or IGT and that the regression of the condition of impaired glycemia to normoglycemia seems to be helpful in delaying the development of T2DM. Flanchs et al. showed in a review that the beneficial effects of *n*-3 PUFAs on insulin sensitivity and glucose metabolism in people with IR are dependent on factors such as disease progression and age [29]. In this study, we found a significant positive effect of *n*-3 PUFA supplementation on glycemic control (glucose and glycosylated hemoglobin), but more studies are needed to test this hypothesis because most of the beneficial effects have been shown in epidemiologic studies based on a habitual fish diet consumed for years [28].

As expected, there were significant reductions in leptin serum levels and hence in leptin/adiponectin ratio, which has been demonstrated to be related to obesity and T2DM [29]. Contrary to expectation, adiponectin did not increase significantly, while resistin increased significantly. Our results are not in line with the results observed in similar studies of supplementation with *n*-3 PUFAs in diabetes [8] and in healthy subjects with a high consumption of fish, which has shown significant increases in adiponectin serum levels after various supplementation periods [30]. As the changes in adipokine profile were similar in both groups, we cannot affirm that higher doses of *n*-3 PUFAs would have led to a decrease in leptin and leptin/adiponectin ratio because there was no lead tendency toward lower leptin concentrations in subjects with the *n*-3 PUFA supplement than in subjects with the placebo.

Our study population showed higher basal adiponectin and leptin serum levels than have been reported in other similar studies, for example, in German [31], Finnish [32], Japanese [8], Asian Indian [33], and Arabic diabetic populations [34], which is likely to be due to ethnicity. Resistin showed similar results compared with serum resistin levels of Egyptians and Japanese although slightly lower [35,36].

It has been demonstrated that weight reduction increases plasma adiponectin concentrations and improves IR [10], but in this study, possibly because there were no significant changes in body weight, there were no significant increases in serum adiponectin levels. In a study with *ob/ob* mice, the administration of recombinant adiponectin, even after the development of diabetes, significantly ameliorated hyperglycemia [37], and it has been reported that serum adiponectin levels correlate inversely with IR [5]. Plasma adiponectin levels have also been demonstrated to be negatively correlated to IR [4], but in this study, we did not find a negative correlation because adiponectin (non-significant) and HOMA-IR increased.

Leptin correlates directly with adipose tissue mass; [5] however, we did not observe a significant reduction in body weight, BMI, and body fat, despite the reduction in serum leptin levels. When we used a bivariate correlation analysis, we found that serum leptin levels showed a positive correlation with BMI ($R = 0.353$ and $p = 0.009$) and body fat percentage ($R = 0.518$ and $p = 0.000$), which is in line with the results of a similar study [5].

Leptin/adiponectin ratio showed a significant reduction in both groups related to the significant decrease in leptin levels. Leptin/adiponectin ratio was a useful measure of IR in non-diabetic white adults [38], but we did not observe a positive correlation between HOMA-IR and leptin serum levels; despite the reduction in this ratio, there was no reduction in HOMA-IR. However, these findings suggest the use of the leptin/adiponectin ratio as a useful tool to detect IR. On the other hand, resistin has been linked to obesity and IR since its discovery [12], but our results are not consistent with these findings because we found a weak negative correlation between resistin levels and HOMA-IR ($R = -0.274$ and $p = 0.045$).

Obesity is the most significant factor contributing to IR and T2DM [39], and although our patients were not obese, we found a weak but significant positive correlation between body fat percentage and HOMA-IR ($R = 0.275$ and $p = 0.046$). This factor might explain the significant increase in HOMA-IR in both groups because there was a non-significant increase in body fat percentage.

Our results are not in accordance with those of Yamamoto et al., who showed in a supplementation study with EPA in hyperlipidemic patients that IR determined by the HOMA-IR was significantly improved in the supplemented group, compared with the placebo [21]. In our study, both groups showed an increase in HOMA-IR, more studies are therefore necessary to evaluate only the EPA effect in the IR of individuals with T2DM.

Our data show an overall improvement in the lipid profile through the atherogenic index in the *n*-3 PUFA supplemented group, with an overall deterioration in the placebo group. Derosa et al. found an increase in HDL-cholesterol and a decrease in triacylglycerides after 18 months of supplementation with *n*-3 PUFA, in patients with impaired glucose metabolism [23]. While in subjects with type 2 diabetes supplemented with DHA-rich fish oil, Mansoori et al. found a decrease in triacylglycerides independently of their initial values [27]. However, several trials of supplementation with *n*-3 PUFA have not found an effect on lipid profile in adults with T2DM [40,41].

Non-HDL-cholesterol has been recommended as a sensitive proxy of the atherogenic metabolic lipid status; importantly, its values in our study population showed a non-significant decrease in the supplemented group but a highly significant increase in the placebo group. This may be considered a protective effect of *n*-3 PUFA supplementation on the lipid metabolic deterioration caused by T2DM [15,16].

With respect to diet analysis, our results are in line with those of a previous study of this group that showed that a Mexican population with T2DM had a very low intake of *n*-3 PUFAs and a high consumption of lipids, particularly saturated fatty acids [42]. According to the recommendations of the Mexican Official Standard NOM-015-SSA2-2010, for prevention, treatment, and control of diabetes mellitus [43], the mean daily energy intake of all groups was adequate, though protein and *n*-3 PUFA intake in both groups and carbohydrate intake in FOG were lower than recommendations, while the total lipid intake and saturated fatty acid intake were higher than recommendations in FOG.

It is well known that the quality of dietary fat is a key determinant of IR and that saturated and trans fatty acids decrease insulin secretion and worsen insulin sensitivity [10]; a factor which could explain the higher increase in HOMA-IR in FOG because of their higher intake of saturated fatty acids.

The quality of fat may have a significant influence on adiponectin concentrations. The data from 13 studies in a systematic review showed a modest and significant effect of *n*-3 PUFA supplementation on adiponectin concentrations [44]. Because of the very low intake of *n*-3 PUFAs in both our groups, we may not have been able to observe significant changes in adiponectin levels. *In vitro* human adipocyte studies found that EPA and DHA (100 μM) treatment for 48 h, increases adiponectin secretion, and that only EPA led to higher cellular adiponectin being introduced into the adipocytes, suggesting that the regulation of adiponectin by *n*-3 PUFAs is dose- and time-dependent and that it can be affected by the maturation stage of adipocytes [9]. However, another study of supplementation with *n*-3 PUFAs in Mexican children and adolescents with obesity and insulin resistance, showed that for *n*-3 PUFAs, the duration of treatment is not associated with the effects observed and that the dosage could be more important, which in this case would suggest that in our study the *n*-3 PUFA dose we used can be considered low [45].

It has been demonstrated that diets high in fish and flaxseed oil lower the serum phospholipid ratio of omega-6/omega-3 fatty acids and that *n*-3 PUFAs are beneficial in patients affected by inflammatory diseases. The omega 6/omega 3 ratio is of importance in health and disease; during the Paleolithic period of human evolution, there was a different balance between *n*-6 and *n*-3, but the last 150 years have seen a significant increase, as in Western diets this ratio is now in the range of 15–20:1 [46]. Because of the low intake of *n*-3 PUFAs and the increased amounts of the *n*-6 PUFA linoleic acid (and high levels found in plasma phospholipids to be published elsewhere) in our study population, the omega 6/omega 3 ratios were of 11:1 and of 13:1 in FOG and PG, respectively, very similar to Western diets [47].

Although we found a beneficial effect of EPA + DHA supplementation on waist circumference, glucose, glycosylated hemoglobin, leptin, and leptin/adiponectin ratio in this population, these beneficial effects may not have been due to the supplement alone because we observed similar results in some of these parameters between patients who took the *n*-3 PUFA supplement and those that took the placebo. Similarly, there were significant increases in resistin, serum insulin, and HOMA-IR in both groups. It is possible that some of the beneficial effects observed in both groups were due to metformin and that the combined use of *n*-3 PUFA and metformin gave rise to better outcome measures. However, the significant increase in monounsaturated fatty acids and protein in the placebo group may also have contributed to the decrease in glycosylated hemoglobin, leptin, and leptin/adiponectin ratio and the increase in resistin, insulin, and HOMA-IR in this group. Interestingly, Schwingshack et al., 2001, and McAllan et al., 2014, have reported that macronutrient quality and composition, i.e. monounsaturated fat and protein can affect some of the parameters we have measured (leptin and glycosylated hemoglobin) and in the same direction we observed for the placebo group [48,49].

5. Conclusions

Additional research is required to fully understand the associated mechanisms between *n*-3 PUFA-rich fish oil consumption and adipokine secretion/expression. The small sample size and use of metformin may have limited our findings as well as the use of a relatively low dose of *n*-3 PUFAs, so larger studies with higher doses of *n*-3 PUFAs are required to confirm and extend our findings. It would be important to measure serum levels of other adipokines related to IR and T2DM, such as visfatin and apelin, to determine if the beneficial effects of PUFA *n*-3 are sustained after the cessation of therapy and to determine if negative effects on insulin sensitivity are actually caused by the supplement. The different effects of EPA and DHA observed in some studies highlight the need to study their actions separately.

In summary and despite the limitations, our study is the first to report serum concentrations of adiponectin, resistin, and leptin and show a beneficial effect of *n*-3 PUFA supplementation on waist circumference, glucose, glycosylated hemoglobin, leptin, and leptin/adiponectin ratio and lipid profile in a group of Mexican individuals with T2DM. Supplementation with *n*-3 PUFA and *n*-3 PUFA combined with metformin both warrant further investigation in Mexican T2DM.

Acknowledgments: The project from which this article derives was funded by the Consejo Nacional de Ciencia y Tecnología (CONACyT), Scientific Development Proposals for the Attention of National Problems No. 212946. México.

Author Contributions: R.V.-R., A.L.G.-L., B.E.M.-C., and L.S.H. participated in the design and implementation of the study protocol. M.G.J.-C., R.V.-R., A.L.G.-L., and B.E.M.-C. underwent all the fieldwork, biochemical and anthropometric measurements. All authors participated in data analysis, contributed in writing the manuscript, and read and approved the final version. The present manuscript is part of the Master in Health Sciences research thesis of M.G.J.-C.

Conflicts of Interest: The authors declare no conflict of interest. The founding sponsors had no role in the design of the study; in the collection, analyses, or interpretation of data; in the writing of the manuscript; or in the decision to publish the results.

References

1. Whiting, D.R.; Guariguata, L.; Weil, C.; Shaw, J. IDF Diabetes Atlas: Global estimates of the prevalence of diabetes for 2011 and 2030. *Diabetes Res. Clin. Pract.* **2011**, *94*, 311–321. [CrossRef] [PubMed]
2. Gutiérrez, J.P.; Rivera-Dommarco, J.; Shamah-Levy, T.; Villalpando-Hernández, S.; Franco, A.C.-N.L.; Romero-Martínez, M.H.-Á.M. Encuesta Nacional de Salud y Nutrición 2012. Resultados Nacionales (Internet). Cuernavaca Morelos, México. 2012. Available online: http://ensanut.insp.mx/informes/ENSANUT2012ResultadosNacionales.pdf (accessed on 5 June 2014).
3. Kwon, H.; Pessin, J.E. Adipokines mediate inflammation and insulin resistance. *Front. Endocrinol.* **2013**, *4*, 71. [CrossRef] [PubMed]
4. Rabe, K.; Lehrke, M.; Parhofer, K.G.; Broedl, U.C. Adipokines and insulin resistance. *Mol. Med.* **2008**, *14*, 741–751. [CrossRef] [PubMed]
5. Catalán, V.; Gómez-Ambrosi, J.; Rodríguez, A.; Salvador, J.; Frühbeck, G. Adipokines in the treatment of diabetes mellitus and obesity. *Expert Opin. Pharmacother.* **2009**, *10*, 239–254. [CrossRef] [PubMed]
6. Zhang, M.; Zhao, X.; Li, M.; Cheng, H.; Hou, D.; Wen, Y.; Katherine, C.; Mi, J. Abnormal adipokines associated with various types of obesity in Chinese children and adolescents. *Biomed. Environ. Sci.* **2011**, *24*, 12–21. [PubMed]
7. Hampe, L.; Radjainia, M.; Xu, C.; Harris, P.W.; Bashiri, G.; Goldstone, D.C.; Brimble, M.A.; Wang, Y.; Mitra, A.K. Regulation and quality control of adiponectin assembly by endoplasmic reticulum chaperone ERp44. *J. Biol. Chem.* **2015**, *290*, 18111–18123. [CrossRef] [PubMed]
8. Nomura, S.; Shouzu, A.; Omoto, S.; Inami, N.; Ueba, T.; Urase, F.; Maeda, Y. Effects of eicosapentaenoic acid on endothelial cell-derived microparticles, angiopoietins and adiponectin in patients with type 2 diabetes. *J. Atheroscler. Thromb.* **2009**, *2*, 83–90. [CrossRef]
9. Martínez-Fernández, M.L.; Laiglesia, L.M.; Huerta, A.E.; Martínez, J.A.; Moreno-Aliaga, M.J. Omega-3 fatty acids and adipose tissue function in obesity and metabolic syndrome. *Prostaglandins Other Lipid Mediat.* **2015**, *121*, 24–41. [CrossRef] [PubMed]
10. Bhaswant, M.; Poudyal, H.; Brown, L. Mechanisms of enhanced insulin secretion and sensitivity with *n*-3 unsaturated fatty acids. *J. Nutr. Biochem.* **2015**, *26*, 571–584. [CrossRef] [PubMed]
11. Son, Y.M.; Ahn, S.M.; Kim, G.R.; Moon, Y.S.; Kim, S.H.; Park, Y.M.; Lee, W.K.; Min, T.S.; Han, S.H.; Yun, C.H. Resistin enhances the expansion of regulatory T cells through modulation of dendritic cells. *BMC Immunol.* **2010**, *11*, 33. [CrossRef] [PubMed]
12. Jamaluddin, M.S.; Weakley, S.M.; Yao, Q.; Chen, C. Resistin: Functional roles and therapeutic considerations for cardiovascular disease. *Br. J. Pharmacol.* **2012**, *165*, 622–632. [CrossRef] [PubMed]
13. Subramanian, S.; Chait, A. Hypertriglyceridemia secondary to obesity and diabetes. *Biochim. Biophys. Acta* **2012**, *1821*, 819–825. [CrossRef] [PubMed]
14. Wu, L.; Parhofer, K.G. Diabetic dyslipidemia. *Metabolism* **2014**, *63*, 1469–1479. [CrossRef] [PubMed]
15. Kuryan, R.E.; Jacobson, M.S.; Frank, G.R. Non-HDL-cholesterol in an adolescent diabetes population. *J. Clin. Lipidol.* **2014**, *8*, 194–198. [CrossRef] [PubMed]
16. Ram, N.; Ahmed, B.; Hashmi, F.; Jabbar, A. Importance of measuring non-HDL cholesterol in type 2 diabetes patients. *J. Pak. Med. Assoc.* **2014**, *64*, 124–128. [PubMed]
17. Nettleton, J.A.; Katz, R. *n*-3 long-chain polyunsaturated fatty acids in type 2 diabetes: A Review. *J. Am. Diet. Assoc.* **2005**, *105*, 428–440. [CrossRef] [PubMed]
18. Wu, J.H.-Y.; Cahill, L.E.; Mozaffarian, D. Effect of fish oil on circulating adiponectin: A systematic review and meta-analysis of randomized controlled trials. *J. Clin. Endocrinol. Metab.* **2013**, *98*, 2451–2459. [CrossRef] [PubMed]

19. Kamat, S.G.; Roy, R. Evaluation of the effect of *n*-3 PUFA-rich dietary fish oils on lipid profile and membrane fluidity in alloxan-induced diabetic mice (*Mus musculus*). *Mol. Cell. Biochem.* **2016**, *416*, 117–129. [CrossRef] [PubMed]

20. Christou, G.A.; Rizos, E.C.; Mpechlioulis, A.; Penzo, C.; Pacchioni, A.; Nikas, D.N. Confronting the residual cardiovascular risk beyond statins: The role of fibrates, omega-3 fatty acids, or niacin, in diabetic patients. *Curr. Pharm. Des.* **2014**, *20*, 3675–3688. [CrossRef] [PubMed]

21. Yamamoto, T.; Kajikawa, Y.; Otani, S.; Yamada, Y.; Takemoto, S.; Hirota, M.; Ikeda, M.; Iwagaki, H.; Saito, S.; Fujiwara, T. Protective effect of eicosapentaenoic acid on insulin resistance in hyperlipidemic patients and on the postoperative course of cardiac surgery patients: The possible involvement of adiponectin. *Acta Med. Okayama* **2014**, *68*, 349–361. [PubMed]

22. Malekshahi, M.A.; Saedisomeolia, A.; Djalali, M.; Djazayery, A.; Pooya, S.; Sojoudi, F. Efficacy of omega-3 fatty acid supplementation on serum levels of tumour necrosis factor alpha, C-reactive protein and interleukin-2 in type 2 diabetes mellitus patients. *Singap. Med. J.* **2012**, *53*, 615–619.

23. Derosa, G.; Cicero, A.F.; D'Angelo, A.; Borghi, C.; Maffioli, P. Effects of *n*-3 PUFAs on fasting plasma glucose and insulin resistance in patients with impaired fasting glucose or impaired glucose tolerance. *Biofactors* **2016**, *42*, 316–322. [PubMed]

24. Vargas, M.L.; Almario, R.U.; Buchan, W.; Kim, K.; Karakas, S.E. Metabolic and endocrine effects of long chain vs. essential omega-3 polyunsaturated fatty acids in polycystic ovary syndrome. *Metabolism* **2011**, *60*, 1711–1718. [CrossRef] [PubMed]

25. Mohammadi, E.; Rafraf, M.; Farzadi, L.; Asghari-Jafarabadi, M.; Sabour, S. Effects of omega-3 fatty acids supplementation on serum adiponectin levels and some metabolic risk factors in women with polycystic ovary syndrome. *Asia Pac. J. Clin. Nutr.* **2012**, *21*, 511–518. [PubMed]

26. Karlström, B.E.; Järvi, A.E.; Byberg, L.; Berglund, L.G.; Vessby, B.O. Fatty fish in the diet of patients with type 2 diabetes: Comparison of the metabolic effects of foods rich in *n*-3 and *n*-6 fatty acids. *Am. J. Clin. Nutr.* **2011**, *94*, 26–33. [CrossRef] [PubMed]

27. Mansoori, A.; Sotoudeh, G.; Djalali, M.; Eshraghian, M.R.; Keramatipour, M.; Nasli-Esfahani, E.; Shidfar, F.; Alvandi, E.; Toupchian, O.; Koohdani, F. Effect of DHA-rich fish oil on PPARγ target genes related to lipid metabolism in type 2 diabetes: A randomized, double-blind, placebo-controlled clinical trial. *J. Clin. Lipidol.* **2015**, *9*, 770–777. [CrossRef] [PubMed]

28. Hendrich, S. (*n*-3) Fatty acids: clinical trials in people with type 2 diabetes. *Adv. Nutr.* **2010**, *1*, 3–7. [CrossRef] [PubMed]

29. Flachs, P.; Rossmeisl, M.; Kopecky, J. The effect of *n*-3 fatty acids on glucose homeostasis and insulin sensitivity. *Physiol. Res.* **2014**, *63*, S93–S118. [PubMed]

30. Al-Hamodi, Z.; AL-Habori, M.; Al-Meeri, A.; Saif-Ali, R. Association of adipokines, leptin/adiponectin ratio and C-reactive protein with obesity and type 2 diabetes mellitus. *Diabetol. Metab. Syndr.* **2014**, *6*, 99. [CrossRef] [PubMed]

31. Lara, J.J.; Economou, M.; Wallace, A.M.; Rumley, A.; Lowe, G.; Slater, C.; Caslake, M.; Sattar, N.; Lean, M.E. Benefits of salmon eating on traditional and novel vascular risk factors in young, non-obese healthy subjects. *Atherosclerosis* **2007**, *193*, 213–221. [CrossRef] [PubMed]

32. Stirban, A.; Nandrean, S.; Götting, C.; Stratmann, B.; Tschoepe, D. Effects of *n*-3 polyunsaturated fatty acids (PUFAs) on circulating adiponectin and leptin in subjects with type 2 diabetes mellitus. *Horm. Metab. Res.* **2014**, *46*, 490–492. [CrossRef] [PubMed]

33. Saltevo, J.; Kautiainen, H.; Vanhala, M. Gender differences in adiponectin and low-grade inflammation among individuals with normal glucose tolerance, prediabetes, and type 2 diabetes. *Gend. Med.* **2009**, *6*, 463–470. [CrossRef] [PubMed]

34. Snehalatha, C.; Mukesh, B.; Simon, M.; Viswanathan, V.; Haffner, S.M.; Ramachandran, A. Plasma adiponectin is an independent predictor of type 2 diabetes in Asian Indians. *Diabetes Care* **2003**, *26*, 3226–3229. [CrossRef] [PubMed]

35. Alfadda, A.A. Circulating adipokines in healthy versus unhealthy overweight and obese subjects. *Int. J. Endocrinol.* **2014**, *2014*, 170434. [CrossRef] [PubMed]

36. Azab, N.; Abdel-Aziz, T.; Ahmed, A.; El-deen, I.M. Correlation of serum resistin level with insulin resistance and severity of retinopathy in type 2 diabetes mellitus. *J. Saudi Chem. Soc.* **2016**, *20*, 272–277. [CrossRef]

37. Tokuyama, Y.; Osawa, H.; Ishizuka, T.; Onuma, H.; Matsui, K.; Egashira, T.; Makino, H.; Kanatsuka, A. Serum resistin level is associated with insulin sensitivity in Japanese patients with type 2 diabetes mellitus. *Metabolism* **2007**, *56*, 693–698. [CrossRef] [PubMed]

38. Deng, Y.; Scherer, P.E. Adipokines as novel biomarkers and regulators of the metabolic syndrome. *Ann. N. Y. Acad. Sci.* **2010**, *1212*, E1–E19. [CrossRef] [PubMed]

39. Finucane, F.M.; Luan, J.; Wareham, N.J.; Sharp, S.J.; O'Rahilly, S.; Balkau, B.; Flyvbjerg, A.; Walker, M.; Hojlund, K.; Nolan, J.J.; et al. Correlation of the leptin: Adiponectin ratio with measures of insulin resistance in non-diabetic individuals. *Diabetologia* **2009**, *52*, 2345–2349. [CrossRef] [PubMed]

40. Müllner, E.; Plasser, E.; Brath, H.; Waldschütz, W.; Forster, E.; Kundi, M.; Wagner, K.H. Impact of polyunsaturated vegetable oils on adiponectin levels, glycaemia and blood lipids in individuals with type 2 diabetes: a randomised, double-blind intervention study. *J. Hum. Nutr. Diet.* **2014**, *27*, 468–478. [CrossRef] [PubMed]

41. Wong, C.Y.; Yiu, K.H.; Li, S.W.; Lee, S.; Tam, S.; Lau, C.P.; Tse, H.F. Fish-oil supplement has neutral effects on vascular and metabolic function but improves renal function in patients with Type 2 diabetes mellitus. *Diabet. Med.* **2010**, *27*, 54–60. [CrossRef] [PubMed]

42. Via, M.A.; Mechanick, J.I. Nutrition in Type 2 Diabetes and the Metabolic Syndrome. *Med. Clin. N. Am.* **2016**, *100*, 1285–1302. [CrossRef] [PubMed]

43. Guadarrama-López, A.L.; Valdés-Ramos, R.; Kaufer-Horwitz, M.; Harbige, L.S.; Contreras, I.; Martínez-Carrillo, B.E. Relationship between fatty acid habitual intake and early inflammation biomarkers in individuals with and without type 2 diabetes in Mexico. *Endocr. Metab. Immune Disord. Drug Targets* **2015**, *15*, 234–241. [CrossRef] [PubMed]

44. NORMA Oficial Mexicana NOM-015-SSA2-2010, Para la Prevención, Tratamiento y Control de la Diabetes Mellitus. Available online: http://www.salud.gob.mx/unidades/cdi/nom/m015ssa24.html (accessed on 5 June 2014).

45. Von Frankenberg, A.D.; Silva, F.M.; de Almeida, J.C.; Piccoli, V.; do Nascimento, F.V.; Sost, M.M.; Leitao, C.B.; Remonti, L.L.; Umpierre, D.; Reis, A.F.; et al. Effect of dietary lipids on circulating adiponectin: A systematic review with meta-analysis of randomised controlled trials. *Br. J. Nutr.* **2014**, *112*, 1235–1250. [CrossRef] [PubMed]

46. Juárez-López, C.; Klünder-Klünder, M.; Madrigal-Azcárate, A.; Flores-Huerta, S. Omega-3 polyunsaturated fatty acids reduce insulin resistance and triglycerides in obese children and adolescents. *Pediatr. Diabetes* **2013**, *14*, 377–383. [CrossRef] [PubMed]

47. Simopoulos, A.P. The importance of the Omega-6/Omega-3 fatty acid ratio in cardiovascular disease and other chronic diseases. *Exp. Biol. Med.* **2008**, *233*, 674–688. [CrossRef] [PubMed]

48. Schwingshackl, L.; Strasser, B.; Hoffmann, G. Effects of Monounsaturated Fatty Acids on Glycaemic Control in Patients with Abnormal Glucose Metabolism: A Systematic Review and Meta-Analysis. *Ann. Nutr. Metab.* **2011**, *58*, 290–296. [CrossRef] [PubMed]

49. McAllan, L.; Skuse, P.; Cotter, P.D.; O' Connor, P.; Cryan, J.F.; Ross, R.P.; Fitzgerald, G.; Roche, H.M.; Nilaweera, K.N. Protein Quality and the Protein to Carbohydrate Ratio within a High Fat Diet Influences Energy Balance and the Gut Microbiota in C57BL/6J Mice. *PLoS ONE* **2014**, *9*, e88904. [CrossRef] [PubMed]

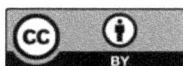

MDPI

Article

Carbohydrates from Sources with a Higher Glycemic Index during Adolescence: Is Evening Rather than Morning Intake Relevant for Risk Markers of Type 2 Diabetes in Young Adulthood?

Tanja Diederichs [1], Christian Herder [2,3], Sarah Roßbach [1], Michael Roden [2,3,4], Stefan A. Wudy [5], Ute Nöthlings [1], Ute Alexy [1,*] and Anette E. Buyken [1,6]

1   IEL-Nutritional Epidemiology, DONALD Study, Rheinische Friedrich-Wilhelms-University Bonn, Heinstueck 11, 44225 Dortmund, Germany; tdiederi@uni-bonn.de (T.D.); srossbac@uni-bonn.de (S.R.); noethlings@uni-bonn.de (U.N.); anette.buyken@uni-paderborn.de (A.E.B.)
2   Institute for Clinical Diabetology, German Diabetes Center, Leibniz Center for Diabetes Research at Heinrich Heine University Düsseldorf, Düsseldorf, Auf'm Hennekamp 65, 40225 Düsseldorf, Germany; christian.herder@ddz.uni-duesseldorf.de (C.H.); michael.roden@ddz.uni-duesseldorf.de (M.R.)
3   German Center for Diabetes Research (DZD), Ingolstädter Landstr. 1, 85764 München-Neuherberg, Germany
4   Department of Endocrinology and Diabetology, Medical Faculty, Heinrich Heine University Düsseldorf, Moorenstraße 5, 40225 Düsseldorf, Germany
5   Pediatric Endocrinology and Diabetology, Laboratory for Translational Hormone Analytics, Peptide Hormone Research Unit, Center of Child and Adolescent Medicine, Justus Liebig University Giessen, Feulgenstraße 10-12, 35392 Gießen, Germany; Stefan.Wudy@paediat.med.uni-giessen.de
6   Institute of Nutrition, Consumption and Health, Faculty of Natural Sciences, University Paderborn, Warburger Straße 100, 33098 Paderborn, Germany
*   Correspondence: alexy@uni-bonn.de; Tel.: +49-231-792210-16; Fax: +49-231-711581

Received: 11 April 2017; Accepted: 7 June 2017; Published: 10 June 2017

Abstract: Background: This study investigated whether glycemic index (GI) or glycemic load (GL) of morning or evening intake and morning or evening carbohydrate intake from low- or higher-GI food sources (low-GI-CHO, higher-GI-CHO) during adolescence are relevant for risk markers of type 2 diabetes in young adulthood. **Methods:** Analyses included DOrtmund Nutritional and Anthropometric Longitudinally Designed (DONALD) study participants who had provided at least two 3-day weighed dietary records (median: 7 records) during adolescence and one blood sample in young adulthood. Using multivariable linear regression analyses, estimated morning and evening GI, GL, low-GI-CHO (GI < 55) and higher-GI-CHO (GI ≥ 55) were related to insulin sensitivity ($N = 252$), hepatic steatosis index (HSI), fatty liver index (FLI) (both $N = 253$), and a pro-inflammatory-score ($N = 249$). **Results:** Morning intakes during adolescence were not associated with any of the adult risk markers. A higher evening GI during adolescence was related to an increased HSI in young adulthood ($p = 0.003$). A higher consumption of higher-GI-CHO in the evening was associated with lower insulin sensitivity ($p = 0.046$) and an increased HSI ($p = 0.006$), while a higher evening intake of low-GI-CHO was related to a lower HSI ($p = 0.009$). Evening intakes were not related to FLI or the pro-inflammatory-score (all $p > 0.1$). **Conclusion:** Avoidance of large amounts of carbohydrates from higher-GI sources in the evening should be considered in preventive strategies to reduce the risk of type 2 diabetes in adulthood.

Keywords: glycaemic index; glycaemic load; daytime; adolescence; type 2 diabetes mellitus

1. Introduction

Diets low in glycemic index (GI) or glycemic load (GL) are related to a lower risk of developing type 2 diabetes mellitus [1,2]. Their preferred use has hence been advocated particularly during periods of physiological insulin resistance, such as puberty [3]. This is supported by our recent observations linking a higher dietary GI/GL during puberty to a lower insulin sensitivity and increased liver enzyme activities [4] as well as increased levels of interleukin-(IL)-6 [5] in young adulthood, i.e., metabolic markers indicating an increased risk of developing type 2 diabetes in later life [6].

Recent discussions on preventive procedures also account for chronobiological aspects of metabolism [7]. This originates from the observation that extreme circadian (circa dies (lat.) = about 24 h) misalignment—as experienced during shiftwork—enhances the risk of type 2 diabetes among adults [8]. In a subsample from a Finnish population-based study, behavioral traits towards eveningness (based on a questionnaire assessing morningness-eveningness) were linked to notably higher odds for type 2 diabetes [9]. Persons with a late chronotype (i.e., those with a preference for a delayed timing of sleep on free days, i.e., without social obligations) are at particular risk of experiencing mild, but chronic misalignment resulting from the discrepancy between their circadian clock and socially determined, fixed schedules [10]. Misalignment may extend to their dietary behavior if it does not match metabolic processes, most of which follow a circadian rhythm [7]. Hence, dietary misalignment can emerge due to a discrepancy between the biological and the social timing or result from a general mismatch of dietary intake to metabolic circadian rhythmicity, e.g., to the decrease in insulin sensitivity over the day [11,12]. It is conceivable that adolescents are vulnerable to dietary misalignment since adolescence is characterized by a pronounced "lateness" in chronotype, i.e., a preference for a delayed timing of sleep on free days [13], which may be exacerbated by the physiological insulin resistance occurring during adolescence [14]. We hence hypothesize that recurring postprandial glycemic excursions elicited by carbohydrate-containing foods with a higher GI are particularly detrimental in evening hours and will have longer-term downstream adverse effects on adult metabolic health. It is possible that these are specific to either the *relative* glycemic response to the carbohydrate-containing foods consumed in evening hours, i.e., their GI [15], to their estimated postprandial glucose and insulin responses (i.e., their GL) and/or the intake of carbohydrates from low-GI (GI < 55) or higher-GI (GI ≥ 55, thus including sources with moderate- as well as high-GI) sources (low-GI-CHO, higher-GI-CHO).

Therefore, the aim of our current analysis was to separately examine the habitual dietary GI and GL of morning and evening intake during adolescence as well as morning and evening low-GI-CHO and higher-GI-CHO intake for prospective associations with risk markers of type 2 diabetes in young adulthood. Primary outcome measures comprised established risk parameters (insulin sensitivity, hepatic steatosis index (HSI), fatty liver index (FLI) and a pro-inflammatory score). Newly emerging risk markers of type 2 diabetes (fetuin A, fibroblast growth factor 21 (FGF-21) [16], interleukin-1 receptor antagonist (IL-1ra) and omentin [17]) were considered as secondary outcomes.

2. Methods

2.1. DONALD Study

The DONALD (DOrtmund Nutritional and Anthropometric Longitudinally Designed) study is an ongoing, open cohort study conducted in Dortmund, Germany, that was previously described [18]. In brief, since 1985, detailed data on diet, growth, development, and metabolism between infancy and early adulthood have been collected from approximately 1550 healthy children. Each year, 30–35 infants are newly recruited and first examined at the ages of three or six months. Participants regularly return to the study center thereafter; assessment during adolescence is scheduled annually. Since 2005, participants aged 18+ years are requested to provide a fasting blood sample in addition to the regular examination. The study was approved by the Ethics Committee of the University of Bonn (project identification code: 098/06, date of approval 21 June 2006); all examinations are performed with written consent from the parents and/or the participants.

2.2. Dietary Assessment

Nutritional data are assessed by 3-day weighed dietary records on three consecutive days. Participants are free to choose the days of recording. Dietary records include information on the timing of meal consumption. Parents and/or participants are instructed by dietitians to weigh all consumed foods and beverages, including leftovers, to the nearest 1 g. To this end, they receive regularly calibrated electronic food scales (initially Soehnle Digita 8000 (Leifheit AG, Nassau, Germany), now WEDO digi 2000 (Werner Dorsch GmbH, Muenster/Dieburg, Germany)). When exact weighing is not possible, semi-quantitative measures (e.g., number of spoons) are allowed. Moreover, information on recipes and on the types and brands of food items consumed is requested. The dietary records are collected as well as reviewed by the dietitians and analyzed using the continuously updated in-house nutrient database LEBTAB [19]. It includes information from standard nutrient tables, product labels, or recipe simulations based on the listed ingredients and nutrients.

2.3. Blood Analysis

Venous blood samples are drawn after an overnight fast, centrifuged at 4 °C and frozen at −80 °C in the DONALD Study Center. Fasting plasma glucose was determined on a Roche/Hitachi Cobas c 311 analyzer (Basel, Switzerland). Plasma insulin concentration was measured at the Laboratory for Translational Hormone Analytics of the University of Giessen using an immunoradiometric assay (IRMA, DRG Diagnostics, Marburg, Germany). All other measurements were performed at the German Diabetes Center with assay characteristics as described [5,20–22]: plasma activities of alanine-aminotransferase (ALT), aspartate-aminotransferase (AST), gamma-glutamyltransferase (GGT), plasma triglycerides (TG) and plasma high-sensitivity C-reactive protein (hsCRP) with the Roche/Hitachi Cobas c311 analyzer (Roche diagnostics, Mannheim, Germany), plasma high-sensitivity interleukin-(IL)-6 using the Human IL-6 Quantikine HS, plasma adiponectin with the Human Total Adiponectin/Acrp30 Quantikine ELISA, serum leptin with the Leptin Quantikine ELISA, serum interleukin-1 receptor antagonist (IL-1ra) with the Human IL-1ra/IL-1F3 ELISA, plasma fibroblast growth factor (FGF-21) with the Human FGF-21 kits all from R & D Systems (Wiesbaden, Germany), serum IL-18 using the Human IL-18 ELISA kit from MBL (Nagoya, Japan), and plasma chemerin with the Human Chemerin ELISA, plasma omentin-1 with the Human Omentin-1 ELISA, plasma chemerin with the Human Chemerin ELISA and plasma fetuin-A with the Human Fetuin-A ELISA kits from BioVendor (Brno, Czech Republic).

Insulin sensitivity was assessed using the updated HOMA2 sensitivity (in %) based on fasting insulin and blood glucose [23]. Indices of hepatic steatosis were calculated as follows:

Hepatic steatosis index (HSI):

- $HSI = 8 \times ALT/AST + BMI$

  (+2, if female; +2, if diabetes mellitus, but not applied, as the DONALD study excludes participants with chronic disease) [24],
- Fatty liver index (FLI):

  $FLI = e^x/(1 + e^x) \times 100$

  with $x = 0.953 \times \ln(TG) + 0.139 \times BMI + 0.718 \times \ln(GGT) + 0.053 \times$ waist circumference $- 15.745$ [25].

To estimate associations with chronic low-grade inflammation a pro-inflammatory score of established inflammation markers—assumed to be more predictive of inflammation than single markers [26]—was obtained by averaging inflammation markers, that were standardized (z) by sex (mean = 0, SD = 1) beforehand. To align anti-inflammatory adiponectin in the pro-inflammatory score it was multiplied by −1:

Pro-inflammatory score = (z-hsCRP + z-IL-6 + z-IL18 + z-chemerin + z-adiponectin $\times$ (−1) + z-leptin)/6.

2.4. Anthropometric Data

Anthropometric measurements are performed by trained nurses according to standard procedures, with the participants dressed only in underwear and barefoot. Standing height is measured to the nearest 0.1 cm (digital stadiometer: Harpenden Ltd., Crymych, UK) and body weight to the nearest 0.1 kg (electronic scale: model 753 E; Seca, Hamburg, Germany). Waist circumference is measured at the midpoint between the lower rib and the iliac crest to the nearest 0.1 cm. Measurements of skinfold thicknesses are taken on the right side of the body at the biceps, triceps, subscapular and suprailiac sites to the nearest 0.1 mm (Holtain caliper: Holtain Ltd., Crymych, UK).

From these measures, adolescent body mass index (BMI, kg/m^2) and its sex- and age-specific SD-scores (SDS) were calculated using current German BMI standards [27]. The prevalence of overweight in adolescence was calculated using standards of the International Obesity TaskForce (IOTF) [28]. Percent body fat (%BF) in adolescence and adulthood was estimated using the Slaughter [29] and the Durnin-Womersley equations [30], respectively. From these, body fat mass (kg) was calculated [(%BF× body mass)/100] and related to the square of height to obtain fat mass index (FMI, kg/m^2).

2.5. Family Characteristics

On a child's admission to the study, information on gestational characteristics and birth anthropometrics are abstracted from a standardized document (Mutterpass), given to all pregnant women in Germany. Moreover, parents are interviewed concerning the child's early life data as well as family and socio-economic characteristics at regular intervals. Additionally, parents are regularly weighed and measured using the same equipment used for participants.

2.6. Definition of Morning and Evening Intake

The definition of morning and evening was described in earlier analyses [31,32]. Briefly, for each age (year), the time between the end of the night and 11 a.m. and the time between 6 p.m. and the start of the night, respectively, was used to define morning and evening.

For estimation of morning and evening GI and GL as well as morning and evening carbohydrate intake from low- or higher-GI food sources, each carbohydrate containing food recorded in the corresponding day-time window was assigned a published GI value [33,34], based on glucose as reference food and according to a standardized procedure [35]. Carbohydrate content of each food consumed in the morning or in the evening was then multiplied by the food's GI to obtain the GL of the corresponding day-time window. Subsequently, overall morning/evening GI was obtained by dividing morning/evening GL by morning/evening carbohydrate intake. To distinguish carbohydrates from low- and higher-GI food sources, a value of 55 (cutoff proposed for low-GI foods [34]) was chosen for categorization. Accordingly, morning and evening carbohydrate intake from low-GI sources (low-GI-CHO (GI < 55) in g) and from moderate- or high-GI sources (higher-GI-CHO (GI ≥ 55) in g) was calculated.

2.7. Study Sample

Due to the open-cohort design of the study, many subjects have not yet reached young adulthood, when blood samples are taken. At the time of this analysis $N = 414$ young adults had provided at least one fasting blood sample, in which risk markers of type 2 diabetes were quantified. As only term (gestational age 37–42 weeks) singletons with a minimum birth weight of 2500 g were included in the analyses, sample size was reduced to $N = 397$. To allow estimation of morning and evening GI, GL, low-GI-CHO and higher-GI-CHO during adolescence (girls: 9–15 years, boys: 10–16 years), at least two 3-day weighed dietary records from three consecutive days were required ($N = 298$). Participants, who were identified to consistently underreport their energy intake were excluded from the study ($N = 12$, resulting in $N = 286$). In line with earlier publications [4,5] 'consistent underreporting' was defined to be present, when more than half of the available food records per participant were implausible. A 3-day weighed dietary record was considered implausible, when the total energy intake documented was inadequate in relation to the basal metabolic rate (estimated from Schofield equations [36]) using cut-offs from Goldberg et al. [37] modified for children and adolescents [38]. Finally, anthropometric measurements from adolescence and young adulthood as well as data on relevant covariates were required, resulting in analyses samples of $N = 253$ for liver steatosis outcomes, $N = 252$ for insulin sensitivity and $N = 249$ for inflammation-related outcomes. Sample sizes for insulin sensitivity and inflammation outcomes were lower because of fasting glucose concentrations below the threshold for calculation of HOMA2 sensitivity (reflecting hypoglycemia) or insufficient amounts of blood were available for determination of analytes.

2.8. Statistical Analysis

SAS procedures (SAS version 9.2, SAS Institute, Cary, NC, USA) were used for data analysis. p-values < 0.05 were considered significant. Tests for interaction indicated no sex differences for the primary outcomes, except for the relevance of evening GL for the pro-inflammatory score. Since stratified analyses for this association yielded similar non-significant results for males and females, all associations are from pooled analyses.

Characteristics of the study population are presented as medians (25th, 75th percentiles) for continuous variables and as absolute (relative) frequencies for categorical variables.

The prospective associations of morning and evening GI, GL, low-GI-CHO and higher-GI-CHO with the risk markers of type 2 diabetes were analyzed using multivariable linear regression models. To achieve normal distribution in the outcome variables, they were transformed prior to analysis using log, double-log, square root or reciprocal transformations, depending on the outcome. In addition, individual outliers which substantially interfered with normal distribution or regression modeling were winsorized, i.e., outliers were replaced by the sex-specifically closest value fitting a normal distribution. The procedure concerned IL-6 ($N = 4$), adiponectin ($N = 1$) and IL-1ra ($N = 2$). Exposures were energy-adjusted for morning and evening energy intake, respectively—except for dietary GI-using the residual method [39]. To account for sex- and age-dependent differences in nutritional intake, all variables were standardized (mean = 0, SD = 1) by sex and age (year) and averaged over the time period of adolescence. Crude models (model A) included the exposure variable as well as sex and age at blood withdrawal in adulthood. In a further step, adjusted models (model B) were constructed by individual examination of potentially influencing covariates and hierarchical inclusion [40] of those which substantially modified the exposure's regression coefficient by $\geq$10% [41] or independently predicted the outcome variable [42]. Potential confounding covariates considered for inclusion in the different hierarchical levels were (1) early life characteristics (gestational weight gain (kg), mother's age at birth (years), duration of pregnancy (weeks) and birth weight (g), first-born child (yes/no), full breastfeeding ($\geq$4 months yes/no)), (2) family and socio-economic characteristics (parental diabetes (yes/no), maternal overweight ($\geq$25 kg/m^2 yes/no), maternal educational status ($\geq$12 year of schooling yes/no), smoking in the household (yes/no)), (3) baseline characteristics (adolescent BMI-SDS, intake of saturated fatty acids (SFA, E%) and intake of animal protein (E%)). To ensure comparability, models were adjusted identically according to the strongest exposure-outcome associations for closely related outcomes (i.e., for (i) insulin sensitivity, (ii) hepatic steatosis markers (HSI, FLI, fetuin A, FGF-21) and (iii) inflammatory markers (pro-inflammatory score, IL-1ra, omentin)). For significant associations (model B), we additionally ran conditional models including waist circumferences to examine whether the observed associations are partly attributable to effects of carbohydrate nutrition on body composition. As HSI and FLI do by definition already include adult BMI and/or waist circumference, no conditional models were run for these outcomes.

3. Results

Characteristics of the study population at baseline and in young adulthood are shown in Tables 1 and 2, respectively (see Section 2.7. for selection of the sample). During adolescence, the GI and GL as well as the relative contribution of carbohydrates from low- or higher-GI sources were broadly comparable between morning and evening intake. Note that the carbohydrate content of morning intake was higher than the carbohydrate content of evening intake. In young adulthood, median age at blood withdrawal was 21 years (range 18–39 years).

Overall, **morning** GI and GL as well as morning carbohydrate intake from low- or higher-GI sources were not related to insulin sensitivity (Table S1), the primary hepatic steatosis outcomes HSI and FLI (Tables S2 and S3) or the pro-inflammatory score (Table 3, top) in young adulthood (all $p > 0.1$). Of note, low-GI-CHO intake during the morning was related to HSI in model A ($p = 0.041$), however, upon further adjustment this association was no longer statistically significant (Table S2, model B, $p = 0.24$). Morning exposures were neither related to the secondary outcomes fetuin A (Table S4), FGF-21 (Table S5), and IL-1ra (Table S6) (all $p > 0.08$). However, a higher morning GI during adolescence was associated with an increased level of the secondary outcome omentin in young adulthood ($p = 0.011$, Table S7); an association that persisted in the conditional model adjusting for adult waist circumference ($p = 0.003$).

In contrast, a higher **evening** carbohydrate intake from higher-GI sources during adolescence was associated with lower insulin sensitivity in young adulthood ($p = 0.046$, Figure 1). Additional adjustment for waist circumference rendered this association non-significant ($p = 0.11$). A higher evening GI ($p = 0.003$) and a higher evening higher-GI-CHO intake ($p = 0.006$) were related to an increased HSI, whereas higher evening low-GI-CHO intake ($p = 0.009$) was associated with a lower HSI (Figure 2). Similarly, a higher evening GL ($p = 0.005$) and higher evening higher-GI-CHO intake ($p = 0.029$) were associated with increased concentrations of the secondary outcome fetuin A (Table S4); neither of these relations was explained by adult waist circumference ($p = 0.006$ and $p = 0.040$ respectively). No prospective associations of evening intakes were observed with the primary outcomes FLI (Table S3) and the pro-inflammatory score (Table 3, bottom), or with the secondary outcomes FGF-21 (Table S5), IL-1ra (Table S6) and omentin (Table S7) (all $p > 0.01$).

Table 1. Baseline sample characteristics [1] ($N = 252$).

General Characteristics	
Sex ♀ (n (%))	130 (51.6)
Mean age (years)	12.4 (12.0; 13.0)
Early Life Factors	
Gestational weight gain (kg)	12 (10; 15)
Mothers age at gestation (years)	30.6 (28.2; 33.3)
Birth weight (g)	3450 (3130; 3810)
Duration of gestation (weeks)	40 (39; 41)
First born child (n (%))	152 (60.3)
Fully breastfed, $\geq$4 months (n (%))	124 (49.2)
Family Characteristics	
Parental diabetes (n (%))	9 (3.6)
Maternal overweight, $\geq$25 kg/m^2 (n (%))	101 (40.1)
Maternal educational status, $\geq$12 years of schooling (n (%))	136 (54.0)
Smoking in the household (n (%))	72 (28.6)
Body Composition during Adolescence [2]	
BMI (kg/m^2)	18.6 (16.8; 20.2)
BMI Standard Deviation Score	−0.13 (−0.87; 0.37)
FMI (kg/m^2)	3.2 (2.4; 4.5)
Overweight (n (%)) [3]	31 (12.3)
Nutrition Parameters during Adolescence [2]	
Number of 3-day dietary records per participant	7 (6; 7)
Daily energy intake (kcal)	1922 (1658; 2158)
Total carbohydrates (E% [4])	51.0 (48.4; 54.3)
Total protein (E% [4])	13.0 (12.0; 14.1)
Animal protein (E% [4])	8.1 (7.2; 9.1)
Total fat (E% [4])	35.9 (32.9; 38.1)
SFA (E% [4])	15.7 (14.1; 17.1)

Table 1. *Cont.*

Nutrition Parameters during Adolescence [2]	
Energy intake **before 11 a.m.** (kcal)	506 (418; 603)
Energy intake **before 11 a.m.** (E% [4])	26.7 (22.7; 30.7)
GI	56.2 (53.6; 58.8)
GL (g)	38.0 (32.5; 47.1)
Carbohydrates with low-GI [5] (E% [6])	21.2 (16.8; 26.6)
Carbohydrates with higher-GI [5] (E% [6])	32.6 (26.8; 37.3)
Total carbohydrates (E% [6])	54.5 (49.9; 59.6)
Total protein (E% [6])	12.0 (10.6; 13.6)
Animal protein (E% [6])	6.8 (5.3; 8.4)
Total fat (E% [6])	32.7 (28.3; 36.3)
SFA (E% [6])	15.0 (12.7; 17.6)
Energy intake **after 6 p.m.** (kcal)	580 (471; 691)
Energy intake **after 6 p.m.** (E% [4])	30.3 (26.7; 34.1)
GI	56.6 (54.3; 59.2)
GL (g)	40.2 (31.5; 49.1)
Carbohydrates with low-GI [5] (E% [6])	18.6 (14.7; 23.1)
Carbohydrates with higher-GI [5] (E% [6])	30.2 (24.8; 34.0)
Total carbohydrates (E% [6])	48.7 (44.8; 52.9)
Total protein (E% [6])	14.0 (12.3; 15.3)
Animal protein (E% [6])	9.0 (7.3; 10.5)
Total fat (E% [6])	37.1 (33.5; 40.5)
SFA (E% [6])	15.6 (14.3; 17.5)

Values are n (%) for categorical variables or medians (25th, 75th percentiles) for continuous variables. [1] General characteristics are shown for the sample used for diabetic risk markers only (N = 252), since samples used for risk marker of hepatic steatosis (N = 253) and inflammation (N = 249) are very similar; [2] mean over six years (♀: 9–15 years, ♂: 10–16 years); [3] includes overweight and obesity as defined by IOTF in Cole 2000 [28]; [4] % of daily energy intake; [5] distinction between carbohydrate intake from low- and higher-GI food sources with a GI of 55 as cut-off; [6] % of energy intake before 11 a.m./after 6 p.m. BMI—body mass index, FMI—fat mass index, GL—glycemic load, GI—glycemic index, SFA—saturated fatty acids.

Table 2. Sample characteristics for young adulthood [1].

	N	Value
General Characteristic		
Mean age at blood withdrawal (years)	252	21.0 (18.1; 24.0)
Lifestyle		
Alcohol consumption (g) [2]	197	0.3 (0.0; 6.0)
Smokers (n (%))	237	65 (27.4)
Body composition		
BMI (kg/m^2)	252	22.1 (20.6; 24.6)
FMI (kg/m^2)	252	5.7 (3.8; 7.2)
Overweight (n (%)) [3]	252	55 (21.8)
Waist circumference (cm)	252	75.9 (70.8; 80.9)
Risk markers of type 2 diabetes		
HOMA2 sensitivity (%)	252	77.1 (61.2; 99.0)
Hepatic steatosis index (HSI)	253	29.8 (27.8; 32.8)
Fatty liver index (FLI)	253	7.3 (4.6; 15.4)
Fetuin A (mg/L)	253	273 (241; 306)
FGF-21 (pg/mL)	253	83.4 (39.7; 156.6)
Pro-inflammatory score	249	−0.11 (−0.38; 0.32)
IL-1ra (pg/mL)	249	218 (169; 295)
Omentin (ng/mL)	249	379 (317; 458)

Values are n (%) for categorical variables and median (25th, 75th percentiles) for continuous variables. [1] General characteristics are shown for the sample used for diabetic risk markers only (N = 252), since samples used for risk marker of hepatic steatosis (N = 253) and inflammation (N = 249) are very similar; [2] estimation is based on N = 197 participants who had provided a 3-day weighed dietary record in young adulthood; [3] including all BMI $\geq$ 25.0; BMI—body mass index, FGF-21—*Fibroblast growth factor 21*, FMI—fat mass index, HOMA2—updated homeostasis model assessment for insulin sensitivity, IL-1ra—Interleukin 1 receptor antagonist.

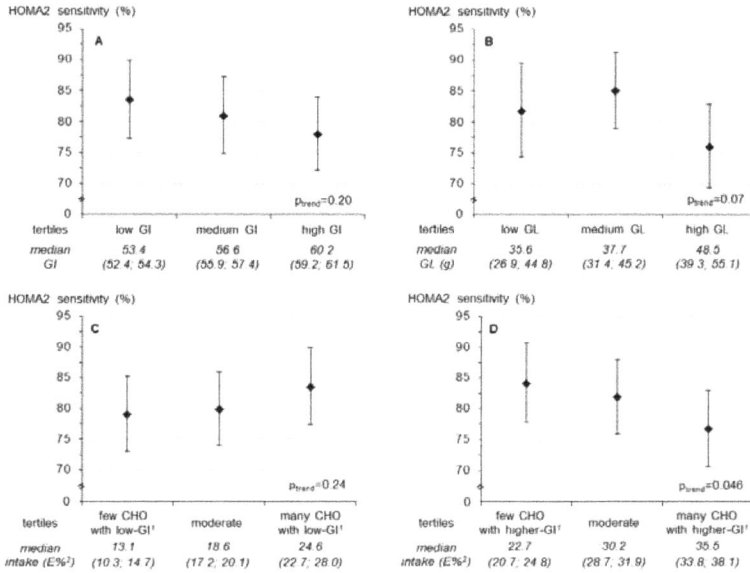

Figure 1. Predicted least square means (95% confidence interval) of **HOMA2 sensitivity** by tertiles of (**A**) glycemic index (GI) after 6 p.m., (**B**) glycemic load (GL) after 6 p.m., (**C**) intake of low-GI-CHO [1] after 6 p.m. and (**D**) intake of higher-GI-CHO [1] after 6 p.m. Values are least-square means for tertiles obtained from linear regression models. *p*-values are based on models using the continuous exposure variables. Models were adjusted for first born child (yes/no), baseline BMI-SDS, baseline evening intake of saturated fatty acids and animal protein (N = 252). Values below the figure refer to median intakes (25th; 75th percentiles) in each tertile of the respective exposure. [1] Distinction between carbohydrate intake from low- and higher-GI food sources with a GI of 55 as cut-off; [2] % of energy intake after 6 p.m.

Table 3. Prospective relation of GI and GL of morning (before 11 a.m.) and evening (after 6 p.m.) intake as well as morning and evening intake from low- and higher-GI food sources during adolescence to **pro-inflammatory score** in young adulthood (N = 249).

	Predicted Means [1] of Pro-Inflammatory Score by Exposure Tertiles (Exposures: Morning and Evening GI, GL, Low-GI-CHO, Higher-GI-CHO)			*p* for Trend [2]
	Low Exposure (T1)	Average Exposure (T2)	High Exposure (T3)	
	MORNING			
Glycemic Index (GI)				
Median GI	52.2 (50.2; 53.8)	56.2 (55.2; 57.0)	59.5 (58.5; 60.6)	
Model A [3]	−0.10 (−0.22; 0.03)	−0.03 (−0.15; 0.10)	−0.04 (−0.16; 0.08)	0.15
Model B [4]	−0.10 (−0.21; 0.02)	−0.04 (−0.16; 0.08)	−0.02 (−0.13; 0.10)	0.18
Glycemic Load (GL)				
Median GL	35.7 (30.4; 41.6)	35.9 (30.4; 42.9)	45.4 (37.1; 53.9)	
Model A [3]	−0.08 (−0.20; 0.04)	−0.02 (−0.14; 0.10)	−0.06 (−0.18; 0.06)	0.40
Model B [4]	−0.11 (−0.23; 0.02)	0.00 (−0.12; 0.12)	−0.05 (−0.17; 0.08)	0.27
CHO with low-GI [5]				
Median low-GI-CHO (E%)	15.4 (12.4; 17.3)	21.4 (19.5; 23.3)	28.8 (26.5; 32.7)	
Model A [3]	0.01 (−0.12; 0.14)	−0.05 (−0.17; 0.08)	−0.13 (−0.25; 0.00)	0.16
Model B [4]	−0.01 (−0.13; 0.11)	−0.03 (−0.14; 0.09)	−0.11 (−0.23; 0.00)	0.39
CHO with higher-GI [5]				
Median higher-GI-CHO (E%)	25.0 (22.5; 27.2)	32.9 (31.0; 34.3)	38.6 (36.5; 42.8)	
Model A [3]	−0.15 (−0.26; −0.03)	−0.06 (−0.18; 0.07)	0.04 (−0.08; 0.17)	0.06
Model B [4]	−0.14 (−0.25; −0.02)	−0.04 (−0.16; 0.08)	0.03 (−0.10; 0.15)	0.12

Table 3. *Cont.*

	Predicted Means [1] of Pro-Inflammatory Score by Exposure Tertiles *(Exposures: Morning and Evening GI, GL, Low-GI-CHO, Higher-GI-CHO)*			*p* for Trend [2]
	Low Exposure (T1)	Average Exposure (T2)	High Exposure (T3)	
	EVENING			
Glycemic Index (GI)				
Median GI	*53.3 (52.4; 54.3)*	*56.6 (55.9; 57.4)*	*60.2 (59.1; 61.5)*	
Model A [3]	0.04 (−0.09; 0.17)	−0.05 (−0.17; 0.08)	−0.15 (−0.27; −0.03)	0.30
Model B [4]	0.01 (−0.11; 0.13)	−0.04 (−0.16; 0.08)	−0.12 (−0.23; 0.00)	0.75
Glycemic Load (GL)				
Median GL	*34.4 (26.9; 44.8)*	*37.1 (31.3; 44.6)*	*48.5 (40.0; 55.1)*	
Model A [3]	−0.01 (−0.14; 0.12)	−0.17 (−0.29; −0.05)	0.02 (−0.10; 0.15)	0.66
Model B [4]	−0.05 (−0.18; 0.09)	−0.13 (−0.24; −0.01)	0.03 (−0.10; 0.16)	0.46
CHO with low-GI [5]				
Median low-GI-CHO (E%)	*13.1 (10.3; 14.7)*	*18.5 (17.2; 20.0)*	*24.6 (22.8; 28.2)*	
Model A [3]	−0.07 (−0.19; 0.06)	−0.06 (−0.18; 0.06)	−0.04 (−0.16; 0.09)	0.56
Model B [4]	−0.05 (−0.17; 0.08)	−0.06 (−0.18; 0.06)	−0.05 (−0.17; 0.07)	0.84
CHO with higher-GI [5]				
Median higher-GI-CHO (E%)	*22.5 (20.8; 24.9)*	*30.2 (28.8; 32.0)*	*35.4 (33.7; 38.1)*	
Model A [3]	−0.09 (−0.21; 0.03)	−0.07 (−0.19; 0.05)	0.00 (−0.12; 0.13)	0.69
Model B [4]	−0.11 (−0.23; 0.01)	−0.06 (−0.17; 0.06)	0.02 (−0.10; 0.14)	0.44

Values in italic refer to median intakes (25th, 75th percentiles) in each tertile of the respective exposure. [1] Model-values are least square means (95% confidence intervals) of pro-inflammatory score; [2] *p*-values for models are based on linear regression analyses using continuous exposure variables; [3] Model A (crude model) adjusted for sex and age at blood withdrawal; [4] Model B additionally adjusted for gestational weight gain, maternal educational status (≥12 years of schooling yes/no), baseline BMI-SDS, baseline morning or evening intake of animal protein; [5] Distinction between carbohydrate intake from low- and higher-GI food sources with a GI of 55 as cut-off.

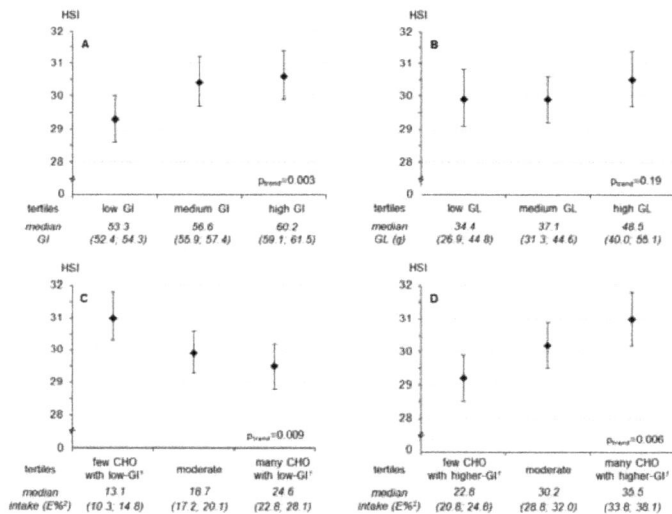

Figure 2. Predicted least square means (95% confidence interval) of **hepatic steatosis index (HSI)** by tertiles of (**A**) glycemic index (GI) after 6 p.m., (**B**) glycemic load (GL) after 6 p.m., (**C**) intake of low-GI-CHO [1] after 6 p.m. and (**D**) intake of higher-GI-CHO [1] after 6 p.m. Values are least-square means for tertiles obtained from linear regression models. *p*-values are based on models using the continuous exposure variables. Models were adjusted for sex, age at blood withdrawal, gestational weight gain, duration of pregnancy and birth weight, maternal educational status (≥12 years of schooling yes/no), maternal overweight (≥25 kg/m[2] yes/no), baseline BMI-SDS, and baseline evening intake of saturated fatty acids (*N* = 253). Values below the figure refer to median intakes (25th; 75th percentiles) in each tertile of the respective exposure. [1] Distinction between carbohydrate intake from low- and higher-GI food sources with a GI of 55 as cut-off; [2] % of energy intake after 6 p.m.

4. Discussion

The present study provides novel evidence that adverse longer-term metabolic effects of recurring postprandial glycemic excursions may be specific to evening carbohydrate consumption. Specifically, adolescents who habitually consumed more carbohydrates from higher-GI food sources in the evening had a lower insulin sensitivity and a higher HSI in young adulthood. By contrast, such adverse prospective associations were not observed for morning intakes. The absence of associations with the pro-inflammatory score suggests that day-time specific intake pattern in adolescence may not be of longer-term relevance for low-grade inflammation among young, healthy adults.

Our observation linking evening higher-GI-CHO to insulin sensitivity is in line with our hypothesis that evening rather than morning intake of higher-GI foods is potentially detrimental for risk factors of type 2 diabetes. A diurnal pattern of insulin sensitivity has been confirmed for both healthy persons [11] and participants with prediabetes [12]. The observed decrease in insulin sensitivity over the course of the day offers a plausible mechanism for our results. In line with our findings, a recent study measuring 20-h day-time profiles from 6 healthy volunteers (4 females, 2 males) reported that estimated postprandial insulin sensitivity was lowest when participants consumed 60% of their daily energy intake in the form of high-GI foods at supper [43]. In an earlier study from the same group, 8-h daytime profiles were collected from 17 middle-aged men with overweight or obesity and at least one cardiac risk factor [44]. Results revealed higher postprandial glucose and insulin responses following high-GI lunch and afternoon tea, but not high-GI breakfast compared to the corresponding low-GI meals. Upon adherence to the assigned diet over 24 days, postprandial insulin resistance had increased in the high-GI diet group compared to the low-GI diet group; thus, there was no metabolic adaptation to the high-GI diet. Our results expand on these findings in that they suggest that higher-GI-CHO habitually consumed in the evening by adolescents may have longer-term adverse consequences for adult insulin sensitivity. Our conditional model suggests that this association may be partly mediated by adult body composition. This is supported by the fact that lower glycogen synthesis over night was observed in subjects with diabetes mellitus type 2 compared to insulin-sensitive subjects [45], so that high evening higher-GI-CHO intake may shift glucose metabolites to de-novo lipogenesis and subsequent fat storage among adolescents experiencing physiological insulin resistance. Hence, future studies should also address the relevance of higher-GI-CHO consumed in the evening for body composition.

Glucose metabolism is closely linked to fatty acid metabolism; therefore insulin resistance and accumulation of fat in the liver are tightly interrelated [46]. Two studies, although heterogeneous in their methods (intervention vs observational study, extreme (dietary GI 32 vs. 84) vs. habitual low/high-GI diets and determination of liver steatosis severity by ^{1}H magnetic resonance spectroscopy and liver ultrasonography scanning, respectively), suggest that the dietary GI may be related to liver function [47,48]. However, it should be noted that imaging methods as used in these studies are time- and cost-intensive and therefore often infeasible in observational studies.

Our study used validated indices, which are preferable over the use of single liver enzyme activities in that they include more than one metabolic parameter predictive of hepatic steatosis. Our results extend existing evidence [47,48] suggesting that a higher-GI diet and an increased intake of higher-GI-CHO are both of longer-term relevance for hepatic steatosis and that these associations are specific to evening intakes.

It is important to note that HSI was shown to reflect the presence as well as the degree of hepatic steatosis [24]. The cut-off value to rule-out hepatic steatosis is 30, while the cut-off value to postulate the presence of hepatic steatosis is 36. In our healthy sample, only those in the lowest tertile of higher-GI-CHO intake had HSI levels clearly below 30, whereas those in the middle and highest tertiles had mean HSI values between 30 and 31 (Figure 2).

Similarly, albeit non-significant associations were observed with the FLI. Both HSI and FLI have similar efficacy to detect steatosis compared to an imaging method and were described as appropriate surrogate markers for epidemiological studies [49]. The two main differences between HSI and FLI are that the latter considers the activity of GGT instead of ALT and AST activities as well as TG and waist circumference in addition to BMI. In an earlier analysis of ours, dietary GI during adolescence had been related to both GGT and ALT in young adulthood [4], but a recent meta-analysis does not support an independent effect of the GI-level of diets on TG concentrations [50]. Therefore, the FLI could by definition be less responsive to the exposures under consideration in the present analysis. Yet, chance must be considered as a possible explanation as well. However, it was noted that results for fetuin A—one of our secondary outcomes, which is closely related to hepatic steatosis [16]—are in line with the findings for HSI and were independent of waist circumference.

We did not observe a relation of morning or evening GI, GL, or intake of low-GI-CHO or higher-GI-CHO to the pro-inflammatory score. In an earlier study of ours, a higher dietary GL as well as higher daily intakes of higher-GI-CHO during adolescence were associated with increased levels of IL-6, but not with hs-CRP, IL-18 or adiponectin in young adulthood [5]. Individual analyses of parameters which are included in the score confirmed these results for the current sample, albeit without an indication of a day-time specificity: Both a higher morning and a higher evening GL as well as higher intakes of morning and evening higher-GI-CHO were associated with increased adult levels of IL-6 (data not shown).

Conversely, a day-time specificity emerged for omentin. Here, higher morning GI during adolescence was associated with increased young adult omentin levels. The association was unaffected by additional adjustment for adult waist circumference. Consistent with our results, data from healthy normal weight children showed higher insulin levels and lower insulin sensitivity in children in the highest as compared to the lowest tertile of omentin [51]. As omentin is discussed to exert anti-inflammatory actions [17], we speculate that our findings may reflect an upregulation due to a habitual counter-regulatory omentin increase in response to regular pro-inflammatory signals. Indeed, a high-GI diet—regularly provoking postprandial glycemic spikes—induces increased oxidative stress [52]. In terms of the day-time specificity, it is worth noting that postprandial glycemic spikes following high GI meals are highest after breakfast compared to lunch and tea times [44].

If confirmed by other studies, our findings have several potential implications: First, the time of day when higher-GI foods are consumed is of relevance, so that a shift in focus is needed from 'what we eat' also to 'when do we eat what'. Second, our observations are based on habitual dietary intake data and reveal that the analyzed population consumed on average more than half of their morning and evening carbohydrates from higher-GI food sources, which translates into a third of their morning and evening energy intake from higher-GI food sources. Of note, those who consumed less than a quarter of their evening energy intake from higher-GI-CHO (i.e., those in the lowest tertile) had a mean HSI below 30. Hence, our data suggest that reducing higher-GI-CHO intake from a third to a quarter of energy intake in the evening offers preventive potential for adult type 2 diabetes risk. Third, the absence of a relation with morning GI, GL, low-GI-CHO or higher-GI-CHO does not justify a recommendation to shift high evening intake of high-GI foods to morning hours, as there is a possibility of adverse longer-term effects for chronic subclinical inflammation in response to habitual postprandial spikes induced in the morning. Moreover, due to the fact that the delay in chronotype (i.e., the preference for a delayed timing of sleep on free days) peaks approximately at the age of 20 years [13], encouraging morning food intake may augment circadian misalignment and would therefore be counterproductive for metabolic health in adolescents and young adults.

Our study is limited by the availability of one blood sample in young adulthood only; the use of surrogate markers of diabetes risk instead of hard end points can be considered as further limitation. However, our population was too young to have established type 2 diabetes. Moreover, it needs to be assumed that the analyzed outcomes themselves follow individual circadian rhythms [53,54] so that measurement of risk markers takes place in blood samples potentially withdrawn during the acrophase (i.e., the maximum value of one rhythm cycle) of one parameter and the bathyphase (i.e., the minimum value of one rhythm cycle) of another parameter. However, withdrawing all blood samples at the approximately same day-time, i.e., during morning hours in our study, results in a standardization of all outcome parameters to day-time. Consequently, differences in the circadian rhythm between the analytes do not affect the calculated indices (HOMA2 sensitivity, HSI, FLI, pro-inflammatory score). Concerning our dietary predictors, the GI concept is still contentious. Recent criticism relates to methodological aspects [55] and GI extrapolation to mixed meals [56]. However, the validity of dietary GI has been demonstrated repeatedly using different methodological approaches [15,57] and ISO-standardization will further reduce methodological errors in measuring the GI of foods [58]. It could be criticized that we excluded only participants who regularly under-reported their energy intake from our analyses. However, exclusion of under-reporters is controversial [59] and it should be noted that in our study only a further $N = 77$ participants had ever underreported their energy intake in any of their protocols (median: 7 protocols). Additional exclusion of these participants did not affect our results. Only the association of higher-GI-CHO with HOMA2 sensitivity was attenuated towards a trend ($p = 0.08$), which is likely attributable to the lower number of participants included in this sensitivity analysis (data not shown). Overall, our results could be subject to concerns about multiple testing. However, three separate sets of primary outcomes were considered (insulin sensitivity, hepatic steatosis, subclinical chronic inflammation) and different mechanisms are discussed for the relevance of GI, GL or CHO from low- or higher-GI sources for these outcomes. Moreover, we abstained from stressing and/or discussing findings that tended to be associated (p-values between 0.05 and <0.1). Generally, the DONALD population is characterized by a socio-economic status that is above average [18], so that extremes in nutritional behavior might not be represented. Consequently, a selection bias is likely introduced. However, the relatively homogeneous sample decreases the vulnerability of the results to residual confounding.

The overall strengths of the study are its prospective design and the detailed repeated dietary data including day-time specific nutritional information during adolescence. Due to the recruitment of study participants during infancy and the annually repeated data collection, 3-day weighed dietary records are documented by participants accustomed to the procedure. Moreover, availability of data on several important potential confounders, i.e., early-life characteristics, anthropometrics, familial and socio-economic factors strengthen our analyses.

5. Conclusions

In conclusion, our data suggest that young adult insulin sensitivity and hepatic steatosis markers are responsive to higher evening, but not morning intakes of higher-GI-CHO during adolescence, whereas there was no association with adult subclinical inflammation. Avoidance of large amounts of higher-GI-CHO in the evening and/or their replacement by low-GI-CHO during adolescence may present a promising preventive strategy to reduce risk of type 2 diabetes in adulthood.

Supplementary Materials: The following are available online at www.mdpi.com/2072-6643/9/6/591/s1. Table S1: Prospective relation of GI and GL of morning (before 11 a.m.) intake as well as morning carbohydrate intake from low- and higher-GI food sources during adolescence to HOMA2 sensitivity in young adulthood ($N = 252$), Table S2: Prospective relation of GI and GL of morning (before 11 a.m.) intake as well as morning carbohydrate intake from low- and higher-GI food sources during adolescence to hepatic steatosis index (HSI) in young adulthood ($N = 253$), Table S3: Prospective relation of GI and GL of morning (before 11 a.m.) and evening (after 6 p.m.) intake as well as morning and evening intake from low- and higher-GI food sources during adolescence to fatty liver index (FLI) in young adulthood ($N = 253$), Table S4: Prospective relation of GI and GL of morning (before 11 a.m.) and evening (after 6 p.m.) intake as well as morning and evening intake from low- and higher-GI food sources during adolescence to fetuin A (mg/L) in young adulthood ($N = 253$), Table S5: Prospective relation of GI and GL of morning (before 11 a.m.) and evening (after 6 p.m.) intake as well as morning and evening intake from low- and higher-GI food sources during adolescence to fibroblast growth factor 21 (FGF-21, pg/mL) in young adulthood ($N = 253$), Table S6: Prospective relation of GI and GL of morning (before 11 a.m.) and evening (after 6 p.m.) intake as well as morning and evening intake from low- and higher-GI food sources during adolescence to interleukin 1 receptor antagonist (IL-1ra, pg/mL) in young adulthood ($N = 249$), Table S7: Prospective relation of GI and GL of morning (before 11 a.m.) and evening (after 6 p.m.) intake as well as morning and evening intake from low- and higher-GI food sources during adolescence to omentin (ng/mL) in young adulthood ($N = 249$).

Acknowledgments: This research project is funded by the German Research Foundation (Bu1807/3-1). The DONALD Study is supported by the Ministry of Science and Research of North Rhine Westphalia, Germany. With respect to the co-authorship of C.H. and M.R., the following applies: The German Diabetes Center is funded by the German Federal Ministry of Health and the Ministry of Innovation, Science, Research and Technology of the State North Rhine-Westphalia. Their participation in this project was supported in part by a grant from the German Federal Ministry of Education and Research to the German Center for Diabetes Research (DZD e.V.). We thank the staff of the DONALD study for carrying out the anthropometric measurements as well as for collecting and coding dietary records and all participants of the study for providing their data.

Author Contributions: A.E.B., U.A., C.H.: conceived the project; T.D.: conducted the statistical analysis and wrote the manuscript; A.E.B.: supervised the study, provided detailed assistance in the drafting process and had primary responsibility for the final content; C.H., M.R., S.A.W.: supervised laboratory measurements of blood analytes; all authors: made substantial contributions and read and approved the final manuscript.

Conflicts of Interest: A.E.B. is a member of the International Carbohydrate Quality Consortium. All other authors declare no conflicts of interest. The funding sponsor had no role in the design of the study; in the collection, analyses, or interpretation of data; in the writing of the manuscript, and in the decision to publish the results.

References

1. Bhupathiraju, S.N.; Tobias, D.K.; Malik, V.S.; Pan, A.; Hruby, A.; Manson, J.E.; Willett, W.C.; Hu, F.B. Glycemic index, glycemic load, and risk of type 2 diabetes: Results from 3 large US cohorts and an updated meta-analysis. *Am. J. Clin. Nutr.* **2014**, *100*, 218–232. [CrossRef] [PubMed]
2. Augustin, L.S.A.; Kendall, C.W.C.; Jenkins, D.J.A.; Willett, W.C.; Astrup, A.; Barclay, A.W.; Bjorck, I.; Brand-Miller, J.C.; Brighenti, F.; Buyken, A.E.; et al. Glycemic index, glycemic load and glycemic response: An International Scientific Consensus Summit from the International Carbohydrate Quality Consortium (ICQC). *Nutr. Metab. Cardiovasc. Dis.* **2015**, *25*, 795–815. [CrossRef] [PubMed]
3. Buyken, A.E.; Mitchell, P.; Ceriello, A.; Brand-Miller, J. Optimal dietary approaches for prevention of type 2 diabetes: A life-course perspective. *Diabetologia* **2010**, *53*, 406–418. [CrossRef] [PubMed]
4. Goletzke, J.; Herder, C.; Joslowski, G.; Bolzenius, K.; Remer, T.; Wudy, S.A.; Roden, M.; Rathmann, W.; Buyken, A.E. Habitually higher dietary glycemic index during puberty is prospectively related to increased risk markers of type 2 diabetes in younger adulthood. *Diabetes Care* **2013**, *36*, 1870–1876. [CrossRef] [PubMed]
5. Goletzke, J.; Buyken, A.E.; Joslowski, G.; Bolzenius, K.; Remer, T.; Carstensen, M.; Egert, S.; Nothlings, U.; Rathmann, W.; Roden, M.; et al. Increased intake of carbohydrates from sources with a higher glycemic index and lower consumption of whole grains during puberty are prospectively associated with higher IL-6 concentrations in younger adulthood among healthy individuals. *J. Nutr.* **2014**, *144*, 1586–1593. [CrossRef] [PubMed]
6. Saponaro, C.; Gaggini, M.; Gastaldelli, A. Nonalcoholic fatty liver disease and type 2 diabetes: Common pathophysiologic mechanisms. *Curr. Diabetes Rep.* **2015**, *15*, 607. [CrossRef] [PubMed]
7. Bailey, S.M.; Udoh, U.S.; Young, M.E. Circadian regulation of metabolism. *J. Endocrinol.* **2014**, *222*, R75–R96. [CrossRef] [PubMed]
8. Scheer, F.A.J.L.; Hilton, M.F.; Mantzoros, C.S.; Shea, S.A. Adverse metabolic and cardiovascular consequences of circadian misalignment. *Proc. Natl. Acad. Sci. USA* **2009**, *106*, 4453–4458. [CrossRef] [PubMed]
9. Merikanto, I.; Lahti, T.; Puolijoki, H.; Vanhala, M.; Peltonen, M.; Laatikainen, T.; Vartiainen, E.; Salomaa, V.; Kronholm, E.; Partonen, T. Associations of chronotype and sleep with cardiovascular diseases and type 2 diabetes. *Chronobiol. Int.* **2013**, *30*, 470–477. [CrossRef] [PubMed]
10. Roenneberg, T.; Allebrandt, K.V.; Merrow, M.; Vetter, C. Social jetlag and obesity. *Curr. Boil.* **2012**, *22*, 939–943. [CrossRef] [PubMed]
11. Saad, A.; Dalla Man, C.; Nandy, D.K.; Levine, J.A.; Bharucha, A.E.; Rizza, R.A.; Basu, R.; Carter, R.E.; Cobelli, C.; Kudva, Y.C.; et al. Diurnal pattern to insulin secretion and insulin action in healthy individuals. *Diabetes* **2012**, *61*, 2691–2700. [CrossRef] [PubMed]
12. Sonnier, T.; Rood, J.; Gimble, J.M.; Peterson, C.M. Glycemic control is impaired in the evening in prediabetes through multiple diurnal rhythms. *J. Diabetes Complicat.* **2014**, *28*, 836–843. [CrossRef] [PubMed]
13. Roenneberg, T.; Kuehnle, T.; Pramstaller, P.P.; Ricken, J.; Havel, M.; Guth, A.; Merrow, M. A marker for the end of adolescence. *Curr. Boil.* **2004**, *14*, R1038–R1039. [CrossRef] [PubMed]
14. Goran, M.I.; Gower, B.A. Longitudinal study on pubertal insulin resistance. *Diabetes* **2001**, *50*, 2444–2450. [CrossRef] [PubMed]

15. Kochan, A.M.; Wolever, T.M.S.; Chetty, V.T.; Anand, S.S.; Gerstein, H.C.; Sharma, A.M. Glycemic index predicts individual glucose responses after self-selected breakfasts in free-living, abdominally obese adults. *J. Nutr.* **2012**, *142*, 27–32. [CrossRef] [PubMed]

16. Iroz, A.; Couty, J.-P.; Postic, C. Hepatokines: Unlocking the multi-organ network in metabolic diseases. *Diabetologia* **2015**, *58*, 1699–1703. [CrossRef] [PubMed]

17. Herder, C.; Carstensen, M.; Ouwens, D.M. Anti-inflammatory cytokines and risk of type 2 diabetes. *Diabetes Obes. Metab.* **2013**, *15*, 39–50. [CrossRef] [PubMed]

18. Kroke, A.; Manz, F.; Kersting, M.; Remer, T.; Sichert-Hellert, W.; Alexy, U.; Lentze, M.J. The DONALD Study. History, current status and future perspectives. *Eur. J. Nutr.* **2004**, *43*, 45–54. [CrossRef] [PubMed]

19. Sichert-Hellert, W.; Kersting, M.; Chahda, C.; Schäfer, R.; Kroke, A. German food composition database for dietary evaluations in children and adolescents. *J. Food Compos. Anal.* **2007**, *20*, 63–70. [CrossRef]

20. Herder, C.; Bongaerts, B.W.C.; Rathmann, W.; Heier, M.; Kowall, B.; Koenig, W.; Thorand, B.; Roden, M.; Meisinger, C.; Ziegler, D. Association of subclinical inflammation with polyneuropathy in the older population: KORA F4 study. *Diabetes Care* **2013**, *36*, 3663–3670. [CrossRef] [PubMed]

21. Herder, C.; Ouwens, D.M.; Carstensen, M.; Kowall, B.; Huth, C.; Meisinger, C.; Rathmann, W.; Roden, M.; Thorand, B. Adiponectin may mediate the association between omentin, circulating lipids and insulin sensitivity: Results from the KORA F4 study. *Eur. J. Endocrinol.* **2015**, *172*, 423–432. [CrossRef] [PubMed]

22. Hatziagelaki, E.; Herder, C.; Tsiavou, A.; Teichert, T.; Chounta, A.; Nowotny, P.; Pacini, G.; Dimitriadis, G.; Roden, M. Serum Chemerin Concentrations Associate with Beta-Cell Function, but Not with Insulin Resistance in Individuals with Non-Alcoholic Fatty Liver Disease (NAFLD). *PLoS ONE* **2015**, *10*, e0124935. [CrossRef] [PubMed]

23. Wallace, T.M.; Levy, J.C.; Matthews, D.R. Use and abuse of HOMA modeling. *Diabetes Care* **2004**, *27*, 1487–1495. [CrossRef] [PubMed]

24. Lee, J.-H.; Kim, D.; Kim, H.J.; Lee, C.-H.; Yang, J.I.; Kim, W.; Kim, Y.J.; Yoon, J.-H.; Cho, S.-H.; Sung, M.-W.; et al. Hepatic steatosis index: A simple screening tool reflecting nonalcoholic fatty liver disease. *Dig. Liver Dis.* **2010**, *42*, 503–508. [CrossRef] [PubMed]

25. Bedogni, G.; Bellentani, S.; Miglioli, L.; Masutti, F.; Passalacqua, M.; Castiglione, A.; Tiribelli, C. The Fatty Liver Index: A simple and accurate predictor of hepatic steatosis in the general population. *BMC Gastroenterol.* **2006**, *6*, 33. [CrossRef] [PubMed]

26. Calder, P.C. Feeding the immune system. *Proc. Nutr. Soc.* **2013**, *72*, 299–309. [CrossRef] [PubMed]

27. Robert-Koch-Institut. *Beiträge zur Gesundheitsberichterstattung des Bundes: Referenzperzentile für anthropometrische Maßzahlen und Blutdruck aus der Studie zur Gesundheit von Kindern und Jugendlichen in Deutschland* (KiGGS) 2003 bis 2006, 1st ed.; Robert-Koch-Institut: Berlin, Germany, 2011.

28. Cole, T.J.; Bellizzi, M.C.; Flegal, K.M.; Dietz, W.H. Establishing a standard definition for child overweight and obesity worldwide: International survey. *BMJ* **2000**, *320*, 1240–1243. [CrossRef] [PubMed]

29. Slaughter, M.H.; Lohman, T.G.; Boileau, R.A.; Horswill, C.A.; Stillman, R.J.; van Loan, M.D.; Bemben, D.A. Skinfold equations for estimation of body fatness in children and youth. *Hum. Boil.* **1988**, *60*, 709–723.

30. Durnin, J.V.; Womersley, J. Body fat assessed from total body density and its estimation from skinfold thickness: Measurements on 481 men and women aged from 16 to 72 years. *Br. J. Nutr.* **1974**, *32*, 77–97. [CrossRef] [PubMed]

31. Rossbach, S.; Diederichs, T.; Bolzenius, K.; Herder, C.; Buyken, A.E.; Alexy, U. Age and time trends in eating frequency and duration of nightly fasting of German children and adolescents. *Eur. J. Nutr.* **2016**. [CrossRef]

32. Diederichs, T.; Rossbach, S.; Herder, C.; Alexy, U.; Buyken, A.E. Relevance of Morning and Evening Energy and Macronutrient Intake during Childhood for Body Composition in Early Adolescence. *Nutrients* **2016**, *8*, 716. [CrossRef] [PubMed]

33. University of Sydney (Sydney, Australia). The Official Website of the Glycemic Index and GI Database. Available online: http://www.glycemicindex.com.

34. Atkinson, F.S.; Foster-Powell, K.; Brand-Miller, J.C. International tables of glycemic index and glycemic load values: 2008. *Diabetes Care* **2008**, *31*, 2281–2283. [CrossRef] [PubMed]

35. Buyken, A.E.; Dettmann, W.; Kersting, M.; Kroke, A. Glycaemic index and glycaemic load in the diet of healthy schoolchildren: Trends from 1990 to 2002, contribution of different carbohydrate sources and relationships to dietary quality. *BJN* **2005**, *94*, 796–803. [CrossRef]

36. Schofield, W.N. Predicting basal metabolic rate, new standards and review of previous work. *Hum. Nutr. Clin. Nutr.* **1985**, *39*, 5–41. [PubMed]

37. Goldberg, G.R.; Black, A.E.; Jebb, S.A.; Cole, T.J.; Murgatroyd, P.R.; Coward, W.A.; Prentice, A.M. Critical evaluation of energy intake data using fundamental principles of energy physiology: 1. Derivation of cut-off limits to identify under-recording. *Eur. J. Clin. Nutr.* **1991**, *45*, 569–581. [PubMed]

38. Sichert-Hellert, W.; Kersting, M.; Schoch, G. Underreporting of energy intake in 1 to 18 year old German children and adolescents. *Z. Ernahrungswiss.* **1998**, *37*, 242–251. [CrossRef] [PubMed]

39. Willett, W.C.; Howe, G.R.; Kushi, L.H. Adjustment for total energy intake in epidemiologic studies. *Am. J. Clin. Nutr.* **1997**, *65*, 1220S–1228S; discussion 1229S–1231S. [PubMed]

40. Victora, C.G.; Huttly, S.R.; Fuchs, S.C.; Olinto, M.T. The role of conceptual frameworks in epidemiological analysis: A hierarchical approach. *Int. J. Epidemiol.* **1997**, *26*, 224–227. [CrossRef] [PubMed]

41. Maldonado, G.; Greenland, S. Simulation study of confounder-selection strategies. *Am. J. Epidemiol.* **1993**, *138*, 923–936. [CrossRef] [PubMed]

42. Kirkwood, B.R.; Sterne, J.A.C. *Essential Medical Statistics*, 2nd ed.; Blackwell Science: Malden, MA, USA, 2003; pp. 315–342.

43. Morgan, L.M.; Shi, J.-W.; Hampton, S.M.; Frost, G. Effect of meal timing and glycaemic index on glucose control and insulin secretion in healthy volunteers. *Br. J. Nutr.* **2012**, *108*, 1286–1291. [CrossRef] [PubMed]

44. Brynes, A.E.; Mark Edwards, C.; Ghatei, M.A.; Dornhorst, A.; Morgan, L.M.; Bloom, S.R.; Frost, G.S. A randomised four-intervention crossover study investigating the effect of carbohydrates on daytime profiles of insulin, glucose, non-esterified fatty acids and triacylglycerols in middle-aged men. *Br. J. Nutr.* **2003**, *89*, 207–218. [CrossRef] [PubMed]

45. Krssak, M.; Brehm, A.; Bernroider, E.; Anderwald, C.; Nowotny, P.; Dalla Man, C.; Cobelli, C.; Cline, G.W.; Shulman, G.I.; Waldhausl, W.; et al. Alterations in postprandial hepatic glycogen metabolism in type 2 diabetes. *Diabetes* **2004**, *53*, 3048–3056. [CrossRef] [PubMed]

46. Sanders, F.W.B.; Griffin, J.L. De novo lipogenesis in the liver in health and disease: More than just a shunting yard for glucose. *Biol. Rev. Camb. Philos. Soc.* **2016**, *91*, 452–468. [CrossRef] [PubMed]

47. Valtuena, S.; Pellegrini, N.; Ardigo, D.; Del Rio, D.; Numeroso, F.; Scazzina, F.; Monti, L.; Zavaroni, I.; Brighenti, F. Dietary glycemic index and liver steatosis. *Am. J. Clin. Nutr.* **2006**, *84*, 136–142. [PubMed]

48. Bawden, S.; Stephenson, M.; Falcone, Y.; Lingaya, M.; Ciampi, E.; Hunter, K.; Bligh, F.; Schirra, J.; Taylor, M.; Morris, P.; et al. Increased liver fat and glycogen stores after consumption of high versus low glycaemic index food: A randomized crossover study. *Diabetes Obes. Metab.* **2017**, *19*, 70–77. [CrossRef] [PubMed]

49. Kahl, S.; Strassburger, K.; Nowotny, B.; Livingstone, R.; Kluppelholz, B.; Kessel, K.; Hwang, J.-H.; Giani, G.; Hoffmann, B.; Pacini, G.; et al. Comparison of liver fat indices for the diagnosis of hepatic steatosis and insulin resistance. *PLoS ONE* **2014**, *9*, e94059. [CrossRef] [PubMed]

50. Goff, L.M.; Cowland, D.E.; Hooper, L.; Frost, G.S. Low glycaemic index diets and blood lipids: A systematic review and meta-analysis of randomised controlled trials. *Nutr. Metab. Cardiovasc. Dis.* **2013**, *23*, 1–10. [CrossRef] [PubMed]

51. Prats-Puig, A.; Bassols, J.; Bargallo, E.; Mas-Parareda, M.; Ribot, R.; Soriano-Rodriguez, P.; Berengui, A.; Diaz, M.; de Zegher, F.; Ibanez, L.; et al. Toward an early marker of metabolic dysfunction: Omentin-1 in prepubertal children. *Obesity* **2011**, *19*, 1905–1907. [CrossRef] [PubMed]

52. Hu, Y.; Block, G.; Norkus, E.P.; Morrow, J.D.; Dietrich, M.; Hudes, M. Relations of glycemic index and glycemic load with plasma oxidative stress markers. *Am. J. Clin. Nutr.* **2006**, *84*, 70–76. [PubMed]

53. Rivera-Coll, A.; Fuentes-Arderiu, X.; Díez-Noguera, A. Circadian Rhythms of Serum Concentrations of 12 Enzymes of Clinical Interest. *Chronobiol. Int.* **2009**, *10*, 190–200. [CrossRef]

54. Rahman, S.A.; Castanon-Cervantes, O.; Scheer, F.A.J.L.; Shea, S.A.; Czeisler, C.A.; Davidson, A.J.; Lockley, S.W. Endogenous circadian regulation of pro-inflammatory cytokines and chemokines in the presence of bacterial lipopolysaccharide in humans. *Brain Behav. Immun.* **2015**, *47*, 4–13. [CrossRef] [PubMed]

55. Matthan, N.R.; Ausman, L.M.; Meng, H.; Tighiouart, H.; Lichtenstein, A.H. Estimating the reliability of glycemic index values and potential sources of methodological and biological variability. *Am. J. Clin. Nutr.* **2016**, *104*, 1004–1013. [CrossRef] [PubMed]

56. Meng, H.; Matthan, N.R.; Ausman, L.M.; Lichtenstein, A.H. Effect of macronutrients and fiber on postprandial glycemic responses and meal glycemic index and glycemic load value determinations. *Am. J. Clin. Nutr.* **2017**, *105*, 842–853. [CrossRef] [PubMed]

57. Fabricatore, A.N.; Ebbeling, C.B.; Wadden, T.A.; Ludwig, D.S. Continuous glucose monitoring to assess the ecologic validity of dietary glycemic index and glycemic load. *Am. J. Clin. Nutr.* **2011**, *94*, 1519–1524. [CrossRef] [PubMed]

58. International Organization for Standardization. *Food Products—Determination of the Glycaemic Index (GI) and Recommendation for Food Classification (ISO 26642:2010)*; ISO: Geneva, Switzerland, 2010.

59. Castro-Quezada, I.; Ruano-Rodriguez, C.; Ribas-Barba, L.; Serra-Majem, L. Misreporting in nutritional surveys: Methodological implications. *Nutr. Hospitalaria* **2015**, *31*, 119–127.

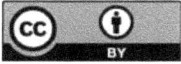

Article

PREVIEW: Prevention of Diabetes through Lifestyle Intervention and Population Studies in Europe and around the World. Design, Methods, and Baseline Participant Description of an Adult Cohort Enrolled into a Three-Year Randomised Clinical Trial

Mikael Fogelholm [1,*], Thomas Meinert Larsen [2], Margriet Westerterp-Plantenga [3], Ian Macdonald [4], J. Alfredo Martinez [5,6], Nadka Boyadjieva [7], Sally Poppitt [8], Wolfgang Schlicht [9], Gareth Stratton [10], Jouko Sundvall [11], Tony Lam [12], Elli Jalo [1], Pia Christensen [2], Mathijs Drummen [3], Elizabeth Simpson [4], Santiago Navas-Carretero [5,6], Teodora Handjieva-Darlenska [7], Roslyn Muirhead [13], Marta P. Silvestre [8], Daniela Kahlert [14], Laura Pastor-Sanz [2], Jennie Brand-Miller [13] and Anne Raben [2]

[1] Department of Food and Environmental Sciences, University of Helsinki, 00014 Helsinki, Finland; elli.jalo@helsinki.fi

[2] Department of Nutrition, Exercise and Sports, Faculty of Science, University of Copenhagen, Rolighedsvej 30, Frederiksberg C, DK-1958 Copenhagen, Denmark; tml@nexs.ku.dk (T.M.L.); piach@nexs.ku.dk (P.C.); laura.pastor@adm.ku.dk (L.P.-S.); ara@nexs.ku.dk (A.R.)

[3] Department of Human Biology, Maastricht University, P.O. Box 616, 6200 MD Maastricht, The Netherlands; m.westerterp@maastrichtuniversity.nl (M.W.-P.); m.drummen@maastrichtuniversity.nl (M.D.)

[4] School of Life Sciences, Faculty of Medicine and Health Sciences, University of Nottingham, Nottingham NG7 2UH, UK; Ian.Macdonald@nottingham.ac.uk (I.M.); liz.simpson@nottingham.ac.uk (E.S.)

[5] Center for Nutrition Research, University of Navarra, 31008 Pamplona, Spain; jalfmtz@unav.es (J.A.M.); snavas@unav.es (S.N.-C.)

[6] CIBERobn, Instituto de Salud Carlos III, 28029 Madrid, Spain

[7] Department of pharmacology and toxicology, Medical University of Sofia, 1431 Sofia, Bulgaria; nadkaboyadjieva@gmail.com (N.B.); teodorah@abv.bg (T.H.-D.)

[8] Human Nutrition Unit, School of Biological Sciences, University of Auckland, Auckland 1024, New Zealand; s.poppitt@auckland.ac.nz (S.P.); m.silvestre@auckland.ac.nz (M.P.S.)

[9] Department of Exercise and Health Sciences, University of Stuttgart, 70569 Stuttgart, Germany; wolfgang.schlicht@inspo.uni-stuttgart.de

[10] School of Sport and Exercise Sciences, A.STEM Research Centre, Swansea University, Swansea SA1 8EN, UK; g.stratton@swansea.ac.uk

[11] National Institute for Health and Welfare THL, 00300 Helsinki, Finland; jouko.sundvall@thl.fi

[12] NetUnion sarl, Ave des Figuires 20, 1007 Lausanne, Switzerland; lam@netunion.com

[13] Charles Perkins Centre, University of Sydney, Sydney 2006, Australia; roslyn.muirhead@sydney.edu.au (R.M.); jennie.brandmiller@sydney.edu.au (J.B.-M.)

[14] Department of Health Science, University of Education Schwäbisch Gmünd, 73525 Gmünd, Germany; daniela.kahlert@ph-gmuend.de

*   Correspondence: mikael.fogelholm@helsinki.fi; Tel.: +358-503180302

Received: 14 May 2017; Accepted: 16 June 2017; Published: 20 June 2017

Abstract: Type-2 diabetes (T2D) is one of the fastest growing chronic diseases worldwide. The PREVIEW project has been initiated to find the most effective lifestyle (diet and physical activity) for the prevention of T2D, in overweight and obese participants with increased risk for T2D. The study is a three-year multi-centre, 2×2 factorial, randomised controlled trial. The impact of a high-protein, low-glycaemic index (GI) vs. moderate protein, moderate-GI diet in combination with moderate or high-intensity physical activity on the incidence of T2D and the related clinical end-points are investigated. The intervention started with a two-month weight reduction using a low-calorie diet, followed by a randomised 34-month weight maintenance phase comprising four treatment arms. Eight intervention centres are participating (Denmark, Finland, United Kingdom, The Netherlands, Spain, Bulgaria, Australia, and New Zealand). Data from blood specimens, urine, faeces, questionnaires, diaries, body composition assessments, and accelerometers are collected at months 0, 2, 6, 12, 18, 24, and 36. In total, 2326 adults were recruited. The mean age was 51.6 (SD 11.6) years, 67% were women. PREVIEW is, to date, the largest multinational trial to address the prevention of T2D in pre-diabetic adults through diet and exercise intervention. Participants will complete the final intervention in March, 2018.

Keywords: diet; protein; carbohydrate; glycaemic index; physical activity; obesity

---

1. Introduction

Type-2 diabetes (T2D) is a disease associated with serious comorbidities, including microvascular (retinopathy, nephropathy, neuropathy) and macrovascular (cardiovascular) events [1]. The estimated global prevalence is approximately 8% and a prediction suggests that this will increase by 55% up to the year 2035 [2,3]. An important risk factor for T2D is obesity (BMI > 30 kg/m^2) predicting a more than 10-fold increase in incidence compared to normal weight [4]. Weight gain during adulthood is also an independent risk factor for T2D [5], as are genetic inheritance, unhealthy dietary habits, and insufficient physical activity [6–8].

Long-term studies have shown benefits of a lifestyle intervention (diet and exercise), on T2D incidence in China [9], USA [10], and Finland [11]. Lifestyle change (diet, physical activity, weight loss) may reduce the incidence of T2D by 28–59% [12]. The American Diabetes Prevention Program (DPP) [13], the Finnish Diabetes Prevention Study (DPS) [14], and the Chinese Da Qing Diabetes Prevention Study [15] were all designed to produce weight loss by prescribing a higher carbohydrate (CHO) (>50 percent of energy (E%) from CHO), low-fat (<30 E%) diet approach, which reflected the understanding of a prudent diet 20 years ago. No attention was paid to glycaemic index (GI), per se, and, to date, no studies have investigated the role of GI for prevention of type-2 diabetes.

Other dietary prescriptions that produce significant and sustainable weight loss may also be effective in T2D prevention. Current international recommendations include lower ranges for CHO intake [16] and a recommendation to choose lower GI foods [17]. A combination of lower CHO (45 E%), higher protein, together with lower GI, might be the optimal diet for prevention of T2D [18], perhaps related to sustained weight loss as shown in medium term trials [19]. To date these hypotheses have not been tested in large trials of long duration [20].

The program for physical activity in the trials described above followed the international public health recommendations, that is, a total of approximately 150 min per week of moderate-intensity aerobic activities or 75 min of vigorous intensity activity [10,14]. A question, not examined in earlier studies, is whether the metabolic responses are different between higher- and lower-intensity exercise programs. Moderate-intensity exercise relies relatively more on fat oxidation, whereas vigorous-intensity exercise relies more on CHO oxidation and use of intramuscular substrates [21]. Houmard et al. found that total exercise time, not intensity or exercise energy expenditure, was associated with the greatest improvement of insulin sensitivity in obese participants [22]. However, the hypothesis that physical activity with different intensity levels may differentially affect T2D prevention has yet to be tested in any large-scale intervention.

Since obesity is a strong risk factor for T2D, any successful prevention program should be able to prevent weight regain in individuals after a significant weight loss. The high heterogeneity of dietary intervention design prevents firm conclusions being drawn regarding preferred macronutrient composition [23]. Notably a recent multi-centre trial 'DiOGenes' (Diet, Obesity, and Genes) identified a higher-protein, moderate-CHO, and low-GI diet as superior to other diets of varying macronutrient composition in preventing weight regain over six months [19] and in a smaller subset over 12 months [24], after two months of rapid weight loss.

Despite the evidence that a lifestyle program combining prudent diet, increased physical activity and weight loss reduces the risk for T2D in susceptible individuals [12], important details remain unanswered. These include the long-term effects and sustainability of diets higher in protein with a lower glycaemic load, combined with the effects of higher intensity exercise. The present paper describes PREVention of diabetes through lifestyle Intervention and population studies in Europe and around the World (PREVIEW), a large multi-centre international randomised controlled trial in adults designed to answer these questions.

2. Methods

2.1. Aims of the Study

The aim is to determine the effects and interactions of two diets and two physical activity programmes on the prevention of T2D in overweight, pre-diabetic adults, who have undergone a short period of significant weight loss. Our primary hypothesis is that a higher protein, lower CHO/low GI diet (based on the DiOGenes study [19]) will be superior in preventing T2D when compared with a moderate protein, higher CHO/moderate GI diet (based on the DPS and DPP studies [10,14]). We also hypothesise that high-intensity physical activity will be superior compared to moderate-intensity physical activity [25].

Each participant receives one of the two dietary programs, and one of the two physical activity programs, thus, we have four groups (high protein diet and high-intensity physical activity; moderate protein diet and high-intensity physical activity; high protein diet and moderate-intensity physical activity; moderate-protein diet and moderate-intensity physical activity). The majority of outcomes will be analysed by using these four arms. The primary endpoint and statistical power calculations are based on a two-arm design (diets compared against each other).

2.2. Primary and Secondary Endpoints

The primary endpoint is incidence of T2D in high vs. moderate protein diet measured over a 36-month intervention period, based on the WHO criteria [26] of either (i) oral glucose tolerance test (OGTT) with fasting plasma glucose (FPG) > 7.0 mmol/L and/or 2-h post prandial (75 g glucose load) plasma glucose $\geq$11.1 mmol/L; or (ii) T2D diagnosed by a medical doctor between the clinical investigation days (CID) of PREVIEW, by using random plasma glucose $\geq$11.1 mmol/L in the presence of symptoms of diabetes, OGTT, or glycated haemoglobin (HbA1c). Asymptomatic individuals with a single abnormal value will have to repeat the test within 2–4 weeks to confirm the T2D diagnosis. The secondary endpoints include changes in HbA1c, body weight, body mass index (BMI), waist, and thigh circumference, body composition, insulin sensitivity, including Matsuda Index [27], glucose tolerance assessed by the area under the curve during OGTT, blood pressure, serum lipids, C-reactive protein, liver enzymes, perceived quality of life and work ability, habitual well-being, sleep, chronic stress, and subjective appetite sensations.

Other endpoints assessed by sub-group studies include liver fat content using magnetic resonance imaging (MRI) and proton magnetic resonance spectroscopy (H-MRS); colorectal cancer risk assessed from faecal markers; gut microbiome community assessment from faecal collections; maximal oxygen uptake capacity (VO_2 max); urine metabolite profiles using metabolomic techniques and food reward outcomes.

2.3. Study Setting and Design

The PREVIEW intervention study for adult participants has eight study sites: University of Copenhagen (Denmark), University of Helsinki (Finland), University of Maastricht (The Netherlands), University of Nottingham (UK), University of Navarra (Spain), Medical University of Sofia (Bulgaria), University of Sydney (Australia), and University of Auckland (New Zealand).

The 36-month intervention consists of two phases (Figure 1): a two-month period of rapid weight reduction achieved using a commercial low-calorie diet (about 800 kcal/day), followed by a 34-month randomised lifestyle (diet and physical activity) intervention phase for weight loss maintenance.

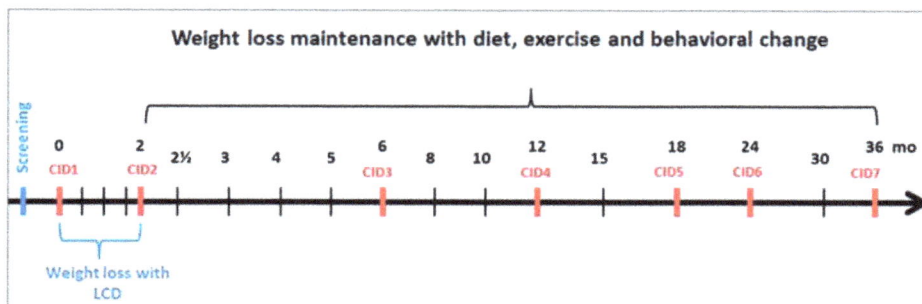

Figure 1. PREVIEW intervention: the general study design.

Clinical investigation days (CID) are conducted throughout the intervention, from CID1 (baseline) to CID7 (end of trial). At CID visits, anthropometry, blood tests, and questionnaires are performed and collection of completed diet records, accelerometers, and 24-h urine samples is done. Adverse (AE) and serious adverse events (SAE) and concomitant medications are recorded. In addition, a total of 17 group visits, leaded by instructors, are held throughout the trial to support lifestyle modification.

The CID assessments and group visits are conducted within University settings or associated Clinics. Participants follow the diet and physical activity counselling advice in a "real-life" setting without daily supervision from researchers.

2.4. Participants, Recruitment, and Randomisation

The inclusion criteria were: age 25–70 years (from mid-2013 to mid-2014 individuals aged 25–45 and 55–70 years were enrolled, and from mid-2014 onwards additionally age-group 45–54 years); BMI > 25 kg/m^2; pre-diabetes confirmed by an OGTT using the American Diabetes Association (ADA) criteria (13): (i) increased fasting glucose (IFG), with venous plasma glucose concentration of 5.6–6.9 mmol/L when fasted; and/or (ii) impaired glucose tolerance (IGT), with venous plasma glucose concentration of 7.8–11.0 mmol/L at 2 h after oral administration of standard 75 g glucose dose, and fasting plasma glucose <7.0 mmol/L. The main exclusion criteria were T2D, and any illness and/or medication with known or potential effect on compliance (e.g., unable to follow the physical activity program) or the main outcomes. A complete list of inclusion and exclusion criteria is presented as Supplementary Table S1.

Participants were recruited using multiple methods across the eight study sites, e.g., newspaper advertisements, newsletters, radio and television advertisements/interviews, and direct contact with primary and occupational health care providers. Interested individuals were contacted for the pre-screening. In the interview, inclusion and exclusion criteria were queried, including the Finnish Diabetes Risk Score [28] assessment. Potential participants were given written and oral information. Signed informed consent was required prior to commencement of laboratory screening.

The laboratory screening comprised measurements of weight, height, resting blood pressure, electrocardiography (in those aged 55 years or more), and an OGTT. A fasting blood sample was collected from the ante-cubital vein for later assessment of full inclusion and exclusion criteria, whilst glucose concentration was immediately analysed at each study site (HemoCue™, Angelholm, Sweden; Reflotron™, Roche diagnostics, Switzerland; or EML105 Radiometer, Copenhagen). Participants were then given a standard glucose drink (75 g glucose, dissolved in 300 mL water), which they had to take within 3–5 min, and a second venous blood sample was collected after 2 h. No other food or drinks or smoking were allowed and participants were required to remain sedentary during the test. The 0 and 2 h glucose concentration were used to identify those with pre-diabetes. Potentially eligible participants had fasting blood samples analysed to assess safety with haemoglobin, creatinine and alanine (ALT)/aspartate transaminase (AST).

Upon confirmation of eligibility, participants were enrolled into the trial and randomised to one of the four treatment groups. Randomisation was stratified by gender and age group (25–45, 46–54, and 55–70 years of age), and sequentially assigned from each stratum to different interventions, hence, securing an even distribution of gender and age group over the four intervention arms in each centre.

2.5. Description of Interventions

2.5.1. Low-Calorie Diet (LCD)

The trial started with a two-month (eight-week) weight reduction program using a commercial LCD, with a requirement to lose $\geq$ 8% initial body weight in order to continue to the weight maintenance phase. The LCD consisted of 3.4 MJ (800 kcal), 15–20 E% fat, 35–40 E% protein (84 g protein), and 45–50 E% CHO. The daily diet comprised of 4 × 40 g Cambridge Weight Plan® meal replacement sachets (Cambridge Weight Plan Ltd., Corby, UK), three of which were dissolved in 250 mL low fat milk ,or similar lactose-free alternatives, and one in 250 mL water. Energy-free drinks were permitted. Moreover, a maximum of 400 g of non-starchy, low-CHO vegetables, such as lettuce, asparagus, broccoli, celery, cucumber, mushrooms, radish, tomato, and watercress could be consumed.

During the LCD, participants attended group visits at weeks 2, 4, 6, and 8. Body weight, AE, SAE, and concomitant medications were recorded, LCD sachets dispensed, and dietary and behavioural instructions given. No specific instructions on physical activity were given during the LCD weight-reduction phase. Upon completion of the two months (CID2), participants who failed to reach the target weight reduction (i.e., $\geq$ 8% of initial body weight) were excluded from the intervention.

2.5.2. Weight Maintenance Phase: Intervention Diets

The two intervention diets are described in Table 1. The moderate protein (MP) diet is based on the DPS-dietary advice [14] aiming to reach a moderate protein (15 E%) and higher CHO (55 E%) macronutrient distribution with at least moderate dietary GI (>56), following current recommendations for prevention of T2D [17]. The (HP) diet has a higher protein (25 E%) and moderate CHO (45 E%) distribution with lower dietary GI (<50), based on the most successful weight-loss maintenance diet in the DiOGenes study [19]. Protein intake is higher and CHO intake is lower than the recommended range for prevention of T2D [16,17].

Both intervention diets are moderate in fat (30 E%) and the target macronutrient profile and food choices are supported by evidence for prevention of weight gain and/or T2D [8,23]. Notably, increased intake of sugar-rich foods or refined grains is not encouraged as a means to reach the higher CHO level, nor is increased consumption of red meat encouraged within the higher protein diet.

The diets are consumed ad libitum with respect to energy, with no provision of an individual target for daily energy intake. Self-monitoring of total energy consumption is not required. However, participants are instructed about controlling portion sizes of specific food types in order to achieve the macronutrient and GI prescriptions, and in self-monitoring and adjustment of portion sizes in general, in order to maintain their body weight loss. They are also encouraged to follow a regular meal pattern. Additional weight reduction is allowed, but without anything other than adherence to the maintenance diet and physical activity regimens.

The participants are given examples of daily eating plans with foods in appropriate proportions to reflect the macronutrient and GI requirements of the two interventions. A food-exchange list assists in self-selected variety, whilst preserving the required macronutrient and GI levels. Cooking books (one for each diet) with recipes suitable for all countries were specifically prepared for PREVIEW.

Table 1. Description of the PREVIEW dietary interventions.

	Higher Protein (25 E% [a]) Moderate Carbohydrate (45 E%) Low GI [b] (≤50) Diet	Moderate Protein (15 E%) Higher Carbohydrate (55 E%) Medium GI (≥56) Diet
Comparison between the groups	• Protein intake higher • Carbohydrate intake lower • GI lower	• Protein intake lower • Carbohydrate intake higher • GI medium
Food items with increased use (relative to the other group)	• Whole-grain cereals with low GI • Pasta • Low-fat dairy products • Poultry • Fish • Legumes	• Whole-grain cereals with moderate/high GI, e.g., bread • Potatoes, sweet potatoes, couscous, rice • Bananas
Similar use	• Most fruits and vegetables • Vegetable oils, margarine • Red meat (decreased in both) • Sugar-sweetened beverages (decreased in both)	

[a] E%, percentage of energy; [b] GI, glycaemic index.

2.5.3. Weight Maintenance Phase: Physical Activity Programmes

The trial has two physical activity interventions with a similar target for energy expenditure (>4.2 MJ/week, >1000 kcal/week), comprising high-intensity (HI) exercise or moderate-intensity (MI) exercise, as shown in Table 2. Measured heart rate using a heart rate monitor or wrist palpation, and/or perceived exertion using the Borg scale [29], are the principal methods of controlling the intensity. The participants may choose from several exercise options with similar level of metabolic turnover (energy expenditure divided by resting metabolic rate, i.e., MET values). The specific advice is based on the U.S. Centres for Disease Control and Prevention (CDC) recommendations of 75 min high-intensity (HI) or 150 min moderate-intensity (MI) physical activity weekly [30]. We developed a leaflet and other written instruction materials for the two PA groups. Physical activity is generally not supervised by the PREVIEW team, but participants are allowed to join supervised exercise groups of their own choice.

Table 2. Description of the physical activity interventions.

	High-Intensity Physical Activity (HI)	Moderate-Intensity Physical Activity (MI)
Heart rate	• 76–90% HRmax [a] or 61–80% HRR [b]	• 60–75% HRmax or 45–60% HRR
Examples of activities (these may vary depending on the fitness level of the participant)	• Bicycling, vigorous effort • Strenuous ball games • Aerobics with very vigorous effort, e.g., with extra weights • Jogging > 8 km/h • Swimming, vigorous effort • Cross-country skiing	• Bicycling, moderate effort • Leisurely ball games • Most conditioning exercises (aerobic, power yoga, etc.) • Brisk walking (4–6 km/h) • Swimming, recreational • Downhill skiing
Weekly duration (in total)	• at least 75 min	• at least 150 min
Recommended weekly frequency	• 2–3 times	• 3–5 times
Daily duration (guideline)	• 25–40 min	• 30–50 min (may be broken down into shorter sessions)
Additional exercises	• Muscle conditioning exercises, by using own weight: twice weekly at home, 15–20 min per session. • Stretching: twice weekly, 15–20 min per session	

[a] HRmax = max heart rate, defined as 220—age (220 in children under 16 years of age); [b] HRR = heart rate reserve, defined as the difference between measured resting HR and estimated HRmax.

A critical issue in PREVIEW is that many participants may be morbidly obese (BMI > 40) and, therefore, their ability to cope with a high-intensity exercise program is likely to be limited, and even risky. We addressed this point during the recruitments by specifically asking about perceived competence in coping with our program, and by ECG in all volunteers aged >55 years. Moreover, significant weight reduction ($\geq$ 8% of baseline body weight) during the first two months' LCD period will also simultaneously decrease the cardiovascular risks. The flexibility of our exercise program (only target energy expenditure is specified, the modes of exercise are due to the participant) is also likely to improve safety and adherence.

2.5.4. Group Visits and the Behavioural Modification Program

Group visits (8–12 individuals), are conducted throughout the three year intervention to deliver the behaviour modification information in relation to diet and physical activity [31]. There are 17 group visits, each 1–2 h, with decreasing frequency as the trial progresses. The behaviour modification programme is developed based on theories and evidence from health psychology and behaviour change [32–34]. For example, participants' beliefs about the consequences of behaviour (i.e., outcome expectancies), their intention to change their behaviour in the long run, and their belief in their ability to achieve the behaviour change goals (self-efficacy) are relevant predictors of successful behaviour change. Counsellors may apply respective behaviour change techniques [35] that are scheduled to common stages of behaviour change [36].

At the beginning of the weight-maintenance phase (i.e., month 2), the participants are instructed on how to plan, to start, and to follow the physical activity programme. In the group sessions, the participants are also instructed on basic principles of increasing physical activity and in motivational and self-regulative behaviour techniques to overcome barriers to exercise and behaviour modification. Stretching and home-based muscle-conditioning exercises are also supervised in a group-based session accompanied with written educational material [31].

2.6. Collection of Data and Description of Analyses

Data are collected from biological specimens (blood, urine, faecal), self-administered records and questionnaires, and an activity-monitoring device (ActiGraph GT3X accelerometer; ActiGraph, Pensacola, FL, USA) (see Table 3 with a description of timing). The CIDs are scheduled for a specific week and the aim is to make the measurements as precisely as scheduled. To accommodate as complete a data collection as possible we allow the following visit windows: month 2: -3 to +5 days; month 6: ±1 weeks; month 12: ±2 weeks; the remaining measurement points: ±4 weeks.

Blood samples are initially stored locally at -80 °C, then transported and analysed centrally at the National Institution for Health and Welfare (THL) in Helsinki, Finland. Diet records are analysed at each site using local food composition data and software. If available, local GI data for individual food items are used, and when not available, generic global GI data are used. Accelerometer data are downloaded at local sites, and collated and analysed centrally at the Swansea University, Wales, UK.

All questionnaires used in PREVIEW were prepared in English, then translated into the local language in Finland, Denmark, The Netherlands, Spain, and Bulgaria using authorized translators. A second authorized translator then back-translated the local versions to English, with this iterative process repeated until a final version of sufficient quality was obtained.

Table 3. Overview of main data collection methods at different clinical investigation days (CID) in PREVIEW.

Outcome	Data Collection Method	Assessment Time-Points (Month)						
		0	2	6	12	18	24	36
		CID1	CID2	CID3	CID4	CID5	CID6	CID7
Glucose tolerance/diagnosis of T2D	75 g oral glucose tolerance test	×		×	×		×	×
Blood chemistry (lipid metabolism, glucose metabolism, inflammation markers, etc.)	Fasting venous blood specimen	×	×	×	×	×	×	×
Urinary nitrogen	24-h urine collection	×		×	×		×	×
Risk markers for colon cancer (e.g., Short Chain Fatty Acids)	3-day faecal collection [a]	×			×			
Gut microbiota	Faecal spot sample [a]	×			×			
Weight, height, BMI and anthropometrics	Weight; height (week 0 and 156); waist and hip circumference	×	×	×	×	×	×	×
Body composition	Body composition by DXA, BodPod or Bioelectrical impedance (BIA)	×	×	×	×		×	×
Blood pressure and resting heart rate	Resting blood pressure and heart rate	×	×	×	×	×	×	×
Nutrient intakes, dietary GI and food consumption	4-day food record	×		×	×		×	×
Physical activity	7-day accelerometer, 7-day physical activity log, Baecke questionnaire	×		×	×		×	×
Maximal oxygen uptake	VO_2 max test by ergometer or treadmill [b]	×		×			×	
Psycho-social mediators and moderators health behaviour	Several questionnaires (listed with references in Supplementary Table S2)	×	×	×	×		×	×
Eating behaviour	Three Factor Eating Questionnaire (TFEQ)	×	×	×	×		×	×
Sleeping	Epworth Sleepiness Scale (ESS), Pittsburgh Sleep Quality Index (PSQI)	×	×	×	×		×	×
Stress and mood	Perceived Stress Scale (PSS), Profile of Mood Scale (POMS)	×	×	×	×		×	×
Quality of life	WHO Quality of Life questionnaire	×			×		×	×
Work ability	Work Ability Index questionnaire	×			×		×	×
Cost-effectiveness	Questionnaire designed by the PREVIEW research group	×			×		×	×

[a] In a subgroup (*n* = 250) in Helsinki and Auckland; [b] In a subgroup (*n* = 120) in Copenhagen, Maastricht, Navarra and Nottingham.

2.7. Data Management

All data are stored in a central project database at the University of Copenhagen. The central database ensures standardized handling and storing of data and the possibility for easy extraction and delivery of data both within and after the official project period (2013–2018).

Currently, the database receives input from four data sources on a regular basis: (1) All immediate data measured (e.g., anthropometrics, blood glucose) and interviewed (e.g., use of medication) during the CIDs and entered into OpenClinica server (electronic case report form); (2) data on social-cognitive determinants of behaviour, on cultural and socio-demographics, as well as socio-economic components, are collected by the questionnaire delivery platform (QDP), designed for PREVIEW by NetUnion. The participants enter their own data into the QDP. A paper version of the questionnaires is also available; (3) physical activity is reported using the Baecke inventory, and an electronic physical activity log (PAL), designed by Swansea University, University of Stuttgart, and implemented by NetUnion; (4) the Central Lab at the National Institute for Health and Welfare (THL) enters all laboratory analyses into the data hub. Data from analyses of the ActiGraph data accelerometers, from food diaries, and from the maximal oxygen uptake (VO_2 max) analyses are imported from all sites.

2.8. Governance and Quality Management

The intervention trial is led by Prof. Fogelholm at the University of Helsinki, in collaboration with the project coordinator, Prof. Raben at the University of Copenhagen. In this large, international multi-centre trial, we are collaborating intensively to ensure data collection of high-quality and consistency of the intervention across all sites.

Specific working groups were formed with relevant site representatives. The purpose of these working groups is to discuss and agree on questions related to dietary topics, physical activity, data management, and other methodological and medical issues.

During the recruitment phase, principal investigators from each centre participated in a monthly teleconference, which continues at regular intervals throughout the intervention.

The core personnel for each site meet annually at a three-day general assembly for the full PREVIEW consortium. PREVIEW has a website [37] with both public access and a restricted area for the PREVIEW researchers.

An electronic trial master file with relevant documents has been designed and is maintained by the University of Copenhagen within the private part of the PREVIEW website. All written study material is uploaded and made available at the PREVIEW website private area, including the protocol and amendments, standard operating procedures (SOPs), and instruction materials for the intervention subjects, in order ensure that comparable methods are followed across individual sites. The SOPs are reviewed and revised as needed and also new SOPs are prepared, if necessary.

Representatives from each intervention site participated in two training sessions, each of 2–3 days duration, in 2013. One session focussed on the main study protocol, the CID protocols, and all outcome measurements (University of Copenhagen). The other session focused on instructor training in group counselling (behaviour change) methods (University of Stuttgart). Attendees then trained their local staff.

2.9. Statistical Power and Basic Analyses

The anticipated three-year incidence of T2D in the PREVIEW trial is 21%, based on data from the Finnish DPS and US DPP [10,11]. The power calculation was derived for comparison of the two dietary interventions (HP vs. MP).

It was hypothesized that a risk reduction of one quarter (1/4) in the MP group would reduce the incidence of T2D incidence from 21% to 16%, and that a risk reduction of one half (1/2) in the HP group would reduce the incidence of T2D from 21% to 10.5%. Consequently, the sample size required to detect this difference in T2D incidence (16% vs. 10.5%) was at least 649 per diet group or 1298 participants in total (for a two-sided comparison with a power (1-ß) of 80% and $p < 0.05$), with a 10% drop-out during the first 10 months from month 2 (CID2) onwards, and another 20% drop-out between months 12 (CID4) and 36 (CID7). Thus, the number of participants needed for the intervention was 1802. To allow an estimated drop-out of 25% as a result of failure to lose >8% of initial body weight during the two-month LCD period, the number of participants required to be enrolled into PREVIEW was initially estimated to be 2403.

The primary data are analysed statistically using the principle of 'intention-to-treat' (ITT cohort) and also as a completers' cohort. A 'completer' is defined as a participant who has remained in the trial for the full three year intervention period, or who has been diagnosed with T2D before the end of the intervention.

The primary outcome in the adults' trial is incidence of T2D. For statistical analysis assessing the effect of the two diets on the T2D is a 'semi-parametric Cox proportional hazards regression model'. Missing data are addressed using hot-deck imputation. Missing covariate information is addressed using multiple imputation. Sensitivity analyses (e.g., complete-case analyses without drop-outs) will be carried out to assess if censoring was informative or non-informative.

For statistical analysis of the continuous secondary outcomes (e.g., blood chemistry, anthropometrics, etc.) a 'linear mixed model' is used. For the categorical outcomes (e.g., sex, educational attainment, proportion of subjects maintaining a defined weight loss, etc.), the type of statistical analysis is 'logistic' or 'ordinal mixed-effects model'. The parameter of interest is the difference in odds ratio between the intervention groups. Although the main statistical analyses will be done by using the entire cohort, one of the most important stratified analyses will use an age-group (e.g., above and below 65 years) stratification. By comparing older against younger participants we might obtain new insight on whether dietary protein content in this respect has different effects on, e.g., body composition, weight, and clinical variables.

2.10. Ethical Issues

The study protocol and amendments were reviewed and approved by local Human Ethics Committees at all study sites. The work of PREVIEW is carried out in full compliance with the relevant requirements of the latest version of the Declaration of Helsinki (59th WMA General Assembly, Seoul, Korea, October 2008), and the ICH-GCP, The International Conference on Harmonisation (ICH) for Good Clinical Practice to the extent that this is possible and relevant. All participants provided written informed consent prior to commencing screening procedures in clinic. All information obtained during the trial is handled according to local regulations and the European Directive 95/46/CE (directive on protection of individuals with regard to the processing of personal data and on the free movement of such data). The trial is registered with ClinicalTrials.gov, NCT01777893.

3. Results

As PREVIEW is an on-going trial, only results obtained from participant screening and baseline phases are presented here. Screening was conducted from June 2013 to February 2015. On average, 35% of the pre-screened individuals were eligible for the laboratory screening. Further, 43% of the screened participants were found to be eligible for the trial. In total, 2326 overweight, pre-diabetic adults were enrolled and randomised into the trial. This was 97% of the original pre-specified target (Figure 2). Approximately half of the participants were 55–70 years at baseline (Table 4).

Baseline characteristics from blood biochemistry and anthropometric assessments are shown assigned to each intervention group in Table 5. The basic characteristics of the groups are similar. A notable feature of the participants is that the mean baseline fasting glucose concentration was approximately at the mid of the eligibility range, whereas the mean 2-h glucose concentration was at the lower cut-off point. According to the OGTT laboratory data, 1389 (62%) of all participants had increased fasting glucose at baseline, 506 (23%) had impaired glucose tolerance and 286 (13%) had both of these pre-diabetic indicators. At baseline (CID1), 25 participants (1%)—who all had been diagnosed with pre-diabetes at screening—were not diagnosed with pre-diabetes anymore. The prevalence of pre-diabetes described above were not significantly different between the four study groups.

Table 4. Number and age distribution of participants recruited for the PREVIEW intervention trial.

Site	Pre-Screened	Screened	Randomised (n)	Men (n)	Women (n)	Age 25–45 Years (n)	Age 46–54 Years (n)	Age 55–70 Years (n)	Mean Age Years (SD)
UCPH	2061	908	379	159	220	86	62	233	54.2 (10.9)
HEL	1269	633	289	88	201	39	33	221	58.2 (8.9)
UM	675	553	203	94	109	42	17	145	56.6 (10.0)
UNOTT	3914	979	264	102	162	95	42	133	51.6 (12.0)
UNAV	1740	732	307	93	214	145	82	93	47.5 (10.6)
MU	1190	488	368	87	281	190	7	158	47.8 (12.0)
UNSYD	3108	595	195	56	139	59	36	102	53.0 (10.8)
UOA	1654	584	321	77	244	156	47	103	47.0 (11.4)
Total	15,611	5472	2326	756	1570	812	326	1188	51.6 (11.6)

Abbreviations for study sites: UCPH = University of Copenhagen (Denmark); HEL = University of Helsinki (Finland); UM = Maastricht University (The Netherlands); UNOTT = University of Nottingham (UK); UNAV = University of Navarra (Spain); MU = Medical University of Sofia (Bulgaria); UNSYD = University of Sydney (Australia); UOA = University of Auckland (New Zealand).

Table 5. Number of participants, age, anthropometric results, blood chemistry, and blood pressure for all intervention groups, assessed at baseline (CID1) before weight reduction. The results are shown as the mean (±SD).

	HP: Higher Protein (25 E%) Moderate Carbohydrate (45 E%) Low GI (≤50) Diet		MP: Moderate Protein (15 E%) Higher Carbohydrate (55 E%) Medium GI (≥56) Diet	
	Moderate-Intensity Physical Activity	High-Intensity Physical Activity	Moderate-Intensity Physical Activity	High-Intensity Physical Activity
No. (men/women)	556 (184/372)	556 (177/379)	559 (180/379)	553 (179/374)
Age, years	51.6 ± 11.5	51.8 ± 11.7	51.4 ± 11.2	51.4 ± 11.8
Anthropometrics				
Height, cm	168 ± 9	168 ± 9	168 ± 9	168 ± 10
Weight, kg	99.3 ± 20.8	100.6 ± 21.0	101.6 ± 22.6	98.7 ± 20.9
Body Mass Index, kg/m^2	35.1 ± 6.5	35.6 ± 6.7	35.7 ± 6.6	35.0 ± 6.4
Waist circumference, cm	109.6 ± 15.2	111.0 ± 15.3	111.1 ± 15.4	109.6 ± 14.5
Hip circumference, cm	117.6 ± 14.5	118.8 ± 14.8	119.2 ± 13.9	117.8 ± 13.8
Body fat (% of weight)	43.0 ± 7.5	43.5 ± 7.5	43.5 ± 7.9	43.1 ± 7.8
Blood chemistry and blood pressure				
fP-glucose, mmol/L	6.2 ± 0.8	6.2 ± 0.6	6.2 ± 0.7	6.2 ± 0.8
2hP-glucose, mmol/L	7.8 ± 2.3	7.7 ± 2.25	7.5 ± 2.2	7.7 ± 2.1
fP-insulin, mU/L	13.6 ± 7.9	14.0 ± 8.7	13.2 ± 7.7	13.1 ± 7.2
HbA1c, mmol/mol	36.6 ± 3.9	36.8 ± 3.9	36.7 ± 4.2	36.7 ± 4.0
Cholesterol, mmol/L	5.2 ± 1.0	5.1 ± 1.0	5.3 ± 1.0	5.1 ± 1.0
LDL cholesterol, mmol/L	3.3 ± 0.9	3.2 ± 0.8	3.3 ± 0.9	3.2 ± 0.8
HDL cholesterol, mmol/L	1.3 ± 0.3	1.3 ± 0.3	1.3 ± 0.3	1.3 ± 0.3
Triglycerides, mmol/L	1.5 ± 0.8	1.5 ± 0.7	1.5 ± 0.9	1.5 ± 0.8
CRP, mg/L	5.3 ± 6.3	6.0 ± 8.7	5.2 ± 5.1	5.1 ± 7.5
Systolic BP, mmHg	128.5 ± 15.6	129.7 ± 16.2	128.7 ± 16.3	129.3 ± 15.5
Diastolic BP, mmHg	78.2 ± 10.9	77.6 ± 11.2	78.4 ± 11.5	78.3 ± 10.7

GI = glycaemic index; BP = blood pressure.

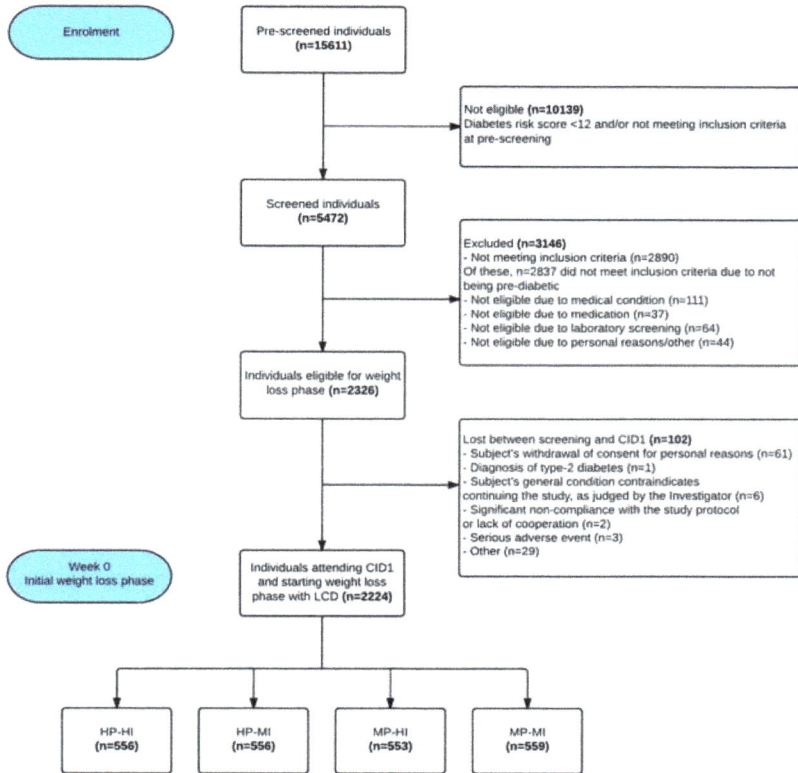

Figure 2. PREVIEW intervention: the subjects' flowchart.

4. Discussion

To our knowledge, PREVIEW is the first trial of its kind comparing two potentially effective interventions, a novel higher protein/low GI diet vs. current best practice moderate protein, higher CHO/moderate GI diet, in order to determine whether there is a more efficient lifestyle strategy to prevent T2D. Moreover, previous studies have neither used an effective weight-loss phase by LCD as a start of the intervention, nor a multi-country design.

Our inclusion criteria for "pre-diabetes" differed from the Finnish DPS. Here, IGT was an unconditional requirement without limits for IFG [14]. In the US DPP, both IGT and IFG were required [38] and the lower limit for IFG was 5.3 mmol/L (vs. 5.6 mmol/L in PREVIEW). It is unclear if the differences in diagnostic criteria between these studies have any major effects on the outcome. In addition to the diagnostic cut-offs, per se, and the distribution of results within the diagnostic criteria (i.e., above the lower and below the upper cut-off points) may have an effect on the outcome [39]. In PREVIEW, a majority of the subjects were eligible due to higher fasting blood glucose, rather than impaired glucose tolerance (higher 2-h value). A small proportion (1%) were no longer diagnosed with pre-diabetes at baseline. This may be explained by change of method (HemoCue™ or Reflotron™ at screening, or the laboratory assessment at baseline), to normal day-to-day variance in the assessed variables, or to a change in lifestyle after being accepted as a participant to PREVIEW. For future studies of T2D prevention, a single measurement of HbA1c, which is becoming the standard clinical practice in many countries may save both time and costs [40]. Still, there remains some controversy as to the utility of HbA1c when compared with standard OGTT as a diagnostic tool [41].

PREVIEW is a much larger trial than both the Finnish DPS (n = 522) [11] and Chinese Da Qing study (n = 577) [9], although smaller than the DPP (n = 3234) [10]. However, in the DPP a third of the participants received 'Metformin' in addition to dietary advice; hence, the number of participants without medical treatment, but adhering to lifestyle intervention (diet and physical activity) was 2161, which is similar to PREVIEW. Of the above interventions, the geographical and ethnic variation is greatest in PREVIEW. The age-range of participants in DPP and DPS was 33–67 years, slightly narrower than in PREVIEW, but the mean age of participants is similar across the studies (50–55 years). The large proportion of older participants in PREVIEW, (>55 years), was expected since the risk for T2D increases with age [2], and due to the growing health consciousness of this age group, many of whom are retired and have the time to participate in a demanding intervention. The smaller proportion of middle age-adults is also explained by later initiation of recruitment in this age group, compared with younger and older participants. In general, finding an adequate number of pre-diabetic subjects was a real challenge in most countries, given the "hidden" status of this condition. Thus, recruitment took about three times as long as planned from the beginning of the project.

One major challenge in PREVIEW is related to adherence to the diet and physical activity programs. The HP-diet is novel and, with the higher protein content, also somewhat outside the current boundaries of nutritional guidelines [42,43]. Whether the HP diet results in better adherence than the MP diet with high CHO and whole-grain cereal intakes is one of the key interests in PREVIEW. Nutrient intakes and food consumption patterns will be assessed in PREVIEW by repeated 4-d diet-records. The poor accuracy of dietary assessment is well known [44], but it is expected that the difference in dietary protein and CHO intakes should be sufficiently large to be detected using this method. Moreover, protein intake is verified using 24 h urinary nitrogen excretion [45].

It may be more difficult to create a verifiable difference for GI than for protein-to-CHO ratio. Whilst GI values of foods have been shown to provide a good summary of postprandial glycaemia [46], difficulties in attributing GI values to foods for which there are no validated data available may add to the variability [47], particularly in a multi-centre intervention such as PREVIEW. In DiOGenes, the reported observed difference in mean dietary GI was small (56 vs. 60 units) [19] which increases the requirements of precision.

The physical activity intervention in PREVIEW is not a supervised training programme. Participants are expected to integrate activity into their daily lives and use local opportunities to achieve their goals. To improve adherence, there is flexibility with the type of activities chosen. A combination of measures of physical activity is used to analyse the compliance to the type of intervention and our methods allow a description of activities that were used to achieve this.

It is probable that the HI-program will be more challenging in the long-term. Warming-up, cooling-down, muscular conditioning exercises, and stretching are carefully explained to the participants in order to decrease the risk for injuries. It should be noted that the HI-program in PREVIEW is not high-intensity interval-training (HIIT). While there are some data on potential benefits from HIIT on cardiovascular function and glucose metabolism [48], we considered the data on feasibility and long-term maintenance of this kind of training still too limited.

In addition to good compliance of the programmes, keeping the drop-out rate as low as possible will be challenging. Frequent contact with the research staff is one way to reduce the drop-out rate. However, PREVIEW has been planned to study how behavioural change is realized under 'real-life' conditions and, hence, the fading visit design where group visits are infrequent during years two and three of the intervention. Adherence is encouraged through a number of practices, including use of specific behavioural change techniques [31], such as implementation intentions, or Facebook groups, one for each randomised group, to promote attendance at group visits and CIDs. In addition, the sites can also conduct general information lectures, physical activity sessions, and/or send a newsletter to the participants, once or twice a year.

Compared to DPS and DPP studies, a particular feature of PREVIEW is related to the different settings in which the intervention is conducted, including not only genetic background, but also attitudes, norms, and socio-economic features. Although the participating countries are well-developed, considerable variations exist, e.g., regarding food attitudes and habits, as well as traditions of practicing physical activity.

The unique feature in the PREVIEW intervention is the direct comparison of two potentially efficacious diet and physical activity intervention programs. Hence, PREVIEW has a clear potential to identify a recommended optimal diet and physical activity programme to prevent T2D, a programme which is also suitable across different countries. It is also possible, however, that PREVIEW data will demonstrate that there are several, equally efficacious alternatives. Clearly, both answers are important from a public health viewpoint.

Supplementary Materials: The following are available online at www.mdpi.com/2072-6643/9/6/632/s1, Table S1: Inclusion and exclusion criteria in the PREVIEW screening, Table S2: Questionnaires on moderators, mediators, behaviour, and social environment.

Acknowledgments: This study has received grants from the EU 7th Framework Programme (FP7-KBBE-2012), grant agreement No. 312057; the New Zealand Health Research Council, grant No. 14/191; and the NHMRC-EU Collaborative Grant, Australia. All LCD products were provided by Cambridge Weight Plan®, UK. This sponsorship is highly appreciated. We want to acknowledge, particularly, the following medical and scientific experts, who have helped us in building up the study: Arne Astrup (Copenhagen, Denmark), Stephen Collagiuri (Sydney, Australia), Peter Mansell (Nottingham, UK), and the PREVIEW Scientific Advisory Board, Louise Dye (Leeds, UK), Richard L. Atkinson (Richmond, VA, USA), Boyd Swinburn (Auckland, New Zealand), Lauren Lissner, (Gothenburg, Sweden), and Grethe Andersen (Copenhagen, Denmark). Moreover, we want to acknowledge the great staff who have worked and are currently working for PREVIEW, e.g., study nurses, lab technicians, nutritionists, physical activity experts, trainees, and post- and under-graduate students, involved in the recruitment of all participants and in planning and initiating the weight-reduction phase and intervention.

Author Contributions: A.R., J.B.-M. and M.F.M. were responsible for the initial study conception. T.M.L., M.W.-P., I.M., J.A.M.H., S.P., W.S., G.S., J.S., T.L., T.H.-D., D.K., J.B.-M. and A.R. were involved in development of the study design. All authors, but particularly E.J., P.C., M.D., E.S., S.N.-C., N.B., R.M., M.P.S. and L.P.-S. were involved in the development of the practical implementation of the study. M.F.M. wrote the draft version of the manuscript and all authors were involved in critically revising the paper. All authors have also seen and accepted the submitted version.

Conflicts of Interest: The authors declare no conflict of interest. The funding sponsors had no role in the design of the study; in the collection, analyses, or interpretation of data; in the writing of the manuscript, and in the decision to publish the results.

References

1. American Diabetes Association. Standards of medical care in diabetes—2011. *Diabetes Care* **2011**, *34* (Suppl. 1), S11–S61.

2. Guariguata, L.; Whiting, D.R.; Hambleton, I.; Beagley, J.; Linnenkamp, U.; Shaw, J.E. Global estimates of diabetes prevalence for 2013 and projections for 2035. *Diabetes Res. Clin. Pract.* **2014**, *103*, 137–149. [CrossRef] [PubMed]

3. Tamayo, T.; Rosenbauer, J.; Wild, S.H.; Spijkerman, A.M.W.; Baan, C.; Forouhi, N.G.; Herder, C.; Rathmann, W. Diabetes in Europe: An update. *Diabetes Res. Clin. Pract.* **2014**, *103*, 206–217. [CrossRef] [PubMed]

4. Guh, D.P.; Zhang, W.; Bansback, N.; Amarsi, Z.; Birmingham, C.L.; Anis, A.H. The incidence of co-morbidities related to obesity and overweight: A systematic review and meta-analysis. *BMC Public Health* **2009**, *9*, 88. [CrossRef] [PubMed]

5. Morimoto, Y.; Schembre, S.M.; Steinbrecher, A.; Erber, E.; Pagano, I.; Grandinetti, A.; Kolonel, L.N.; Maskarinec, G. Ethnic differences in weight gain and diabetes risk: The Multiethnic Cohort Study. *Diabetes Metab.* **2011**, *37*, 230–236. [CrossRef] [PubMed]

6. Aune, D.; Norat, T.; Leitzmann, M.; Tonstad, S.; Vatten, L.J. Physical activity and the risk of type 2 diabetes: A systematic review and dose-response meta-analysis. *Eur. J. Epidemiol.* **2015**, *30*, 529–542. [CrossRef] [PubMed]

7. Bhupathiraju, S.N.; Tobias, D.K.; Malik, V.S.; Pan, A.; Hruby, A.; Manson, J.E.; Willett, W.C.; Hu, F.B. Glycemic index, glycemic load, and risk of type 2 diabetes: Results from 3 large US cohorts and an updated meta-analysis. *Am. J. Clin. Nutr.* **2014**, *100*, 218–232. [CrossRef] [PubMed]

8. Ley, S.H.; Hamdy, O.; Mohan, V.; Hu, F.B. Prevention and management of type 2 diabetes: Dietary components and nutritional strategies. *Lancet* **2014**, *383*, 1999–2007. [CrossRef]

9. Li, G.; Zhang, P.; Wang, J.; An, Y.; Gong, Q.; Gregg, E.W.; Yang, W.; Zhang, B.; Shuai, Y.; Hong, J.; et al. Cardiovascular mortality, all-cause mortality, and diabetes incidence after lifestyle intervention for people with impaired glucose tolerance in the Da Qing Diabetes Prevention Study: A 23-year follow-up study. *Lancet Diabetes Endocrinol.* **2014**, *2*, 474–480. [CrossRef]

10. Knowler, W.C.; Barrett-Connor, E.; Fowler, S.E.; Hamman, R.F.; Lachin, J.M.; Walker, E.A.; et al. Reduction in the incidence of type 2 diabetes with lifestyle intervention or metformin. *N. Engl. J. Med.* **2002**, *346*, 393–403. [PubMed]

11. Tuomilehto, J.; Lindström, J.; Eriksson, J.G.; Valle, T.T.; Hämäläinen, H.; Ilanne-Parikka, P.; Keinänen-Kiukaanniemi, S.; Laakso, M.; Louheranta, A.; Rastas, M.; et al. Prevention of type 2 diabetes mellitus by changes in lifestyle among subjects with impaired glucose tolerance. *N. Engl. J. Med.* **2001**, *344*, 1343–1350. [CrossRef] [PubMed]

12. Walker, K.Z.; O'Dea, K.; Gomez, M.; Girgis, S.; Colagiuri, R. Diet and exercise in the prevention of diabetes. *J. Hum. Nutr. Diet.* **2010**, *23*, 344–352. [CrossRef] [PubMed]

13. Mayer-Davis, E.J.; Sparks, K.C.; Hirst, K.; Costacou, T.; Lovejoy, J.C.; Regensteiner, J.G.; Hoskin, M.A.; Kriska, A.M.; Bray, G.A.; Diabetes Prevention Program Research Group. Dietary intake in the diabetes prevention program cohort: Baseline and 1-year post randomization. *Ann. Epidemiol.* **2004**, *14*, 763–772. [CrossRef] [PubMed]

14. Eriksson, J.; Lindström, J.; Valle, T.; Aunola, S.; Hämäläinen, H.; Ilanne-Parikka, P.; Keinänen-Kiukaanniemi, S.; Laakso, M.; Lauhkonen, M.; Lehto, P.; et al. Prevention of Type II diabetes in subjects with impaired glucose tolerance: The Diabetes Prevention Study (DPS) in Finland. Study design and 1-year interim report on the feasibility of the lifestyle intervention programme. *Diabetologia* **1999**, *42*, 793–801. [CrossRef] [PubMed]

15. Pan, X.R.; Li, G.W.; Hu, Y.H.; Wang, J.X.; Yang, W.Y.; An, Z.X.; Hu, Z.X.; Lin, J.; Xiao, J.Z.; Cao, H.B.; et al. Effects of diet and exercise in preventing NIDDM in people with impaired glucose tolerance. The Da Qing IGT and Diabetes Study. *Diabetes Care* **1997**, *20*, 537–544. [CrossRef] [PubMed]

16. Mann, J.I.; De Leeuw, I.; Hermansen, K.; Karamanos, B.; Karlström, B.; Katsilambros, N.; Riccardi, G.; Rivellese, A.A.; Rizkalla, S.; Slama, G.; et al. Evidence-based nutritional approaches to the treatment and prevention of diabetes mellitus. *Nutr. Metab. Cardiovasc. Dis.* **2004**, *14*, 373–394. [CrossRef]

17. Ajala, O.; English, P.; Pinkney, J. Systematic review and meta-analysis of different dietary approaches to the management of type 2 diabetes. *Am. J. Clin. Nutr.* **2013**, *97*, 505–516. [CrossRef] [PubMed]

18. Buyken, A.E.; Mitchell, P.; Ceriello, A.; Brand-Miller, J. Optimal dietary approaches for prevention of type 2 diabetes: A life-course perspective. *Diabetologia* **2010**, *53*, 406–418. [CrossRef] [PubMed]

19. Larsen, T.M.; Dalskov, S.-M.; van Baak, M.; Jebb, S.A.; Papadaki, A.; Pfeiffer, A.F.H.; Martinez, J.A.; Handjieva-Darlenska, T.; Kunešová, M.; Pihlsgård, M.; et al. Diets with high or low protein content and glycemic index for weight-loss maintenance. *N. Engl. J. Med.* **2010**, *363*, 2102–2113. [CrossRef] [PubMed]

20. Astrup, A.; Raben, A.; Geiker, N. The role of higher protein diets in weight control and obesity-related comorbidities. *Int. J. Obes.* **2015**, *39*, 721–726. [CrossRef] [PubMed]

21. Romijn, J.A.; Coyle, E.F.; Sidossis, L.S.; Gastaldelli, A.; Horowitz, J.F.; Endert, E.; Wolfe, R.R. Regulation of endogenous fat and carbohydrate metabolism in relation to exercise intensity and duration. *Am. J. Physiol.* **1993**, *265 Pt 1*, E380–E391. [PubMed]

22. Houmard, J.A.; Tanner, C.J.; Slentz, C.A.; Duscha, B.D.; McCartney, J.S.; Kraus, W.E. Effect of the volume and intensity of exercise training on insulin sensitivity. *J. Appl. Physiol.* **2004**, *96*, 101–106. [CrossRef] [PubMed]

23. Fogelholm, M.; Anderssen, S.; Gunnarsdottir, I.; Lahti-Koski, M. Dietary macronutrients and food consumption as determinants of long-term weight change in adult populations: A systematic literature review. *Food Nutr. Res.* **2012**, *56*. [CrossRef] [PubMed]

24. Aller, E.E.J.G.; Larsen, T.M.; Claus, H.; Lindroos, A.K.; Kafatos, A.; Pfeiffer, A.; Martinez, J.A.; Handjieva-Darlenska, T.; Kunesova, M.; Stender, S.; et al. Weight loss maintenance in overweight subjects on ad libitum diets with high or low protein content and glycemic index: The DIOGENES trial 12-month results. *Int. J. Obes.* **2014**, *38*, 1511–1517. [CrossRef] [PubMed]

25. Watt, M.J.; Heigenhauser, G.J.; Spriet, L.L. Effects of dynamic exercise intensity on the activation of hormone-sensitive lipase in human skeletal muscle. *J. Physiol.* **2003**, *547 Pt 1*, 301–308. [CrossRef] [PubMed]

26. WHO. Definition and Diagnosis of Diabetes Mellitus and Intermediate Hyperglycaemia. Available online: http://www.who.int/diabetes/publications/diagnosis_diabetes2006/en/ (accessed on 19 July 2017).

27. Matsuda, M.; DeFronzo, R.A. Insulin sensitivity indices obtained from oral glucose tolerance testing: Comparison with the euglycemic insulin clamp. *Diabetes Care* **1999**, *22*, 1462–1470. [CrossRef] [PubMed]

28. Silventoinen, K.; Pankow, J.; Lindström, J.; Jousilahti, P.; Hu, G.; Tuomilehto, J. The validity of the Finnish Diabetes Risk Score for the prediction of the incidence of coronary heart disease and stroke, and total mortality. *Eur. J. Cardiovasc. Prev. Rehabil.* **2005**, *12*, 451–458. [CrossRef] [PubMed]

29. Borg, G.A. Psychophysical bases of perceived exertion. *Med. Sci. Sports Exerc.* **1982**, *14*, 377–381. [CrossRef] [PubMed]

30. 2008 Physical Activity Guidelines for Americans. Available online: http://www.health.gov/paguidelines/guidelines/ (accessed on 19 July 2017).

31. Kahlert, D.; Unyi-Reicherz, A.; Stratton, G.; Meinert Larsen, T.; Fogelholm, M.; Raben, A.; Schlicht, W. PREVIEW Behavior Modification Intervention Toolbox (PREMIT): A Study Protocol for a Psychological Element of a Multicenter Project. *Front. Psychol.* **2016**, *7*, 1136. [CrossRef] [PubMed]

32. Michie, S.; Abraham, C.; Whittington, C.; McAteer, J.; Gupta, S. Effective techniques in healthy eating and physical activity interventions: A meta-regression. *Health Psychol.* **2009**, *28*, 690–701. [CrossRef] [PubMed]

33. Greaves, .C.J.; Sheppard, K.E.; Abraham, C.; Hardeman, W.; Roden, M.; Evans, P.H.; Schwarz, P.; IMAGE Study Group. Systematic review of reviews of intervention components associated with increased effectiveness in dietary and physical activity interventions. *BMC Public Health* **2011**, *11*, 119. [CrossRef] [PubMed]

34. Olander, E.K.; Fletcher, H.; Williams, S.; Atkinson, L.; Turner, A.; French, D.P. What are the most effective techniques in changing obese individuals' physical activity self-efficacy and behaviour: A systematic review and meta-analysis. *Int. J. Behav. Nutr. Phys. Act.* **2013**, *10*, 29. [CrossRef] [PubMed]

35. Michie, S.; Richardson, M.; Johnston, M.; Abraham, C.; Francis, J.; Hardeman, W.; Eccles, M.P.; Cane, J.; Wood, C.E. The behavior change technique taxonomy (v1) of 93 hierarchically clustered techniques: Building an international consensus for the reporting of behavior change interventions. *Ann. Behav. Med.* **2013**, *46*, 81–95. [CrossRef] [PubMed]

36. Prochaska, J.O.; DiClemente, C.C. Stages of change in the modification of problem behaviors. *Prog. Behav. Modif.* **1992**, *28*, 183–218. [PubMed]

37. PREVIEW. Available online: http://previewstudy.com (accessed on 19 July 2017).

38. The Diabetes Prevention Program: Baseline characteristics of the randomized cohort. The Diabetes Prevention Program Research Group. *Diabetes Care* **2000**, *23*, 1619–1629.

39. Edelstein, S.L.; Knowler, W.C.; Bain, R.P.; Andres, R.; Barrett-Connor, E.L.; Dowse, G.K.; Haffner, S.M.; Pettitt, D.J.; Sorkin, J.D.; Muller, D.C.; et al. Predictors of progression from impaired glucose tolerance to NIDDM: An analysis of six prospective studies. *Diabetes* **1997**, *46*, 701–710. [CrossRef] [PubMed]

40. Saudek, C.D.; Herman, W.H.; Sacks, D.B.; Bergenstal, R.M.; Edelman, D.; Davidson, M.B. A new look at screening and diagnosing diabetes mellitus. *J. Clin. Endocrinol. Metab.* **2008**, *93*, 2447–2453. [CrossRef] [PubMed]

41. Malkani, S.; Mordes, J.P. Implications of using hemoglobin A1C for diagnosing diabetes mellitus. *Am. J. Med.* **2011**, *124*, 395–401. [CrossRef] [PubMed]

42. Nordic Nutrition Recommendations Project Group. *Nordic Nutrition Recommendations 2012. Integrating Nutrition and Physical Activity*, 5th ed.; Nordic Council of Ministers: Copenhagen, Denmark, 2014.

43. Dietary Guidelines for Americans. Available online: http://www.cnpp.usda.gov/DietaryGuidelines (accessed on 19 July 2017).

44. Dhurandhar, N.V.; Schoeller, D.; Brown, A.W.; Heymsfield, S.B.; Thomas, D.; Sørensen, T.I.A.; Speakman, J.R.; Jeansonne, M.; Allison, D.B.; Energy Balance Measurement Working Group. Energy balance measurement: When something is not better than nothing. *Int. J. Obes.* **2015**, *39*, 1109–1113. [CrossRef] [PubMed]

45. Corella, D.; Ordovás, J.M. Biomarkers: Background, classification and guidelines for applications in nutritional epidemiology. *Nutr. Hosp.* **2015**, *31* (Suppl. 3), 177–188. [PubMed]

46. Brand-Miller, J.C.; Stockmann, K.; Atkinson, F.; Petocz, P.; Denyer, G. Glycemic index, postprandial glycemia, and the shape of the curve in healthy subjects: Analysis of a database of more than 1000 foods. *Am. J. Clin. Nutr.* **2009**, *89*, 97–105. [CrossRef] [PubMed]

47. Whelan, W.J.; Hollar, D.; Agatston, A.; Dodson, H.J.; Tahal, D.S. The glycemic response is a personal attribute. *IUBMB Life* **2010**, *62*, 637–641. [CrossRef] [PubMed]
48. Ramos, J.S.; Dalleck, L.C.; Tjonna, A.E.; Beetham, K.S.; Coombes, J.S. The impact of high-intensity interval training versus moderate-intensity continuous training on vascular function: A systematic review and meta-analysis. *Sports Med.* **2015**, *45*, 679–692. [CrossRef] [PubMed]

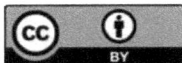

nutrients

MDPI

Article

Glucose and Lipid Dysmetabolism in a Rat Model of Prediabetes Induced by a High-Sucrose Diet

Ana Burgeiro [1,†], Manuela G. Cerqueira [1,†], Bárbara M. Varela-Rodríguez [1], Sara Nunes [1,2], Paula Neto [3], Frederico C. Pereira [1,2], Flávio Reis [1,2,*] and Eugénia Carvalho [1,4,5,6,*]

[1] Center of Neuroscience and Cell Biology (CNC) and CNC.IBILI Research Consortium, University of Coimbra, 3004-504 Coimbra, Portugal; burgeiroana@gmail.com (A.B.); manuela.g.cerqueira@gmail.com (M.G.C.); biobvr00@udc.es (B.M.V.-R.); sara_nunes20@hotmail.com (S.N.); fredcp@ci.uc.pt (F.C.P.)

[2] Laboratory of Pharmacology and Experimental Therapeutics, Institute for Biomedical Imaging and Life Sciences (IBILI), Faculty of Medicine, University of Coimbra, 3000-548 Coimbra, Portugal

[3] Service of Anatomical Pathology, Coimbra University Hospital Centre (CHUC), 3000-075 Coimbra, Portugal; anahepafr@gmail.com

[4] The Portuguese Diabetes Association (APDP), 1250-203 Lisbon, Portugal

[5] Department of Geriatrics, University of Arkansas for Medical Sciences, Little Rock, AR 72202, USA

[6] Arkansas Children's Hospital Research Institute, Little Rock, AR 72202, USA

[*] Correspondence: freis@fmed.uc.pt (F.R.); ecarvalh@cnc.uc.pt (E.C.); Tel.: +351-239-480-053 (F.R.); +351-239-820-190 (E.C.)

[†] These authors contributed equally to this work.

Received: 2 April 2017; Accepted: 14 June 2017; Published: 21 June 2017

Abstract: Glucotoxicity and lipotoxicity are key features of type 2 diabetes mellitus, but their molecular nature during the early stages of the disease remains to be elucidated. We aimed to characterize glucose and lipid metabolism in insulin-target organs (liver, skeletal muscle, and white adipose tissue) in a rat model treated with a high-sucrose (HSu) diet. Two groups of 16-week-old male Wistar rats underwent a 9-week protocol: HSu diet ($n = 10$)—received 35% of sucrose in drinking water; Control ($n = 12$)—received vehicle (water). Body weight, food, and beverage consumption were monitored and glucose, insulin, and lipid profiles were measured. Serum and liver triglyceride concentrations, as well as the expression of genes and proteins involved in lipid biosynthesis were assessed. The insulin-stimulated glucose uptake and isoproterenol-stimulated lipolysis were also measured in freshly isolated adipocytes. Even in the absence of obesity, this rat model already presented the main features of prediabetes, with fasting normoglycemia but reduced glucose tolerance, postprandial hyperglycemia, compensatory hyperinsulinemia, as well as decreased insulin sensitivity (resistance) and hypertriglyceridemia. In addition, impaired hepatic function, including altered gluconeogenic and lipogenic pathways, as well as increased expression of acetyl-coenzyme A carboxylase 1 and fatty acid synthase in the liver, were observed, suggesting that liver glucose and lipid dysmetabolism may play a major role at this stage of the disease.

Keywords: high-sucrose diet; prediabetes; glucose; lipid; metabolism; hypertriglyceridemia

1. Introduction

Type 2 diabetes mellitus (T2DM) has become an epidemic of noncommunicable diseases, with 415 million people worldwide currently living with diabetes [1]. According to the International Diabetes Federation, about 5 million people died from DM in 2015 and the estimates indicate that there will be about 642 million people living with DM by 2040. In addition, there are about 318 million adults with impaired glucose tolerance (IGT), which puts them at high risk for the disease.

Prediabetes (or intermediate hyperglycemia) already displays metabolic alterations and is a high risk state for developing T2DM. According to the American Diabetes Association, prediabetes is distinguished by having impaired fasting glucose (IFG) (100–125 mg/dL glucose), IGT (140–199 mg/dL glucose 2 h after a 75-g oral glucose tolerance test), and glycated hemoglobin (HbA1c) levels between 5.7–6.4%. The prevalence of prediabetes is rapidly increasing with over 470 million people projected with prediabetes by 2030 [2]. This likely anticipates increased morbidity, mortality, and healthcare costs in the near future with DM management. Thus, preventing the progression of IGT and/or IFG to T2DM is the most rational and effective way to combat the DM epidemic and lessen healthcare costs. However, before we can succeed, we need to unravel glucose and lipid metabolism at this stage of the disease.

Diets enriched in sugars including the intake of sugar-sweetened beverages have been consistently linked to the increased risk of hypertriglyceridemia, obesity, T2DM, and cardiovascular disease [3]. A central feature of T2DM is hyperglycemia, as a result of excessive hepatic glucose production, insulin resistance, and deficient secretion of pancreatic insulin. An often overlooked feature is the relationship between glucose and lipids, whose fluxes are indeed closely interlinked through the intersection of metabolic pathways at the acetyl-CoA formation [4]. Impairment of one pathway can indirectly have a major impact on another [4,5]. Molecular and metabolic abnormalities in insulin action, such as peripheral tissues (muscle, liver, and adipose tissues) insulin resistance, together with minor defects in insulin secretion, can be clearly identified before the development of obesity or hyperglycemia. These factors contribute to the increased fatty acid influx into the liver and muscle causing accumulation of toxic lipid metabolites. Particularly, chronically increased levels of plasma nonesterified fatty acids (NEFA) and triglyceride (TG)-rich lipoproteins impair lipid metabolism, a process referred to as lipotoxicity [6]. Furthermore, when the NEFA supply exceeds metabolic capacity, lipids accumulate in peripheral tissues, such as liver and muscle, inducing organ dysfunction [6]. Several recent lines of evidence show that the typical dyslipidemia in T2DM patients, characterized by elevated TGs, low high density lipoprotein cholesterol (HDL-c), and the predominance of small-dense low density lipoprotein (LDL) particles, may not only be the consequence of diabetes but may also cause disturbances of glucose metabolism. In fact, hypertriglyceridemia leads to elevated levels of free fatty acids (FFAs), which contribute to insulin resistance and β-cell dysfunction, putatively by impairing the molecular mechanisms linking insulin receptors with glucose transporters, as well as by directly damaging β-cells. Moreover, hypertriglyceridemia and elevated FFAs can contribute to inflammation, which boosts insulin resistance and β-cell dysfunction [4–7]. In addition, low HDL-c could also influence low-grade inflammation and affect glucose metabolism, thus contributing to diabetes [8]. Collectively, lipotoxicity and glucotoxicity are associated to the progression of DM and its micro- and macrovascular complications [5,9]. However, the nature of glucose and lipid deregulation in the prediabetic state remains to be elucidated.

Therefore, we aim to evaluate glucose and lipid metabolism in a prediabetic rat model, induced by a high-sucrose (HSu) diet [10,11], focusing on the main insulin-target organs: liver, skeletal muscle, and white adipose tissue.

2. Materials and Methods

2.1. Animals and Diets

Male Wistar rats (16 week-old; Charles River Laboratories, Barcelona, Spain) were housed, two per cage, under controlled conditions (12 h light/dark cycle schedule and controlled temperature (22 ± 1 °C) and humidity). After an adaptation period of 1 week, rats were randomly divided into two groups (2 animals per cage) and submitted to a 9-week protocol: (1) control—receiving tap water as vehicle; (2) Hsu—receiving 35% sucrose (S0389; Sigma-Aldrich, St. Louis, MO, USA) in the drinking water. All animals were fed standard rat chow, containing 60% of carbohydrates, 16.1% of protein, 3.1% of lipids, 3.9% of fibers, and 5.1% of minerals (AO4 Panlab, Barcelona, Spain), ad libitum (except during fasting periods). Body weight, food, and beverage consumption were monitored every two days and presented as weekly variation per rat (which is the mean of the two rats per cage). All experiments were conducted in accordance with the European Union (EU) Legislation for the protection of animals used for scientific purposes "Animals (Scientific Procedures) Act", Directive 2010/63/EU, and with the National and Local Authorities, under authorization of the Organ Responsible for Animal Welfare of Faculty of Medicine of Coimbra University (07/2016).

2.2. Chemicals

Collagenase type II was from Roche (Lisbon, Portugal). D-[[^{14}C(U)]-glucose (250 mCi/mmol/L) was from Scopus Research BV (Wageningen, The Netherlands). Human insulin, Actrapid, was kindly supplied by Novo Nordisk A/S (Paço de Arcos, Portugal). N-heptane was from Merck-&-Co., Inc. (Whitehouse Station, NJ, USA). Optiphase Hisafe was from PerkinElmer, Inc. (Waltham, MA, USA). RNeasy® MiniKits were from QIAGEN Sciences (Germantown, MD, USA). High Capacity cDNA Reverse Transcriptase kits were from Applied Biosystems (Forest City, CA, USA). PCR primers were designed using Beacon Designer software and synthesized by IDT-Integrated DNA Technologies, Inc. (BVBA, Leuven, Belgium). SYBRGreen Supermix was from Quanta Biosciences (Gaithersburg, MA, USA). All other reagents were from Sigma (St. Louis, MO, USA). ECF reagent was from GE Healthcare (Little Chalfont, UK).

2.3. Metabolic Characterization

Metabolic characterization was performed as previously described [10] and is detailed in the supplemental material. This included a glucose tolerance test (GTT), an insulin tolerance test (ITT), fasting insulin levels, and insulin resistance (evaluated by the homeostatic model assessment of insulin resistance HOMA-IR index), as well as serum TG to HDL-c ratio (TG/HDL-c), TG-glucose (TyG) index, as well as fed and fasted alanine aminotransferase [6] and aspartate aminotransferase (AST) assessment. Caloric intake was calculated based on the daily food intake, and in HSu-treated animals, the energy related to sucrose consumption was also calculated.

2.4. Blood and Tissues Collection

After a 9-week treatment, blood and tissues (liver, skeletal muscle—from the posterior thigh of the rat leg—and epididymal adipose tissue) were snap frozen and stored at −80 °C. Details are available in the supplemental material.

2.5. Liver Pathology and Triglyceride Content

Liver TG were extracted and quantified as previously reported [12]. Briefly, 50 mg of liver samples were homogenized in 0.5 mL of chlorophorm/methanol (2:1) and incubated for 3 h with agitation at 4 °C. 300 µL of milliQ water were then added to the homogenate and centrifuged (13,000 rpm for 20 min, room temperature). The organic phase was transferred to a clean Eppendorf tube, allowed to evaporate at 4 °C, and finally stored at −20 °C. Liver TG quantification was performed with a specific commercial kit from Spinreact. Colorimetric determination was performed in a spectrophotometer (SPECTRAmax PLUS384, Molecular Devices, Sunnyvale, CA, USA) at a wavelength of 505 nm or 490 nm after TG resuspension in 500 µL of chloroform. Intensity of the formed color was proportional to TG concentration in each sample. Oil red O staining of liver frozen sections was performed to evaluate lipid deposition, according to previously described methodology [13]. Liver pathology was assessed by hematoxylin and eosin (H&E) in paraffin-embedded sections fixed with paraformaldehyde at the moment of sample collection. Data analysis was performed in a blind fashion by a pathologist.

2.6. Cell Size and Weight, Glucose Uptake, and Lipolysis in Isolated Epididymal Adipocytes

Epididymal adipocyte size and weight, insulin-stimulated D-[[^{14}C(U)]-glucose uptake, and isoproterenol-stimulated lipolysis in isolated adipocytes were performed as previously described [14,15]. Briefly, for the insulin-stimulated glucose uptake, the isolated adipocytes were diluted ten times and were stimulated or not with human insulin (1000 μU/mL), for 10 min, at 37 °C, in a shaking water-bath. Subsequently, 0.86 μM D-[[^{14}C(U)]-glucose was added to the medium and the accumulation of glucose followed for 30 min. The cell suspension was then transferred to pre-chilled tubes, containing silicone oil, allowing cells to be separated from the buffer by centrifugation. Cell-associated radioactivity was determined by liquid scintillation counting, which allowed us to calculate the rate of transmembranar glucose transport, according to the formula: cellular clearance of medium glucose = (c.p.m. cells × volume)/(c.p.m. medium × cell number × time).

For isoproterenol-stimulated lipolysis, the isolated adipocytes were diluted ten times and were incubated in the presence or absence of insulin (1000 μU/mL), in a shaking water bath, at 37 °C, for 60 min. The medium was also supplemented or not with isoproterenol (1 μM). Following incubation, cells were separated from the medium by centrifugation and glycerol levels were measured in the medium using an assay kit (Zen Bio, Inc., Research Triangle Park, NC, USA). Further details are available in the supplemental material.

2.7. Liver, Skeletal Muscle, and Adipose Tissue Gene and Protein Expression

Total RNA from liver, skeletal muscle, and epididymal adipose tissue was extracted, and cDNA synthesis and relative mRNA levels for glucose transporter-1(Glut1), -2 (Slc2a2), and -4 (Glut4), phosphoenolpyruvate carboxykinase (Pepck), glucose-6-phosphatase (G6pc), acetyl-CoA carboxylase 1 (Acc1), fatty acid synthase (Fasn), diglyceride acyltransferase (Dgat1), carbohydrate-responsive element-binding protein (Mlxipl/Chrebp), sterol regulatory element-binding transcription factor 1 (Srebf1), and hormone-sensitive lipase (Hsl) were measured (by real time-PCR), as previously described [16]. Protein extraction and Western blot analysis of GLUT1, GLUT2, GLUT4, PEPCK, G6PC, ACC1, FASN, DGAT1, ChREBP, SREBP, and HSL were performed as previously described [14,15]. The supplemental material details the protocols and lists the primer sequences (Table S1) and antibodies (Table S2) used.

2.8. Statistical Analysis

Results were expressed as mean ± standard error of the mean, using GraphPad Prism, version 6 (GraphPad Software, San Diego, CA, USA). Student's *t*-test for normally distributed data or the Mann Whitney test for non-normally distributed data were performed when two groups were considered. One-way or two-way ANOVA, followed by Tukey post hoc test, for multiple comparisons, was used as appropriate. Repeated measures ANOVA, followed by the Tukey post-hoc test, was used to assess the differences between groups and between basal and insulin-stimulated glucose uptake. Differences were considered significant when * $p \leq 0.05$, ** $p \leq 0.01$, *** $p \leq 0.001$, or **** $p \leq 0.0001$.

3. Results

3.1. HSu Diet Increases Beverage Consumption and Caloric Intake, Maintaining Body Weight

During 9 weeks of treatment, the body weight evolution was identical in HSu-treated and control rats (Figure 1A). However, HSu-treated animals had a higher beverage (35% sucrose) consumption but a lower food ingestion (Figure 1B,C). This behavior translated to an increased total caloric intake, mainly from carbohydrates, with a lower calorie consumption from proteins and lipids, when compared with the control animals ((Figure 1D–G).

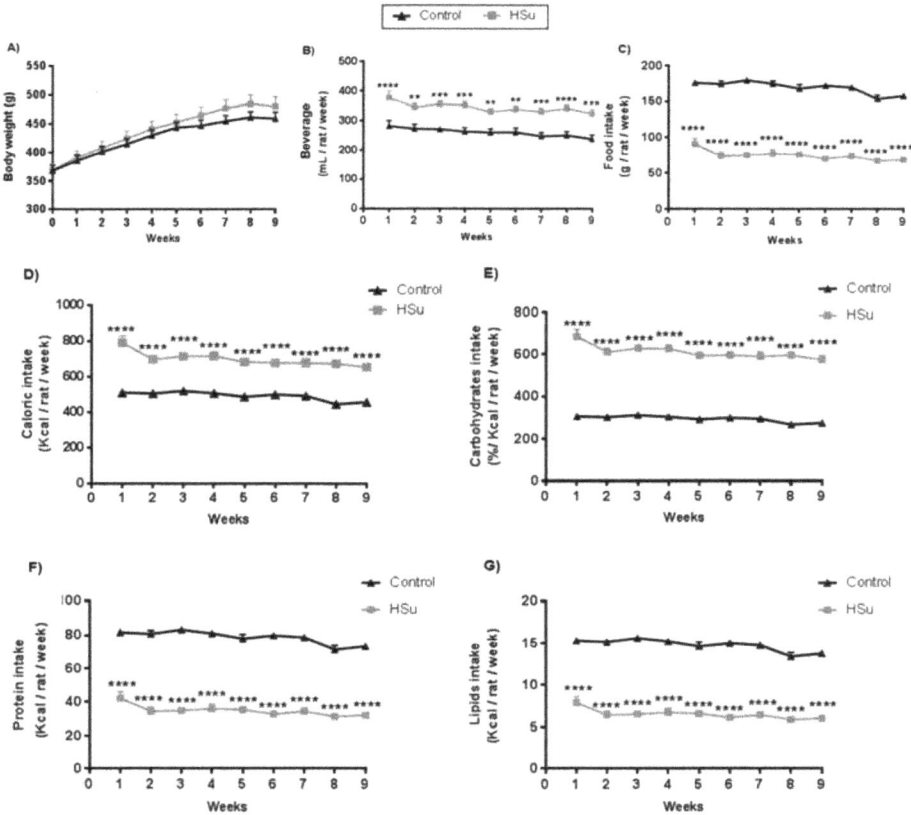

Figure 1. Evolution of body weight (**A**), beverage (**B**) and food (**C**) intake, as well as total caloric consumption (**D**) and caloric intake related with carbohydrates (**E**), protein (**F**), and lipids (**G**), throughout the 9 weeks of treatment. Control ($n = 12$) and HSu ($n = 10$). ** $p < 0.01$, *** $p < 0.001$, **** $p < 0.0001$.

3.2. HSu Diet Increases Serum Triglyceride Levels and Impairs Liver Function

The serum TG content in HSu-treated rats was significantly higher than in control animals in the fed state. Also, fed HSu-treated rats presented higher TG concentrations than in fasted HSu animals (Figure 2A). However, no significant differences were found in liver TG levels (Figure 2B). Regardless of the nutritional status (fasted or fed), serum ALT levels were reduced in the HSu-treated rats (Figure 2C); however, no significant differences were found in serum AST levels (Figure 2D). In addition, the liver weight/body weight ratio was increased in HSu-treated animals (Figure 2E).

Despite markers of impaired liver function, no changes in liver structure were found when analyzed by H&E histology (Figure 3(A1,A2)). Oil red O staining showed a slight deposition of lipids in the HSu-treated animals, when compared with the control ones (Figure 3(B1,B2)), respectively.

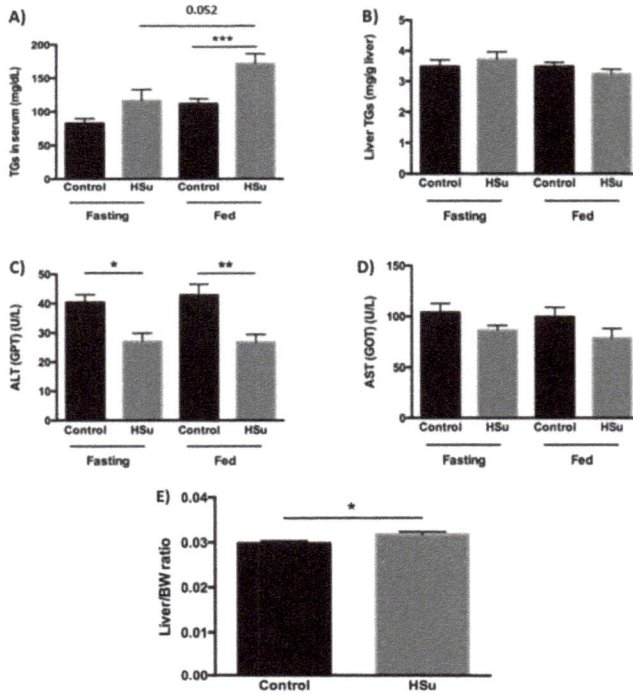

Figure 2. Serum (**A**) and liver (**B**) triglyceride (TG) content, serum alanine aminotransferase (ALT) (**C**) and aspartate aminotransferase (AST) (**D**) levels, as well as liver weight/body weight ratio (**E**) at the end of treatment. Control (n = 12) and HSu (n = 10). * $p < 0.05$, ** $p < 0.01$, *** $p < 0.001$.

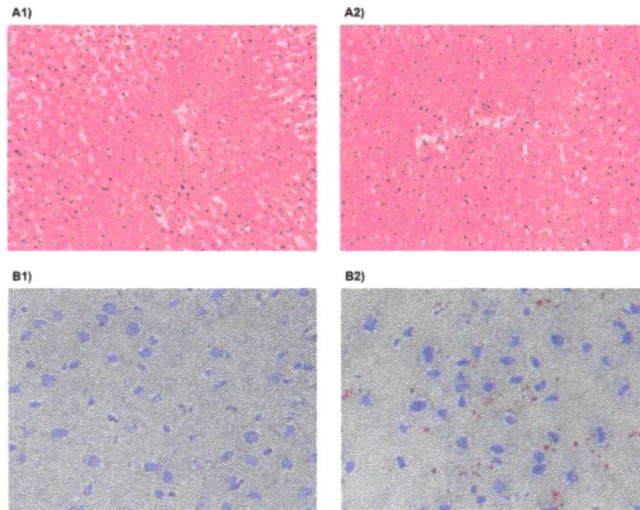

Figure 3. Liver (**A1,A2**) Hematoxylin and Eosin (H&E) staining ($\times 200$) and (**B1,B2**) Oil red O staining ($\times 400$) in control (1) and HSu-treated (2) rats. Six sections per group were measured.

3.3. HSu Diet Impairs Glucose Tolerance and Causes Insulin Resistance

Although both groups showed similar fasting glucose levels (Figure 4A,C,E), the HSu-treated rats had significantly slower glucose excursion during a GTT (2 g/kg body weight of glucose), compared to control animals (Figure 4A,B), revealing glucose intolerance. Blood glucose levels were significantly elevated in the HSu-treated rats, 120 min after an insulin injection (0.75 U/kg body weight of insulin) (Figure 4C,D). In addition, serum fasting insulin concentration was significantly elevated in HSu-treated animals (Figure 4F). Moreover, TG/HDL-c ratio, TyG and HOMA-IR indexes, known markers of insulin resistance, were significantly elevated in the HSu-treated rats, compared to the controls (Figure 4G–I).

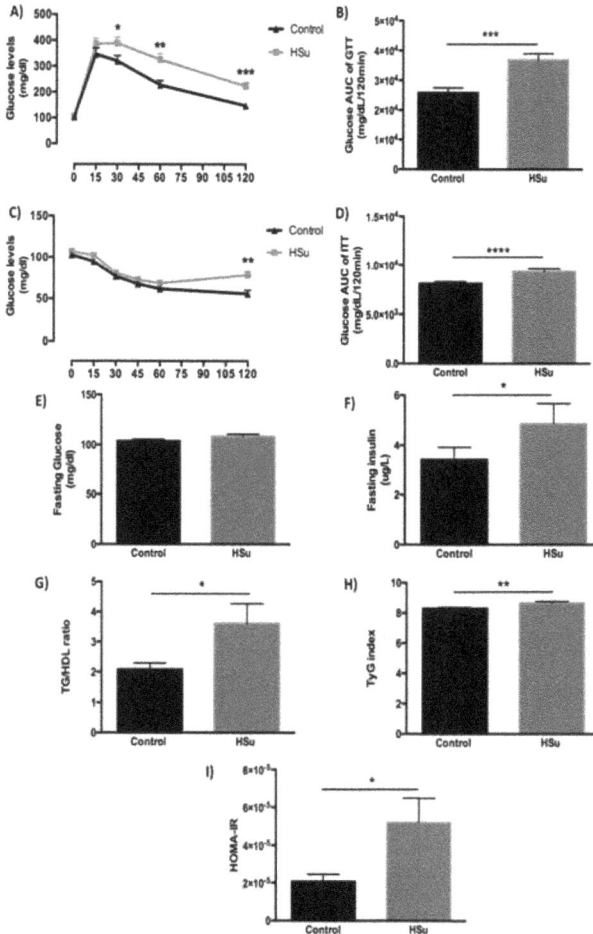

Figure 4. Glucose tolerance test (GTT) and area under the curve (**A,B**), insulin tolerance test (ITT) and area under the curve (**C,D**), fasting glucose (**E**) and insulin (**F**) levels, as well as insulin resistance markers: triglycerides to high density lipoprotein cholesterol (TG/HDL-c) ratio (**G**), triglyceride glucose (TyG) index (**H**) and homeostatic model assessment of insulin resistance (HOMA-IR) index (**I**) at the end of treatment. Control ($n = 12$) and HSu ($n = 10$). * $p < 0.05$, ** $p < 0.01$, *** $p < 0.001$, and **** $p \leq 0.0001$.

3.4. HSu Diet Increases Fat Mass While the Insulin-Stimulated Glucose Uptake in Adipocytes Is Impaired

The epididymal fat pad weight/body weight ratio was significantly higher in the HSu-treated rats when compared to the controls (Figure 5A), while fat cell diameter and weight were unchanged between the groups (Figure 5C,D). Insulin-stimulated glucose uptake was measured in freshly isolated adipocytes. Basal glucose uptake was not significantly different between groups ($p > 0.05$). Adipocytes responded to the stimulatory effect of insulin in the uptake of glucose in both groups (Control − Basal = 20.31 ± 2.59 vs. Insulin = 35.88 ± 4.22, $p < 0.001$; HSu − Basal = 8.55 ± 1.09 vs. Insulin = 17.48 ± 1.16, $p < 0.001$); however, the insulin-stimulated glucose uptake was significantly reduced in adipocytes from HSu-treated rats compared to the controls (17.48 ± 1.16 vs. 35.88 ± 4.22, $p < 0.01$, respectively) (Figure 5B).

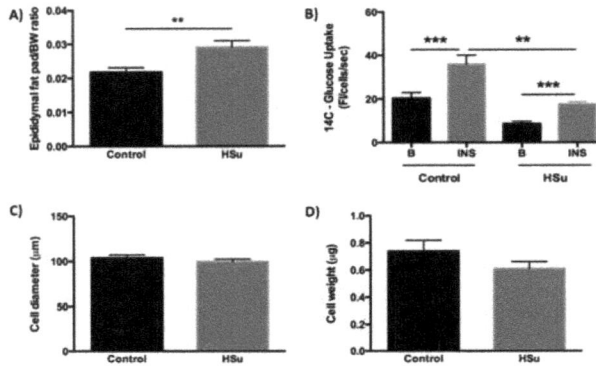

Figure 5. Epididymal fat pad weight/bw ratio (**A**), insulin-stimulated D-[[^{14}C(U)]-glucose uptake in isolated adipocytes (**B**), and adipocyte diameter (**C**) and weight (**D**) at the end of treatment. Control (n = 12) and HSu (n = 10). ** $p < 0.01$, *** $p < 0.001$.

3.5. HSu Diet Decreased GLUT1 but Increased G6Pase Levels in Liver

The gene and protein levels of mediators of glucose uptake and gluconeogenesis were quantified in liver, skeletal muscle (posterior thigh of the leg), and epididymal adipose tissue. There were no changes in glucose transporter gene levels in all tissues, in the fed state (Figure 6A). Moreover, GLUT1 protein levels were reduced in HSu-treated rats versus controls, with no change in GLUT2 expression, in the liver. In addition, no differences were found in either GLUT1 or GLUT4 protein levels in skeletal muscle or epididymal adipose tissue. To assess hepatic gluconeogenesis, PEPCK and G6Pase gene and protein levels were evaluated. While there was no alteration in gene expression, there was a significant increase in only G6Pase protein levels in the HSu-treated group (Figure 6B).

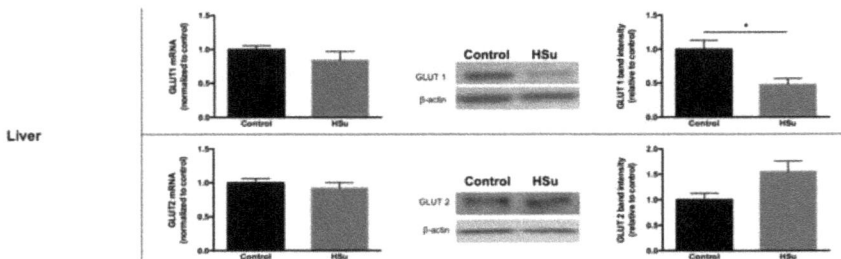

Figure 6. *Cont.*

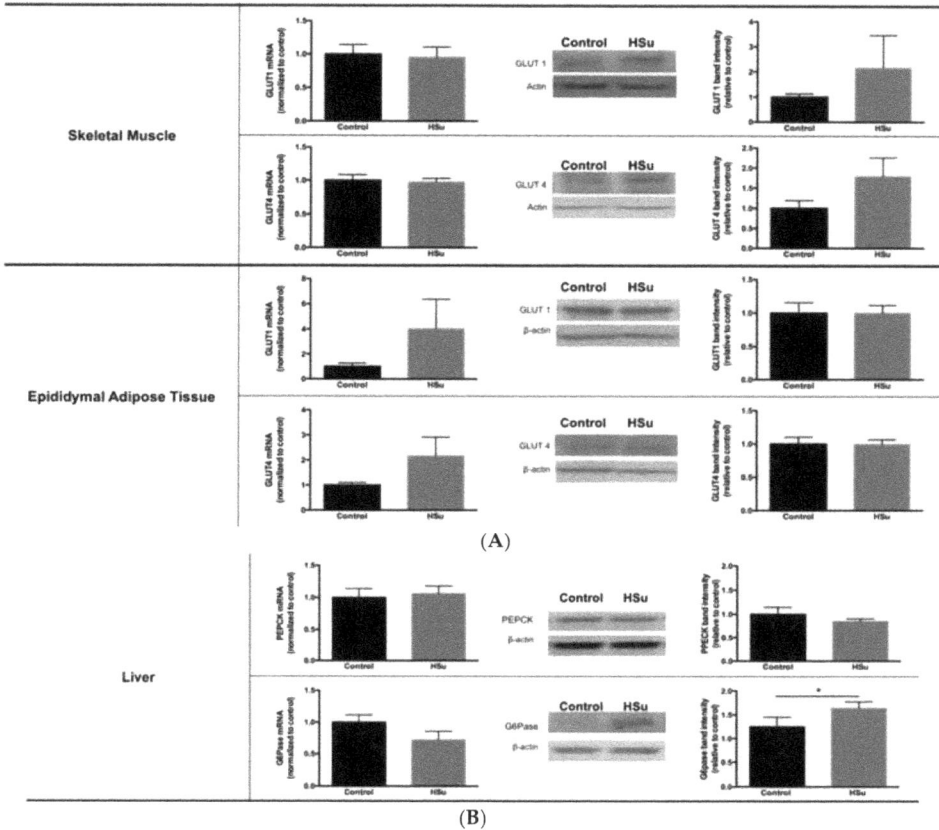

Figure 6. (**A**) Glucose transporters. (**B**) Gluconeogenesis. Gene and protein levels of glucose transporters (**A**) in liver, skeletal muscle (posterior thigh of the leg), and epididymal adipose tissue. Gene and protein levels of mediators of hepatic gluconeogenesis (**B**). Control (*n* = 12) and HSu (*n* = 10). * $p \leq 0.05$.

3.6. HSu Diet Increases Hepatic Lipid Biosynthesis, without Alterations in Lipolysis

Gene and protein levels of ACC1, FASN, and DGAT1, that play a major role in lipid biosynthesis in the liver and in fat, were analyzed, together with SREBP and ChREBP. Increased protein levels of ACC1, FASN, and SREBP were observed in the liver of HSu-treated animals, without changes in gene levels (Figure 7A). In addition, in adipose tissue, both gene and protein levels for ChREBP were increased in the HSu-treated rats, without further changes on the other measured mediators (Figure 7A).

Isoproterenol-stimulated lipolysis was performed to measure TG hydrolysis into glycerol and free fatty acids, and to evaluate the antilipolytic effect of insulin in isolated adipocytes (Figure 7(B1)). Both groups responded similarly to the stimulatory effect of isoproterenol (Control: 0.66 ± 0.11; HSu: 0.50 ± 0.08) versus basal (Control: 0.30 ± 0.03; HSu: 0.22 ± 0.03) and insulin levels (Control: 0.34 ± 0.04; HSu: 0.24 ± 0.03). Even though there is a tendency for an antilipolytic effect of insulin after isoproterenol stimulation (Control: 0.50 ± 0.05; HSu: 0.39 ± 0.05), it does not reach significance. Moreover, gene and protein expression levels for HSL were not different between the two groups (Figure 7(B2)).

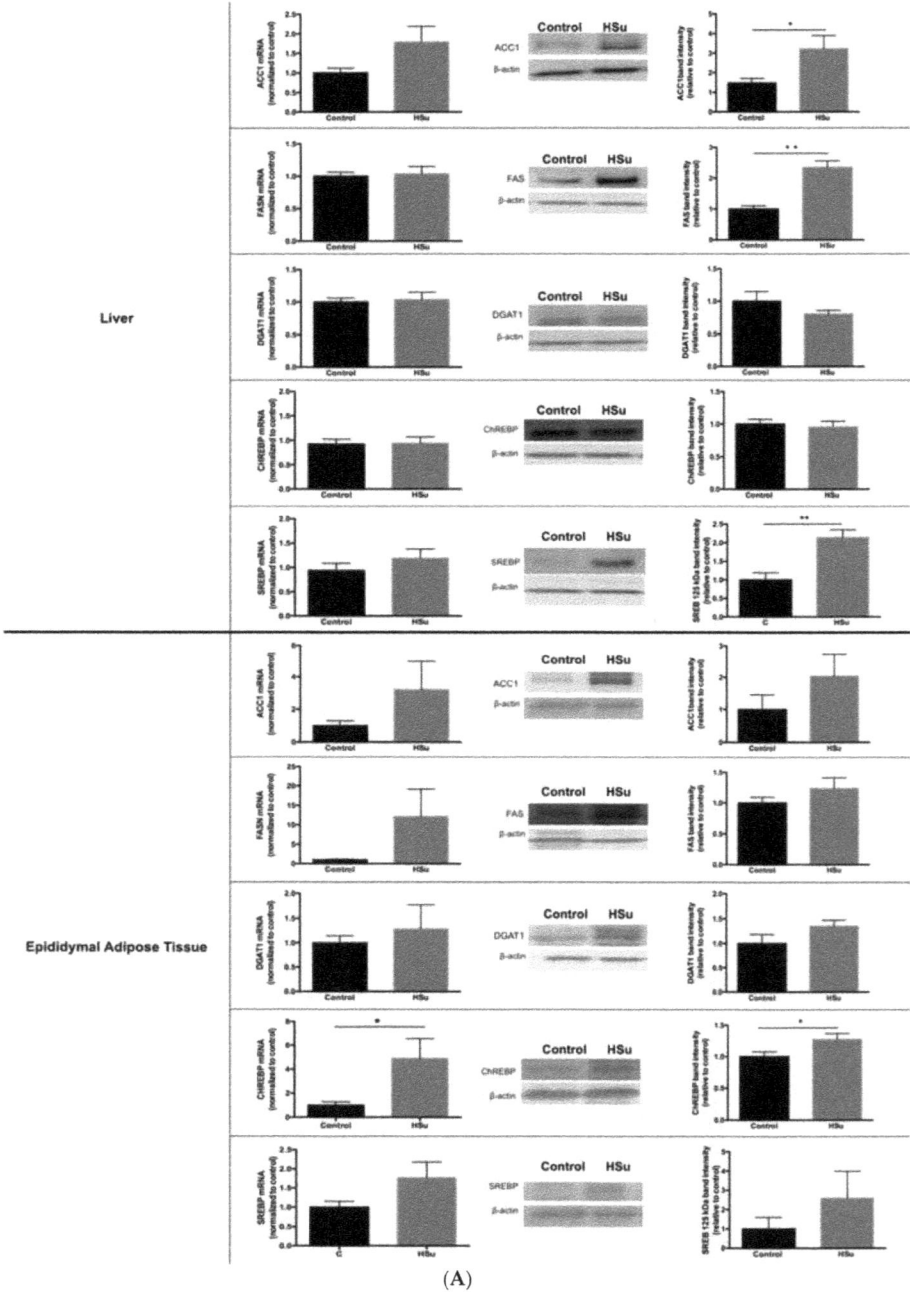

(A)

Figure 7. *Cont.*

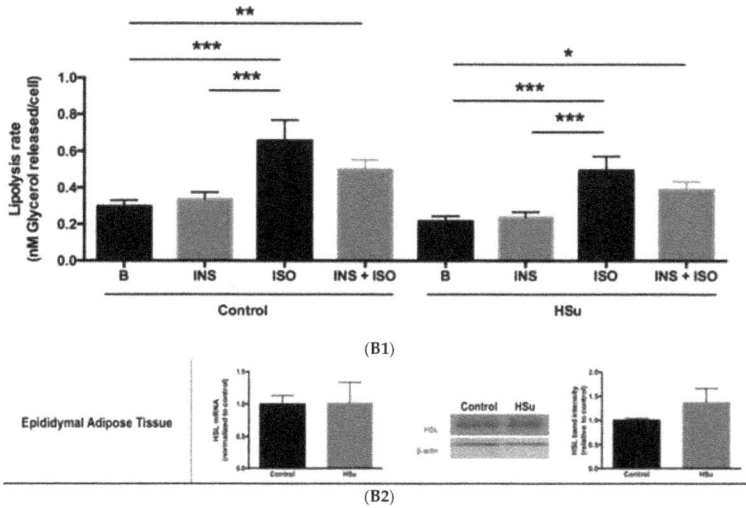

Figure 7. (**A**) Lipid biosynthesis. (**B1,B2**) Lipolysis. (**B1**) Isoproterenol-stimulated lipolysis. (**B2**) Hormone-sensitive lipase gene and protein. Gene and protein levels of mediators of lipid biosynthesis (**A**) in liver and epididymal adipose tissue. Isoproterenol-stimulated lipolysis (**B1**) and HSL gene and protein levels (**B2**) in epididymal adipose tissue. Control ($n = 12$) and HSu ($n = 10$). * $p \leq 0.05$, ** $p < 0.01$, and *** $p < 0.001$.

4. Discussion

The novel findings from this study indicate that a high-sugar diet induces early glucose and lipid dysmetabolism, in the absence of weight gain, only after 9 weeks of treatment. HSu-treated animals developed impaired insulin-stimulated glucose uptake and reduced insulin sensitivity (resistance), together with decreased GLUT1 but increased G6Pase protein levels in the liver. These metabolic changes are paralleled by fed hyperglycemia and hypertriglyceridemia.

Throughout the 9-week treatment, the HSu-treated group had lower food consumption but higher beverage (35% sucrose) and caloric intake, while maintaining body weight, as previously described [17–19]. Similar body weight might have been maintained due to: first, differences in digestion and absorption may have modified the amount of 'bioavailable' energy, affecting the actual positive energy balance; second, the composition of weight gain (fat mass and lean mass) might be different, as the energy cost of protein deposition is higher than that of adipose tissue. In fact, we observed that HSu-treated animals have a greater adiposity translated by an increased epididymal fat pad weight/body weight ratio. Moreover, dietary protein content was suggested to be a critical determinant of weight gain during ad libitum feeding [20].

This prediabetic animal model presented low food intake, which is enriched in 16.1% protein, and increased fluid intake of sucrose-enriched water, in agreement with previous studies [18]. This means that HSu-treated animals ingested a smaller amount of protein and a greater amount of carbohydrates, which can be translated by higher fat mass and smaller lean mass, which allowed the maintenance of body weight. This suggestion might be further confirmed by performing an in vivo non-invasive ecographic magnetic resonance imaging (Echo-MRI) analysis to assess whole body fat, lean, free water, and total water masses.

Indeed, epididymal fat pad weight/body weight ratio was significantly higher in HSu-treated rats. Moreover, high-protein diets are known to reduce adiposity/lipogenesis in the context of high carbohydrate consumption in Western diets [21]. In fact, high-sucrose diets may increase adiposity by stimulating liver lipogenesis [22].

After 9 weeks of treatment, the HSu-treated group had higher serum TG levels, in agreement with previous reports [18,23–25], together with increased lipid deposition in the hepatic tissue, viewed by the Oil Red O staining. In addition, ALT levels were significantly reduced in HSu-treated rats, while a significant increase in the liver weight/body weight ratio was observed, suggesting altered liver function, without liver lesion at this stage of impaired metabolism. The strongest hypothesis to explain the reduced liver function and ALT low levels is malnutrition or an altered nutritional pattern. This prediabetes model had lower food consumption (constituted by 16.1% protein) and increased fluid intake (sucrose-enriched water). Thus, the low serum ALT levels, indicative of liver dysfunction, observed in the HSu-treated rats might be caused by a diet poor in essential nutrients/macromolecules (including proteins and lipids), i.e., malnutrition.

This prediabetes model presented impaired glucose homeostasis. Already at the early stages of the disease, there were initial metabolic deregulations, evidenced by alterations in glucose tolerance during the GTT and ITT, as well as the glucose and insulin levels, indicative of insulin resistance, in agreement with other studies [18,26,27]. At this stage, although fasting glucose levels are maintained within normal values (normoglycemia), due to compensatory hyperinsulinemia, there is already some degree of glucose intolerance and peripheral insulin resistance, in agreement with other reports [18,28–30].

Insulin resistance was demonstrated not only by the increased HOMA-IR index but also by augmented TG/HDL-c ratio and the TyG index, which have previously been used as surrogate measures of impaired insulin sensitivity in obese adolescents with normoglycemia, in prediabetes, as well as in T2DM [31].

In an attempt to explain the glucose, insulin, and lipid dysmetabolism in this model at the prediabetic stage, we assessed possible alterations in glucose and lipid metabolism in fat. Accordingly with previous studies [18], the HSu diet increased fat mass, which is closely linked to the development of severe peripheral IR and prediabetes [32,33]. Moreover, under the fed state, the HSu diet impaired insulin-induced glucose uptake in isolated adipocytes, confirming that visceral adiposity is strongly associated with impaired glucose uptake and IR [34]. Additionally, under IGT, adipocytes are resistant to insulin, and its effectiveness may be impaired, contributing to postprandial hyperglycemia in prediabetic states. Furthermore, the decrease in hepatic GLUT1 in the HSu-treated rats might be mediated by the hyperinsulinemia observed in this animal model [35], although supplementary confirmation of this hypothesis could be achieved by evaluating GLUT1 expression under fasting conditions. On the other hand, both GLUT2 (in the liver) and GLUT4 protein levels (in the adipose tissue and skeletal muscle), were unchanged. The translocation of both GLUT2 and GLUT4 to the plasma membrane is mediated by insulin; however, under IR conditions, this process is impaired [36,37], leading to decreased insulin-stimulated glucose uptake in hepatocytes (mostly by GLUT2), while increasing postprandial blood glucose levels. Even though we did not measure translocation of glucose transporters in this study, it may be possible that these processes are impaired, thus also contributing to the increased postprandial blood glucose levels.

Another factor that may also be contributing to the postprandial hyperglycemia observed in this animal model is that high sucrose consumption increased gluconeogenesis, as previously reported [38]. However, under IGT and/or IR conditions, the derangement of hepatic glucose handling, indicated by changes in GLUT1 and G6Pase may at least in part lead to postprandial hyperglycemia in prediabetic states [39]. Furthermore, in this animal model of IR, insulin may not inhibit the de novo glucose production by the liver, leading therefore to elevated gluconeogenesis, resulting in elevated blood glucose levels in the fed state, as previously reported [35], as well as altered glucose tolerance during a GTT.

Furthermore, the HSu diet increased liver lipid biosynthesis. Our results show that ACC1 and FASN enzymes, as well as the transcription factor SREBP expression levels were increased in the liver of HSu-treated rats, in agreement with previous studies [40–44]. The perturbed liver lipid metabolism that was observed might explain the hypertriglyceridemia present in this prediabetic animal model. In addition, high sucrose consumption may also be contributing to hypertriglyceridemia due to the increased ChREBP gene and protein levels observed in fat [45]. However, the HSu diet did not induce changes in the isoproterenol-stimulated lipolysis in isolated adipocytes, and the HSL protein levels were not different. HSL lipolytic activity is regulated by reversible phosphorylation on five critical residues [46]. Therefore the absence of alterations in lipolysis suggest that HSL phosphorylation was not changed by the HSu diet. Finally, insulin did not show a significant antilipolytic effect at these insulin concentrations. However, it is important to note that we used supra-physiological insulin concentrations (1000 μU/mL), in order to evoke a sustained respond to study the impact of the treatment. Testing physiological insulin concentrations are warranted in both control and HSu animals in future research. In addition, there are other aspects for the forthcoming studies that could consolidate this model, namely lipid profiling of FPLC-separated lipoprotein fractions, quantification of FFA levels, as well as the estimation of VLDL secretion. Furthermore, the impact of the HSu diet on leptin serum levels and on leptin receptor expression would be of interest.

Overall, our study shows that nine week of HSu-diet, which mimics at least in part Western diets [10,11,47], can lead to impaired hepatic glucose and lipid metabolism, typical features of T2DM, already present in this prediabetic model, even in the absence of obesity. This animal model of diet-induced prediabetes shows reduced glucose tolerance, postprandial hyperglycemia, hyperinsulinemia, reduced insulin sensitivity (resistance), and hypertriglyceridemia, together with impaired gluconeogenesis and lipogenesis (Figure 8).

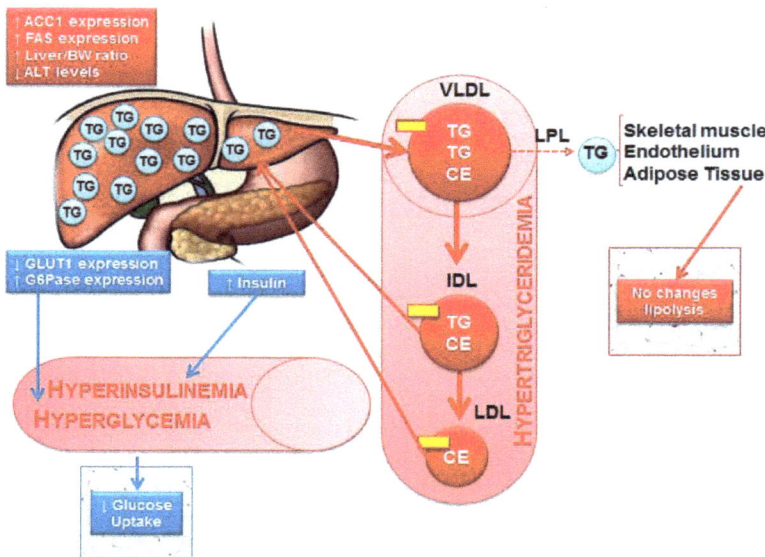

Figure 8. A molecular model describing insulin resistance and prediabetes development after a HSu diet. HSu diet increases serum triglyceride (TG) accumulation and triggers liver lipogenesis, inducing hypertriglyceridemia and interfering with liver function. However, no alterations were observed in lipolysis. The HSu diet alters hepatic proteins involved in basal glucose uptake and gluconeogenesis and impairs the insulin-stimulated glucose uptake in adipocytes, leading to impaired glucose homeostasis and increased IR markers. Legend: ▬ Apolipoprotein; CE—Cholesterol ester; IDL—Intermediate-density protein; LDL—Low-density lipoprotein; LDL—Lipoprotein lipase; TG—Triglycerides; VLDL—Very low-density lipoprotein.

This study should be viewed as an important wake up call for the lifestyle that the general population have been gradually adopting, by consuming large amounts of simple sugars in soft drinks [48]. Importantly, exaggerated consumption of these drinks has been associated with an increased risk for T2DM development by about 26% if the average intake is one/two cans a day, or even more [49]. This feeding behavior is one of the main causes of the uncontrolled increase of IR, T2DM, and associated complications, such as coronary heart disease [50,51].

5. Conclusions

This animal model of prediabetes induced by high-sucrose consumption presents liver glucose and lipid dysmetabolism. It is expected that new insights of impaired metabolism at this early stage of the disease might contribute to disclosing new therapeutic targets and strategies to counteract prediabetes and hinder the natural course of T2DM progression.

Supplementary Materials: The following are available online at www.mdpi.com/2072-6643/9/6/638/s1, Supplemental methods; Table S1: Primer sequences for RT-PCR; Table S2: Antibodies used for Western blotting.

Acknowledgments: The authors kindly thank Novo Nordisk A/S for the human insulin (Actrapid), as well as funding support from: SPD/GIFT award, European Foundation for the Study of Diabetes (EFSD), EXCL/DTP-PIC/0069/2012, CNC.IBILI Strategic Project 2015-UID/NEU/04539/2013 funded by the Portuguese Foundation for Science and Technology (FCT) and by FEDER through Operational Programme Competitiveness Factors (COMPETE): FCOMP-01-0124-FEDER-028417 and POCI-01-0145-FEDER-007440,, SFRH/BD/109017/2015 (Sara Nunes PhD scholarship by FCT) as well as Centro 2020 Regional Operational Programmes (CENTRO-01-0145-FEDER-000012: HealthyAging2020 and CENTRO-01-0145-FEDER-000008: BrainHealth 2020). E.C. is partly supported by NIH P30AG028718 and NIH RO1 AG033761.

Author Contributions: A.B., F.C.P., F.R. and E.C. designed the study. All authors participated in rat housing/feeding and/or in the analytical assays. P.N. performed the histopathological analysis. A.B., M.C., B.M.V.-R. and S.N. performed statistical analyses. A.B. and M.C. prepared figures and drafted the manuscript. A.B., F.C.P., F.R. and E.C. edited and revised the manuscript. All authors read and approved the final version.

Conflicts of Interest: The authors declare no conflict of interest.

References

1. Lau, D.C.; Teoh, H. Current and emerging pharmacotherapies for weight management in prediabetes and diabetes. *Can. J. Diabetes* **2015**, *39* (Suppl. S5), S134–S141. [CrossRef] [PubMed]
2. Tabak, A.G.; Herder, C.; Rathmann, W.; Brunner, E.J.; Kivimaki, M. Prediabetes: A high-risk state for diabetes development. *Lancet* **2012**, *379*, 2279–2290. [CrossRef]
3. Malik, V.S.; Hu, F.B. Fructose and Cardiometabolic Health: What the Evidence from Sugar-Sweetened Beverages Tells Us. *J. Am. Coll. Cardiol.* **2015**, *66*, 1615–1624. [CrossRef] [PubMed]
4. Parhofer, K.G. Interaction between glucose and lipid metabolism: More than diabetic dyslipidemia. *Diabetes Metab. J.* **2015**, *39*, 353–362. [CrossRef] [PubMed]
5. Erion, D.M.; Park, H.J.; Lee, H.Y. The role of lipids in the pathogenesis and treatment of type 2 diabetes and associated co-morbidities. *BMB Rep.* **2016**, *49*, 139–148. [CrossRef] [PubMed]
6. Van Raalte, D.H.; van der Zijl, N.J.; Diamant, M. Pancreatic steatosis in humans: Cause or marker of lipotoxicity? *Curr. Opin. Clin. Nutr. Metab. Care* **2010**, *13*, 478–485. [CrossRef] [PubMed]
7. Rachek, L.I. Free fatty acids and skeletal muscle insulin resistance. *Prog. Mol. Biol. Transl. Sci.* **2014**, *121*, 267–292. [PubMed]
8. Drew, B.G.; Rye, K.A.; Duffy, S.J.; Barter, P.; Kingwell, B.A. The emerging role of HDL in glucose metabolism. *Nat. Rev. Endocrinol.* **2012**, *8*, 237–245. [CrossRef] [PubMed]
9. Cusi, K. The role of adipose tissue and lipotoxicity in the pathogenesis of type 2 diabetes. *Curr. Diabetes Rep.* **2010**, *10*, 306–315. [CrossRef] [PubMed]
10. Nunes, S.; Soares, E.; Fernandes, J.; Viana, S.; Carvalho, E.; Pereira, F.C.; Reis, F. Early cardiac changes in a rat model of prediabetes: Brain natriuretic peptide overexpression seems to be the best marker. *Cardiovasc. Diabetol.* **2013**, *12*, 44. [CrossRef] [PubMed]

11. Soares, E.; Prediger, R.D.; Nunes, S.; Castro, A.A.; Viana, S.D.; Lemos, C.; De Souza, C.M.; Agostinho, P.; Cunha, R.A.; Carvalho, E.; et al. Spatial memory impairments in a prediabetic rat model. *Neuroscience* **2013**, *250*, 565–577. [CrossRef] [PubMed]

12. Silva, A.M.; Martins, F.; Jones, J.G.; Carvalho, R. 2H2O incorporation into hepatic acetyl-CoA and de novo lipogenesis as measured by Krebs cycle-mediated 2H-enrichment of glutamate and glutamine. *Magn. Reson. Med.* **2011**, *66*, 1526–1530. [CrossRef] [PubMed]

13. Kho, M.C.; Lee, Y.J.; Park, J.H.; Kim, H.Y.; Yoon, J.J.; Ahn, Y.M.; Tan, R.; Park, M.C.; Cha, J.D.; Choi, K.M.; et al. Fermented red ginseng potentiates improvement of metabolic dysfunction in metabolic syndrome rat models. *Nutrients* **2016**, *8*, E369. [CrossRef] [PubMed]

14. Pereira, M.J.; Palming, J.; Rizell, M.; Aureliano, M.; Carvalho, E.; Svensson, M.K.; Eriksson, J.W. mTOR inhibition with rapamycin causes impaired insulin signalling and glucose uptake in human subcutaneous and omental adipocytes. *Mol. Cell. Endocrinol.* **2012**, *355*, 96–105. [CrossRef] [PubMed]

15. Pereira, M.J.; Palming, J.; Rizell, M.; Aureliano, M.; Carvalho, E.; Svensson, M.K.; Eriksson, J.W. The immunosuppressive agents rapamycin, cyclosporin A and tacrolimus increase lipolysis, inhibit lipid storage and alter expression of genes involved in lipid metabolism in human adipose tissue. *Mol. Cell. Endocrinol.* **2013**, *365*, 260–269. [CrossRef] [PubMed]

16. Burgeiro, A.; Fuhrmann, A.; Cherian, S.; Espinoza, D.; Jarak, I.; Carvalho, R.A.; Loureiro, M.; Patrício, M.; Antunes, M.; Carvalho, E. Glucose uptake and lipid metabolism are impaired in epicardial adipose tissue from heart failure patients with or without diabetes. *Am. J. Physiol. Endocrinol. Metab.* **2016**, *310*, E550–E564. [CrossRef] [PubMed]

17. Ritze, Y.M.; Bardos, G.; D'Haese, J.G.; Ernst, B.; Thurnheer, M.; Schultes, B.; Bischoff, S.C. Effect of high sugar intake on glucose transporter and weight regulating hormones in mice and humans. *PLoS ONE* **2014**, *9*, e101702. [CrossRef] [PubMed]

18. Lirio, L.M.; Forechi, L.; Zanardo, T.C.; Batista, H.M.; Meira, E.F.; Nogueira, B.V.; Mill, J.G.; Baldo, M.P. Chronic fructose intake accelerates non-alcoholic fatty liver disease in the presence of essential hypertension. *J. Diabetes Complicat.* **2016**, *30*, 85–92. [CrossRef] [PubMed]

19. Glendinning, J.I.; Breinager, L.; Kyrillou, E.; Lacuna, K.; Rocha, R.; Sclafani, A. Differential effects of sucrose and fructose on dietary obesity in four mouse strains. *Physiol. Behav.* **2010**, *101*, 331–343. [CrossRef] [PubMed]

20. Galgani, J.; Ravussin, E. Energy metabolism, fuel selection and body weight regulation. *Int. J. Obes.* **2008**, *32* (Suppl. S7), S109–S119. [CrossRef] [PubMed]

21. Chaumontet, C.; Even, P.C.; Schwarz, J.; Simonin-Foucault, A.; Piedcoq, J.; Fromentin, G.; Azzout-Marniche, D.; Tomé, D. High dietary protein decreases fat deposition induced by high-fat and high-sucrose diet in rats. *Br. J. Nutr.* **2015**, *114*, 1132–1142. [CrossRef] [PubMed]

22. Borsheim, E.; Bui, Q.U.; Tissier, S.; Cree, M.G.; Rønsen, O.; Morio, B.; Ferrando, A.A.; Kobayashi, H.; Newcomer, B.R.; Wolfe, R.R. Amino acid supplementation decreases plasma and liver triacylglycerols in elderly. *Nutrition* **2009**, *25*, 281–288. [CrossRef] [PubMed]

23. Simental-Mendia, L.E.; Rodriguez-Moran, M.; Guerrero-Romero, F. The hypertriglyceridemia is associated with isolated impaired glucose tolerance in subjects without insulin resistance. *Endocr. Res.* **2015**, *40*, 70–73. [CrossRef] [PubMed]

24. Ram, J.; Snehalatha, C.; Nanditha, A.; Selvam, S.; Shetty, S.A.; Godsland, I.F.; Johnston, D.G.; Ramachandran, A. Hypertriglyceridaemic waist phenotype as a simple predictive marker of incident diabetes in Asian-Indian men with prediabetes. *Diabet. Med.* **2014**, *31*, 1542–1549. [CrossRef] [PubMed]

25. Daly, M.E.; Vale, C.; Walker, M.; Alberti, K.G.; Mathers, J.C. Dietary carbohydrates and insulin sensitivity: A review of the evidence and clinical implications. *Am. J. Clin. Nutr.* **1997**, *66*, 1072–1085. [PubMed]

26. Giorelli Gde, V.; Matos, L.N.; Saado, A.; Soibelman, V.L.; Dias, C.B. No association between 25-hydroxyvitamin D levels and prediabetes in Brazilian patients. A cross-sectional study. *Sao Paulo Med. J.* **2015**, *133*, 73–77. [CrossRef] [PubMed]

27. Jenkins, N.T.; Hagberg, J.M. Aerobic training effects on glucose tolerance in prediabetic and normoglycemic humans. *Med. Sci. Sports Exerc.* **2011**, *43*, 2231–2240. [CrossRef] [PubMed]

28. Fiorini, F.; Raffa, M.; Patrone, E.; Castelluccio, A. Glucose metabolism and chronic renal insufficiency. *Arch. Ital. Urol. Androl.* **1994**, *66*, 51–56. [PubMed]

29. Pagliassotti, M.J.; Prach, P.A.; Koppenhafer, T.A.; Pan, D.A. Changes in insulin action, triglycerides, and lipid composition during sucrose feeding in rats. *Am. J. Physiol.* **1996**, *271*, R1319–R1326. [PubMed]

30. Dutta, K.; Podolin, D.A.; Davidson, M.B.; Davidoff, A.J. Cardiomyocyte dysfunction in sucrose-fed rats is associated with insulin resistance. *Diabetes* **2001**, *50*, 1186–1192. [CrossRef] [PubMed]

31. Mohd Nor, N.S.; Lee, S.; Bacha, F.; Tfayli, H.; Arslanian, S. Triglyceride glucose index as a surrogate measure of insulin sensitivity in obese adolescents with normoglycemia, prediabetes, and type 2 diabetes mellitus: Comparison with the hyperinsulinemic-euglycemic clamp. *Pediatr. Diabetes* **2016**, *17*, 458–465. [CrossRef] [PubMed]

32. Weiss, R.; Dufour, S.; Taksali, S.E.; Tamborlane, W.V.; Petersen, K.F.; Bonadonna, R.C.; Boselli, L.; Barbetta, G.; Allen, K.; Rife, F.; et al. Prediabetes in obese youth: A syndrome of impaired glucose tolerance, severe insulin resistance, and altered myocellular and abdominal fat partitioning. *Lancet* **2003**, *362*, 951–957. [CrossRef]

33. Neeland, I.J.; Turer, A.T.; Ayers, C.R.; Powell-Wiley, T.M.; Vega, G.L.; Farzaneh-Far, R.; Grundy, S.M.; Khera, A.; McGuire, D.K.; de Lemos, J.A. Dysfunctional adiposity and the risk of prediabetes and type 2 diabetes in obese adults. *JAMA* **2012**, *308*, 1150–1159. [CrossRef] [PubMed]

34. Kim, G.; Jo, K.; Kim, K.J.; Lee, Y.H.; Han, E.; Yoon, H.J.; Wang, H.J.; Kang, E.S.; Yun, M. Visceral adiposity is associated with altered myocardial glucose uptake measured by (18)FDG-PET in 346 subjects with normal glucose tolerance, prediabetes, and type 2 diabetes. *Cardiovasc. Diabetol.* **2015**, *14*, 148. [CrossRef] [PubMed]

35. Tal, M.; Kahn, B.B.; Lodish, H.F. Expression of the low Km GLUT-1 glucose transporter is turned on in perivenous hepatocytes of insulin-deficient diabetic rats. *Endocrinology* **1991**, *129*, 1933–1941. [CrossRef] [PubMed]

36. Tobin, V.; Le Gall, M.; Fioramonti, X.; Stolarczyk, E.; Blazquez, A.G.; Klein, C.; Prigent, M.; Serradas, P.; Cuif, M.H.; Magnan, C.; et al. Insulin internalizes GLUT2 in the enterocytes of healthy but not insulin-resistant mice. *Diabetes* **2008**, *57*, 555–562. [CrossRef] [PubMed]

37. Carvalho, E.; Rondinone, C.; Smith, U. Insulin resistance in fat cells from obese Zucker rats—Evidence for an impaired activation and translocation of protein kinase B and glucose transporter 4. *Mol. Cell. Biochem.* **2000**, *206*, 7–16. [CrossRef] [PubMed]

38. Basu, R.; Barosa, C.; Jones, J.; Dube, S.; Carter, R.; Basu, A.; Rizza, R.A. Pathogenesis of prediabetes: Role of the liver in isolated fasting hyperglycemia and combined fasting and postprandial hyperglycemia. *J. Clin. Endocrinol. Metab.* **2013**, *98*, E409–E417. [CrossRef] [PubMed]

39. Dinneen, S.F. The postprandial state: Mechanisms of glucose intolerance. *Diabet. Med.* **1997**, *14* (Suppl. S3), S19–S24. [CrossRef]

40. Ryu, M.H.; Cha, Y.S. The effects of a high-fat or high-sucrose diet on serum lipid profiles, hepatic acyl-CoA synthetase, carnitine palmitoyltransferase-I, and the acetyl-CoA carboxylase mRNA levels in rats. *J. Biochem. Mol. Biol.* **2003**, *36*, 312–318. [CrossRef] [PubMed]

41. Bruckdorfer, K.R.; Khan, I.H.; Yudkin, J. Fatty acid synthetase activity in the liver and adipose tissue of rats fed with various carbohydrates. *Biochem. J.* **1972**, *129*, 439–446. [CrossRef] [PubMed]

42. Agheli, N.; Kabir, M.; Berni-Canani, S.; Petitjean, E.; Boussairi, A.; Luo, J.; Bornet, F.; Slama, G.; Rizkalla, S.W. Plasma lipids and fatty acid synthase activity are regulated by short-chain fructo-oligosaccharides in sucrose-fed insulin-resistant rats. *J. Nutr.* **1998**, *128*, 1283–1288. [PubMed]

43. Im, S.S.; Kang, S.Y.; Kim, S.Y.; Kim, H.I.; Kim, J.W.; Kim, K.S.; Ahn, Y.H. Glucose-stimulated upregulation of GLUT2 gene is mediated by sterol response element-binding protein-1c in the hepatocytes. *Diabetes* **2005**, *54*, 1684–1691. [CrossRef] [PubMed]

44. Ducluzeau, P.H.; Perretti, N.; Laville, M.; Andreelli, F.; Vega, N.; Riou, J.P.; Vidal, H. Regulation by insulin of gene expression in human skeletal muscle and adipose tissue. Evidence for specific defects in type 2 diabetes. *Diabetes* **2001**, *50*, 1134–1142. [CrossRef] [PubMed]

45. Herman, M.A.; Peroni, O.D.; Villoria, J.; Schön, M.R.; Abumrad, N.A.; Blüher, M.; Klein, S.; Kahn, B.B. A novel ChREBP isoform in adipose tissue regulates systemic glucose metabolism. *Nature* **2012**, *484*, 333–338. [CrossRef] [PubMed]

46. Lampidonis, A.D.; Rogdakis, E.; Voutsinas, G.E.; Stravopodis, D.J. The resurgence of Hormone-Sensitive Lipase (HSL) in mammalian lipolysis. *Gene* **2011**, *477*, 1–11. [CrossRef] [PubMed]

47. Bouchard-Mercier, A.; Rudkowska, I.; Lemieux, S.; Couture, P.; Vohl, M.C. The metabolic signature associated with the Western dietary pattern: A cross-sectional study. *Nutr. J.* **2013**, *12*, 158. [CrossRef] [PubMed]

48. Hu, F.B. Resolved: There is sufficient scientific evidence that decreasing sugar-sweetened beverage consumption will reduce the prevalence of obesity and obesity-related diseases. *Obes. Rev.* **2013**, *14*, 606–619. [CrossRef] [PubMed]

49. Malik, V.S.; Popkin, B.M.; Bray, G.A.; Despres, J.P.; Willett, W.C.; Hu, F.B. Sugar-sweetened beverages and risk of metabolic syndrome and type 2 diabetes: A meta-analysis. *Diabetes Care* **2010**, *33*, 2477–2483. [CrossRef] [PubMed]
50. Fung, T.T.; Malik, V.; Rexrode, K.M.; Manson, J.E.; Willett, W.C.; Hu, F.B. Sweetened beverage consumption and risk of coronary heart disease in women. *Am. J. Clin. Nutr.* **2009**, *89*, 1037–1042. [CrossRef] [PubMed]
51. Lana, A.; Rodriguez-Artalejo, F.; Lopez-Garcia, E. Consumption of sugar-sweetened beverages is positively related to insulin resistance and higher plasma leptin concentrations in men and non overweight women. *J. Nutr.* **2014**, *144*, 1099–1105. [CrossRef] [PubMed]

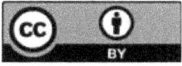

![nutrients](nutrients logo)

MDPI

Review

Nuts and Dried Fruits: An Update of Their Beneficial Effects on Type 2 Diabetes

Pablo Hernández-Alonso [1,2], Lucía Camacho-Barcia [1,2], Mònica Bulló [1,2,*] and Jordi Salas-Salvadó [1,2,*]

[1] Human Nutrition Unit, Biochemistry and Biotechnology Department, Faculty of Medicine and Health Sciences, University Hospital of Sant Joan de Reus, IISPV, Universitat Rovira i Virgili, St/Sant Llorenç 21, 43201 Reus, Spain; pablo1280@gmail.com (P.H.-A.); marialucia.camacho@urv.cat (L.C.-B.)
[2] CIBERobn Physiopathology of Obesity and Nutrition, Instituto de Salud Carlos III, 28029 Madrid, Spain
* Correspondence: monica.bullo@urv.cat (M.B.); jordi.salas@urv.cat (J.S.-S.);
  Tel.: +34-977-759-312 (M.B.); +34-977-759-311 (J.S.-S.)

Received: 24 May 2017; Accepted: 22 June 2017; Published: 28 June 2017

Abstract: Nuts and dried fruit are essential foods in the Mediterranean diet. Their frequent consumption has been associated with the prevention and/or the management of such metabolic conditions as type 2 diabetes (T2D), metabolic syndrome and cardiovascular diseases. Several previous reviews of epidemiological studies and clinical trials have evaluated the associations of nuts and/or dried fruit with various metabolic disorders. However, no reviews have focused on the mechanisms underlying the role of nuts and/or dried fruit in insulin resistance and T2D. This review aims to report nut and dried-fruit nutritional interventions in animals and humans, and to focus on mechanisms that could play a significant role in the prevention and treatment of insulin resistance and T2D.

Keywords: diabetes; nuts; dried fruits; insulin resistance; mechanisms; clinical trials

1. Introduction

Nuts and traditional dried fruit (i.e., with no added sugar) are key food categories in the Mediterranean diet and other regional diets [1]. Several prospective studies, clinical trials and research in animals have reported beneficial effects after nut consumption [2]. However, the benefits of dried fruits (DF), mainly raisins, have been less explored [3].

Over time, food consumption has varied. More than 30 years ago, the consumption of nuts and DF was discouraged because of their high fat and sugar content, respectively. However, at the beginning of the 1990s, several randomized clinical trials (RCT) and animal experiments demonstrated their potential beneficial effect on cardiovascular diseases (CVD). Nuts and DF contain various macro and micronutrients together with other important bioactive compounds that may synergically contribute to modulate specific metabolic diseases such as hypercholesterolemia, hypertension and type 2 diabetes (T2D) (reviewed in [3,4]). Even so, the specific role of nuts and DF in the development and progression of insulin resistance (IR) and T2D are still controversial.

In this review, we focus on the role of nuts and DF in the prevention and treatment of T2D. We summarize published in vivo, in vitro, epidemiological and clinical studies, and we review the potential mechanisms that could explain the beneficial role of nut consumption on glucose and insulin metabolism, both of which are altered in T2D and in other glucose-impaired states. Given that the present article is not a systematic review, we may not have identified some studies and publication bias should be acknowledged. However, all authors independently conducted the literature search.

1.1. Nuts and Dried Fruits: The Concept

1.1.1. Nuts

Nuts have been part of the human diet since prehistoric times [5,6]. They are an independent food group and are one of the cornerstones of the Mediterranean diet (MedDiet) [7]. According to the botanical definition, a nut is simply a dried fruit with one seed (rarely two) in which the ovary walls are very hard (stony or woody) at maturity, and the seed is unattached or free within the ovary wall. However, the word "nut" is commonly used to refer to any large, oily kernel in a shell that can be eaten as food. In this review, we use the term "nuts" to refer to almonds, Brazil nuts, cashews, hazelnuts, macadamias, peanuts, pecans, pine nuts, pistachios and walnuts. Although peanuts are actually classified as legumes because of their similar nutrient composition and their proven cardiovascular health benefits, they are commonly regarded as being a nut.

1.1.2. Dried Fruits

To extend their shelf life, fresh fruits are processed by various techniques to become DFs [3]. Dried fruits are a concentrated form of fresh fruits with a lower moisture content. Fruits can be dried whole (e.g., apricots, berries and grapes), in halves, or in slices (e.g., kiwis, mangoes and papayas). In this form, they are easy to store and distribute, they can be available throughout the year, and they are a healthier alternative to salty or sugary snacks. Apples, apricots, currants, dates, figs, peaches, pears, prunes, and raisins are referred to as "conventional" or "traditional" DFs. Meanwhile, such fruits as blueberries, cranberries, cherries, strawberries and mangoes are commonly infused with different types of sugar solution (or fruit juice) concentrate before drying [8] so are not included in the aforementioned category. Moreover, we have also excluded dried tomato because although it is botanically a berry-type fruit, it is culinary considered a vegetable and it shares nutrient composition with this food category.

1.2. Nutritional Composition of Nuts and Dried Fruits

Nuts and DFs are a matrix of important bioactive compounds such as Vitamins (Vitamin E, niacin, choline and/or folic acid), minerals (magnesium, potassium, calcium and/or phosphorus), phenolic compounds, carotenoids and/or phytosterols [9]. Importantly, some nuts and DFs are among the 50 foods with the highest antioxidant capacity [10] and are also a known source of bioactive compounds, including plant sterols [11]. Pistachios are particularly rich in β-carotenes which have been widely associated with a protective T2D role [12,13]. In addition, pistachios are the only nuts that contain significant amounts of lutein and zeaxanthin [9]. Sun-dried raisins retain the minerals and most of the phytochemicals and antioxidants of the grape, including its resveratrol [14,15]. In fact, sun-drying enhances the antioxidant content of raisins. Because of the dehydration process, phytonutrients are more concentrated in raisins than in grapes. However, the concentration of some compounds is decreased by the sun-drying process in DFs and by dry roasting techniques in nuts [9]. Polyphenols and tocopherols from nuts and DF have proved to be rapidly accessible in the stomach, thus maximizing the possibility of absorption in the upper small intestine, and contributing to the beneficial relation between nut and DF consumption and health-related outcomes [8,16].

However, their macronutrient compositions are quite different, which means that their energy contents are also quite different. Nuts contain a high amount of total fat (Range (Re): 43.9–78.8%) with a high amount of unsaturated fat (monounsaturated fatty acids (MUFA) + polyunsaturated fatty acids (PUFA), Re: 31.6–62.4%), a relatively low amount of carbohydrates (CHOs) (Re: 11.7–30.2%) and vegetable protein (Re: 7.9–25.8%) (Table 1).

Conversely, DFs are mainly composed of CHOs (Re: 61.3–72.8%). They have a low content of protein (Re: 0.17–4.08%) and a fat content of less than 1% (Table 2). Importantly, both foods also contain a considerable amount of dietary fiber. Overall, their unique and varied nutrient composition makes them key foods to counteract various metabolic diseases.

Table 1. Nutrient composition of nuts (per 100 g of raw nut).

Nutrient	Almonds	Brazil Nuts [b]	Cashews	Hazelnuts	Macadamias	Peanuts	Pecans	Pine Nuts [b]	Pistachios	Walnuts [c]
Energy, Kcal	579	659	553	628	718	567	691	673	560	654
Water, g	4.4	3.4	5.2	5.3	1.4	6.5	3.5	2.3	4.4	4.1
Fat, g	49.9	67.1	43.9	60.8	75.8	49.2	72.0	68.4	45.3	65.2
SFA, g	3.8	16.1	7.8	4.5	12.1	6.3	6.2	4.9	5.9	6.1
MUFA, g	31.6	23.9	23.8	45.7	58.9	24.4	40.8	18.8	23.3	9.0
PUFA, g	12.3	24.4	7.8	7.9	1.5	15.6	21.6	34.1	14.4	47.2
Protein, g	21.2	14.3	18.2	15.0	7.9	25.8	9.2	13.7	20.2	15.2
CHO, g	21.6	11.7	30.2	16.7	13.8	16.1	13.9	13.1	27.2	13.7
Fiber, g	12.5	7.5	3.3	9.7	8.6	8.5	9.6	3.7	10.6	6.7
Ca, mg	269	160	37	114	85	92	70	16	105	98
Mg, mg	270	376	292	163	130	168	121	251	121	158
Na, mg	1	3	12	0	5	18	0	2	1	2
K, mg	733	659	660	680	368	705	410	597	1025	441
P, mg	481	725	593	290	188	376	277	575	490	346
Lutein-Zeaxanthin, µg	1	0	22	92	NA	0	17	9	2903	9
β-Carotene, µg	1	0	0	11	NA	0	29	17	305	12
α-Carotene, µg	0	0	0	3	NA	0	0	0	10	0
Phytosterols [a], mg	197	123.5	151	122	116	NA	158.8	236.1	214	110.2
Total phenols, mg	287	244	137	687	126	406	1284	32	867	1576
Vitamin E (α-tocopherol), mg	25.6	5.7	0.9	15.0	0.5	8.3	1.4	9.3	2.9	0.7

Nutrient information is taken from the United States Department of Agriculture (USDA) Nutrient Database Standard Reference, Release 28 [9]. CHO, carbohydrates; MUFA, monounsaturated fatty acids; NA: not available; PUFA, polyunsaturated fatty acids; SFA, saturated fatty acids. [a] Phytosterols, are the sum of stigmasterol, campesterol, β-sitosterol and other phytosterols; [b] dry roasted; [c] English variety.

Table 2. Nutrient composition of dried fruits (per 100 g).

Nutrient	Apples [a]	Apricots [a]	Currants (Zante)	Cranberries [b]	Dates [c]	Figs	Peaches [a]	Pears [a]	Plums/Prunes	Raisins [d]
Energy, Kcal	243	241	283	308	282	249	239	262	240	299
Water, g	31.76	30.89	19.21	15.79	20.53	30.05	31.80	26.69	30.92	15.43
Fat, g	0.32	0.51	0.27	1.09	0.39	0.93	0.76	0.63	0.38	0.46
CHO, g	65.89	62.64	74.08	82.80	75.03	63.87	61.33	69.70	63.88	79.18
Sugars, g	57.19	53.44	67.28	72.56	63.35	47.92	41.74	62.20	38.13	59.19
Fructose, g	NA	12.47	NA	26.96	19.56	22.93	13.49	NA	12.45	29.68
Protein, g	0.93	3.39	4.08	0.17	2.45	3.30	3.61	1.87	2.18	3.07
Fiber, g	8.7	7.3	6.8	5.3	8.0	9.8	8.2	7.5	7.1	3.7
Ca, mg	14	55	86	9	39	162	28	34	43	50
Fe, mg	1.40	2.66	3.26	0.39	1.02	2.03	4.06	2.10	0.93	1.88
Mg, mg	16	32	41	4	43	68	42	33	41	32
Na, mg	87	10	8	5	2	10	7	6	2	11
K, mg	450	1162	892	49	656	680	996	533	732	749
Cu, mg	0.19	0.34	0.47	0.06	0.21	0.29	0.36	0.37	0.28	0.32
β-carotene, μg	0	2163	43	27	6	6	1074	2	394	0
α-carotene, μg	0	0	1	0	0	0	3	0	57	0
Lutein-Zeaxanthin, μg	0	0	0	138	75	32	559	50	148	0
Vitamin A, IU	0	3604	73	46	10	10	2163	3	781	0
Total phenols, mg GAE/100g [e]	324	248	NA	NA	661	960	283	679	938	1065

Data is for traditional dried fruits which is defined as those with no added sugars, typically sun-dried or dried with minimal processing. Nutrient information is taken from the United States Department of Agriculture (USDA) Nutrient Database Standard Reference, Release 28 [9]. CHO, carbohydrates; GAE, gallic acid equivalents; IU, international unit; NA, not available. [a] Sulfured; [b] sweetened; [c] Deglet noor is the common variety; [d] seedless; [e] Total phenol content was obtained from Alasalvar and Shahidi [8].

1.3. Diet Quality in the Context of Nut and Dried Fruit Consumption

Epidemiological studies conducted in children and adults have demonstrated a significant positive association between nut consumption and diet quality [17,18]. Furthermore, the results of a clinical trial conducted in obese (Ob) subjects (*n* = 124) showed that the nutritional dietary quality of nut consumers (reporting to eat 42 g hazelnuts/day for 12 weeks) was remarkably higher than among other groups consuming chocolate, potato crisps or no additional foods [19]. Moreover, including nuts in energy-restricted diets reduced attrition and increased weight loss, indicating that nuts enhance palatability and compliance with diets without compromising health [20].

Several studies have examined the associations of whole fruit or 100% fruit juice [21] with nutritional or health outcomes such as T2D but there is a lack of studies examining potential links between DF and diet quality. A prospective study conducted in adult participants (*n* = 13,292) in the 1999–2004 National Health and Nutrition Examination Survey (NHANES) demonstrated an association between DF consumption and diet quality [22]. DF consumption was associated with improved nutrient intakes, a higher overall diet quality score, and lower body weight (BW)/adiposity measures [22]. Moreover, in a cross-sectional study in healthy adults (*n* = 797) from Hong Kong, an inverse association has been found between the intake of vegetables, legumes, fruits, dried fruits and Vitamin C and the prevalence of metabolic disorders such as non-alcoholic fatty liver disease (NAFLD) [23].

The 2015 Dietary Guidelines for Americans included the following three healthy dietary patterns: a Healthy US-style Pattern, a Healthy Vegetarian Pattern and a Healthy Mediterranean-style pattern. Fruits, nuts, and seeds play a prominent role in all three of these food-based dietary patterns, which recommend 350–440 g/day of fruit, and 16–28 g/day of nuts and seeds [24].

2. In Vivo and In Vitro Studies

Even though much of the research on nuts, dried fruits and T2D is based on observational studies and human trials, some in vitro and in vivo studies also evaluate their modulatory effect on glucose and insulin metabolism. In this regard, the effect of nuts on glucose and insulin metabolism has been investigated by evaluating nut extracts [25,26] or nuts as a whole [27–29] mainly in mice or rats. However, dried fruit has been investigated—like their non-dried counterparts—mainly in in vitro studies [30–33]. Almost all the research has focused on the extracts from non-edible parts, such as the shell [34], leaves [35,36], stems [37] and roots [38], and very little on the nut or fruit kernel [27–29,39]. However, this review focuses on those studies evaluating specific nutrients (e.g., polyphenols) or edible parts in both traditional nuts and dried fruits with outcomes related to glucose metabolism, IR, and the T2D oxidation/inflammation axis [32,40].

2.1. Nuts

The in vivo studies on nuts and T2D-related parameters are summarized in Table 3. These studies were mainly performed using extracts from peanuts or walnuts. Peanut oil supplementation for 42 days in diabetes-induced rats significantly reduced glucose and glycated hemoglobin (HbA$_{1c}$) concentrations and improved lipid metabolism compared to normal rats [27]. Other researchers have found similar improvements in glycaemia in genotypes of diabetes in rats fed with peanut oil extract [41,42] or peanut aqueous extract [25]. In the case of walnuts, a polyphenol-rich walnut extract (PWE) for 4 weeks significantly decreased urinary 8-hydroxy-2'-deoxyguanosin levels (an in vivo marker of oxidative stress) and improved serum TG in *db/db* mice [26]. Moreover, an HFD with a 21.5% of energy from walnuts tested in mice for 20 weeks significantly reduced TG compared to nut-free HFD and tended to improve glucose and IR [29].

Table 3. Summary of in vivo studies and their characteristics in the context of nut consumption and type 2 diabetes (T2D)-related outcomes.

First Author (Year) [Reference]	Nut (Study Length)	Animal Model Used	Control	Intervention	Glucose and Insulin Metabolism Effects	Other Outcomes
Bilbis, L.S.; et al. (2002) [25]	Aqueous extract of peanut (21 days)	Alloxan-induced diabetic rats (n = 12) and non-diabetic rats (n = 12), divided into 3 equal groups	Non-diabetic with unrestricted standard diet and: (a) water ad libitum; (b) unrestricted access to drinking water and 2 mL of the extract 3 times/day; or (c) free access to the extract as the only drinking water.	Diabetic controls: treated as (a), (b) or (c)	The extract (alone or plus water) decreased FBG in both normal and alloxan-induced diabetic rats.	Significant decrease in serum TG, TC, HDL-C and LDL-C in both normal and alloxan-induced diabetic rats.
Fukuda, T.; et al. (2004) [26]	Polyphenol-rich walnut extract (PWE) (4 weeks)	db/db (n = 15) and C57BL/KsJ-db/db (n = 6) mice	Control db/db mice (n = 8) and C57BL/KsJ-db/+ m mice (n = 6, used for the blank group) were given water.	Experimental db/db mice (n = 7) received oral PWE (200 mg/kg BW)	Significant decrease in the level of urinary 8-hydroxy-2'-deoxyguanosin (in vivo marker of oxidative stress) in PWE-fed mice	Serum TG level was improved after PWE administration
Ramesh, B.; et al. (2006) [27]	Peanut oil (42 days)	Normal (n = 12) and STZ-diabetes induced (n = 18) Wistar rats	G1: Normal rats G3: Diabetic rats	G2: Normal rats + peanut oil diet (2%) G4: Diabetic rats + peanut oil diet (2%) G5: Diabetic rats + GLI (600 µg/kg BW)	Diabetic rats fed with peanut oil significantly reduce glucose, HbA$_{1C}$, and G6Pase and FBP activities	Diabetic rats fed with peanut oil showed a small but significant reduction in TC, VLDL-C, LDL-C and TG and an increase in HDL-C.
Vassiliou, E.K.; et al. (2009) [41]	Peanut oil (21 days)	Male KKA^y (n = 24) mice	KKA ^{y} mice fed with normal diet (11.4% fat)	Diabetic KKA^y + HFD. Diabetic KKA^y + HFD with peanut oil (0.70 mL/day). HFD is 58% fat.	Diabetic mice administered peanut oil had lower glucose levels than animals administered HFD alone.	
Choi, Y.; et al. (2016) [29]	Walnuts (20 weeks)	Male C57BL/6J mice (≥6 mice/group)	Regular rodent chow	HFD (45% energy-derived) with or without walnuts (21.5% energy-derived)	Glucose and insulin resistance tended to improve with walnut supplementation.	Walnut supplementation did not change the HFD-induced increase in BW or VFM. However, dietary walnuts significantly decreased the amounts of hepatic TG observed in HFD-fed mice.
Adewale, O.F.; et al. (2016) [42]	Peanut oil Palm oil (3 weeks)	Normal (n = 12) and alloxan-induced diabetic Wistar rats (n = 36)	Non-diabetic	Diabetic non-supplemented. Diabetic supplemented with PeO or PaO (200 mg/kg/day)	Significant reduction in blood glucose of supplemented groups (PeO + PaO) compared to the diabetic non-supplemented group.	Plasma Vitamins C and E and albumin levels were significantly increased in the supplemented groups versus the diabetic non-supplemented group.

BW, body weight; FBG, fasting blood glucose; FBP, fructose-1,6-bisphosphate; G6Pase, glucose 6-phosphatase; GLI, glibenclamide; HDL-C, high-density lipoprotein cholesterol; HFD, high-fat diet; LDL-C, low-density lipoprotein cholesterol; PaO, palm oil; PeO, peanut oil; PWE, polyphenol-rich walnut extract; STZ, streptozotocin; T2D, type 2 diabetes; TC, total cholesterol; TF, tissue factor; TG, triglycerides; VFM, visceral fat mass; VLDL-C, very low-density lipoprotein.

In vitro assessment of the T2D-related antioxidant and inflammatory capacity of nuts has largely been conducted by examining the ability of extracts to increase the resistance of human plasma or low density lipoprotein (LDL) to oxidation. Extracts of walnut [43], almond and almond skins [44,45], pistachio [46], and hazelnut [47] have been found to increase the lag time oxidation of LDL. However, little research has focused on their in vitro effects on glucose and insulin metabolism. Specifically, a hydro-ethanolic extract of cashew nut and its principal compound, anacardic acid, significantly stimulated glucose uptake in C2C12 muscle cells in a concentration-dependent manner, suggesting that it may be a potential anti-diabetic nutraceutical [48]. Moreover, cytoprotective activity of pistachio extracts (methanolic, water or ethyl acetate) against oxidative (reactive oxygen species formation) and carbonyl stress has also been reported in a T2D model in hepatocytes from rats [49].

2.2. Dried Fruits

Both in vitro and in vivo research has mostly focused on grape. Overman and collaborators showed that a grape powder extract (GPE) significantly attenuated lipopolysaccharide (LPS)-mediated inflammation in macrophages and decreased the capacity of LPS-stimulated human macrophages to inflame adipocytes and cause IR [30]. Moreover, GPE further attenuated tumor necrosis factor-α (TNF-α) mediated inflammation and IR in primary cultures of human adipocytes [31]. Grape polyphenol extract modulated in vitro membrane phospholipid fatty acid (FA) composition but also decreased muscle TG content and increased muscle glucose transporter type 4 (GLUT4) expression in high-fat-high-sucrose diet-fed rats. Overall, it improved insulin resistance status (i.e., HOMA-IR parameter) [50]. This is of considerable importance because the accumulation of muscle TG content and the modification of the muscle phospholipid fatty acid pattern may have an impact on lipid metabolism and increase the risk of developing T2D [51]. Mice fed with grape skin extract showed hypoglycaemic and anti-hyperglycaemic effects (independent of an increase in insulin release) but are probably dependent on an increase in insulin sensitivity resulting from the activation of the insulin-signaling cascade in skeletal muscle [52]. Furthermore, grape seed aqueous extract protected the pancreas against oxidative stress, inflammation and apoptosis-induced damage while preserving pancreatic function at near normal levels in diabetic rats [53].

Other DF extracts have also been evaluated. Treatment with a date fruit extract was effective at decreasing behavioral, neurophysiological, and pathological alterations induced by diabetes in the peripheral nerves of streptozotocin (STZ)-induced diabetic rats (well-characterized animal model of type 1 diabetes) [33]. Moreover, daily consumption of a low- or high-fat diet supplemented with 1% black currant powder extract (with 32% of anthocyanins) for 8 weeks reduced body weight gain and improved glucose metabolism [54].

The beneficial effect of fruit juices and fermented grape juice (i.e., wine) have also been an important focus of research. Schmatz and collaborators investigated the ex vivo effects of a moderate consumption of red wine (RW) and grape juice (GJ), and the in vitro effects of various substances (resveratrol, caffeic acid, gallic acid, quercetin and rutin) on STZ-induced diabetic rats. They demonstrated decreased platelet aggregation in diabetic-induced rats after moderate RW and GJ consumption for 45 days [55]. Similarly, resveratrol increased the hydrolysis of adenosine triphosphate (ATP), while quercetin decreased it in platelets [55]. These results were extended using a wine grape powder supplementation, which prevented hyperglycemia and IR, and reduced oxidative stress in a rat model of metabolic syndrome (MetS) [56].

Specific compounds found in both nuts and DFs were also further investigated. Quercetin and trans-resveratrol are plant polyphenols which have showed a significant reduction of IR and inflammation associated with obesity. Eid et al. showed that quercetin (isolated from lingonberry) exerted an anti-diabetic activity by stimulating adenosine monophosphate-activated protein kinase (AMPK) [40]. Moreover, quercetin also enhanced basal glucose uptake in mouse myoblast C2C12 muscle cells in the absence of insulin [40] via a mechanism which is highly analogous to metformin.

Importantly, quercetin seems to be as effective as or more effective than resveratrol in attenuating TNF-α-mediated inflammation and IR in primary human adipocytes and macrophages [32,57].

3. Epidemiological Studies on Nuts

The relationship between the consumption of different food categories and the incidence or prevalence of metabolic disorders has been explored all over the world. As is shown in Table 4, numerous epidemiological studies have assessed the associations between nut consumption and T2D. However, no studies have been published on the link between DF consumption and risk of T2D.

As far as nuts are concerned, several studies have found an inverse association between the frequency of consumption and the development of this metabolic pathology [58–64]. In the Nurses' Health Study (NHS) and NHS II cohort, the intake of different types of nut was explored [61,64]. Total nut, walnut and peanut butter intake were associated with a lower risk of T2D in women. In the NHS (n = 83,818 female subjects), those with the highest nut consumption (28 g/day; $\geq$5 days a week) had a lower relative risk (RR) of developing T2D (0.73 [95% confidence interval (CI), 0.60–0.89]) than those who never/almost never consume (0.92 [95% CI, 0.85–1.00]) [61]. Results were similar for peanut butter: the RR was 0.79 (95% CI, 0.68–0.91) in those women who had a higher intake (5 times or more a week) than those who never/almost never ate peanut butter [61]. After combining NHS and NHS II cohorts, in a total of 137,953 female subjects, Pan and collaborators found that walnut consumption was inversely associated with risk of T2D [64].

These results are in line with those of a cross-sectional study of 7,210 subjects at high CV risk within the context of the PREvención con DIeta MEDiterránea (PREDIMED) study, where the upper category of nut consumption had a lower prevalence of T2D than the lower category [63]. A recent prospective study also associated the consumption of nuts—higher than 4 times a week—with a lower risk of T2D [60]. A cross-sectional study performed in the context of the National Health and Nutrition Examination Survey (NHANES) established a relation between the homeostatic model assessment of insulin resistance (HOMA-IR) and tree nut consumption. Decreased insulin resistance and lower levels of β-cell function markers were found in the nut consumers than the non-consumers [59]. In a large cohort of the Netherlands Cohort Study (NLCS), the total nut intake was associated to lower T2D cause-specific mortality in men and women [65].

Even though current evidence shows that nuts have a strong protective effect against the progress of T2D, especially in women, some epidemiological studies have not identified this relation [66,67]. The latest systematic review and meta-analysis designed to assess the relation between nut consumption and risk of cancer and T2D was published in 2015. It included five studies that were linked to T2D. After pooling data from studies conducted in both genders, it was found that there was no statistically significant association between nut consumption and risk of developing T2D (RR = 0.98 [95% CI, 0.84–1.14]), even though the heterogeneity was significant [68].

Table 4. Summary of epidemiological studies evaluating nut consumption.

First Author (Year) [Reference]	Study Name (Design)	Number of Subjects	Years of Follow-Up	Exposure	Findings
Jiang, R.; et al. (2002) [61]	NHS (Prospective)	83,818 women	16	≥5 times/week vs. never/almost never	Nut and peanut butter consumption was inversely associated with the risk of incident T2D.
Nettleton, J.A.; et al. (2008) [58]	MESA (Prospective)	5011 men and women	5	Quintiles of low-risk food pattern	High intake of whole grains, fruit, nuts/seeds, and green leafy vegetables was inversely associated to the risk of incident T2D.
Villegas, R.; et al. (2008) [62]	SWHS (Prospective)	64,227 women	4.6	Quintiles of peanut consumption	Consumption of peanuts was associated with a decreased risk of incident T2D.
Kochar, J.; et al. (2010) [67]	PHS I (Prospective)	20,224 men	19.2	≥7 servings of nuts/week vs. rarely or never consumers	No statistically significant association was found between nut consumption and T2D in either lean or overweight/obese subjects.
Ibarrola-Jurado, N.; et al. (2013) [63]	PREDIMED (Cross-sectional)	7210 at high cardiovascular risk	Baseline	<1 serving/week, 1–3 servings/week and >3 servings/week	The upper category of nut consumption had a lower prevalence of T2D than the lowest category.
Pan, A.; et al. (2013) [64]	NHS, NHS II (Prospective)	137,953 women	10	1–3 servings/month, 1 serving/week, and ≥2 servings/week of walnuts vs. never/rarely	Higher walnut consumption is associated with a significantly lower risk of T2D incidence.
O'Neil, C.E.; et al. (2015) [59]	NHANES (Cross-sectional)	14,386 men and women	6	Tree nut consumption compared with no consumption	Tree nut consumption was associated with lower HOMA-IR
Buijsse, B.; et al. (2015) [66]	EPIC-InterAct Study (Case-cohort)	16,154 men and women	12.3 Incident cases of T2D at 6.8	Non-consumers vs. the middle tertile of consumption.	Consumption of nuts and seeds does not modify T2D risk under isocaloric conditions and independent from BMI.
Asghari, G.; et al. (2017) [60]	TLGS (prospective)	1984 men and women	6.2 ± 0.7	≥4 servings/week vs. 1 or <1 serving/week	Nut consumption was associated with a lower risk of T2D incidence.

BMI, body mass index; CVD, cardiovascular disease; HOMA-IR, homeostatic model assessment of insulin resistance; MI, myocardial infarction; T2D, type 2 diabetes. Study name acronyms: EPIC, European Prospective Investigation into Cancer; HPFS, Health Professionals Follow-Up Study; MESA, Multi-Ethnic Study of Atherosclerosis; NHANES, National Health and Nutrition Examination Survey; NHS, Nurses' Health Study; NLCS, Netherlands Cohort Study; PHS, Physicians' Health Study; PREDIMED, PREvención con DIeta MEDiterránea; SCCS, Southern Community Cohort Study; SMHS, Shanghai Men's Health Study; SWHS, Shanghai Women's Health Study; TLGS, Tehran Lipid and Glucose Study.

4. Human Clinical Trials

The effect of nut consumption on glucose and insulin metabolism has also been researched in acute and chronic clinical trials. Acute studies mostly demonstrate a decrease in postprandial glycaemia and hyperinsulinemia after nut consumption. In contrast, chronic randomized clinical trials designed to analyze the effects on glucose metabolism provided controversial results.

4.1. Nuts

4.1.1. Acute Clinical Trials on Nuts

Table 5 summarizes various acute clinical studies of nut consumption, most of which focus on almonds [69–73]. In a randomized crossover trial in healthy subjects, almond intake decreased postprandial glycaemia and insulinaemia [69]. In a dose-response study conducted in healthy individuals, almond intake attenuated the postprandial glycaemic response of white bread [70]. In impaired glucose-tolerant subjects, it was observed that the consumption of almonds with a meal also decreased blood glucose in plasma [71]. In a recent crossover study performed in pre-diabetic subjects, a preload of almonds decreased postprandial glycaemia [73]. In healthy and diabetic individuals, Cohen et al. also showed a 30% reduction in postprandial glycaemia after almond consumption compared with a starchy meal [72].

The effect of pistachio intake on postprandial glycaemia was investigated by Kendall et al. in two randomized studies. In overweight (Ow) healthy subjects, pistachio consumption was reported to have a minimal effect on postprandial glycaemia. When pistachios were included in a carbohydrate meal, the relative glycaemic response (RGR) was attenuated [74]. In a crossover trial with 20 subjects with MetS, postprandial glycaemia decreased after the consumption of pistachios (85 g) compared to white bread. In the same study, a peripheral increase in the glucagon-like peptide-1 (GLP-1) concentrations was also observed after pistachio consumption compared with the consumption of white bread [75].

For peanuts, a randomized crossover trial conducted in 13 healthy subjects reported a decreased postprandial glycaemic response after the consumption of a breakfast containing 63 g of one of the following types of peanuts: raw with skin, roasted without skin and ground-roasted without skin [76]. Similarly, in a parallel study conducted in 65 overweight and obese men, peanut consumption reduced postprandial insulinaemia levels compared to high-oleic peanut consumption [77].

Nut consumption was observed to have similar beneficial effects on glucose and insulin metabolism in the only study to analyze the effect of a mix of nuts (almonds, macadamias, walnuts, pistachios, hazelnuts and pecans). In this study conducted in 10 diabetic and 14 non-diabetic subjects, nut consumption decreased the RGR compared to white bread. Importantly, this study also reported that nut consumption improved short-term glycaemic control in patients with T2D [74].

In summary, nuts seem to have beneficial postprandial glycaemic effects when consumed alone or in combination with high carbohydrate foods, and so may potentially help to prevent and manage impaired glucose states.

Table 5. Summary of acute clinical studies analyzing the effect of nut consumption on postprandial response.

First Author (Year) [Reference]	N° of Subjects (M/F) Type of Subject (Age in Years)	Type of Nut (Study Design)	Control Group	Intervention Group	Glucose and Insulin Metabolism Outcomes	Other Outcomes
Jenkins, D.J.; et al. (2006) [69]	15 (7/8) Healthy subjects (26.3 ± 8.6)	Almonds (crossover)	97 g of white bread	- Almond meal: 60 g almonds +97 g bread - Parboiled rice meal: 68 g cheese and 14 g butter +60 g parboiled rice - Mashed potato meal: 62 g cheese and 16 g butter +68 g mashed potatoes	Almonds decrease postprandial glycaemia and insulinaemia.	Almonds are likely to decrease oxidative damage to serum proteins by decreasing glycaemic excursion and providing antioxidants.
Josse, A.R.; et al. (2007) [70]	9 (7/2) Healthy subjects (27.8±6.9)	Almonds (crossover dose-response study)	White bread	- White bread +30 g almonds - White bread +60 g almonds - White bread +90 g almonds	The 90-g almond meal resulted in a significantly lower GI than the white bread control meal	
Mori, A.M.; et al. (2011) [71]	14 (8/6) IGT (39.3 ± 10.9)	Almonds (crossover)	75 g of available CHO (No almonds)	75 g of available CHO from: - Whole almonds - Almond butter - Defatted almond flour - Almond oil	Whole almonds significantly attenuated second-meal and daylong blood glucose IAUC.	GLP-1 concentrations did not significantly vary between treatments.
Kendall, C.W.; et al. (2011) [74]	10 (3/7) Ow healthy subjects (48.3 ± 6.4)	Pistachios (crossover)	White bread	Study 1: - 28, 56 and 84 g pistachios - 28, 56 and 84 g Study 2: - 56 g of pistachios + different commonly consumed carbohydrate foods (50 g available carbohydrate).	Pistachios consumed alone had a minimal effect on postprandial glycaemia. Pistachios consumed with a carbohydrate meal attenuated the RGR.	
Cohen, A.E. and Johnston, C.S. (2011) [72]	20 (6/14) Healthy subjects (n = 13) and T2D subjects (n = 7) (Healthy: 53.0 ± 3 and T2D: 66.0 ± 3.3)	Almonds (postprandial crossover trial)	No almond meal	28 g almonds enriched meal	The ingestion of almonds immediately before a starchy meal significantly reduced postprandial glycaemia by 30%.	
Kendall, C.W.; et al. (2011) [78]	24 (11/13) Healthy (n = 14) and T2D subjects (n = 10) (Healthy: 36.0 ± 4 and T2D: 68.0 ± 2)	Mixed nuts (i.e., almonds, macadamias, walnuts, pistachios, hazelnuts and pecans) (crossover)	White bread	3 doses of 30, 60 and 90 g of mixed nuts	Nuts improve short-term glycaemic control in patients with T2D.	

Table 5. *Cont.*

First Author (Year) [Reference]	N° of Subjects (M/F) Type of Subject (Age in Years)	Type of Nut (Study Design)	Control Group	Intervention Group	Glucose and Insulin Metabolism Outcomes	Other Outcomes
Reis, C.E.; et al. (2011) [76]	13 (4/9) Healthy subjects (28.5 ± 10)	Peanuts (crossover)	Cheese sandwich	63 g of: - raw peanuts with skin - roasted peanuts without skin - ground-roasted peanuts without skin	The ingestion of ground-roasted peanuts without skin for breakfast leads to a lower CHO intake and reduced postprandial glycaemic response.	
Moreira, A.P.; et al. (2014) [77]	65 men Ow/Ob (Range: 18–50)	Conventional peanuts and high-oleic peanuts (parallel)	56 g biscuit	- 56 g conventional peanuts ($n = 21$) - 56 g high-oleic peanuts ($n = 23$)	Conventional peanut consumption was associated with decreased postprandial insulinaemia, which might be beneficial for saving β-cell function, independently of the influence on LPS concentrations.	
Kendall, C.W.; et al. (2014) [75]	20 (8/12) Subjects with MetS (54.0 ± 8)	Pistachios (crossover)	Control 1: white bread Control 2: (white bread + butter + cheese)	Test meal 1: WB + 85 g of pistachios Test meal 2: 85 g of pistachios	Pistachio consumption reduced postprandial glycaemia compared with white bread.	Pistachio consumption increased GLP-1 levels compared with white bread.
Crouch, M.A. and Slater, R.T. (2016) [73]	20 (13/7) Subjects with pre-diabetes * (Mean: 60.8)	Almonds (crossover)	No almonds	12 units of dry-roasted almonds	A low-calorie almond preload "appetizer" decreased postprandial hyperglycemia.	

Age is shown as mean ± SD unless otherwise stated. BMI, body mass index; CHO, carbohydrate; GLP-1, glucagon-like peptide-1; HbA$_{1c}$, glycated hemoglobin; IAUC, incremental area under the curve; IGT, impaired glucose tolerance; LPS, lipopolysaccharide; MetS, metabolic syndrome; M/F, male/female; Ob, obese; Ow, overweight; RGR, relative glycaemic responses; T2D, type 2 diabetes; WB, white bread. * also include "isolated 1-h glucose > 160 mg/dL".

4.1.2. Chronic Clinical Trials on Nuts

Most of the RCTs have compared nut-enriched diets with control diets in order to analyze their effects on lipid profile, and blood glucose and insulin concentrations as a secondary outcome. However, some, mainly conducted in subjects with T2D [72,79–84], but also in pre-diabetic [85], hyperlipemic [86], overweight/obese [87] and healthy individuals [88], were specifically designed to assess changes in glucose or insulin metabolism after nut consumption (Table 6).

In 2002, Lovejoy and coworkers evaluated the effect of an almond-enriched diet in 20 healthy and 30 T2D subjects in two different studies [79]. Healthy subjects, supplemented with 100 g almonds/day for 4 weeks and advised to reduce their energy intake by an equivalent amount, did not change their insulin sensitivity, whereas their body weight increased and their lipid profile improved. In a second study, subjects with T2D were randomized following a crossover design to one of 4 diets with different fat contents (25% or 37%) with 10% of fat from almonds or from olive or canola oil, with a minimum washout of 2 weeks between periods. Fat source (almond vs. oil) or fat level (high fat vs. low fat) were not observed to have any significant effect on either the glucose or insulin index. In contrast, in a crossover study conducted in 20 Chinese patients with T2D and mild-hyperlipidemia assigned to either a control diet (National Cholesterol Education Program (NCEP) step II diet) or an almond-enriched diet (with almonds replacing the 20% total daily calorie intake) for 4 weeks, a significant decrease in fasting insulin and glucose concentrations together with an improvement of HOMA-IR were reported during the almond phase [80]. In a similar crossover study conducted in 48 diabetic patients who received 50 g/day of pistachios and a pistachio-free diet (12 weeks each period), with an 8-week washout, a significant improvement in fasting blood glucose (FBG) and HbA$_{1c}$ was observed during the pistachio consumption, while no changes in HOMA-IR were reported [83]. Recently, Gulati and coworkers conducted a pre-post intervention study in a group of 50 Asian Indians who consumed 20% of total energy in the form of whole raw almonds for 24 weeks preceded by a control diet free of nuts. Although no changes in FBG were observed during the almond consumption, the authors found a significant reduction in glycosylated hemoglobin, together with an improvement in other T2D risk factors such as waist circumference or inflammation status [84]. To determine whether the beneficial effect of nut consumption on glucose and insulin metabolism could also be extended to pre-diabetic subjects our group conducted a randomized crossover study in 54 pre-diabetic subjects who consumed a pistachio-supplemented diet (55 g pistachio/day) and a control diet (nut-free diet), each for 4 months with a 2-week washout period. We found a beneficial effect of pistachio intake on fasting glucose, insulin, and HOMA-IR. Other cardiometabolic risk markers such as fibrinogen, oxidized LDL, platelet factor 4 and GLP-1 were also modified appropriately during the consumption of pistachios [85].

Changes in fasting glucose or insulin levels, HOMA-IR and glycosylated hemoglobin have also been assessed as secondary outcomes in several clinical feeding trials with different designs (parallel, crossover) and subject characteristics (i.e., healthy, overweight/obese, TD2, MetS), mainly using walnuts and almonds, and with different intervention lengths (from 2 weeks to 2 years). The results obtained are controversial. Although most studies found no improvement in glucose/insulin metabolism [89–103], others reported a significant reduction in FBG levels [89,92,104,105], fasting insulin or insulin resistance [90,92,106,107] and HbA$_{1c}$ [92]. However, a meta-analysis of RCTs including 25 trials with a total of 1,650 particpants who were otherwise healthy or had dyslipidaemia, metabolic syndrome or type 2 diabetes mellitus showed that the consumption of tree nuts led to modest decreases in fasting blood glucose compared with control diet interventions [108].

Table 6. Summary of chronic clinical trials and their characteristics in the context of nut consumption.

First Author (Year) [Reference]	N° of Subjects (M/F) Type of Subjects (Age in Years)	Nut Study Design (Length of the Intervention)	Control Group	Intervention Group(s)	Glucose and Insulin Metabolism Outcomes	Other Outcomes
Lovejoy, J.C.; et al. (2002) [79]	30 (13/17) T2D subjects (mean ± SEM: 53.8 ± 1.9)	Almonds Crossover (1 month per period)	HF-Control LF-Control	HF-HA LF-HA	No significant changes in glycaemia were observed.	Total cholesterol was lowest after the HF-HA diet. HDL-C was significantly decreased after the almond diet; however, no significant effect of fat source on LDL: HDL was reported.
Jenkins, D.J.A.; et al. (2008) [86]	27 (15/12) Hyperlipidemic subjects (64 ± 9)	Almonds Crossover (1 month per period)	147 ± 6 g/day of muffins	Almonds (73 ± 3 g/day) Half portion of almonds (37 ± 2 g/day) plus muffins (75 ± 3 g/day) Isoenergetic (mean, 423 Kcal/day)	No significant changes were observed in FBG, insulin, C-peptide, or HOMA-IR. The 24-h urinary C-peptide output, as a marker of 24-h insulin secretion, was significantly reduced by the half-and full-dose almonds in comparison to the control muffin diet after adjustment for urinary creatinine output.	There were no significant treatment differences in BW.
Claesson, A.L.; et al. 2009 [88]	25 (11/14) Healthy subjects (range: 19–30)	Peanuts Parallel (2 weeks)	Addition of 20 kcal/kg-BW of candy to the regular caloric intake.	Addition of 20 kcal/kg-BW of roasted peanuts to the regular caloric intake.	Plasma-insulin and C-peptide increased in the candy group, but not in the peanut group. FBG was not modified.	Energy intake increased similarly in both groups. BW and WC increased significantly only in the candy group. At the end of the study LDL-C and ApoB/ApoA-1-ratio were higher in the candy group than in the peanut group.
Cohen, A.E.; et al. (2011) [72]	13 (7/6) T2D subjects (66.0 ± 3.3)	Almonds Parallel (3 months)	Nut-free diet	Diet enriched with almonds (28 g, 5 times/week)	Significant reduction of HbA1c in the almond group compared to the nut-free diet group.	Chronic almond ingestion was associated with a reduction in BMI as compared with no change in the nut-free diet group.
Li, S.C.; et al. (2011) [80]	20 (9/11) T2D subjects (Mean: 58)	Almonds Crossover (1 month per period)	NCEP step II diet (control diet); CHO (56 E%), protein (17 E%), and fat (27 E%).	Almonds were added to the control diet to replace 20% of total daily calorie intake.	Compared with subjects in the control diet, those in the almond diet reduced the levels of fasting insulin, FBG, and HOMA-IR.	Almond intake decreased TC, LDL-C, and LDL-C/HDL-C. The almond diet enhanced plasma α-tocopherol level compared with control diet.
Damavandi, R.D.; et al. (2013) [81]	45 (15/33) Medicated T2D subjects (55.68 ± 7.74)	Hazelnuts Parallel (2 months)	Control diet	10% of total daily calorie intake was replaced with hazelnuts	No significant differences in FBG between groups.	No changes in BMI were reported. Significant HDL-C reduction in control group was observed. Although the hazelnut group achieved a greater reduction in TG concentrations than the control group, these changes were non-significant.
Hernández-Alonso, P.; et al. (2014) [85]	54 (29/25) Subjects with Pre-D Mean: 55 (range: 53.4–56.8)	Crossover (4 months per period)	Nut-free diet: the energy intake of other fatty foods, mostly olive oil, was adjusted to compensate for the energy from pistachios included in the PD.	Pistachio diet was supplemented with 2 ounces of pistachio (57 g/day)	FBG, insulin, and HOMA-IR decreased significantly after the chronic pistachio period compared with the nut-free period.	Fibrinogen, oxidized-LDL, and PF-4 significantly decreased under the pistachio period compared to the nut-free period, whereas GLP-1 increased.

Table 6. *Cont.*

First Author (Year) [Reference]	N° of Subjects (M/F) Type of Subjects (Age in Years)	Nut Study Design (Length of the Intervention)	Control Group	Intervention Group(s)	Glucose and Insulin Metabolism Outcomes	Other Outcomes
Lasa, A.; et al. (2014) [82]	191 (77/114) T2D subjects (Mean: 67)	Mixed nuts Parallel (1 year)	LFD	Mediterranean diets supplemented with either virgin olive oil or mixed nuts	Increased values of the adiponectin/leptin ratio and adiponectin/HOMA-IR ratio and decreased values of WC were observed in the three groups.	In both Mediterranean diet groups, but not in the LFD group, this was associated with a significant reduction in BW.
Parham, M.; et al. (2014) [83]	44 (11/33) T2D subjects (Mean: 51)	Pistachios Crossover (3 months per period)	Previous diet without pistachios	Two snacks of 25 g pistachios/day	Marked decrease in HbA$_{1c}$ and FBG concentrations in the pistachio diet group compared with the control group.	There were no overall significant changes in BMI, blood pressure, HOMA-IR, or CRP concentrations.
Le, T.; et al. (2016) [87]	213 women Ow/Ob subjects (Mean: 50)	Walnuts Parallel (1 year)	Control 1: a lower fat (20 E%), higher CHO (65 E%) diet. Control 2: lower CHO (45 E%), higher fat (35 E%) diet	Walnut-enriched diet: high fat (35 E%), lower CHO (45 E%) diet.	Insulin sensitivity and CRP levels improved after walnut-rich diet	TG decreased in all study arms at 6 months. The walnut-rich diet increased HDL-C more than either the lower fat or lower CHO diet. The walnut-rich diet also reduced LDL-C.

Age is shown as mean ± SD unless otherwise stated. Apo, apolipoprotein; BMI, Body mass index; BW, body weight; CHO, carbohydrate; CRP, C-reactive protein; E%, energy percentage; FBG, fasting blood glucose; GLP-1, glucagon-like peptide-1; HA: high almond; HbA$_{1c}$, glycated hemoglobin; HDL-C, high-density lipoprotein cholesterol; HF, high fat; HOMA-IR, homeostatic model assessment of insulin resistance; LDL-C, low-density lipoprotein cholesterol; LF: low fat; LFD, LF diet; M/F, male/female; NCEP, National Cholesterol Education Program; NS, non-significant; Ob, obese; Ow, overweight; PF-4, platelet factor-4; PM, post-menopausal; Pre-D, pre-diabetes; T2D, type 2 diabetes; TC, total cholesterol; TG, triglycerides; WC, waist circumference; WHtR, waist-to-height ratio.

4.2. Dried Fruits

4.2.1. Acute Clinical Trials on Dried Fruits

Less research has been carried out into DFs than into nuts. However, the findings to date point to a beneficial effect of DFs on postprandial glucose regulation and glycaemic control in T2D subjects.

The putative effect of DFs on postprandial glycaemia and insulinaemia has been studied mainly using raisins (Table 7). However, some research into dried plums has also been published.

First, in 1989 Rasmussen and coworkers evaluated in healthy and T2D subjects the postprandial effects of three meals: raw rolled oats, oatmeal porridge, or a mixture of raw rolled oats with raisins, compared to a control glucose ingestion [109]. The substitution of 25% of the starch meal with raisins (i.e., simple sugars) did not affect blood glucose or insulin responses. In addition, a similar glucose and insulin response in both normal and T2D subjects were reported [109]. Other researchers investigated the postprandial effect of raisins consumed alone. When the GI was investigated in three different groups (sedentary, aerobically trained or pre-diabetic subjects), no significant differences were found among groups, even though the GI (55–69) it seemed moderate for aerobically trained adults, and low (GI, ≤55) for the other groups [110]. Kanellos and collaborators found a moderate GI of raisins in healthy and T2D subjects [111], whereas Esfahani et al. found that raisins were low-GI and glycaemic load (GL) foods in healthy subjects [112]. Recently, researchers have found that even though the same available CHO content from raisins and glucose generated a similar postprandial response, raisins significantly modulated the levels of GIP, ghrelin and ghrelin/obestatin ratio, with important implications in terms of appetite regulation and overall insulin secretion [113]. In overweight women, researchers determined that dried plums had a lower plasma glucose and insulin incremental area under the curve (IAUC) than an isoenergetic low-fat cookie meal [114].

Overall, results suggest that raisins have a beneficial postprandial glucose and insulin effect, which may cautiously be extrapolated to other DFs considering their overall macronutrient composition.

Table 7. Summary of acute clinical studies analyzing the effect of dried fruit consumption on postprandial response.

First Author (Year) [Reference]	N° of Subjects (M/F) Type of Subject (Age in Years)	Dried Fruit (Study Design)	Control Group	Intervention Group(s)	Glucose and Insulin Metabolism Outcomes	Other Outcomes
Rasmussen, O.; et al. (1989) [109]	20 (9/11) Healthy (n = 11) and T2D subjects (n = 9) (Healthy: 30 ± 2; T2D subjects: 67 ± 2)	Raisins (crossover)	75 g (healthy) or 50 g (T2D) of CHO	Raw rolled oats; oatmeal porridge or a mixture of raw rolled oats with raisins	Substitution of 25% of the starch meal with raisins (simple sugars) did not affect blood glucose or insulin responses	In normal and T2D subjects, the three meals produce similar glucose and insulin response curves.
Kim, Y.; et al. (2008) [110]	10 S; 11 AT and 10 Pre-D (S (25.7 ± 1.3), AT (23.1 ± 1.0), Pre-D (50.0 ± 2.6))	Raisins (crossover)	50 g of available CHO from glucose	50 g of available CHO from raisins	NS differences among groups. The GI of raisins seemed lower (≤55) in the S and P groups compared to moderate (GI, 56–69) in the A group. The insulinaemic index of raisins was not different among groups.	
Furchner-Evanson, A.; et al. (2010) [114]	19 women ow subjects (39.2 ± 0.7)	Dried plums (crossover)	White bread (238 Kcal)	Dried plums (238 Kcal) Low-fat cookies (238 Kcal)	Dried plums elicited lower plasma glucose and insulin IAUC than low-fat cookies.	The satiety index IAUC was greater for the dried plums than low-fat cookies, and tended to promote a greater plasma ghrelin AOC
Kanellos, P.T.; et al. (2013) [111]	30 (17/13) Healthy and T2D subjects (n = 15 each) (Healthy: 25.9 ± 0.8; T2D: 63.2 ± 1.7)	Corinthian raisins (crossover)	50 g of glucose	74 g of Corinthian raisins; 50 g of available CHO	Significantly different glucose peaks between raisins and glucose in healthy and in diabetic subjects. Glycaemic and insulinaemic responses were decreased after raisin consumption compared to glucose ingestion.	
Esfahani, A.; et al. (2014) [112]	10 (4/6) Healthy subjects (39 ± 11)	Raisins (crossover)	108 g of white bread; 50 g available CHO (consumed on two separate occasions)	R50: 69 g raisins; 50 g available CHO R20: 28 g raisins; 20 g available CHO	The raisin meals, R50 and R20, resulted in significantly reduced postprandial glucose and insulin responses compared with white bread	Raisins were determined to be low in GI, GL and insulinaemic index.
Kaliora, A.C.; et al. (2017) [113]	10 Healthy normo-weight subjects (26.3 ± 0.8)	Raisins (crossover)	50 g of glucose	74 g of raisins; 50 g of available CHO	At 60 min, glucose and insulin levels were maximum in both groups.	GIP was lower after raising intake compared to glucose intake at 60 and 120 min postprandially. Ghrelin was lower after raisin intake compared to glucose intake at 120 and at 180 min post-ingestion. No differences were reported for GLP-1, apelin or obestatin in either trial.

Age is shown as mean ± SD unless otherwise stated. AT, aerobically trained; AOC, area over the curve; CHO, carbohydrates; GI, glycaemic index; GL, glycaemic load; GLP-1, glucagon-like peptide-1; IAUC, incremental area under the curve; M/F, male/female; NS, non-significant; ow, overweight; Pre-D, pre-diabetic; S, sedentary; T2D, type 2 diabetes; WB, white bread.

4.2.2. Chronic Clinical Trials on Dried Fruits

The study of the beneficial effects of chronic DF consumption also focuses on raisins (Table 8). Randomized clinical trials have been conducted in healthy [115], overweight or obese [116,117], T2D subjects [118,119], or a combination of the three [120]. In a 6-week parallel trial in healthy subjects, Puglisi et al. included 150 g/day of raisins into subjects' habitual diet or increased their physical activity (or combined them both). Neither FPG nor insulin levels were different among groups or compared to baseline. However, the inflammation status reported by plasma TNF-α significantly decreased in the raisin intervention [115].

The results for overweight or obese subjects do not show a significant improvement in glucose or insulin levels after the consumption of raisins [116] or dried plums [117]. However, these studies are only short (2 weeks) which makes it impossible to analyze the chronic effect. In fact, in a parallel study conducted in Ow/Ob subjects, comparing raisin consumption (270 Kcal/day) with a snack (300 Kcal/day) for 12 weeks, researchers [120] found that even though FGP or insulin were not affected by either intervention, HbA$_{1c}$ levels and postprandial glucose levels had been reduced by raisin consumption by the end of the trial. This suggests a beneficial effect of raisin consumption on glycaemic control in Ow/Ob subjects with pre-D. Importantly, raisin intake also improved systolic blood pressure (SBP) and diastolic blood pressure (DBP) and had a null effect on body weight [120].

Two studies have been conducted in individuals with T2D. A parallel study comparing the consumption of 36 g of raisins versus the habitual diet free of raisins or grapes for 24 weeks did not find any change in either body weight or in glycaemic control and lipid profile, but the total antioxidant capacity increased and the DBP decreased after raisin consumption [118]. Likewise, the consumption of raisins as a snack (84 g/day, 270 Kcal/day) for 12 weeks significantly reduced the postprandial glucose response in T2D subjects compared to an alternative snack (300 Kcal/day) for 12 weeks. A non-significant trend to a reduction in fasting glucose and HbA$_{1c}$ was also observed in the same group of raisin consumers [119].

The results of DF consumption on glycaemia/insulinaemia point to a beneficial effect. However, novel acute and long-term RCTs assessing other types of DF should be carried out in order to corroborate and expand what is known about raisins.

Table 8. Summary of chronic clinical trials and their characteristics in the context of dried fruit consumption.

First Author (Year) [Reference]	N° of Subjects (M/F) Type of Subject (Age in Years)	Study Design (Length of the Intervention)	Control Group	Intervention Group(s)	Glucose and Insulin Metabolism Outcomes	Other Outcomes
Puglisi, M.J.; et al. (2008) [115]	34 (17/17 PM) Healthy (range: 50–70)	Raisin Parallel (6 weeks)	Walk (increase in the steps taken per day)	150 g/day of raisins. Walk + 150 g/day of raisins	Changes in FBG and insulin values did not differ among intervention groups or from baseline. Plasma TNF-α decreased in the raisin group but no differences were reported between groups.	Plasma TC and LDL-C decreased in all the intervention groups.
Rankin, J.W.; et al. (2008) [116]	17 (8/9) Ow (26.5 ± 7.6)	Raisin Crossover (2 weeks per period)	Jelly candy (264 Kcal/day)	90 g/day raisins (264 Kcal/day)	NS changes in FBG or markers of inflammation or endothelial dysfunction after the raisin intervention.	Fasting protein-free ORAC was modestly higher after the raisin intervention than the jelly candy intervention.
Howarth, L.; et al. (2010) [117]	26 women Ow/Ob (range: 25–54)	Dried plums Crossover (2 weeks per period)	Low-fat cookies (200 Kcal/day)	Dried plums (200 Kcal/day)	No changes were found in plasma glucose or insulin levels in any intervention.	Plasma TG concentration was unchanged by dried plum consumption and was higher after the consumption of low-fat cookies. Incorporation of dried plums or low-fat cookies into the diet did not alter energy intake or BW.
Anderson, J.W.; et al. (2014) [120]	46 (21/25) Ow/Ob with Pre-D or at T2D risk. (snack (mean: 61.1), raisins (mean: 60.3))	Raisins Parallel (12 weeks)	Snacks (300 Kcal/day)	84 g/day of raisins (270 Kcal/day)	Fasting HbA$_{1c}$ levels were significantly reduced after raisin intake, whereas FBG and insulin levels were not significantly affected by the intake of raisins or snacks. Postprandial glucose levels were significantly reduced by raisin intake vs. snacks.	Raisin intake was associated with reductions in SBP and DBP. BW did not significantly change within or between groups.
Kanellos, P.T.; et al. (2014) [118]	48 (25/23) T2D (raisins (63.7 ± 6.3), control (63 ± 8.5))	Corinthian raisins Parallel (24 weeks)	Usual diet avoiding grapes and raisins	36 g/day of Corinthian raisins	BW, glycaemic control, and lipid profile were not changed in either arm of the intervention. Patients in the CR arm reduced their DBP and increased their total antioxidant potential compared with baseline values and the control group.	No change in CRP was observed. A significant difference in plasma circulating p-hydroxybenzoic acid was observed between groups at the end of the trial.
Bays, H.; et al. (2015) [119]	46 (19/27) T2D (mean: 58)	Dark raisins Parallel (12 weeks)	Snack group (300 Kcal/day)	84 g/day of dark raisins group (270 Kcal/day)	Compared to the snack group, those who consumed raisins reduced their postprandial glucose levels, and an NS trend to a reduction in fasting glucose and HbA$_{1c}$. NS changes in BW, fasting insulin, HOMA-IR or lipid profile between intervention groups.	Compared to alternative processed snacks, those who consumed raisins had a significant reduction in SBP but not a significant reduction in DBP.

Age is shown as mean ± SD unless otherwise stated. BW, body weight; CRP, C-reactive protein; DBP, diastolic blood pressure; FBG, fasting blood glucose; HbA$_{1c}$, glycated hemoglobin; HOMA-IR, homeostatic model assessment of insulin resistance; LDL-C, low-density lipoprotein cholesterol; M/F, male/female; NS, non-significant; Ob, obese; ORAC, oxygen radical absorbance capacity; Ow, overweight; pre-D, pre-diabetes; PM, postmenopausal women; SBP, systolic blood pressure; T2D, type 2 diabetes; TC, total cholesterol; TG, triglycerides; TNF-α, tumor necrosis factor-α.

5. Potential Mechanisms Linking Nut and Dried Fruit Consumption to Glucose and Insulin Metabolism

5.1. Nut- and Dried Fruit-Related Nutrients and Their Role in Glucose and Insulin Metabolism

Fiber Content in Nuts and Dried Fruits

Both nuts and DFs are high in dietary fiber [9]. Diets rich in complex CHO and fiber are associated with increased insulin sensitivity and reduced plasma insulin levels, promoting better glycaemic control in diabetic patients [121]. Soluble fiber increases gastric distension, viscosity in the gastrointestinal tract, and slower absorption of macronutrients [122]. As a consequence, the speed of CHO absorption and the concentration of postprandial glucose tend to be lower after the ingestion of fiber-rich foods than foods or meals poor in fibers [123].

Fiber is resistant to enzymatic digestion in the small intestine and thus susceptible to fermentation by bacteria in the colon. It produces short chain fatty acids (SCFA, e.g., acetate, propionate and butyrate) which reduce the production of hepatic glucose and stimulate the secretion of GLP-1 [124,125]. Incretins such as GLP-1 and gastric inhibitory polypeptide (GIP) stimulate the secretion of insulin by β-cells and promote the proliferation of these cells, favoring the maintenance of normal blood glucose levels [125]. The secretion of GLP-1—which is mainly performed by enteroendocrine L-cells of the gastrointestinal tract -is partly mediated by monosaccharides, peptides and amino-acids, MUFA and PUFA as well as by SCFA. Therefore, the positive influence of GLP-1 on blood glucose homeostasis, appetite sensations, and food intake provides a strong rationale for its therapeutic potential in the nutritional management of T2D and obesity [126].

Overall fiber contained in nuts and DFs is also able to decrease postprandial glycaemic levels and this could be a strategy for increasing insulin sensitivity which improves T2D and several other CV risk factors for chronic diseases [74,127].

Carbohydrate Content—Glycaemic Index of Nuts and Dried Fruits

It should be noted that nuts are relatively low in CHO (approximately 15% of the total energy) whereas DFs have a high amount of CHO (60–80%). Nuts have a low glycaemic index and therefore increase the blood glucose level less and require less insulin secretion, thus favoring the control of T2D. However, because DFs are high in carbohydrates and fiber, their specific GI has been the object of considerable study. The GI of raisins was first evaluated in three heterogeneous groups of subjects (aerobically trained, sedentary or pre-diabetic) and was described between 49 and 69, therefore corresponding to the low-to-moderate GI foods [110]. However, later studies have reported that raisins are in the low GI category in healthy subjects (a GI of 49.4 and an insulinemic index of 47.1) [15]. This suggests a favorable postprandial glucose and insulin response [112], that could be explained by the high proportion of fructose that DFs contain.

Overall, the inclusion of both nuts and DFs in a balanced diet may reduce the overall glycaemic index of the diet, with benefits to glycaemic and insulinemic control in both healthy and T2D subjects [128].

Fat Content in Nuts

The high content of MUFA and PUFA in nuts seems to enhance the reduction of IR, thus consequently reducing the risk of developing T2D [129–131]. However, the mechanisms by which these fatty acids (FA) affect insulin sensitivity are not yet fully understood [132]. It is believed, however, that the FAs present in the phospholipids of different cell membranes are affected by the type of fatty acid intake, thus affecting insulin sensitivity. The different unsaturated FAs that are part of the cell membrane influence the action of insulin via affecting the binding or affinity of insulin to its cellular receptor [133]. It is hypothesized that a higher unsaturation of FA in the cell membrane facilitates the movement of the glucose receptor to the cell surface, thus increasing insulin sensitivity [134].

In addition, as we have seen, unsaturated fatty acids act through the stimulation of GLP-1 secretion, thus improving the efficiency of β-cells. SFA and MUFA act on the lipogenic gene expression, while PUFA inhibit the expression of these genes, partly by binding and activating nuclear receptors, such as those activated by peroxisome proliferators (PPAR) [131]. It has been suggested that the activation of PPAR has a therapeutic role in the treatment of T2D, because it induces fatty acid clearance by the adipose tissue, decreasing its plasma levels and thus increasing insulin sensitivity in the muscle [135].

Mineral Content in Nuts and Dried Fruits

Nuts contain relatively high quantities of different minerals such as potassium, magnesium and calcium, whereas DF contains more moderate quantities (mainly potassium, magnesium and boron). Magnesium has been associated with beneficial effects on glycaemic control [136]. Low magnesium levels have been implicated in IR development [124]. In fact, kidneys lose the ability to retain magnesium in periods of acute hyperglycemia. It is excreted in the urine, leading to low mineral blood levels. It has been shown that correcting this depletion improves response and insulin action. Magnesium deficiency also interferes with the reactions that use or produce ATP, thus altering the enzyme cascade involved in the CHO metabolism and favoring the development of T2D [137].

Therefore, the minerals present in nuts and DF could explain the relationship observed between magnesium intake and the lower risk of developing T2D and other chronic diseases [138,139].

Other Bioactive Compounds in Nuts and Dried Fruits

The other bioactive compounds contained in nuts and DF could partially explain their protective anti-oxidant and anti-inflammatory properties [2] and their implication in glucose and insulin metabolism (and therefore in T2D). Significant evidence suggests that polyphenol-rich diets have the ability to protect against diabetes [140]. It appears that anthocyanins (or anthocyanin-rich foods) are inversely associated to the risk of T2D, but there is no association for other polyphenol subclasses [141,142]. Dietary polyphenols have some benefits for T2D: they protect pancreatic β-cells against glucose toxicity and they have anti-inflammatory and anti-oxidant effects, among other things. Quercetin is a member of the flavonoid class of polyphenols which is abundant in such foods as fruits, vegetables, nuts and seeds [143]. Several in vitro studies have sought to elucidate the mechanisms behind the antidiabetic properties of quercetin: for example the inhibition of the α-amylase and α-glucosidase activities, and the prevention of the lipid peroxidation of pancreatic tissue homogenates [144]. Moreover, ellagic acid (EA) is another polyphenol which naturally occurs in some fruits, such as berries (strawberries and red and black raspberries), nuts, and pomegranates [145]. There is emerging in vitro evidence that EA may ameliorate symptoms of chronic metabolic diseases—by decreasing chronic inflammation at the expression level—which include dyslipidemia, IR and T2D [146–148]. Despite the growing amount of information on EA, a definitive mechanism of action has not been established. This may be attributed to the complexity of EA metabolism, which is governed by various factors [145].

A growing body of evidence suggests that dietary agents and the non-nutrient components of fruits, vegetables and nuts can affect epigenetic processes related to T2D [149,150]. Epigenetics generally refers to heritable and reversible changes affecting gene expression and chromatin organization that are not due to alterations in the DNA sequence [151,152]. No specific data is available on the role of nuts and DFs in T2D epigenetics. However, dietary polyphenol resveratrol—most abundant in the skin of grapes and raisins, but also found in peanuts and cranberries [153]—and other phytochemicals (e.g., curcumin) have proved to be effective agents against cancer and to act through epigenetic mechanisms that affect the global epigenome [154,155]. However, future studies are needed to determine the biological importance of the altered tissue-specific DNA methylation in T2D resulting from nutritional modifications [152].

5.2. Cellular and Molecular Mechanisms Linking Nut and Dried Fruit Consumption and the Prevention and/or Management of T2D/IR

Gene Expression

Some studies have analyzed the effect of nut and DF consumption on changes in the gene expression of particular cells and/or tissues and its relationship with glucose and insulin metabolism or T2D. In particular, a crossover study conducted in pre-diabetic subjects consuming pistachio for 4 months reported a downregulation of interleukin-6 (*IL-6*) and resistin (*RETN*) genes in leukocytes, whereas the pistachio diet led to a lower significant increase of solute carrier family 2 member 4 (*SLC2A4*, codifying GLUT4) [85]. Consistent with this attenuation in the expression of glucose transporters, leukocytes significantly reduced the uptake of glucose following pistachio consumption, suggesting a decrease in the cell hyperactivity described in T2D.

To our knowledge no published studies have evaluated gene expression after the consumption of DF. However, a translational study conducted in 120 healthy young subjects has shown that individuals in the highest tertile of fruit and vegetable consumption had statistically lower values of the expression of some pro-inflammatory marker genes such as intercellular adhesion molecule-1 (ICAM-1), IL-6 and TNF-α, in peripheral blood mononuclear cells (PBMC) [156].

Therefore, these results shed new light on the nutrient-gene interactions in nuts and DFs. However, further research is needed.

MicroRNAs

The modulatory role of nuts and DF on the expression of genes related to inflammation, oxidative stress and glucose metabolism can also be mediated by the effect of nutrients on microRNAs. MicroRNAs (miRNAs) are RNA molecules that belong to a family of small non-coding RNAs with 20 to 25 nucleotides [157,158] that post-transcriptionally and negatively regulate gene expression.

Research into the nutritional modulation of miRNA is still in its infancy and few studies have assessed whether a specific dietary pattern, food, supplements or a particular nutrient can influence miRNA levels [159]. In humans, consumption of grape extract rich in resveratrol, and Vitamin supplementation modulated specific miRNAs towards a healthier status [160]. Similarly, a PUFA-enriched diet including almonds and walnuts was effective at modifying several miRNAs [161]. More recently, pistachio consumption in pre-diabetic subjects significantly diminished the levels of miR-375 and miR-192, both related to the glucose and insulin metabolism [162]. However, there is still much to discover about the exact mechanisms linking miRNAs with the glucose and insulin metabolism and the dietary modulation of miRNA expression.

Microbiota and Metabolomic Modulation

In recent years, many studies have pointed out that the gut microbiome might make an important contribution to the development of insulin resistance and T2D. Several mechanisms related to the composition of gut microbes—including changes in bowel permeability, endotoxemia and interaction with bile acids—may contribute to the onset of insulin resistance. On the other hand, it is well established that long-term dietary patterns and shorter-term dietary variation influence gut microbiota composition [163]. Many potential prebiotic components can be present in a particular food. For example, the fermentation of fiber from nuts and DF to beneficial end-products (e.g., butyric acid) and the biotransformation of phytochemicals (i.e., tocopherols, phytosterols, and phenolic compounds) are associated with the transition to a healthier microbiota composition [2,164].

There is little information on the putative effect of nuts and DF on microbiota modulation. In fact, only two publications have evaluated the effect of nut consumption (almonds and pistachios) on changes in microbiota. Mandalari et al. conducted an in vitro study with almond skins and they found that almond fiber significantly altered the composition of gut bacteria, specifically *Bifidobacteria*, thus showing that almond skins had a potential prebiotic use [165]. Some years later, Ukhanova and collaborators carried out two separate crossover feeding trials with nuts and pistachios, and showed that they both significantly affected microbiota modulation [166]. However, a greater prebiotic effect was found after pistachio intake. In fact, pistachio increased the number of butyrate-producing bacteria, which are potentially beneficial, whereas the numbers of *Bifidobacteria* were not affected by the consumption of either nut [166].

Recently, dietary polyphenols have been found to be involved in gut microbiota dysbiosis processes which may lead to a reduction of fat storage, inflammation and IR (reviewed in [167]). In fact, a cranberry extract also altered the gut microbiome of mice by increasing mucin-degrading bacteria, a potential link to reverse the dysbiosis and metabolic inflammation underlying T2D [168].

Very few studies have been made on metabolomic modulation after nut and DF intake. Of the studies that have been made, some have evaluated changes in metabolites after a chronic consumption of nuts. They showed a modulation in the levels of metabolites such as raffinose, (12Z)-9,10-dihydroxyoctadec-12-enoate, sucrose, together with some modulations of plasma amino acids and fatty acids [169], and a modulation of gut-related metabolites and cis-aconitate, an intermediate of tricarboxylic acid [170], after pistachio consumption.

Therefore, several specific nutrients—together with their synergic effects—in both nuts and DFs may explain their beneficial role in glucose and insulin metabolism, which helps to prevent or maintain T2D (Figure 1).

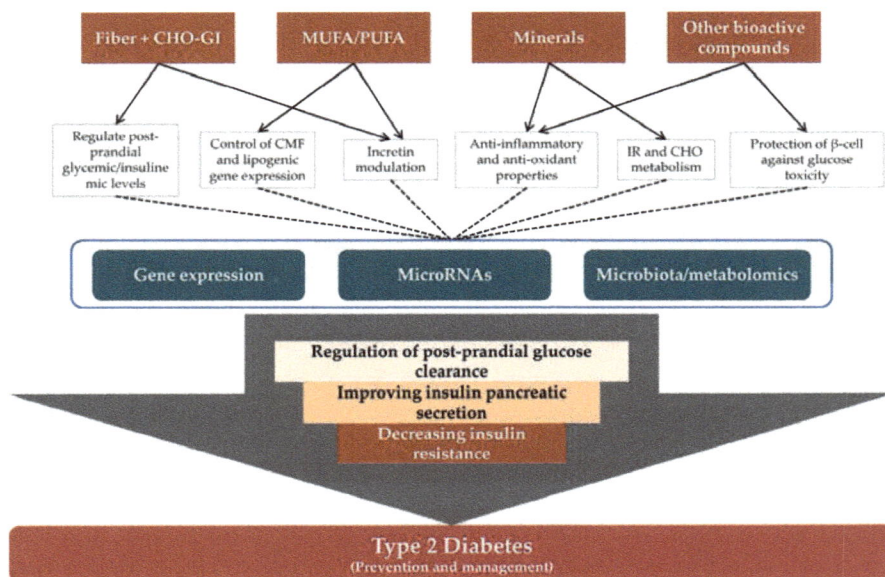

Figure 1. Role of nutrients from nuts and dried fruits in glucose and insulin metabolism, and cellular and molecular mechanisms related to T2D/IR. CHO, carbohydrate; CMF, cellular membrane fluidity; GI, glycaemic index; IR, insulin resistance; MUFA, monounsaturated fatty acid; PUFA, polyunsaturated fatty acid; T2D, type 2 diabetes.

6. Concluding Remarks

Undoubtedly, the specific composition of nuts and dried fruits means that they can be used to efficiently counteract metabolic diseases such as type 2 diabetes. Their unique profile of macronutrients, micronutrients and other bioactive compounds may explain the beneficial effects observed in clinical and epidemiological studies. However, the exact mechanisms by which they modulate glucose and insulin metabolism and influence T2D have yet to be fully discovered. They contain fiber, fat, minerals and other bioactive molecules that modulate several gene mechanisms at the cellular and molecular level. This may explain some of their beneficial effects. However, further basic and translational research is needed in order to extend their positive health benefits and to find novel mechanisms and targets to explain their contribution to the management of type 2 diabetes.

Acknowledgments: We thank Carles Munné and Susana Segura (Universitat Rovira i Virgili) for their help as editor assistance. Lucía Camacho-Barcia is the recipient of a pre-doctoral fellowship from the Generalitat de Catalunya's Department of Universities (FI-DGR 2017).

Author Contributions: Pablo Hernández-Alonso, Lucía Camacho-Barcia, Mònica Bulló and Jordi Salas-Salvadó designed the review. Pablo Hernández-Alonso, Lucía Camacho-Barcia and Mònica Bulló performed the bibliographical search. Pablo Hernández-Alonso, Lucía Camacho-Barcia, Mònica Bulló and Jordi Salas-Salvadó wrote the first draft of the manuscript, and all authors contributed to the editing of the manuscript. All authors approved the final manuscript.

Conflicts of Interest: Pablo Hernández-Alonso, Lucía Camacho-Barcia and Mònica Bulló have nothing to declare. Jordi Salas-Salvadó is a nonpaid member of the Scientific Advisory Council of the International Nut Council.

Abbreviations

AMPK	adenosine monophosphate-activated protein kinase
AT	aerobically trained
ATP	adenosine triphosphate
AOC	area over the curve
Apo	apolipoprotein
BMI	body mass index
BW	body weight
C	cholesterol
CHO	carbohydrate
CI	confidence interval
CMF	cellular membrane fluidity
CRP	C-reactive protein
CVD	cardiovascular disease
DF	dried fruit
EA	ellagic acid
EPIC	European Prospective Investigation into Cancer
FA	fatty acid
FBG	fasting blood glucose
FBP	fructose-1,6-bisphosphatase
G6Pase	glucose 6-phosphatase
GAE	gallic acid equivalents
GI	glycaemic index
GIP	gastric inhibitory polypeptide
GL	glycaemic load
GJ	grape juice
GLI	glibenclamide
GLP-1	glucagon-like peptide-1
GLUT	glucose transporter type
GPE	grape powder extract
HA	high almond
HbA_{1c}	glycated hemoglobin
HDL	high-density lipoprotein
HF	high fat
HFD	high-fat diet
HOMA-IR	homeostatic model assessment of insulin resistance
HPFS	Health Professionals Follow-Up Study
IAUC	incremental area under the curve
ICAM-1	intercellular adhesion molecule-1

IGT	impaired glucose tolerance
IL-6	interleukin-6
IR	insulin resistance
LDL	low-density lipoprotein
LF	low-fat
LPS	lipopolysaccharide
MedDiet	Mediterranean diet
MESA	Multi-Ethnic Study of Atherosclerosis
MetS	metabolic syndrome
MI	myocardial infarction
miRNA and miR	microRNA
M/F	male/female
MUFA	monounsaturated fatty acids
NA	not available
NAFLD	non-alcoholic fatty liver disease
NCEP	National Cholesterol Education Program
NHANES	National Health and Nutrition Examination Survey
NHS	Nurses' Health Study
NLCS	Netherlands Cohort Study
NS	non-significant
Ob	obese
ORAC	oxygen radical absorbance capacity
Ow	overweight
PBMC	peripheral blood mononuclear cell
PF-4	platelet factor-4
PHS	Physicians' Health Study
PM	post-menopausal
PPAR	peroxisome proliferator-activated receptors
pre-D	pre-diabetes
PREDIMED	PREvención con DIeta MEDiterránea
PUFA	polyunsaturated fatty acids
PWE	polyphenol-rich walnut extract
Re	range
RETN	resistin
RCT	randomized clinical trial
RGR	relative glycaemic responses
RR	relative risk
RW	red wine
ROS	reactive oxygen species
S	sedentary
SBP	systolic blood pressure
SCCS	Southern Community Cohort Study
SCFA	short chain fatty acids
SFA	saturated fatty acids
SLC2A4	solute carrier family 2 member 4
SMHS	Shanghai Men's Health Study
STZ	streptozotocin
SWHS	Shanghai Women's Health Study
T2D	type 2 diabetes
TC	total cholesterol
TF	tissue factor
TG	triglycerides
TLGS	Tehran Lipid and Glucose Study
TNF-α	tumor necrosis factor-α
USDA	United States Department of Agriculture
VFM	visceral fat mass
WB	white bread
WC	waist circumference
WHtR	*waist-to-height ratio*

References

1. Widmer, R.J.; Flammer, A.J.; Lerman, L.O.; Lerman, A. The Mediterranean diet, its components, and cardiovascular disease. *Am. J. Med.* **2015**, *128*, 229–238. [CrossRef] [PubMed]
2. Ros, E. Health Benefits of Nut Consumption. *Nutrients* **2010**, *2*, 652–682. [CrossRef] [PubMed]
3. Chang, S.K.; Alasalvar, C.; Shahidi, F. Review of dried fruits: Phytochemicals, antioxidant efficacies, and health benefits. *J. Funct. Foods* **2016**, *21*, 113–132. [CrossRef]
4. Ros, E. Nuts and CVD. *Br. J. Nutr.* **2015**, *113* (Suppl.), S111–S120. [CrossRef] [PubMed]
5. Casas-Agustench, P.; Salas-Huetos, A.; Salas-Salvadó, J. Mediterranean nuts: Origins, ancient medicinal benefits and symbolism. *Public Health Nutr.* **2011**, *14*, 2296–2301. [CrossRef] [PubMed]
6. Salas-Salvadó, J.; Casas-Agustench, P.; Salas-Huetos, A. Cultural and historical aspects of Mediterranean nuts with emphasis on their attributed healthy and nutritional properties. *Nutr. Metab. Cardiovasc. Dis.* **2011**, *21* (Suppl. 1), S1–S6. [CrossRef] [PubMed]
7. Sofi, F. The Mediterranean diet revisited: Evidence of its effectiveness grows. *Curr. Opin. Cardiol.* **2009**, *24*, 442–446. [CrossRef] [PubMed]
8. Alasalvar, C.; Shahidi, F. Composition, phytochemicals, and beneficial health effects of dried fruits: An overview. In *Dried Fruits: Phytochemicals and Health Effects*; Wiley-Blackwell: Oxford, UK, 2013; pp. 372–392.
9. US Department of Agriculture, Agricultural Research Service, Nutrient Data Laboratory. USDA National Nutrient Database for Standard Reference, Release 28 (revised), Version Current: May 2015. Available online: http://www.ars.usda.gov/ba/bhnrc/ndl (accessed on 3 March 2017).
10. Halvorsen, B.L.; Carlsen, M.H.; Phillips, K.M.; Bøhn, S.K.; Holte, K.; Jacobs, D.R.; Blomhoff, R. Content of redox-active compounds (ie, antioxidants) in foods consumed in the United States. *Am. J. Clin. Nutr.* **2006**, *84*, 95–135. [PubMed]
11. Phillips, K.M.; Ruggio, D.M.; Ashraf-Khorassani, M. Phytosterol composition of nuts and seeds commonly consumed in the United States. *J. Agric. Food Chem.* **2005**, *53*, 9436–9445. [CrossRef] [PubMed]
12. Montonen, J.; Knekt, P.; Jarvinen, R.; Reunanen, A. Dietary Antioxidant Intake and Risk of Type 2 Diabetes. *Diabetes Care* **2004**, *27*, 362–366. [CrossRef] [PubMed]
13. Sluijs, I.; Cadier, E.; Beulens, J.W.J.; van der A, D.L.; Spijkerman, A.M.W.; van der Schouw, Y.T. Dietary intake of carotenoids and risk of type 2 diabetes. *Nutr. Metab. Cardiovasc. Dis.* **2015**, *25*, 376–381. [CrossRef] [PubMed]
14. Zhao, B.; Hall, C.A. Composition and antioxidant activity of raisin extracts obtained from various solvents. *Food Chem.* **2008**, *108*, 511–518. [CrossRef] [PubMed]
15. Anderson, J.W.; Waters, A.R. Raisin consumption by humans: Effects on glycemia and insulinemia and cardiovascular risk factors. *J. Food Sci.* **2013**, *78*, A11–A17. [CrossRef] [PubMed]
16. Mandalari, G.; Bisignano, C.; Filocamo, A.; Chessa, S.; Sarò, M.; Torre, G.; Faulks, R.M.; Dugo, P. Bioaccessibility of pistachio polyphenols, xanthophylls, and tocopherols during simulated human digestion. *Nutrition* **2013**, *29*, 338–344. [CrossRef] [PubMed]
17. O'Neil, C.E.; Keast, D.R.; Fulgoni, V.L.; Nicklas, T.A. Tree nut consumption improves nutrient intake and diet quality in US adults: An analysis of national health and nutrition examination survey (NHANES) 1999–2004. *Asia Pac. J. Clin. Nutr.* **2010**, *19*, 142–150. [PubMed]
18. O'Neil, C.E.; Keast, D.R.; Nicklas, T.A.; Fulgoni, V.L. Out-of-hand nut consumption is associated with improved nutrient intake and health risk markers in US children and adults: National Health and Nutrition Examination Survey 1999–2004. *Nutr. Res.* **2012**, *32*, 185–194. [CrossRef] [PubMed]
19. Tey, S.L.; Brown, R.; Gray, A.; Chisholm, A.; Delahunty, C. Nuts improve diet quality compared to other energy-dense snacks while maintaining body weight. *J. Nutr. Metab.* **2011**, *2011*, 357350. [CrossRef] [PubMed]
20. McManus, K.; Antinoro, L.; Sacks, F. A randomized controlled trial of a moderate-fat, low-energy diet compared with a low fat, low-energy diet for weight loss in overweight adults. *Int. J. Obes. Relat. Metab. Disord.* **2001**, *25*, 1503–1511. [CrossRef] [PubMed]
21. Bazzano, L.A.; Li, T.Y.; Joshipura, K.J.; Hu, F.B. Intake of fruit, vegetables, and fruit juices and risk of diabetes in women. *Diabetes Care* **2008**, *31*, 1311–1317. [CrossRef] [PubMed]

22. Keast, D.R.; O'Neil, C.E.; Jones, J.M. Dried fruit consumption is associated with improved diet quality and reduced obesity in US adults: National Health and Nutrition Examination Survey, 1999–2004. *Nutr. Res.* **2011**, *31*, 460–467. [CrossRef] [PubMed]

23. Chan, R.; Wong, V.W.-S.; Chu, W.C.-W.; Wong, G.L.-H.; Li, L.S.; Leung, J.; Chim, A.M.-L.; Yeung, D.K.-W.; Sea, M.M.-M.; Woo, J.; et al. Diet-Quality Scores and Prevalence of Nonalcoholic Fatty Liver Disease: A Population Study Using Proton-Magnetic Resonance Spectroscopy. *PLoS ONE* **2015**, *10*, e0139310. [CrossRef] [PubMed]

24. U.S. Department of Health and Human Services and U.S. Department of Agriculture. 2015–2020 Dietary Guidelines for Americans, 8th Edition edDecember 2015. Available online: http://health.gov/dietaryguidelines/2015/guidelines/ (accessed on 10 March 2017).

25. Bilbis, L.S.; Shehu, R.A.; Abubakar, M.G. Hypoglycemic and hypolipidemic effects of aqueous extract of Arachis hypogaea in normal and alloxan-induced diabetic rats. *Phytomedicine* **2002**, *9*, 553–555. [CrossRef] [PubMed]

26. Fukuda, T.; Ito, H.; Yoshida, T. Effect of the walnut polyphenol fraction on oxidative stress in type 2 diabetes mice. *Biofactors* **2004**, *21*, 251–253. [CrossRef] [PubMed]

27. Ramesh, B.; Saravanan, R.; Pugalendi, K. V Effect of dietary substitution of groundnut oil on blood glucose, lipid profile, and redox status in streptozotocin-diabetic rats. *Yale J. Biol. Med.* **2006**, *79*, 9–17. [PubMed]

28. Emekli-Alturfan, E.; Kasikci, E.; Yarat, A. Tissue factor activities of streptozotocin induced diabetic rat tissues and the effect of peanut consumption. *Diabetes Metab. Res. Rev.* **2007**, *23*, 653–658. [CrossRef] [PubMed]

29. Choi, Y.; Abdelmegeed, M.A.; Akbar, M.; Song, B.-J.J. Dietary walnut reduces hepatic triglyceride content in high-fat-fed mice via modulation of hepatic fatty acid metabolism and adipose tissue inflammation. *J. Nutr. Biochem.* **2016**, *30*, 116–125. [CrossRef] [PubMed]

30. Overman, A.; Bumrungpert, A.; Kennedy, A.; Martinez, K.; Chuang, C.-C.; West, T.; Dawson, B.; Jia, W.; McIntosh, M. Polyphenol-rich grape powder extract (GPE) attenuates inflammation in human macrophages and in human adipocytes exposed to macrophage-conditioned media. *Int. J. Obes. (Lond.)* **2010**, *34*, 800–808. [CrossRef] [PubMed]

31. Chuang, C.-C.; Bumrungpert, A.; Kennedy, A.; Overman, A.; West, T.; Dawson, B.; McIntosh, M.K. Grape powder extract attenuates tumor necrosis factor α-mediated inflammation and insulin resistance in primary cultures of human adipocytes. *J. Nutr. Biochem.* **2011**, *22*, 89–94. [CrossRef] [PubMed]

32. Chuang, C.-C.; Martinez, K.; Xie, G.; Kennedy, A.; Bumrungpert, A.; Overman, A.; Jia, W.; McIntosh, M.K. Quercetin is equally or more effective than resveratrol in attenuating tumor necrosis factor—Mediated inflammation and insulin resistance in primary human adipocytes. *Am. J. Clin. Nutr.* **2010**, *92*, 1511–1521. [CrossRef] [PubMed]

33. Zangiabadi, N.; Asadi-Shekaari, M.; Sheibani, V.; Jafari, M.; Shabani, M.; Asadi, A.R.; Tajadini, H.; Jarahi, M. Date fruit extract is a neuroprotective agent in diabetic peripheral neuropathy in streptozotocin-induced diabetic rats: A multimodal analysis. *Oxid. Med. Cell. Longev.* **2011**, *2011*, 976948. [CrossRef] [PubMed]

34. Porto, L.C.S.; da Silva, J.; Ferraz, A.B.F.; Ethur, E.M.; Porto, C.D.L.; Marroni, N.P.; Picada, J.N. The Antidiabetic and Antihypercholesterolemic Effects of an Aqueous Extract from Pecan Shells in Wistar Rats. *Plant Foods Hum. Nutr.* **2015**, *70*, 414–419. [CrossRef] [PubMed]

35. Tédong, L.; Dzeufiet, P.D.D.; Dimo, T.; Asongalem, E.A.; Sokeng, S.N.; Flejou, J.-F.; Callard, P.; Kamtchouing, P. Acute and subchronic toxicity of Anacardium occidentale Linn (Anacardiaceae) leaves hexane extract in mice. *Afr. J. Tradit. Complement. Altern. Med. AJTCAM* **2006**, *4*, 140–147. [CrossRef] [PubMed]

36. Asgary, S.; Parkhideh, S.; Solhpour, A.; Madani, H.; Mahzouni, P.; Rahimi, P. Effect of ethanolic extract of *Juglans regia* L. on blood sugar in diabetes-induced rats. *J. Med. Food* **2008**, *11*, 533–538. [CrossRef] [PubMed]

37. Ojewole, J.A.O. Laboratory evaluation of the hypoglycemic effect of Anacardium occidentale Linn (Anacardiaceae) stem-bark extracts in rats. *Methods Find. Exp. Clin. Pharmacol.* **2003**, *25*, 199–204. [CrossRef] [PubMed]

38. Egwim, E. Hypoglycemic potencies of crude ethanolic extracts of cashew roots and unripe pawpaw fruits in guinea pigs and rats. *J. Herb. Pharmacother.* **2005**, *5*, 27–34. [CrossRef] [PubMed]

39. Jelodar, G.; Mohsen, M.; Shahram, S. Effect of walnut leaf, coriander and pomegranate on blood glucose and histopathology of pancreas of alloxan induced diabetic rats. *Afr. J. Tradit. Complement. Altern. Med. AJTCAM* **2007**, *4*, 299–305. [CrossRef] [PubMed]

40. Eid, H.M.; Martineau, L.C.; Saleem, A.; Muhammad, A.; Vallerand, D.; Benhaddou-Andaloussi, A.; Nistor, L.; Afshar, A.; Arnason, J.T.; Haddad, P.S. Stimulation of AMP-activated protein kinase and enhancement of basal glucose uptake in muscle cells by quercetin and quercetin glycosides, active principles of the antidiabetic medicinal plant Vaccinium vitis-idaea. *Mol. Nutr. Food Res.* **2010**, *54*, 991–1003. [CrossRef] [PubMed]

41. Vassiliou, E.K.; Gonzalez, A.; Garcia, C.; Tadros, J.H.; Chakraborty, G.; Toney, J.H. Oleic acid and peanut oil high in oleic acid reverse the inhibitory effect of insulin production of the inflammatory cytokine TNF-alpha both in vitro and in vivo systems. *Lipids Health Dis.* **2009**, *8*, 25. [CrossRef] [PubMed]

42. Adewale, O.F.; Isaac, O.; Tunmise, M.T.; Omoniyi, O. Palm oil and ground nut oil supplementation effects on blood glucose and antioxidant status in alloxan-induced diabetic rats. *Pak. J. Pharm. Sci.* **2016**, *29*, 83–87. [PubMed]

43. Anderson, K.J.; Teuber, S.S.; Gobeille, A.; Cremin, P.; Waterhouse, A.L.; Steinberg, F.M. Walnut polyphenolics inhibit in vitro human plasma and LDL oxidation. *J. Nutr.* **2001**, *131*, 2837–2842. [PubMed]

44. Chen, C.-Y.; Milbury, P.E.; Lapsley, K.; Blumberg, J.B. Flavonoids from almond skins are bioavailable and act synergistically with vitamins C and E to enhance hamster and human LDL resistance to oxidation. *J. Nutr.* **2005**, *135*, 1366–1373. [PubMed]

45. Wijeratne, S.S.K.; Abou-Zaid, M.M.; Shahidi, F. Antioxidant polyphenols in almond and its coproducts. *J. Agric. Food Chem.* **2006**, *54*, 312–318. [CrossRef] [PubMed]

46. Gentile, C.; Tesoriere, L.; Butera, D.; Fazzari, M.; Monastero, M.; Allegra, M.; Livrea, M.A. Antioxidant activity of Sicilian pistachio (Pistacia vera L Var. Bronte) nut extract and its bioactive components. *J. Agric. Food Chem.* **2007**, *55*, 643–648. [CrossRef] [PubMed]

47. Shahidi, F.; Alasalvar, C.; Liyana-Pathirana, C.M. Antioxidant phytochemicals in hazelnut kernel (Corylus avellana L) and hazelnut byproducts. *J. Agric. Food Chem.* **2007**, *55*, 1212–1220. [CrossRef] [PubMed]

48. Tedong, L.; Madiraju, P.; Martineau, L.C.; Vallerand, D.; Arnason, J.T.; Desire, D.D.P.; Lavoie, L.; Kamtchouing, P.; Haddad, P.S. Hydro-ethanolic extract of cashew tree (Anacardium occidentale) nut and its principal compound, anacardic acid, stimulate glucose uptake in C2C12 muscle cells. *Mol. Nutr. Food Res.* **2010**, *54*, 1753–1762. [CrossRef] [PubMed]

49. Shahraki, J.; Zareh, M.; Kamalinejad, M.; Pourahmad, J. Cytoprotective Effects of Hydrophilic and Lipophilic Extracts of Pistacia vera against Oxidative Versus Carbonyl Stress in Rat Hepatocytes. *Iran. J. Pharm. Res. IJPR* **2014**, *13*, 1263–1277. [PubMed]

50. Aoun, M.; Michel, F.; Fouret, G.; Schlernitzauer, A.; Ollendorff, V.; Wrutniak-Cabello, C.; Cristol, J.-P.; Carbonneau, M.-A.; Coudray, C.; Feillet-Coudray, C. A grape polyphenol extract modulates muscle membrane fatty acid composition and lipid metabolism in high-fat–high-sucrose diet-fed rats. *Br. J. Nutr.* **2011**, *106*, 491–501. [CrossRef] [PubMed]

51. Weijers, R.N.M. Lipid composition of cell membranes and its relevance in type 2 diabetes mellitus. *Curr. Diabetes Rev.* **2012**, *8*, 390–400. [CrossRef] [PubMed]

52. Soares de Moura, R.; da Costa, G.F.; Moreira, A.S.B.; Queiroz, E.F.; Moreira, D.D.C.; Garcia-Souza, E.P.; Resende, A.C.; Moura, A.S.; Teixeira, M.T. Vitis vinifera L. grape skin extract activates the insulin-signalling cascade and reduces hyperglycaemia in alloxan-induced diabetic mice. *J. Pharm. Pharmacol.* **2012**, *64*, 268–276. [CrossRef] [PubMed]

53. Adam, S.H.; Giribabu, N.; Kassim, N.; Kumar, K.E.; Brahmayya, M.; Arya, A.; Salleh, N. Protective effect of aqueous seed extract of Vitis Vinifera against oxidative stress, inflammation and apoptosis in the pancreas of adult male rats with diabetes mellitus. *Biomed. Pharmacother.* **2016**, *81*, 439–452. [CrossRef] [PubMed]

54. Esposito, D.; Damsud, T.; Wilson, M.; Grace, M.H.; Strauch, R.; Li, X.; Lila, M.A.; Komarnytsky, S. Black Currant Anthocyanins Attenuate Weight Gain and Improve Glucose Metabolism in Diet-Induced Obese Mice with Intact, but Not Disrupted, Gut Microbiome. *J. Agric. Food Chem.* **2015**, *63*, 6172–6180. [CrossRef] [PubMed]

55. Schmatz, R.; Mann, T.R.; Spanevello, R.; Machado, M.M.; Zanini, D.; Pimentel, V.C.; Stefanello, N.; Martins, C.C.; Cardoso, A.M.; Bagatini, M.; et al. Moderate red wine and grape juice consumption modulates the hydrolysis of the adenine nucleotides and decreases platelet aggregation in streptozotocin-induced diabetic rats. *Cell Biochem. Biophys.* **2013**, *65*, 129–143. [CrossRef] [PubMed]

56. Hernández-Salinas, R.; Decap, V.; Leguina, A.; Cáceres, P.; Perez, D.; Urquiaga, I.; Iturriaga, R.; Velarde, V. Antioxidant and anti hyperglycemic role of wine grape powder in rats fed with a high fructose diet. *Biol. Res.* **2015**, *48*, 53. [CrossRef] [PubMed]

57. Overman, A.; Chuang, C.-C.; McIntosh, M. Quercetin attenuates inflammation in human macrophages and adipocytes exposed to macrophage-conditioned media. *Int. J. Obes. (Lond.)* **2011**, *35*, 1165–1172. [CrossRef] [PubMed]

58. Nettleton, J.A.; Steffen, L.M.; Ni, H.; Liu, K.; Jacobs, D.R. Dietary patterns and risk of incident type 2 diabetes in the Multi-Ethnic Study of Atherosclerosis (MESA). *Diabetes Care* **2008**, *31*, 1777–1782. [CrossRef] [PubMed]

59. O'Neil, C.E.; Fulgoni, V.L.; Nicklas, T.A. Tree Nut consumption is associated with better adiposity measures and cardiovascular and metabolic syndrome health risk factors in U.S. Adults: NHANES 2005–2010. *Nutr. J.* **2015**, *14*, 64. [CrossRef] [PubMed]

60. Asghari, G.; Ghorbani, Z.; Mirmiran, P.; Azizi, F. Nut consumption is associated with lower incidence of type 2 diabetes: The Tehran Lipid and Glucose Study. *Diabetes Metab.* **2017**, *43*, 18–24. [CrossRef] [PubMed]

61. Jiang, R.; Manson, J.E.; Stampfer, M.J.; Liu, S.; Willett, W.C.; Hu, F.B. Nut and peanut butter consumption and risk of type 2 diabetes in women. *JAMA* **2002**, *288*, 2554–2560. [CrossRef] [PubMed]

62. Villegas, R.; Gao, Y.-T.T.; Yang, G.; Li, H.-L.L.; Elasy, T.A.; Zheng, W.; Shu, X.O. Legume and soy food intake and the incidence of type 2 diabetes in the Shanghai Women's Health Study. *Am. J. Clin. Nutr.* **2008**, *87*, 162–167. [PubMed]

63. Ibarrola-Jurado, N.; Bulló, M.; Guasch-Ferré, M.; Ros, E.; Martínez-González, M.A.; Corella, D.; Fiol, M.; Wärnberg, J.; Estruch, R.; Román, P.; et al. Cross-sectional assessment of nut consumption and obesity, metabolic syndrome and other cardiometabolic risk factors: The PREDIMED study. *PLoS ONE* **2013**, *8*, e57367. [CrossRef] [PubMed]

64. Pan, A.; Sun, Q.; Manson, J.E.; Willett, W.C.; Hu, F.B. Walnut consumption is associated with lower risk of type 2 diabetes in women. *J. Nutr.* **2013**, *143*, 512–518. [CrossRef] [PubMed]

65. van den Brandt, P.A.; Schouten, L.J. Relationship of tree nut, peanut and peanut butter intake with total and cause-specific mortality: A cohort study and meta-analysis. *Int. J. Epidemiol.* **2015**, *44*, 1038–1049. [CrossRef] [PubMed]

66. Buijsse, B.; Boeing, H.; Drogan, D.; Schulze, M.B.; Feskens, E.J.; Amiano, P.; Barricarte, A.; Clavel-Chapelon, F.; de Lauzon-Guillain, B.; Fagherazzi, G.; et al. Consumption of fatty foods and incident type 2 diabetes in populations from eight European countries. *Eur. J. Clin. Nutr.* **2015**, *69*, 455–461. [CrossRef] [PubMed]

67. Kochar, J.; Gaziano, J.M.; Djoussé, L. Nut consumption and risk of type II diabetes in the Physicians' Health Study. *Eur. J. Clin. Nutr.* **2010**, *64*, 75–79. [CrossRef] [PubMed]

68. Pimpin, L.; Wu, J.H.Y.; Haskelberg, H.; Del Gobbo, L.; Mozaffarian, D. Is Butter Back? A Systematic Review and Meta-Analysis of Butter Consumption and Risk of Cardiovascular Disease, Diabetes, and Total Mortality. *PLoS ONE* **2016**, *11*, e0158118. [CrossRef] [PubMed]

69. Jenkins, D.J.A.; Kendall, C.W.C.; Josse, A.R.; Salvatore, S.; Brighenti, F.; Augustin, L.S.A.; Ellis, P.R.; Vidgen, E.; Rao, A.V. Almonds Decrease Postprandial Glycemia, Insulinemia, and Oxidative Damage in Healthy Individuals. *J. Nutr.* **2006**, *136*, 2987–2992. [PubMed]

70. Josse, A.R.; Kendall, C.W.C.; Augustin, L.S.A.; Ellis, P.R.; Jenkins, D.J.A. Almonds and postprandial glycemia—A dose-response study. *Metabolism* **2007**, *56*, 400–404. [CrossRef] [PubMed]

71. Mori, A.M.; Considine, R.V.; Mattes, R.D.; Wong, J.; Jenkins, D.; Jiang, R.; Manson, J.; Stampfer, M.; Liu, S.; Willett, W.; et al. Acute and second-meal effects of almond form in impaired glucose tolerant adults: A randomized crossover trial. *Nutr. Metab. (Lond.)* **2011**, *8*, 6. [CrossRef] [PubMed]

72. Cohen, A.E.; Johnston, C.S. Almond ingestion at mealtime reduces postprandial glycemia and chronic ingestion reduces hemoglobin A1c in individuals with well-controlled type 2 diabetes mellitus. *Metabolism* **2011**, *60*, 1312–1317. [CrossRef] [PubMed]

73. Crouch, M.A.; Slater, R.T. Almond "Appetizer" Effect on Glucose Tolerance Test (GTT) Results. *J. Am. Board Fam. Med.* **2016**, *29*, 759–766. [CrossRef] [PubMed]

74. Kendall, C.W.C.; Josse, A.R.; Esfahani, A.; Jenkins, D.J.A. The impact of pistachio intake alone or in combination with high-carbohydrate foods on post-prandial glycemia. *Eur. J. Clin. Nutr.* **2011**, *65*, 696–702. [CrossRef] [PubMed]

75. Kendall, C.W.C.; West, S.G.; Augustin, L.S.; Esfahani, A.; Vidgen, E.; Bashyam, B.; Sauder, K.A.; Campbell, J.; Chiavaroli, L.; Jenkins, A.L.; et al. Acute effects of pistachio consumption on glucose and insulin, satiety hormones and endothelial function in the metabolic syndrome. *Eur. J. Clin. Nutr.* **2014**, *68*, 370–375. [CrossRef] [PubMed]

76. Reis, C.E.G.; Bordalo, L.A.; Rocha, A.L.C.; Freitas, D.M.O.; da Silva, M.V.L.; de Faria, V.C.; Martino, H.S.D.; Costa, N.M.B.; Alfenas, R.C. Ground roasted peanuts leads to a lower post-prandial glycemic response than raw peanuts. *Nutr. Hosp.* **2011**, *26*, 745–751. [PubMed]

77. Moreira, A.P.B.; Teixeira, T.F.S.; Alves, R.D.M.; Peluzio, M.C.G.; Costa, N.M.B.; Bressan, J.; Mattes, R.; Alfenas, R.C.G. Effect of a high-fat meal containing conventional or high-oleic peanuts on post-prandial lipopolysaccharide concentrations in overweight/obese men. *J. Hum. Nutr. Diet.* **2016**, *29*, 95–104. [CrossRef] [PubMed]

78. Kendall, C.W.C.; Esfahani, A.; Josse, A.R.; Augustin, L.S.A.; Vidgen, E.; Jenkins, D.J.A. The glycemic effect of nut-enriched meals in healthy and diabetic subjects. *Nutr. Metab. Cardiovasc. Dis.* **2011**, *21* (Suppl. 1), S34–S39. [CrossRef] [PubMed]

79. Lovejoy, J.C.; Most, M.M.; Lefevre, M.; Greenway, F.L.; Rood, J.C. Effect of diets enriched in almonds on insulin action and serum lipids in adults with normal glucose tolerance or type 2 diabetes. *Am. J. Clin. Nutr.* **2002**, *76*, 1000–1006. [PubMed]

80. Li, S.-C.; Liu, Y.-H.; Liu, J.-F.; Chang, W.-H.; Chen, C.-M.; Chen, C.-Y.O. Almond consumption improved glycemic control and lipid profiles in patients with type 2 diabetes mellitus. *Metabolism* **2011**, *60*, 474–479. [CrossRef] [PubMed]

81. Damavandi, R.D.; Eghtesadi, S.; Shidfar, F.; Heydari, I.; Foroushani, A.R. Effects of hazelnuts consumption on fasting blood sugar and lipoproteins in patients with type 2 diabetes. *J. Res. Med. Sci.* **2013**, *18*, 314–321. [PubMed]

82. Lasa, A.; Miranda, J.; Bulló, M.; Casas, R.; Salas-Salvadó, J.; Larretxi, I.; Estruch, R.; Ruiz-Gutiérrez, V.; Portillo, M.P. Comparative effect of two Mediterranean diets versus a low-fat diet on glycaemic control in individuals with type 2 diabetes. *Eur. J. Clin. Nutr.* **2014**, *68*, 767–772. [CrossRef] [PubMed]

83. Parham, M.; Heidari, S.; Khorramirad, A.; Hozoori, M.; Hosseinzadeh, F.; Bakhtyari, L.; Vafaeimanesh, J. Effects of pistachio nut supplementation on blood glucose in patients with type 2 diabetes: A randomized crossover trial. *Rev. Diabet. Stud.* **2014**, *11*, 190–196. [CrossRef] [PubMed]

84. Gulati, S.; Misra, A.; Pandey, R.M. Effect of Almond Supplementation on Glycemia and Cardiovascular Risk Factors in Asian Indians in North India with Type 2 Diabetes Mellitus: A 24–Week Study. *Metab. Syndr. Relat. Disord.* **2017**, *15*, 98–105. [CrossRef] [PubMed]

85. Hernández-Alonso, P.; Salas-Salvadó, J.; Baldrich-Mora, M.; Juanola-Falgarona, M.; Bulló, M. Beneficial Effect of Pistachio Consumption on Glucose Metabolism, Insulin Resistance, Inflammation, and Related Metabolic Risk Markers: A Randomized Clinical Trial. *Diabetes Care* **2014**, *37*, 3098–3105. [CrossRef] [PubMed]

86. Jenkins, D.J.A.; Kendall, C.W.C.; Marchie, A.; Josse, A.R.; Nguyen, T.H.; Faulkner, D.A.; Lapsley, K.G.; Singer, W. Effect of almonds on insulin secretion and insulin resistance in nondiabetic hyperlipidemic subjects: A randomized controlled crossover trial. *Metabolism* **2008**, *57*, 882–887. [CrossRef] [PubMed]

87. Le, T.; Flatt, S.W.; Natarajan, L.; Pakiz, B.; Quintana, E.L.; Heath, D.D.; Rana, B.K.; Rock, C.L. Effects of Diet Composition and Insulin Resistance Status on Plasma Lipid Levels in a Weight Loss Intervention in Women. *J. Am. Heart Assoc.* **2016**, *5*, e002771. [CrossRef] [PubMed]

88. Claesson, A.-L.; Holm, G.; Ernersson, A.; Lindström, T.; Nystrom, F.H. Two weeks of overfeeding with candy, but not peanuts, increases insulin levels and body weight. *Scand. J. Clin. Lab. Invest.* **2009**, *69*, 598–605. [CrossRef] [PubMed]

89. Wien, M.A.; Sabaté, J.M.; Iklé, D.N.; Cole, S.E.; Kandeel, F.R. Almonds vs. complex carbohydrates in a weight reduction program. *Int. J. Obes. Relat. Metab. Disord.* **2003**, *27*, 1365–1372. [CrossRef] [PubMed]

90. Esposito, K.; Marfella, R.; Ciotola, M.; Di Palo, C.; Giugliano, F.; Giugliano, G.; D'Armiento, M.; D'Andrea, F.; Giugliano, D. Effect of a mediterranean-style diet on endothelial dysfunction and markers of vascular inflammation in the metabolic syndrome: A randomized trial. *JAMA* **2004**, *292*, 1440–1446. [CrossRef] [PubMed]

91. Tapsell, L.C.; Gillen, L.J.; Patch, C.S.; Batterham, M.; Owen, A.; Baré, M.; Kennedy, M. Including walnuts in a low-fat/modified-fat diet improves HDL cholesterol-to-total cholesterol ratios in patients with type 2 diabetes. *Diabetes Care* **2004**, *27*, 2777–2783. [CrossRef] [PubMed]

92. Tapsell, L.C.; Batterham, M.J.; Teuss, G.; Tan, S.-Y.; Dalton, S.; Quick, C.J.; Gillen, L.J.; Charlton, K.E. Long-term effects of increased dietary polyunsaturated fat from walnuts on metabolic parameters in type II diabetes. *Eur. J. Clin. Nutr.* **2009**, *63*, 1008–1015. [CrossRef] [PubMed]

93. Ma, Y.; Njike, V.Y.; Millet, J.; Dutta, S.; Doughty, K.; Treu, J.A.; Katz, D.L. Effects of walnut consumption on endothelial function in type 2 diabetic subjects: A randomized controlled crossover trial. *Diabetes Care* **2010**, *33*, 227–232. [CrossRef] [PubMed]

94. Brennan, A.M.; Sweeney, L.L.; Liu, X.; Mantzoros, C.S. Walnut consumption increases satiation but has no effect on insulin resistance or the metabolic profile over a 4-day period. *Obesity (Silver Spring)* **2010**, *18*, 1176–1182. [CrossRef] [PubMed]

95. Wang, X.; Li, Z.; Liu, Y.; Lv, X.; Yang, W. Effects of pistachios on body weight in Chinese subjects with metabolic syndrome. *Nutr. J.* **2012**, *11*, 20. [CrossRef] [PubMed]

96. Katz, D.L.; Davidhi, A.; Ma, Y.; Kavak, Y.; Bifulco, L.; Njike, V.Y. Effects of walnuts on endothelial function in overweight adults with visceral obesity: A randomized, controlled, crossover trial. *J. Am. Coll. Nutr.* **2012**, *31*, 415–423. [CrossRef] [PubMed]

97. Richmond, K.; Williams, S.; Mann, J.; Brown, R.; Chisholm, A. Markers of Cardiovascular Risk in Postmenopausal Women with Type 2 Diabetes Are Improved by the Daily Consumption of Almonds or Sunflower Kernels: A Feeding Study. *ISRN Nutr.* **2013**, *2013*, 1–9. [CrossRef] [PubMed]

98. Tan, S.Y.; Mattes, R.D. Appetitive, dietary and health effects of almonds consumed with meals or as snacks: A randomized, controlled trial. *Eur. J. Clin. Nutr.* **2013**, *67*, 1205–1214. [CrossRef] [PubMed]

99. Liu, J.-F.; Liu, Y.-H.; Chen, C.-M.; Chang, W.-H.; Chen, C.-Y.O. The effect of almonds on inflammation and oxidative stress in Chinese patients with type 2 diabetes mellitus: A randomized crossover controlled feeding trial. *Eur. J. Nutr.* **2013**, *52*, 927–935. [CrossRef] [PubMed]

100. Wu, L.; Piotrowski, K.; Rau, T.; Waldmann, E.; Broedl, U.C.; Demmelmair, H.; Koletzko, B.; Stark, R.G.; Nagel, J.M.; Mantzoros, C.S.; et al. Walnut-enriched diet reduces fasting non-HDL-cholesterol and apolipoprotein B in healthy Caucasian subjects: A randomized controlled cross-over clinical trial. *Metabolism* **2014**, *63*, 382–391. [CrossRef] [PubMed]

101. Wien, M.; Oda, K.; Sabaté, J. A randomized controlled trial to evaluate the effect of incorporating peanuts into an American Diabetes Association meal plan on the nutrient profile of the total diet and cardiometabolic parameters of adults with type 2 diabetes. *Nutr. J.* **2014**, *13*, 10. [CrossRef] [PubMed]

102. Sauder, K.A.; McCrea, C.E.; Ulbrecht, J.S.; Kris-Etherton, P.M.; West, S.G. Effects of pistachios on the lipid/lipoprotein profile, glycemic control, inflammation, and endothelial function in type 2 diabetes: A randomized trial. *Metabolism* **2015**, *64*, 1521–1529. [CrossRef] [PubMed]

103. Njike, V.Y.; Ayettey, R.; Petraro, P.; Treu, J.A.; Katz, D.L. Walnut ingestion in adults at risk for diabetes: Effects on body composition, diet quality, and cardiac risk measures. *BMJ Open Diabetes Res. Care* **2015**, *3*, e000115. [CrossRef] [PubMed]

104. Sari, I.; Baltaci, Y.; Bagci, C.; Davutoglu, V.; Erel, O.; Celik, H.; Ozer, O.; Aksoy, N.; Aksoy, M. Effect of pistachio diet on lipid parameters, endothelial function, inflammation, and oxidative status: A prospective study. *Nutrition* **2010**, *26*, 399–404. [CrossRef] [PubMed]

105. Gulati, S.; Misra, A.; Pandey, R.M.; Bhatt, S.P.; Saluja, S. Effects of pistachio nuts on body composition, metabolic, inflammatory and oxidative stress parameters in Asian Indians with metabolic syndrome: A 24-week, randomized control trial. *Nutrition* **2014**, *30*, 192–197. [CrossRef] [PubMed]

106. Wien, M.; Bleich, D.; Raghuwanshi, M.; Gould-Forgerite, S.; Gomes, J.; Monahan-Couch, L.; Oda, K. Almond consumption and cardiovascular risk factors in adults with prediabetes. *J. Am. Coll. Nutr.* **2010**, *29*, 189–197. [CrossRef] [PubMed]

107. Casas-Agustench, P.; López-Uriarte, P.; Bulló, M.; Ros, E.; Cabré-Vila, J.J.; Salas-Salvadó, J. Effects of one serving of mixed nuts on serum lipids, insulin resistance and inflammatory markers in patients with the metabolic syndrome. *Nutr. Metab. Cardiovasc. Dis.* **2011**, *21*, 126–135. [CrossRef] [PubMed]

108. Mejia, S.B.; Kendall, C.W.C.; Viguiliouk, E.; Augustin, L.S.; Ha, V.; Cozma, A.I.; Mirrahimi, A.; Maroleanu, A.; Chiavaroli, L.; Leiter, L.A.; et al. Effect of tree nuts on metabolic syndrome criteria: A systematic review and meta-analysis of randomised controlled trials. *BMJ Open* **2014**, *4*, e004660. [CrossRef] [PubMed]

109. Rasmussen, O.; Winther, E.; Hermansen, K. Postprandial glucose and insulin responses to rolled oats ingested raw, cooked or as a mixture with raisins in normal subjects and type 2 diabetic patients. *Diabet. Med.* **1989**, *6*, 337–341. [CrossRef] [PubMed]

110. Kim, Y.; Hertzler, S.R.; Byrne, H.K.; Mattern, C.O. Raisins are a low to moderate glycemic index food with a correspondingly low insulin index. *Nutr. Res.* **2008**, *28*, 304–308. [CrossRef] [PubMed]

111. Kanellos, P.T.; Kaliora, A.C.; Liaskos, C.; Tentolouris, N.K.; Perrea, D.; Karathanos, V.T. A study of glycemic response to Corinthian raisins in healthy subjects and in type 2 diabetes mellitus patients. *Plant Foods Hum. Nutr.* **2013**, *68*, 145–148. [CrossRef] [PubMed]

112. Esfahani, A.; Lam, J.; Kendall, C.W.C. Acute effects of raisin consumption on glucose and insulin reponses in healthy individuals. *J. Nutr. Sci.* **2014**, *3*, e1. [CrossRef] [PubMed]

113. Kaliora, A.C.; Kanellos, P.T.; Gioxari, A.; Karathanos, V.T. Regulation of GIP and Ghrelin in Healthy Subjects Fed on Sun-Dried Raisins: A Pilot Study with a Crossover Trial Design. *J. Med. Food* **2017**, *20*, 301–308. [CrossRef] [PubMed]

114. Furchner-Evanson, A.; Petrisko, Y.; Howarth, L.; Nemoseck, T.; Kern, M. Type of snack influences satiety responses in adult women. *Appetite* **2010**, *54*, 564–569. [CrossRef] [PubMed]

115. Puglisi, M.J.; Vaishnav, U.; Shrestha, S.; Torres-Gonzalez, M.; Wood, R.J.; Volek, J.S.; Fernandez, M.L. Raisins and additional walking have distinct effects on plasma lipids and inflammatory cytokines. *Lipids Health Dis.* **2008**, *7*, 14. [CrossRef] [PubMed]

116. Rankin, J.W.; Andreae, M.C.; Oliver Chen, C.-Y.; O'Keefe, S.F. Effect of raisin consumption on oxidative stress and inflammation in obesity. *Diabetes Obes. Metab.* **2008**, *10*, 1086–1096. [CrossRef] [PubMed]

117. Howarth, L.; Petrisko, Y.; Furchner-Evanson, A.; Nemoseck, T.; Kern, M. Snack Selection Influences Nutrient Intake, Triglycerides, and Bowel Habits of Adult Women: A Pilot Study. *J. Am. Diet. Assoc.* **2010**, *110*, 1322–1327. [CrossRef] [PubMed]

118. Kanellos, P.T.; Kaliora, A.C.; Tentolouris, N.K.; Argiana, V.; Perrea, D.; Kalogeropoulos, N.; Kountouri, A.M.; Karathanos, V.T. A pilot, randomized controlled trial to examine the health outcomes of raisin consumption in patients with diabetes. *Nutrition* **2014**, *30*, 358–364. [CrossRef] [PubMed]

119. Bays, H.; Weiter, K.; Anderson, J. A randomized study of raisins versus alternative snacks on glycemic control and other cardiovascular risk factors in patients with type 2 diabetes mellitus. *Phys. Sportsmed.* **2015**, *43*, 37–43. [CrossRef] [PubMed]

120. Anderson, J.W.; Weiter, K.M.; Christian, A.L.; Ritchey, M.B.; Bays, H.E. Raisins Compared with Other Snack Effects on Glycemia and Blood Pressure: A Randomized, Controlled Trial. *Postgrad. Med.* **2014**, *126*, 37–43. [CrossRef] [PubMed]

121. Chandalia, M.; Garg, A.; Lutjohann, D.; von Bergmann, K.; Grundy, S.M.; Brinkley, L.J. Beneficial effects of high dietary fiber intake in patients with type 2 diabetes mellitus. *N. Engl. J. Med.* **2000**, *342*, 1392–1398. [CrossRef] [PubMed]

122. Dikeman, C.L.; Fahey, G.C. Viscosity as Related to Dietary Fiber: A Review. *Crit. Rev. Food Sci. Nutr.* **2006**, *46*, 649–663. [CrossRef] [PubMed]

123. Hopping, B.N.; Erber, E.; Grandinetti, A.; Verheus, M.; Kolonel, L.N.; Maskarinec, G. Dietary fiber, magnesium, and glycemic load alter risk of type 2 diabetes in a multiethnic cohort in Hawaii. *J. Nutr.* **2010**, *140*, 68–74. [CrossRef] [PubMed]

124. Lovejoy, J.C. The impact of nuts on diabetes and diabetes risk. *Curr. Diab. Rep.* **2005**, *5*, 379–384. [CrossRef] [PubMed]

125. Heppner, K.M.; Perez-Tilve, D. GLP-1 based therapeutics: Simultaneously combating T2DM and obesity. *Front. Neurosci.* **2015**, *9*, 92. [CrossRef] [PubMed]

126. Bodnaruc, A.M.; Prud'homme, D.; Blanchet, R.; Giroux, I. Nutritional modulation of endogenous glucagon-like peptide-1 secretion: A review. *Nutr. Metab. (Lond.)* **2016**, *13*, 92. [CrossRef] [PubMed]

127. Brand-Miller, J.; Hayne, S.; Petocz, P.; Colagiuri, S. Low-glycemic index diets in the management of diabetes: A meta-analysis of randomized controlled trials. *Diabetes Care* **2003**, *26*, 2261–2267. [CrossRef] [PubMed]

128. Mirrahimi, A.; Chiavaroli, L.; Srichaikul, K.; Augustin, L.S.A.; Sievenpiper, J.L.; Kendall, C.W.C.; Jenkins, D.J.A. The role of glycemic index and glycemic load in cardiovascular disease and its risk factors: A review of the recent literature. *Curr. Atheroscler. Rep.* **2014**, *16*, 381. [CrossRef] [PubMed]

129. Storlien, L.H.; Baur, L.A.; Kriketos, A.D.; Pan, D.A.; Cooney, G.J.; Jenkins, A.B.; Calvert, G.D.; Campbell, L. V Dietary fats and insulin action. *Diabetologia* **1996**, *39*, 621–631. [CrossRef] [PubMed]

130. Haag, M.; Dippenaar, N.G. Dietary fats, fatty acids and insulin resistance: Short review of a multifaceted connection. *Med. Sci. Monit.* **2005**, *11*, RA359–RA367. [PubMed]

131. Risérus, U.; Willett, W.C.; Hu, F.B. Dietary fats and prevention of type 2 diabetes. *Prog. Lipid Res.* **2009**, *48*, 44–51. [CrossRef] [PubMed]

132. Segal-Isaacson, C.J.; Carello, E.; Wylie-Rosett, J. Dietary fats and diabetes mellitus: Is there a good fat? *Curr. Diabetes Rep.* **2001**, *1*, 161–169. [CrossRef]

133. Rajaram, S.; Sabaté, J. Nuts, body weight and insulin resistance. *Br. J. Nutr.* **2006**, *96* (Suppl. 2), S79–S86. [CrossRef] [PubMed]

134. Kien, C.L. Dietary interventions for metabolic syndrome: Role of modifying dietary fats. *Curr. Diabetes Rep.* **2009**, *9*, 43–50. [CrossRef]

135. Grygiel-Górniak, B. Peroxisome proliferator-activated receptors and their ligands: Nutritional and clinical implications - a review. *Nutr. J.* **2014**, *13*, 17. [CrossRef] [PubMed]

136. Martini, L.A.; Catania, A.S.; Ferreira, S.R. Role of vitamins and minerals in prevention and management of type 2 diabetes mellitus. *Nutr. Rev.* **2010**, *68*, 341–354. [CrossRef] [PubMed]

137. Chaudhary, D.P.; Sharma, R.; Bansal, D.D. Implications of magnesium deficiency in type 2 diabetes: A review. *Biol. Trace Elem. Res.* **2010**, *134*, 119–129. [CrossRef] [PubMed]

138. Lopez-Ridaura, R.; Willett, W.C.; Rimm, E.B.; Liu, S.; Stampfer, M.J.; Manson, J.E.; Hu, F.B. Magnesium intake and risk of type 2 diabetes in men and women. *Diabetes Care* **2004**, *27*, 134–140. [CrossRef] [PubMed]

139. Guasch-Ferré, M.; Bulló, M.; Estruch, R.; Corella, D.; Martínez-González, M.A.; Ros, E.; Covas, M.; Arós, F.; Gómez-Gracia, E.; Fiol, M.; et al. Dietary magnesium intake is inversely associated with mortality in adults at high cardiovascular disease risk. *J. Nutr.* **2014**, *144*, 55–60. [CrossRef] [PubMed]

140. Pandey, K.B.; Rizvi, S.I. Current Understanding of Dietary Polyphenols and their Role in Health and Disease. *Curr. Nutr. Food Sci.* **2009**, *5*, 249–263. [CrossRef]

141. Xiao, J.B.; Högger, P. Dietary polyphenols and type 2 diabetes: Current insights and future perspectives. *Curr. Med. Chem.* **2015**, *22*, 23–38. [CrossRef] [PubMed]

142. Guo, X.; Yang, B.; Tan, J.; Jiang, J.; Li, D. Associations of dietary intakes of anthocyanins and berry fruits with risk of type 2 diabetes mellitus: A systematic review and meta-analysis of prospective cohort studies. *Eur. J. Clin. Nutr.* **2016**, *70*, 1360–1367. [CrossRef] [PubMed]

143. Oboh, G.; Ademosun, A.O.; Ogunsuyi, O.B. Quercetin and Its Role in Chronic Diseases. In *Advances in Experimental Medicine and Biology*; Springer Science+Business Media: Berlin/Heidelberg, Germany, 2016; Volume 929, pp. 377–387.

144. Meng, Y.; Su, A.; Yuan, S.; Zhao, H.; Tan, S.; Hu, C.; Deng, H.; Guo, Y. Evaluation of Total Flavonoids, Myricetin, and Quercetin from Hovenia dulcis Thunb. As Inhibitors of α-Amylase and α-Glucosidase. *Plant Foods Hum. Nutr.* **2016**, *71*, 444–449. [CrossRef] [PubMed]

145. Kang, I.; Buckner, T.; Shay, N.F.; Gu, L.; Chung, S. Improvements in Metabolic Health with Consumption of Ellagic Acid and Subsequent Conversion into Urolithins: Evidence and Mechanisms. *Adv. Nutr.* **2016**, *7*, 961–972. [CrossRef] [PubMed]

146. Yoshimura, Y.; Nishii, S.; Zaima, N.; Moriyama, T.; Kawamura, Y. Ellagic acid improves hepatic steatosis and serum lipid composition through reduction of serum resistin levels and transcriptional activation of hepatic ppara in obese, diabetic KK-Ay mice. *Biochem. Biophys. Res. Commun.* **2013**, *434*, 486–491. [CrossRef] [PubMed]

147. Panchal, S.K.; Ward, L.; Brown, L. Ellagic acid attenuates high-carbohydrate, high-fat diet-induced metabolic syndrome in rats. *Eur. J. Nutr.* **2013**, *52*, 559–568. [CrossRef] [PubMed]

148. Ahad, A.; Ganai, A.A.; Mujeeb, M.; Siddiqui, W.A. Ellagic acid, an NF-κB inhibitor, ameliorates renal function in experimental diabetic nephropathy. *Chem. Biol. Interact.* **2014**, *219*, 64–75. [CrossRef] [PubMed]

149. Karachanak-Yankova, S.; Dimova, R.; Nikolova, D.; Nesheva, D.; Koprinarova, M.; Maslyankov, S.; Tafradjiska, R.; Gateva, P.; Velizarova, M.; Hammoudeh, Z.; et al. Epigenetic alterations in patients with type 2 diabetes mellitus. *Balkan J. Med. Genet.* **2015**, *18*, 15–24. [CrossRef] [PubMed]

150. Paluszczak, J.; Krajka-Kuźniak, V.; Baer-Dubowska, W. The effect of dietary polyphenols on the epigenetic regulation of gene expression in MCF7 breast cancer cells. *Toxicol. Lett.* **2010**, *192*, 119–125. [CrossRef] [PubMed]

151. Holliday, R. Mechanisms for the control of gene activity during development. *Biol. Rev. Camb. Philos. Soc.* **1990**, *65*, 431–471. [CrossRef] [PubMed]

152. Choi, S.-W.; Claycombe, K.J.; Martinez, J.A.; Friso, S.; Schalinske, K.L. Nutritional Epigenomics: A Portal to Disease Prevention. *Adv. Nutr. Int. Rev. J.* **2013**, *4*, 530–532. [CrossRef] [PubMed]

153. Das, D.K.; Mukherjee, S.; Ray, D. Resveratrol and red wine, healthy heart and longevity. *Heart Fail. Rev.* **2010**, *15*, 467–477. [CrossRef] [PubMed]

154. Lee, K.W.; Lee, H.J.; Lee, C.Y. Vitamins, phytochemicals, diets, and their implementation in cancer chemoprevention. *Crit. Rev. Food Sci. Nutr.* **2004**, *44*, 437–452. [CrossRef] [PubMed]

155. Link, A.; Balaguer, F.; Goel, A. Cancer chemoprevention by dietary polyphenols: Promising role for epigenetics. *Biochem. Pharmacol.* **2010**, *80*, 1771–1792. [CrossRef] [PubMed]

156. Hermsdorff, H.H.M.; Zulet, M.Á.; Puchau, B.; Martínez, J.A. Fruit and vegetable consumption and proinflammatory gene expression from peripheral blood mononuclear cells in young adults: A translational study. *Nutr. Metab. (Lond.)* **2010**, *7*, 42. [CrossRef] [PubMed]

157. Ambros, V. The functions of animal microRNAs. *Nature* **2004**, *431*, 350–355. [CrossRef] [PubMed]

158. Ambros, V.; Bartel, B.; Bartel, D.P.; Burge, C.B.; Carrington, J.C.; Chen, X.; Dreyfuss, G.; Eddy, S.R.; Griffiths-Jones, S.; Marshall, M.; et al. A uniform system for microRNA annotation. *RNA* **2003**, *9*, 277–279. [CrossRef] [PubMed]

159. Ross, S.A.; Davis, C.D. The emerging role of microRNAs and nutrition in modulating health and disease. *Annu. Rev. Nutr.* **2014**, *34*, 305–336. [CrossRef] [PubMed]

160. Tomé-Carneiro, J.; Larrosa, M.; Yáñez-Gascón, M.J.; Dávalos, A.; Gil-Zamorano, J.; Gonzálvez, M.; García-Almagro, F.J.; Ruiz Ros, J.A.; Tomás-Barberán, F.A.; Espín, J.C.; et al. One-year supplementation with a grape extract containing resveratrol modulates inflammatory-related microRNAs and cytokines expression in peripheral blood mononuclear cells of type 2 diabetes and hypertensive patients with coronary artery disease. *Pharmacol. Res.* **2013**, *72*, 69–82. [CrossRef] [PubMed]

161. Ortega, F.J.; Cardona-Alvarado, M.I.; Mercader, J.M.; Moreno-Navarrete, J.M.; Moreno, M.; Sabater, M.; Fuentes-Batllevell, N.; Ramírez-Chávez, E.; Ricart, W.; Molina-Torres, J.; et al. Circulating profiling reveals the effect of a polyunsaturated fatty acid-enriched diet on common microRNAs. *J. Nutr. Biochem.* **2015**, *26*, 1095–1101. [CrossRef] [PubMed]

162. Hernández-Alonso, P.; Giardina, S.; Salas-Salvadó, J.; Arcelin, P.; Bulló, M. Chronic pistachio intake modulates circulating microRNAs related to glucose metabolism and insulin resistance in prediabetic subjects. *Eur. J. Nutr.* **2016**. [CrossRef] [PubMed]

163. Conlon, M.A.; Bird, A.R. The Impact of Diet and Lifestyle on Gut Microbiota and Human Health. *Nutrients* **2014**, *7*, 17–44. [CrossRef] [PubMed]

164. Ansell, J.; Parkar, S.; Paturi, G.; Rosendale, D.; Blatchford, P. Modification of the Colonic Microbiota. *Adv. Food Nutr. Res.* **2013**, *68*, 205–217. [PubMed]

165. Mandalari, G.; Faulks, R.M.; Bisignano, C.; Waldron, K.W.; Narbad, A.; Wickham, M.S.J. In vitro evaluation of the prebiotic properties of almond skins (Amygdalus communis L.). *FEMS Microbiol. Lett.* **2010**, *304*, 116–122. [CrossRef] [PubMed]

166. Ukhanova, M.; Wang, X.; Baer, D.J.; Novotny, J.A.; Fredborg, M.; Mai, V. Effects of almond and pistachio consumption on gut microbiota composition in a randomised cross-over human feeding study. *Br. J. Nutr.* **2014**, *111*, 2146–2152. [CrossRef] [PubMed]

167. Anhê, F.F.; Varin, T.V.; Le Barz, M.; Desjardins, Y.; Levy, E.; Roy, D.; Marette, A. Gut Microbiota Dysbiosis in Obesity-Linked Metabolic Diseases and Prebiotic Potential of Polyphenol-Rich Extracts. *Curr. Obes. Rep.* **2015**, *4*, 389–400. [CrossRef] [PubMed]

168. Anhê, F.F.; Roy, D.; Pilon, G.; Dudonné, S.; Matamoros, S.; Varin, T.V.; Garofalo, C.; Moine, Q.; Desjardins, Y.; Levy, E.; et al. A polyphenol-rich cranberry extract protects from diet-induced obesity, insulin resistance and intestinal inflammation in association with increased *Akkermansia* spp. population in the gut microbiota of mice. *Gut* **2015**, *64*, 872–883. [PubMed]

169. Nieman, D.C.; Scherr, J.; Luo, B.; Meaney, M.P.; Dréau, D.; Sha, W.; Dew, D.A.; Henson, D.A.; Pappan, K.L. Influence of pistachios on performance and exercise-induced inflammation, oxidative stress, immune dysfunction, and metabolite shifts in cyclists: A randomized, crossover trial. *PLoS ONE* **2014**, *9*, e113725. [CrossRef] [PubMed]

170. Hernández-Alonso, P.; Cañueto, D.; Giardina, S.; Salas-Salvadó, J.; Cañellas, N.; Correig, X.; Bulló, M. Effect of pistachio consumption on the modulation of urinary gut microbiota-related metabolites in pre-diabetic subjects. *J. Nutr. Biochem.* **2017**, *45*, 48–53. [CrossRef] [PubMed]

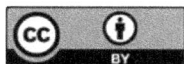

nutrients

MDPI

Article

Integrated Assessment of Pharmacological and Nutritional Cardiovascular Risk Management: Blood Pressure Control in the DIAbetes and LifEstyle Cohort Twente (DIALECT)

Christina M. Gant [1,2,†], S. Heleen Binnenmars [1,2,†], Else van den Berg [2], Stephan J. L. Bakker [2] (ID), Gerjan Navis [2] and Gozewijn D. Laverman [1,2,*]

1   Department of Internal Medicine/Nephrology, Ziekenhuisgroep Twente, Zilvermeeuw 1, 7609 PP Almelo, The Netherlands; c.gant@zgt.nl (C.M.G.); s.h.binnenmars@umcg.nl (S.H.B.)
2   Department of Internal Medicine, Division of Nephrology, University of Groningen, University Medical Center Groningen, Hanzeplein 1, 9713 GZ Groningen, The Netherlands; e.van.den.berg@umcg.nl (E.v.d.B.); s.j.l.bakker@umcg.nl (S.J.L.B.); G.j.navis@umcg.nl (G.N.)
*   Correspondence: g.laverman@zgt.nl; Tel.: +3188-7083079
†   These authors contributed equally.

Received: 15 May 2017; Accepted: 3 July 2017; Published: 6 July 2017

Abstract: Cardiovascular risk management is an integral part of treatment in Type 2 Diabetes Mellitus (T2DM), and requires pharmacological as well as nutritional management. We hypothesize that a systematic assessment of both pharmacological and nutritional management can identify targets for the improvement of treatment quality. Therefore, we analysed blood pressure (BP) management in the DIAbetes and LifEstyle Cohort Twente (DIALECT). DIALECT is an observational cohort from routine diabetes care, performed at the ZGT Hospital (Almelo and Hengelo, The Netherlands). BP was measured for 15 min with one minute intervals. Sodium and potassium intake was derived from 24-hour urinary excretion. We determined the adherence to pharmacological and non-pharmacological guidelines in patients with BP on target (BP-OT) and BP not on target (BP-NOT). In total, 450 patients were included from August 2009 until January 2016. The mean age was 63 ± 9 years, and the majority was male (58%). In total, 53% had BP-OT. In those with BP-NOT, pharmacological management was suboptimal (zero to two antihypertensive drugs) in 62% of patients, and nutritional guideline adherence was suboptimal in 100% of patients (only 8% had a sodium intake on target, 66% had a potassium intake on target, 3% had a sodium-to-potassium ratio on target, and body mass index was <30 kg/m² in 35%). These data show pharmacological undertreatment and a low adherence to nutritional guidelines. Uncontrolled BP is common in T2DM, and our data show a window of opportunity for improving BP control, especially in nutritional management. To improve treatment quality, we advocate to incorporate the integrated monitoring of nutritional management in quality improvement cycles in routine care.

Keywords: Type 2 diabetes mellitus; blood pressure; pharmacological management; nutrition; dietary sodium intake

1. Introduction

Type 2 Diabetes Mellitus (T2DM), with an estimated number of 422 million patients worldwide, is one of the major conditions associated with cardiovascular events and cardiovascular death [1]. Therefore, the prevention of the development and progression of such complications is a main goal in the treatment of T2DM, and evidence-based recommendations to reach this goal are incorporated in treatment guidelines. Treatment consists of pharmacological and non-pharmacological management, the latter consisting in large part of nutritional guidance. Still, cardiovascular complications develop in the majority of T2DM patients, demonstrating the large challenge of adequate treatment [2,3]. One explanation for this could be a failure to reach guideline treatment targets. Indeed, several studies have shown that targets for blood pressure, glycemic control, and Low Density Lipoprotein (LDL) cholesterol are not reached in a large number of patients [4–8].

Pharmacological and nutritional management are often studied as separate entities, despite the fact that both are crucial elements of treatment. We hypothesize that a systematic assessment of both pharmacological and nutritional management can identify targets for the improvement of treatment quality. The DIAbetes and LifEstyle Cohort Twente (DIALECT) cohort study was specifically designed for this purpose. DIALECT is an observational study in T2DM patients in a well-defined region in The Netherlands, and uses validated and detailed real-world data on nutritional habits, pharmacological treatment, and current clinical condition. To obtain non-biased data on individual nutrient intake, 24-hour urine collections were used and stored in a biobank to allow for future analyses [9].

We aim to address how well the targets for blood pressure management are reached, and how this is related to (1) pharmacological management; and (2) nutritional management (i.e., the dietary intake of salt [10,11], potassium [12,13], body mass index (BMI), and alcohol). Moreover, we assessed additional nutritional parameters for which no specific counselling was given, but have been shown to be relevant to cardiovascular risk in diabetic kidney disease (magnesium [14–16] and phosphate [17,18]). Because the presence of diabetic kidney disease implicates different blood pressure targets, we analysed patients without and with renal involvement separately.

2. Materials and Methods

2.1. Study Design and Participants

DIALECT is a prospective cohort study in patients with T2DM, performed in the ZGT Hospital, which is located in Almelo and Hengelo, The Netherlands. It is designed to study pharmacological and non-pharmacological management in a regional T2DM population treated in a secondary health care center. All patients with T2DM and aged 18+ years treated in the outpatient clinic of our hospital were eligible, with the only exclusion criteria being an inability to understand the informed consent procedure, insufficient knowledge of the Dutch language, or a dependency on renal replacement therapy.

This paper reports on the DIALECT-1 population, consisting of the first 450 patients, recruited between September 2009 and January 2016. The inclusion of new patients in DIALECT-2 will be performed until December 2019, or until the number of 850 is reached. The study is performed according to the guidelines of good clinical practice and the Declaration of Helsinki. It has been approved by the local institutional review boards (METC-registration numbers NL57219.044.16 and 1009.68020), and is registered in the Netherlands Trial Register (NTR trial code 5855).

2.2. Study Procedures

Patients were screened for eligibility in the electronic patient file, and subsequently invited for a study visit. At the clinic, all of the information relevant to the medical condition was recorded in a database (Figure 1, Supplementary Table S1). Height, weight, and waist and hip circumference were measured. Body mass index was calculated as weight divided by height squared (kg/m^2), and body surface area was estimated by applying the universally adopted formula of DuBois [19]. Blood pressure was measured in a supine position by an automated device (Dinamap®; GE Medical systems, Milwaukee, WI, USA) for 15 min with a one-minute interval. The mean systolic and diastolic pressure of the last three measurements was used for further analysis.

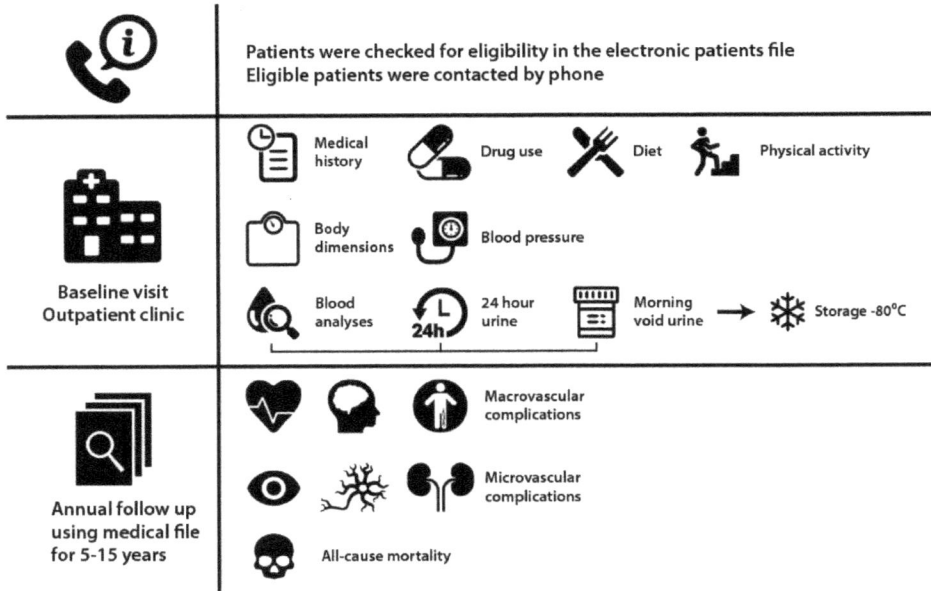

Figure 1. Patient inclusion and data collection.

Physical activity was assessed using the Short Questionnaire to Asses Health enhancing physical activity (SQUASH) questionnaire, which was previously validated in [20]. The 24-hour urinary content of specific substances was measured where possible and appropriate.

Routine laboratory tests were performed in venous blood, including blood count tests, liver function tests, renal function tests, HbA1c, and cholesterol. The estimated glomerular filtration rate (eGFR) was calculated using the Chronic Kidney Disease Epidemiology Collaboration (CKD-EPI) formula [21]. From samples of a 24-hour urine collection, the following parameters were measured: sodium, potassium, creatinine, calcium, phosphate, chloride, albumin, protein, urea, and uric acid excretion. Twenty-four-hour urinary excretion was calculated by multiplying these concentrations with the volume of the 24-hour urine collection. Creatinine clearance was calculated from the 24-hour urine creatinine excretion and the plasma creatinine concentration. For the proper collection of the 24-hour urine sample, patients were instructed to dispose of the first morning void urine, and thereafter collect all urine in the provided canister until the first morning void urine of the next day. In between voids, they were instructed to store the canister in a dark cool place, preferably in a refrigerator. A separate single morning void urine was used to assess the urinary albumin-to-creatinine ratio.

The samples of blood, 24-hour urine collection, and morning void urine were stored in a biobank at −80 degrees Celsius for additional analyses, as specified in Supplementary Table S1.

2.3. Routine Clinical Care

Diabetes care in the Netherlands is standardised, both in the outpatient clinic and at the general practitioner. It consists of three to four outpatient clinic visits per year. The development of albuminuria is assessed yearly using the albumin–creatinine ratio in a single morning void urine. Retinopathy is assessed at one to two year intervals. Neuropathy is assessed yearly using monofilament and vibration tests with a tuning fork.

Lifestyle management in T2DM consists of guidance regarding weight loss, increasing physical activity, and smoking cessation, and of referral to a dietician for dietary guidance on weight loss and the adherence to dietary guidelines, including sodium restriction and stimulating an intake of fruit and vegetables. The frequency of dietary follow-up visits is targeted at the individual goals and needs of patients depending on personal preferences as well as comorbidity. At each doctor visit, target HbA1c and blood pressure are monitored, and pharmacological intervention is adjusted accordingly. Cholesterol levels are monitored yearly. Targets for HbA1c and LDL cholesterol are often individualized; the general targets are <53 mmol/L and <2.5 mmol/L, respectively.

2.4. Definitions

The blood pressure (BP) targets in our analyses were derived from the international guidelines for diabetes management, which have been adopted for use in The Netherlands [22,23]. In patients with diabetic kidney disease, the BP target was set according to the Kidney Diseases Improving Global Outcomes (KDIGO) guidelines, which are internationally acclaimed guidelines for chronic kidney disease, and are also applied in The Netherlands [23]. Patients with diabetic kidney disease without albuminuria (eGFR <60, no albuminuria) had a BP target of ≤140/90 mmHg, while patients with albuminuria and either an eGFR ≥60 mL/min or an eGFR <60 mL/min had a BP target of ≤130/80 mmHg. For patients with T2DM without diabetic kidney disease, the European Association for the Study of Diabetes (EASD) guidelines are used, which stipulate a blood pressure (BP) target of <140/85 mmHg [22]. Accordingly, the patients were grouped by eGFR above or below 60 mL/min and by the presence of albuminuria. Albuminuria was defined as a 24-hour urinary albumin excretion >30 mg/day. As the EASD and KDIGO guidelines for those without albuminuria differ slightly, we performed all of the analyses using the EASD guidelines for those with eGFR <60 and no albuminuria as well. The results were virtually similar, and for the sake of conciseness, the data is not shown.

The targets for nutritional management were set according to the Dutch guidelines when available. The target dietary salt intake was ≤6 g/day [24], and the target dietary potassium intake was set at ≥3.5 g/day, according to best evidence [13]. The target alcohol intake was ≤2 units per day for women, and ≤3 units per day for men. It should be noted that in 2015, the Health Council of The Netherlands changed the guidelines for alcohol consumption to zero units per day; however, our patients were included in the study before the introduction of these new guidelines [25]. The target BMI was <30 kg/m^2. The target for smoking was either no smoking history, or having previously stopped smoking.

The data on dietary intake of salt, potassium, and proteins were derived from 24-hour urinary excretion. For this, it is important to realise that the patients in our cohort were assessed under steady state conditions, in which the net renal excretion of sodium is almost equal to the dietary intake of sodium, with only approximately 5–10% being excreted by other routes (e.g., sweat or feces) [9]. Therefore, 24-hour urinary sodium excretion is considered the gold standard for the assessment of sodium intake [9,26], and dietary salt intake was calculated by multiplying the net 24-hour sodium excretion (in mol/day) with the molar weight of salt (NaCl, 58.44 g/mol). Dietary potassium intake was calculated from urinary potassium excretion under the assumption of a renal excretion rate of 77% [13,27]. Dietary protein intake was calculated from urinary urea nitrogen excretion using the Maroni formula [28]. As the renal excretion of magnesium is lower in patients with a low eGFR, dietary magnesium intake could not be calculated from urinary magnesium excretion with the same formula (using the assumption of an intestinal absorption of 30%) [16]. Therefore, we present the urinary daily excretion of magnesium. Also, while no consensus exists to calculate dietary phosphate intake from the urinary excretion, urinary phosphate excretion does reflect variability in intestinal phosphate uptake [29,30], so we present the urinary excretion values.

2.5. Statistical Analyses

All of the statistical analyses were performed using Statistical Package for the Social Sciences (SPSS), version 23.0. Normally distributed data are presented as mean ± standard deviation. Skewed variables are expressed as median [interquartile range]. Dichotomous variables are presented in number and percentage. First, we divided the population according to the presence of albuminuria and/or a reduced eGFR (<60 mL/min), as in these groups the target BP is different (<140/85 for those without diabetic kidney disease, ≤140/90 mmHg for patients without albuminuria and an eGFR <60 mL/min, and ≤130/80 mmHg for those with albuminuria). Second, we divided the population into two groups, according to the reached blood pressure. These groups are denoted as "Blood pressure on target" (BP-OT) and "Blood pressure not on target" (BP-NOT), respectively. The differences between the groups were analysed using the student *t*-test, one-way ANOVA, the Mann–Whitney U test, the Kruskall–Wallis test, and the Chi Square test when appropriate. To perform a multivariate analysis of the determinants of not on target BP, multivariate logistic regression was used. In order to adjust for age and gender, the differences in nutritional data among the groups were also determined using mixed model analyses with Sidak post-hoc tests.

3. Results

Between September 2009 and January 2016, 1082 eligible patients were identified and invited to participate in the study, of whom 470 were enrolled in the study and performed the baseline visit. The most common causes for not participating in the study were: No interest in research, and inability due to co-morbidity (Figure 2). Twenty patients were excluded after the baseline visit, as in closer analysis their correct diagnosis was Type 1 Diabetes Mellitus instead of Type 2. All of the remaining 450 patients were included in our data analysis.

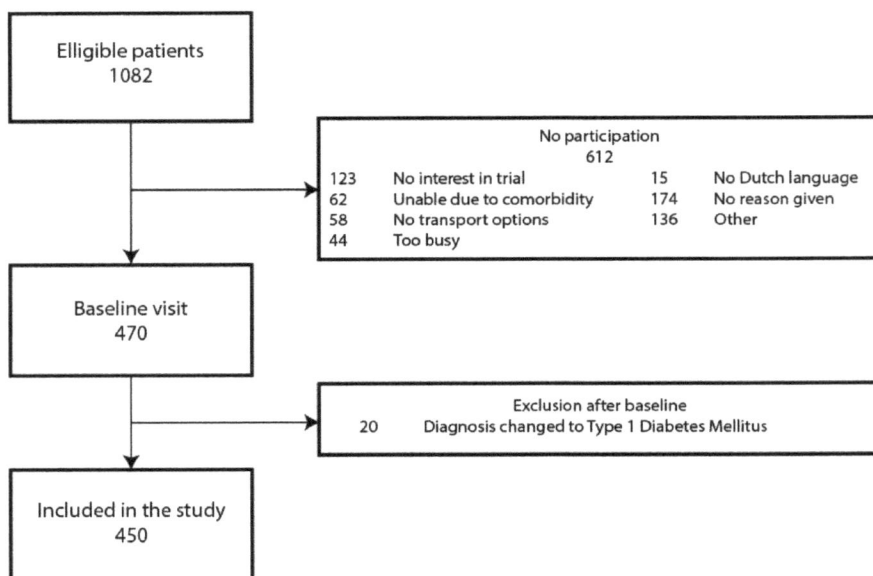

Figure 2. Patient recruitment flowchart.

3.1. Baseline Pharmacological and Nutritional Characteristics

The baseline data are presented in Table 1, by a break-up according to reduced eGFR (<60 mL/min) and the presence of albuminuria. The mean age of the participants was 63 ± 9 years, and was higher in the groups with eGFR <60 (Table 1). There were more men (58%) than women, and men were over-represented in the albuminuria groups (74% and 77% respectively for eGFR ≥60 and <60). The mean BMI was 32.9 ± 6.2 kg/m^2, reflecting a predominantly obese T2DM population, and BMI did not differ among the groups (Table 1).

Table 1. DIALECT-1 Baseline, nutritional, and pharmacological characteristics.

Variable	Total Population	eGFR ≥60		eGFR <60		p-Value
		Albuminuria No	Albuminuria Yes	Albuminuria No	Albuminuria Yes	
Number of patients (% of population)	450	257 (57)	85 (19)	52 (12)	51 (11)	
Patient characteristics						
Age (years)	63 ± 9	61 ± 9	62 ± 8	67 ± 8 *,†	69 ± 7 *,†	<0.001
Male, n (%)	259 (58)	139 (54)	63 (74)	19 (37)	39 (77)	<0.001
Years T2DM (years)	11 (7–18)	11 (7–18)	14 (8–19)	12 (6–17)	10 (6–15)	0.45
Serum HbA1C (mmol/mol)	57 ± 12	58 ± 11	59 ± 13	54 ± 11	57 ± 13	0.15
Insulin use, n (%)	284 (63)	160 (62)	64 (75)	31 (60)	28 (55)	0.07
Systolic blood pressure (mmHg)	139 ± 16	136 ± 15	140 ± 19	131 ± 13 †	139 ± 17	0.009
Diastolic blood pressure (mmHg)	76 ± 9	75 ± 9	76 ± 10	70 ± 9 *,†	75 ± 10 ‡	0.004
BP on target, n (%)	236 (53)	155 (60)	28 (33)	41 (79)	12 (24)	<0.001
Macrovascular disease, n (%)	158 (35)	68 (27)	36 (42)	25 (48)	31 (61)	<0.001
eGFR (mL/min)	84 (62–97)	92 (78–100)	88 (74–99)	47 (36–54)	39 (33–45)	<0.001
Albumin excretion (mg/day)	11 (3–66)	5 (2–11)	94 (62–202)	4 (1–12)	332 (93–661)	<0.001
Pharmacological management						
RAASi, n (%)	296 (67)	152 (59)	63 (74)	39 (75)	42 (82)	0.001
β-blockers, n (%)	207 (46)	100 (39)	37 (44)	36 (69)	33 (65)	<0.001
Thiazide diuretics, n (%)	137 (31)	81 (32)	15 (18)	21 (40)	18 (35)	0.02
Calcium antagonists, n (%)	101 (23)	43 (17)	26 (31)	13 (25)	19 (37)	0.002
Loop diuretics, n (%)	81 (18)	26 (10)	18 (21)	17 (33)	20 (39)	<0.001
Potassium sparing diuretics, n (%)	43 (10)	11 (4)	8 (9)	12 (23)	12 (24)	<0.001
Number of antihypertensives	2 (1–3)	2 (0–3)	2 (1–3)	3 (2–3)	3 (2–4)	<0.001
No antihypertensive therapy, n (%)	83 (19)	65 (25)	12 (14)	1 (2)	2 (4)	<0.001
1 drug, n (%)	101 (23)	61 (24)	17 (20)	6 (12)	6 (12)	
2 drugs, n (%)	106 (24)	57 (22)	28 (33)	13 (25)	11 (22)	
3 drugs, n (%)	91 (20)	44 (17)	15 (18)	21 (40)	12 (24)	
4 drugs, n (%)	56 (13)	24 (9)	10 (12)	8 (15)	13 (26)	
5+ drugs, n (%)	11 (3)	6 (2)	3 (4)	3 (6)	7 (14)	
Hypertension requiring 4+ drugs, n (%)	117 (26)	48 (19)	23 (27)	16 (31)	30 (59)	<0.001
Total number of drugs	7 ± 3	6 ± 3	7 ± 2	8 ± 3 *	9 ± 3 *,†	<0.001

Table 1. *Cont.*

Variable	Total Population	eGFR ≥60		eGFR <60		p-Value
		Albuminuria No	Albuminuria Yes	Albuminuria No	Albuminuria Yes	
Non-pharmacological management						
BMI (kg/m^2)	32.9 ± 6.2	32.9 ± 6.5	32.9 ± 5.4	33.3 ± 6.2	32.3 ± 6.1	0.89
Current smoker, *n* (%)	74 (17)	41 (16)	15 (18)	10 (19)	8 (16)	0.93
Alcohol intake (units per month)	5 (0–30)	5 (0–28)	10 (0–47)	3 (0–24)	12 (0–40)	0.22
25(OH) Vitamin D (nmol/L)	42 ± 20	43 ± 18	37 ± 19	42 ± 26	44 ± 22	0.09
Urinary excretion						
Urinary creatinine excretion (mmol/day)	13.8 ± 4.8	13.9 ± 4.9	14.8 ± 5.4	12.8 ± 4.2	12.8 ± 3.6	0.03
Urinary magnesium excretion (mmol/day)	4.0 ± 2.1	4.1 ± 2.1	4.4 ± 2.3	3.3 ± 1.7 *,†	3.2 ± 1.4 *,†	0.001
Urinary phosphate excretion (mmol/day)	27.5 ± 11.6	28.2 ± 12.2	30.3 ± 12.6	22.7 ± 7.7 *,†	25.0 ± 7.9	0.001
Sodium-to-potassium ratio (mmol/mmol)	2.5 ± 1.0	2.5 ± 1.0	2.8 ± 1.2	2.2 ± 0.7 †	2.3 ± 0.8	0.004
Calculated intake						
Dietary salt intake (g/day)	10.9 ± 4.7	11.0 ± 4.3	12.7 ± 5.6 *	8.7 ± 4.0 *,†	9.7 ± 3.9 †	<0.001
Salt intake ≤6 g/day	53 (12)	26 (10)	5 (6)	15 (29)	7 (14)	<0.001
Dietary potassium intake (g/day)	3.9 ± 1.3	4.0 ± 1.4	4.1 ± 1.1	3.5 ± 1.3	3.6 ± 0.9	0.01
Potassium intake ≥3.5 g/day	290 (66)	173 (69)	62 (73)	27 (53)	29 (59)	0.06
Dietary protein intake (g/day)	92 ± 27	94 ± 28	98 ± 29	80 ± 23 *,†	84 ± 21 †	0.001

* $p < 0.05$ vs. eGFR ≥60/Albuminuria (Alb)−; † $p < 0.05$ vs. eGFR ≥60/Alb+. ‡ $p < 0.05$ vs. eGFR <60/Alb−. Abbreviations: T2DM, Type 2 Diabetes Mellitus; BP, blood pressure.

There was no renal involvement in 57% of the patients (eGFR $\geq$60/Alb$-$; Table 1). Of all of the patients, 30% (n = 136) had albuminuria, either with a preserved (n = 85, eGFR $\geq$60/Alb+) or reduced renal function (n = 51, eGFR <60/Alb+). Fifty-two patients (12%) had a reduced renal function without albuminuria (eGFR <60/Alb$-$). The mean systolic blood pressure was 139 $\pm$ 16 mmHg, and the mean diastolic BP was 76 $\pm$ 9 mmHg. Most of the patients (81%) used one or more antihypertensive drugs. The target BP was reached in 53% of all patients, while 47% had BP not on target. In patients with albuminuria, 33% and 24% reached the target blood pressure in eGFR $\geq$60 and in eGFR <60, respectively (Table 1). Additionally, a blood pressure of $\leq$140/90 mmHg was reached in 48% and 41% of albuminuria patients with an eGFR $\geq$60 and eGFR <60, respectively. The group with albuminuria and eGFR <60 received the largest number of antihypertensive drugs (3 (2–4) drugs, Table 1). Additionally, the number of patients with hypertension requiring 4+ drugs was highest in this group (59%, p < 0.001). In contrast, the antihypertensive drug use in the eGFR $\geq$60/Alb+ group is not higher than in the other groups (2 (1–3) drugs). Patients without chronic kidney disease (CKD) (Table 1, group eGFR $\geq$60/Alb$-$) most commonly used renin-angiotensin-aldosterone-system inhibition (RAASi) (59%), followed by β-blockers (39%), and thiazide diuretics (32%). This was different in those with CKD (groups eGFR $\geq$60/Alb+, eGFR <60/Alb$-$, and eGFR <60/Alb+): RAASi (77%), β-blockers (62%), and Calcium antagonists (31%). There were two patients with an eGFR <60 that used a phosphate binder, one in the Alb$-$ group, and one in the Alb+ group.

The mean dietary salt intake was high, namely, 10.9 g of salt per day, and was considerably higher in the groups with preserved eGFR. When adjusting for age and gender, these differences remained virtually similar (data not shown). In the overall population, only 53 patients (12%) adhered to the dietary guidelines for dietary salt intake, $\leq$6 g/day, and in the eGFR $\geq$60/Alb+ group this percentage was even lower, i.e., 6%. In total, 8% of patients had a salt intake of $\leq$5 g/day as recommended by the WHO. The mean potassium intake was 3.9 $\pm$ 1.3 g/day, and 66% of patients had an intake, as recommended, above 3.5 g/day (Table 1). The mean urinary magnesium excretion was 4.0 $\pm$ 2.1 mmol/day, and as expected was lower in patients with an eGFR <60 mL/min than in those with an eGFR $\geq$ 60mL/min. The mean urinary phosphate excretion was 27.5 $\pm$ 11.6 mmol/day, and the mean calculated dietary protein intake was 92 $\pm$ 27 g/day.

3.2. Pharmacological and Nutritional Management in BP-On Target (BP-OT) and BP-Not On Target (BP-NOT) Groups

Table 2 shows the patients' characteristics by a break-up of BT-OT and BP-NOT. Patients with BP-NOT were more often men (64% vs. 53%, P = 0.018), and had a higher HbA1C (59 $\pm$ 12 vs. 56 $\pm$ 11 mmol/L, P = 0.031). While the presence of albuminuria was a strong predictor of uncontrolled BP (46% vs. 17%, p < 0.001), poor BP control was not associated with an eGFR <60 mL/min (24% vs. 22%).

Patients with BP-OT used loop diuretics more often than those with BP-NOT (Table 2). There were no other differences in the pharmacological treatment between the BP groups; neither in the types of prescribed drugs, nor in the total number of prescribed antihypertensive drugs. Surprisingly, of the patients with BP-NOT, 21% did not use any antihypertensive drug, while 20% used only one, and 21% used two antihypertensive drugs.

Adherence to the recommended nutritional guidelines by a breakup of BP-OT and BP-NOT is shown in Figure 3. In both groups, adherence to the recommended lifestyle guidelines was poor, and the total number of lifestyle targets adhered to did not differ between the groups (3 (2–3) in BP-OT vs. 3 (2–3) in BP-NOT, p = 0.22). In patients with BP-NOT, 8% had a dietary salt intake below the recommended 6 g/day, which was lower than those with BP-OT (15%, p = 0.025). Adherence to the potassium guideline (66% of patients) did not differ among the groups. Only 3% of patients had a sodium-to-potassium ratio $\leq$1.0 in both BP groups. There were only three patients (1%) who adhered to both the recommended intakes of salt and potassium. BMI was $\leq$30 kg/m^2 in 35% of patients, and this proportion did not differ among the BP groups. The smoking and alcohol guidelines were adhered to by 83% and 86% of all patients, and these proportions were not different among the BP groups. We found no differences in the other nutritional factors between the BP-OT and BP-NOT groups (Table 2). In the total population, there was only one patient (with BP-OT) who adhered to all of the lifestyle guidelines simultaneously. There were no differences in lifestyle guidelines adherence between those with zero to two antihypertensives and those with three-plus antihypertensives.

Table 2. DIALECT-1 pharmacological and nutritional management by a breakup of BP on target/not on target.

Variable	BP On Target	BP Not On Target	*p*-Value
Patient characteristics	*n* = 239	*n* = 210	
Age (years)	63 ± 9	63 ± 9	0.36
Male, *n* (%)	126 (53)	134 (64)	0.02
Years T2DM (years)	11 (7–17)	12 (7–18)	0.26
Serum HbA1C (mmol/mol)	56 ± 11	59 ± 12	0.03
Insulin use, *n* (%)	149 (62)	136 (65)	0.60
Systolic blood pressure (mmHg)	125 ± 10	149 ± 13	<0.001
Diastolic blood pressure (mmHg)	70 ± 8	80 ± 9	<0.001
eGFR <60, *n* (%)	53 (22)	51 (24)	0.60
Albuminuria, *n* (%)	40 (17)	95 (46)	<0.001
Pharmacological management			
RAASi, *n* (%)	163 (68)	134 (64)	0.33
β-blockers, *n* (%)	115 (48)	93 (44)	0.42
Thiazide diuretics, *n* (%)	71 (30)	66 (31)	0.69
Calcium antagonists, *n* (%)	50 (21)	52 (25)	0.33
Loop diuretics, *n* (%)	52 (22)	29 (14)	0.03
Potassium sparing diuretics, *n* (%)	22 (9)	21 (10)	0.78
Number of antihypertensives	2 (1–3)	2 (1–3)	0.51
No antihypertensive therapy, *n* (%)	39 (16)	44 (21)	0.85
1 drug, *n* (%)	47 (20)	42 (20)	
2 drugs, *n* (%)	64 (27)	45 (21)	
3 drugs, *n* (%)	50 (21)	43 (21)	
4 drugs, *n* (%)	29 (12)	27 (13)	
5+ drugs, *n* (%)	10 (4)	9 (4)	
Hypertension requiring 4+ drugs, *n* (%)	39 (16)	79 (38)	<0.001
Total number of drugs	7.0 ± 2.6	6.7 ± 2.8	0.30
Non-pharmacological management			
BMI (kg/m^2)	32.8 ± 5.8	32.9 ± 6.7	0.89
Serum 25 (OH) Vitamin D (nmol/L)	43 ± 20	41 ± 20	0.22
Urinary excretion			
Urinary creatinine excretion (mmol/day)	13.6 ± 4.9	14.1 ± 4.7	0.22
Urinary magnesium excretion (mmol/day)	3.9 ± 2.1	4.0 ± 1.9	0.43
Urinary phosphate excretion (mmol/day)	26.9 ± 12.3	28.2 ± 10.7	0.26
Sodium-to-potassium ratio (mmol/mmol)	2.5 ± 1.0	2.5 ± 0.9	0.49
Calculated intake			
Dietary salt intake (g/day)	10.7 ± 4.8	11.1 ± 4.4	0.47
Dietary potassium intake (g/day)	3.8 ± 1.3	4.0 ± 1.2	0.15
Dietary protein intake (g/day)	90 ± 29	93 ± 26	0.29

In the multivariate logistic regression analysis, albuminuria and the use of loop diuretics remained the only significant predictors of BP-NOT (data not shown).

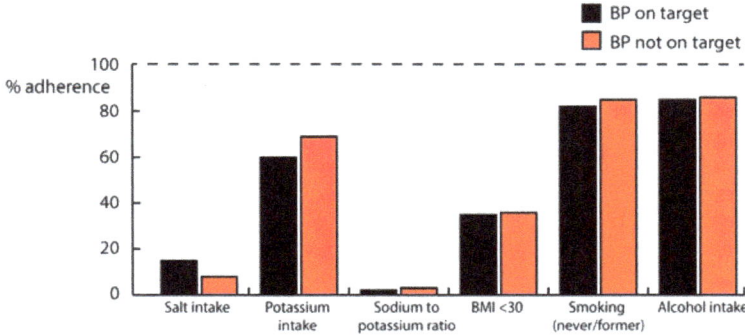

Figure 3. % Adherence to nutritional guidelines, by a breakup of blood pressure on target/not on target. Alcohol intake is self-reported, and the target intake was ≤2 units per day for women and ≤3 units per day for men.

4. Discussion

In this paper, we present the blood pressure management of Type 2 diabetes patients (T2DM), using combined data on pharmacological and nutritional management in a real-life secondary health care setting. As anticipated, the prevalence of hypertension was high, and 81% of patients were on antihypertensives. However, BP control was poor, as the target BP was not reached in 47% of patients. An integrated assessment of pharmacological and nutritional management demonstrated a large window of opportunity for improving BP control in T2DM, both by intensifying antihypertensive drug treatment, and increasing nutritional guideline adherence.

The proportion of patients with their blood pressure on target (BP-OT) in our cohort is in line with findings in other T2DM cohorts [31], as well as diabetic kidney disease cohorts [5,32]. The proportion was lower than found in T2DM patients treated in the primary care setting, in whom adequate blood pressure control was found in 85% of patients [33,34], which may well reflect the referral policy, with more difficult patients being referred to secondary care. In the baseline data of the LEADER-4 trial (a randomized clinical trial in T2DM patients) [31], where 51% of patients had BP-NOT, the antihypertensive use was lower than we report, as about 80% of all patients used zero to two antihypertensive drugs. In diabetic kidney disease studies (i.e., studies with T2DM and either albuminuria and/or eGFR <60), the antihypertensive drug use is mostly in line with our findings, with >90% of patients using antihypertensive drugs, and RAASi being the most frequently used drug [5,32]. In line with our findings, Smits et al. found that RAASi was the most commonly used class of antihypertensive drugs in a Dutch T2DM cohort in primary care, followed by betablockers and diuretics [33]. The number of used antihypertensive drugs they report is largely comparable to our findings, albeit that the use of four to five drugs seems more common in our secondary care cohort. It should be noted that in these studies regarding BP control in a real world setting, data regarding nutrient intake is not available.

An important issue when evaluating the pharmacological management of blood pressure is treatment non-adherence, which reportedly ranges from 31 to 40% in patients with poorly controlled blood pressure [35,36]. Thus, establishing an infrastructure that allows the monitoring of adherence would be of great value. Yet, even assuming a drug-treatment non-adherence rate of 40% in our patients, the non-adherence to lifestyle measures seems to stand out as an additional important target for intervention.

What can be done to improve BP control in T2DM? Our data, and data from other trials, clearly show that true therapy-resistant hypertension, defined as hypertension persisting despite three antihypertensive drugs at maximum tolerable dosage of which one is a diuretic, is not the issue in most patients with BP-NOT. The majority of BP-NOT patients (62%) do not use more than two antihypertensive drugs, illustrating the opportunity for intensifying pharmacological treatment. One promising option in this regard is the removal of excess extracellular fluid with diuretics, especially in those patients with a high salt intake.

Our data show that, especially for nutritional management, there is a large window of opportunity for improvement, as in the total population only one patient adhered to all of the nutritional guidelines simultaneously. This is highly relevant, since lifestyle interventions have the potential to not only reduce BP, but to also reduce the overall cardiovascular risk [11,37–40]. Even though dietary counselling has already been part of their routine care, the mean daily salt intake in our population was almost 11 g/day, roughly twice that of the recommended 6 g/day, and considerably higher than the mean salt intake in the general Dutch population of 8.5 g/day [41]. Previously, Mente et al demonstrated that for each 1-gram increment in estimated sodium excretion, blood pressure was 2/1 mmHg higher, where this slope was more pronounced and steeper in those with hypertension, high-sodium diets (>5g/day), and older persons [42]. Therefore, the most obvious step to improve non-pharmacological management would be to reduce dietary salt intake. This is underscored by a previous study, performed in T2DM patients in the same region, which has shown that, although the aim to reduce dietary salt intake to <6 g/day was not reached, even a relatively modest reduction in salt intake from 12 to 9 g/day can reduce blood pressure by 6/3 mmHg and albuminuria by 42% while under RAASi [43]. Furthermore, reducing salt intake is associated with potentiating the antihypertensive effects of RAASi [44–46].

There is evidence that a combined dietary approach aimed at reducing salt while increasing potassium intake has the potential to improve cardiovascular risk management [12,47]. However, the potassium intake in our patients was generally already above the recommended intake of 3.5 g/day. Therefore, the finding that the sodium-to-potassium ratio was higher than the deemed optimal ratio of 1 mmol/mmol in 97% of patients is primarily determined by high salt intake.

To improve blood pressure control, dietary intervention could also be aimed at reducing body weight. The mean BMI in our cohort was above 30 kg/m². While a relationship between obesity and blood pressure has previously been demonstrated [7,48], we did not find such an association here. This might be due to the fact that we had few participants with a BMI < 25 kg/m², and therefore did not have a large enough dispersion to differentiate between the BP groups. Intentional weight loss has been associated with beneficial effects, both on BP and on other cardiovascular risk factors such as LDL cholesterol and glycemic control [49]. Therefore, even though weight loss is notoriously difficult to achieve, especially in patients on insulin treatment, it should remain a priority in the non-pharmacological treatment of T2DM, and also in secondary health care centres.

Finally, an association between the intake of magnesium and phosphate and blood pressure has been reported previously [14,17,18,50,51]. Here, we did not find differences in urinary magnesium excretion or in urinary phosphate excretion between those with BP-OT and BP-NOT. As the urinary excretion of magnesium and phosphate is lower in those with a low eGFR, these results might be misleading. However, the proportion of patients with a low eGFR was similar in both the BP-OT and BP-NOT groups, making it less likely that differences in the urinary excretion of magnesium and phosphate between the BP groups were masked by differences in urinary excretion due to a low eGFR. In the general population, a continuous relationship between lower magnesium excretion and the risk for hypertension was reported [16]; moreover, patients with a low magnesium intake had a greater risk of developing ischemic heart disease [52]. While no nutritional recommendations are currently available for magnesium to stratify adequate/inadequate intake, in our population approximately 28% of patients had a magnesium excretion below the values associated with ischemic heart disease in the general population. Regarding phosphate intake, population-based studies as well as studies in CKD have shown associations with outcome, albeit not equivocal [53,54], and it has been proposed that excess phosphate intake is a risk factor that is generally overlooked in patients with early stages of CKD by lack of measurements [55]. While more research is needed on the relation between magnesium and phosphate excretion and adverse outcomes, our data illustrate that 24-hour urine, collected to assess the intake of established nutritional targets such as salt and potassium, can simply be used to establish a more complete nutritional profile, which could be useful for future improvements in nutritional studies and counselling.

It should be noted that the adherence to nutritional guidelines was equally poor in the BP-OT and BP-NOT groups. While in the BP-NOT group there is more urgency to adhere to these guidelines, namely to correct BP, the adherence to the guidelines in the BP-OT group should not be overlooked. In regard to salt intake, previously it has been shown that a higher salt intake while under RAASi is associated with worse cardiovascular outcomes, even independent of BP [46]. Furthermore, as stated above, intentional weight loss has many benefits that surpass BP management [49], and therefore can also greatly improve outcomes if BP is already on target. Lastly, in a population-based cohort, low potassium intake has been associated with the occurrence of chronic kidney disease [56].

The DIALECT study has several strengths, including the use of real-world data from a cohort representative of secondary health care in T2DM, at least in the context of the Dutch referral health care setting. Second, we study the integrated role of non-biased data on both pharmacological and non-pharmacological parameters on BP, which is an important approach, as in cardiovascular risk management pharmacological and non-pharmacological interventions go hand in hand. Third, through the use of 24-hour urine collections, we provide objective measurements of dietary intake and several relevant nutrients.

There are also some limitations. An observational study cannot prove causal relationships. Also, there is some risk of response bias, although patient characteristics were similar between those who did and did not participate.

What are the implications of our study? Adequate management equals the sum of measures taken in combination with compliance. Our data on poor nutritional management do not distinguish between a lack of adequate nutritional counselling and a lack of compliance. However, it is well established that sustained lifestyle change is difficult to achieve, demonstrating that currently no modus of adequate counselling and therefore adequate management exists. The question, therefore, is how to establish this. Previous well-designed studies, using interventions of intensive nurse practitioner support and self-management, both did not lead to neither long-standing changes in nutritional habits, nor a reduction of cardiovascular outcomes [57,58]. As alternative approach, improvement strategies as tested for pharmacological management could be considered. In particular, it has been shown that the systematic evaluation of prescription quality as assessed by prescription quality indicators not only improved pharmacological compliance with guidelines, but also patient outcomes [59]. To the best of our knowledge, such approaches have never been developed and tested for nutritional management. As several objective parameters are available, such as the urinary excretion of sodium and potassium, this would be feasible in routine clinical care. Therefore, to improve blood pressure control, in our opinion, the use of nutritional quality indicators may have the potential to improve treatment quality as a whole.

5. Conclusions

Uncontrolled BP is common in T2DM, especially in those with microalbuminuria. An integrated assessment of pharmacological and nutritional management demonstrated a window of opportunity for improving BP treatment, especially in nutritional management. We advocate that incorporating the integrated monitoring of pharmacological and nutritional management in quality control cycles has the potential to improve treatment quality in T2DM.

Supplementary Materials: The following are available online at www.mdpi.com/2072-6643/9/7/709/s1, Table S1: Data collection in DIALECT.

Acknowledgments: We thank Willeke van Kampen, Sanne van Huizen, Anne Davina, Jolien Jaspers, and Manon Harmelink for their contribution to patient inclusion. Furthermore, we would like to thank Bettine Haandrikman for her help with setting up the biobank. Lastly, we would like to thank Job van der Palen and Marloes Vermeer for their support in statistical analyses.

Author Contributions: E.v.d.B., S.J.L.B., G.J.N. and G.D.L. conceived and designed the study. C.M.G., H.B. and E.v.d.B. included patients and performed the measurements. C.M.G. and H.B. analysed the data. S.J.L.B., G.J.N. and G.D.L. contributed materials. C.M.G., H.B., S.J.L.B., G.J.N. and G.D.L. wrote the paper.

Conflicts of Interest: The authors declare no conflict of interest.

References

1. World Health Organization. *Global Report on Diabetes*; WHO Press: Geneva, Switzerland, 2016.
2. Tancredi, M.; Rosengren, A.; Svensson, A.M.; Kosiborod, M.; Pivodic, A.; Gudbjornsdottir, S.; Wedel, H.; Clements, M.; Dahlqvist, S.; Lind, M. Excess Mortality among Persons with Type 2 Diabetes. *N. Engl. J. Med.* **2015**, *373*, 1720–1732. [CrossRef] [PubMed]
3. Fox, C.S.; Coady, S.; Sorlie, P.D.; Levy, D.; Meigs, J.B.; D'Agostino, R.B., Sr.; Wilson, P.W.; Savage, P.J. Trends in Cardiovascular Complications of Diabetes. *JAMA* **2004**, *292*, 2495–2499. [CrossRef] [PubMed]
4. Langsted, A.; Freiberg, J.J.; Nordestgaard, B.G. Extent of Undertreatment and Overtreatment with Cholesterol-Lowering Therapy According to European Guidelines in 92,348 Danes without Ischemic Cardiovascular Disease and Diabetes in 2004–2014. *Atherosclerosis* **2016**, *257*, 9–15. [CrossRef] [PubMed]
5. De Cosmo, S.; Viazzi, F.; Piscitelli, P.; Giorda, C.; Ceriello, A.; Genovese, S.; Russo, G.; Guida, P.; Fioretto, P.; Pontremoli, R.; et al. Blood Pressure Status and the Incidence of Diabetic Kidney Disease in Patients with Hypertension and Type 2 Diabetes. *J. Hypertens.* **2016**, *34*, 2090–2098. [CrossRef] [PubMed]
6. Gorter, K.; van Bruggen, R.; Stolk, R.; Zuithoff, P.; Verhoeven, R.; Rutten, G. Overall Quality of Diabetes Care in a Defined Geographic Region: Different Sides of the Same Story. *Br. J. Gen. Pract.* **2008**, *58*, 339–345. [CrossRef] [PubMed]
7. Baptista, D.R.; Thieme, R.D.; Reis, W.C.; Pontarolo, R.; Correr, C.J. Proportion of Brazilian Diabetes Patients that Achieve Treatment Goals: Implications for Better Quality of Care. *Diabetol. Metab. Syndr.* **2015**, *7*, 113. [CrossRef] [PubMed]
8. Laxy, M.; Knoll, G.; Schunk, M.; Meisinger, C.; Huth, C.; Holle, R. Quality of Diabetes Care in Germany Improved from 2000 to 2007 to 2014, but Improvements Diminished since 2007. Evidence from the Population-Based KORA Studies. *PLoS ONE* **2016**, *11*, e0164704. [CrossRef] [PubMed]
9. McLean, R.M. Measuring Population Sodium Intake: A Review of Methods. *Nutrients* **2014**, *6*, 4651–4662. [CrossRef] [PubMed]
10. WHO. *Guideline: Sodium Intake for Adults and Children*; WHO Press: Geneva, Switzerland, 2012.
11. Fox, C.S.; Golden, S.H.; Anderson, C.; Bray, G.A.; Burke, L.E.; de Boer, I.H.; Deedwania, P.; Eckel, R.H.; Ershow, A.G.; Fradkin, J.; et al. Update on Prevention of Cardiovascular Disease in Adults with Type 2 Diabetes Mellitus in Light of Recent Evidence: A Scientific Statement from the American Heart Association and the American Diabetes Association. *Diabetes Care* **2015**, *38*, 1777–1803. [CrossRef] [PubMed]
12. Filippini, T.; Violi, F.; D'Amico, R.; Vinceti, M. The Effect of Potassium Supplementation on Blood Pressure in Hypertensive Subjects: A Systematic Review and Meta-Analysis. *Int. J. Cardiol.* **2017**, *230*, 127–135. [CrossRef] [PubMed]
13. WHO. *Guideline: Potassium Intake for Adults and Children*; WHO Press: Geneva, Switzerland, 2012.
14. Zhang, X.; Li, Y.; Del Gobbo, L.C.; Rosanoff, A.; Wang, J.; Zhang, W.; Song, Y. Effects of Magnesium Supplementation on Blood Pressure: A Meta-Analysis of Randomized Double-Blind Placebo-Controlled Trials. *Hypertension* **2016**, *68*, 324–333. [CrossRef] [PubMed]
15. Bain, L.K.; Myint, P.K.; Jennings, A.; Lentjes, M.A.; Luben, R.N.; Khaw, K.T.; Wareham, N.J.; Welch, A.A. The Relationship between Dietary Magnesium Intake, Stroke and its Major Risk Factors, Blood Pressure and Cholesterol, in the EPIC-Norfolk Cohort. *Int. J. Cardiol.* **2015**, *196*, 108–114. [CrossRef] [PubMed]
16. Joosten, M.M.; Gansevoort, R.T.; Mukamal, K.J.; Kootstra-Ros, J.E.; Feskens, E.J.; Geleijnse, J.M.; Navis, G.; Bakker, S.J. PREVEND Study Group. Urinary Magnesium Excretion and Risk of Hypertension: The Prevention of Renal and Vascular End-Stage Disease Study. *Hypertension* **2013**, *61*, 1161–1167. [CrossRef] [PubMed]
17. Bozic, M.; Panizo, S.; Sevilla, M.A.; Riera, M.; Soler, M.J.; Pascual, J.; Lopez, I.; Freixenet, M.; Fernandez, E.; Valdivielso, J.M. High Phosphate Diet Increases Arterial Blood Pressure Via a Parathyroid Hormone Mediated Increase of Renin. *J. Hypertens.* **2014**, *32*, 1822–1832. [CrossRef] [PubMed]

18. Mizuno, M.; Mitchell, J.H.; Crawford, S.; Huang, C.L.; Maalouf, N.; Hu, M.C.; Moe, O.W.; Smith, S.A.; Vongpatanasin, W. High Dietary Phosphate Intake Induces Hypertension and Augments Exercise Pressor Reflex Function in Rats. *Am. J. Physiol. Regul. Integr. Comp. Physiol.* **2016**, *311*, R39–R48. [CrossRef] [PubMed]

19. Du Bois, D.; Du Bois, E.F. A Formula to Estimate the Approximate Surface Area if Height and Weight be Known. 1916. *Nutrition* **1989**, *5*, 303–311. [PubMed]

20. Wendel-Vos, G.C.; Schuit, A.J.; Saris, W.H.; Kromhout, D. Reproducibility and Relative Validity of the Short Questionnaire to Assess Health-Enhancing Physical Activity. *J. Clin. Epidemiol.* **2003**, *56*, 1163–1169. [CrossRef]

21. Levey, A.S.; Stevens, L.A.; Schmid, C.H.; Zhang, Y.L.; Castro, A.F., 3rd; Feldman, H.I.; Kusek, J.W.; Eggers, P.; Van Lente, F.; Greene, T.; et al. A New Equation to Estimate Glomerular Filtration Rate. *Ann. Intern. Med.* **2009**, *150*, 604–612. [CrossRef] [PubMed]

22. Authors/Task Force Members; Ryden, L.; Grant, P.J.; Anker, S.D.; Berne, C.; Cosentino, F.; Danchin, N.; Deaton, C.; Escaned, J.; Hammes, H.P.; et al. ESC Guidelines on Diabetes, Pre-Diabetes, and Cardiovascular Diseases Developed in Collaboration with the EASD: The Task Force on Diabetes, Pre-Diabetes, and Cardiovascular Diseases of the European Society of Cardiology (ESC) and Developed in Collaboration with the European Association for the Study of Diabetes (EASD). *Eur. Heart J.* **2013**, *34*, 3035–3087. [PubMed]

23. Kidney Disease: Improving Global Outcomes (KDIGO) Blood Pressure Work Group. KDIGO Clinical Practice Guideline for the Management of Blood Pressure in Chronic Kidney Disease. *Kidney Int. Suppl.* **2012**, *2*, 337–414.

24. Kromhout, D.; Spaaij, C.J.; de Goede, J.; Weggemans, R.M. The 2015 Dutch Food-Based Dietary Guidelines. *Eur. J. Clin. Nutr.* **2016**, *70*, 869–878. [CrossRef] [PubMed]

25. Gezondheidsraad. *Richtlijnen Goede Voeding 2015*; Gezondheidsraad: The Hague, The Netherlands, 2015.

26. Bock, H.A.; Stein, J.H. Diuretics and the Control of Extracellular Fluid Volume: Role of Counterregulation. *Semin. Nephrol.* **1988**, *8*, 264–272. [PubMed]

27. Holbrook, J.T.; Patterson, K.Y.; Bodner, J.E.; Douglas, L.W.; Veillon, C.; Kelsay, J.L.; Mertz, W.; Smith, J.C., Jr. Sodium and Potassium Intake and Balance in Adults Consuming Self-Selected Diets. *Am. J. Clin. Nutr.* **1984**, *40*, 786–793. [PubMed]

28. Maroni, B.J.; Steinman, T.I.; Mitch, W.E. A Method for Estimating Nitrogen Intake of Patients with Chronic Renal Failure. *Kidney Int.* **1985**, *27*, 58–65. [CrossRef] [PubMed]

29. Newsome, B.; Ix, J.H.; Tighiouart, H.; Sarnak, M.J.; Levey, A.S.; Beck, G.J.; Block, G. Effect of Protein Restriction on Serum and Urine Phosphate in the Modification of Diet in Renal Disease (MDRD) Study. *Am. J. Kidney Dis.* **2013**, *61*, 1045–1046. [CrossRef] [PubMed]

30. Block, G.A.; Wheeler, D.C.; Persky, M.S.; Kestenbaum, B.; Ketteler, M.; Spiegel, D.M.; Allison, M.A.; Asplin, J.; Smits, G.; Hoofnagle, A.N.; et al. Effects of Phosphate Binders in Moderate CKD. *J. Am. Soc. Nephrol.* **2012**, *23*, 1407–1415. [CrossRef] [PubMed]

31. Petrie, J.R.; Marso, S.P.; Bain, S.C.; Franek, E.; Jacob, S.; Masmiquel, L.; Leiter, L.A.; Haluzik, M.; Satman, I.; Omar, M.; et al. LEADER-4: Blood Pressure Control in Patients with Type 2 Diabetes and High Cardiovascular Risk: Baseline Data from the LEADER Randomized Trial. *J. Hypertens.* **2016**, *34*, 1140–1150. [CrossRef] [PubMed]

32. Halimi, J.M.; Joly, D.; Combe, C.; Choukroun, G.; Dussol, B.; Fauvel, J.P.; Quere, S.; Fiquet, B. Blood Pressure and Proteinuria Control Remains a Challenge in Patients with Type 2 Diabetes Mellitus and Chronic Kidney Disease: Experience from the Prospective Observational ALICE-PROTECT Study. *BMC Nephrol.* **2016**, *17*, 135. [CrossRef] [PubMed]

33. Smits, K.P.; Sidorenkov, G.; Kleefstra, N.; Bouma, M.; Meulepas, M.; Voorham, J.; Navis, G.; Bilo, H.J.; Denig, P. Development and Validation of Prescribing Quality Indicators for Patients with Type 2 Diabetes. *Int. J. Clin. Pract.* **2017**, *71*. [CrossRef] [PubMed]

34. Walraven, I.; Mast, M.R.; Hoekstra, T.; Jansen, A.P.; Rauh, S.P.; Rutters, F.R.; van der Heijden, A.A.; Elders, P.J.; Moll, A.C.; Polak, B.C.; et al. Real-World Evidence of Suboptimal Blood Pressure Control in Patients with Type 2 Diabetes. *J. Hypertens.* **2015**, *33*, 2091–2098. [CrossRef] [PubMed]

35. Vrijens, B.; Antoniou, S.; Burnier, M.; de la Sierra, A.; Volpe, M. Current Situation of Medication Adherence in Hypertension. *Front. Pharmacol.* **2017**, *8*, 100. [CrossRef] [PubMed]

36. De Jager, R.L.; de Beus, E.; Beeftink, M.M.; Sanders, M.F.; Vonken, E.J.; Voskuil, M.; van Maarseveen, E.M.; Bots, M.L.; Blankestijn, P.J. SYMPATHY Investigators. Impact of Medication Adherence on the Effect of Renal Denervation: The SYMPATHY Trial. *Hypertension* **2017**, *69*, 678–684. [CrossRef] [PubMed]

37. Dunkler, D.; Kohl, M.; Heinze, G.; Teo, K.K.; Rosengren, A.; Pogue, J.; Gao, P.; Gerstein, H.; Yusuf, S.; Oberbauer, R.; et al. Modifiable Lifestyle and Social Factors Affect Chronic Kidney Disease in High-Risk Individuals with Type 2 Diabetes Mellitus. *Kidney Int.* **2015**, *87*, 784–791. [CrossRef] [PubMed]

38. Knowler, W.C.; Barrett-Connor, E.; Fowler, S.E.; Hamman, R.F.; Lachin, J.M.; Walker, E.A.; Nathan, D.M. Diabetes Prevention Program Research Group. Reduction in the Incidence of Type 2 Diabetes with Lifestyle Intervention Or Metformin. *N. Engl. J. Med.* **2002**, *346*, 393–403. [PubMed]

39. Bibbins-Domingo, K.; Chertow, G.M.; Coxson, P.G.; Moran, A.; Lightwood, J.M.; Pletcher, M.J.; Goldman, L. Projected Effect of Dietary Salt Reductions on Future Cardiovascular Disease. *N. Engl. J. Med.* **2010**, *362*, 590–599. [CrossRef] [PubMed]

40. Wong, M.M.; Arcand, J.; Leung, A.A.; Thout, S.R.; Campbell, N.R.; Webster, J. The Science of Salt: A Regularly Updated Systematic Review of Salt and Health Outcomes (December 2015–March 2016). *J. Clin. Hypertens. (Greenwich)* **2017**, *19*, 322–332. [CrossRef] [PubMed]

41. Hendriksen, M.; Etemad, Z.; van den Bogaard, C.H.; van der A, D.L. *Salt, Iodine and Potassium Intake among Adults in Doetinchem in 2015*; RIVM Report 2016–0081; Rijksinstituut voor Volksgezondheid en Milieu: Bilthoven, The Netherlands, 2016.

42. Mente, A.; O'Donnell, M.J.; Rangarajan, S.; McQueen, M.J.; Poirier, P.; Wielgosz, A.; Morrison, H.; Li, W.; Wang, X.; Di, C.; et al. Association of Urinary Sodium and Potassium Excretion with Blood Pressure. *N. Engl. J. Med.* **2014**, *371*, 601–611. [CrossRef] [PubMed]

43. Kwakernaak, A.J.; Krikken, J.A.; Binnenmars, S.H.; Visser, F.W.; Hemmelder, M.H.; Woittiez, A.J.; Groen, H.; Laverman, G.D.; Navis, G. Holland Nephrology Study (HONEST) Group. Effects of Sodium Restriction and Hydrochlorothiazide on RAAS Blockade Efficacy in Diabetic Nephropathy: A Randomised Clinical Trial. *Lancet Diabetes Endocrinol.* **2014**, *2*, 385–395. [CrossRef]

44. Lambers Heerspink, H.J.; de Borst, M.H.; Bakker, S.J.; Navis, G.J. Improving the Efficacy of RAAS Blockade in Patients with Chronic Kidney Disease. *Nat. Rev. Nephrol.* **2013**, *9*, 112–121. [CrossRef] [PubMed]

45. Vogt, L.; Waanders, F.; Boomsma, F.; de Zeeuw, D.; Navis, G. Effects of Dietary Sodium and Hydrochlorothiazide on the Antiproteinuric Efficacy of Losartan. *J. Am. Soc. Nephrol.* **2008**, *19*, 999–1007. [CrossRef] [PubMed]

46. Lambers Heerspink, H.J.; Holtkamp, F.A.; Parving, H.H.; Navis, G.J.; Lewis, J.B.; Ritz, E.; de Graeff, P.A.; de Zeeuw, D. Moderation of Dietary Sodium Potentiates the Renal and Cardiovascular Protective Effects of Angiotensin Receptor Blockers. *Kidney Int.* **2012**, *82*, 330–337. [CrossRef] [PubMed]

47. Kieneker, L.M.; Gansevoort, R.T.; Mukamal, K.J.; de Boer, R.A.; Navis, G.; Bakker, S.J.; Joosten, M.M. Urinary Potassium Excretion and Risk of Developing Hypertension: The Prevention of Renal and Vascular End-Stage Disease Study. *Hypertension* **2014**, *64*, 769–776. [CrossRef] [PubMed]

48. Adeniyi, O.V.; Yogeswaran, P.; Longo-Mbenza, B.; Ter Goon, D. Uncontrolled Hypertension and its Determinants in Patients with Concomitant Type 2 Diabetes Mellitus (T2DM) in Rural South Africa. *PLoS ONE* **2016**, *11*, e0150033. [CrossRef] [PubMed]

49. Zomer, E.; Gurusamy, K.; Leach, R.; Trimmer, C.; Lobstein, T.; Morris, S.; James, W.P.; Finer, N. Interventions that Cause Weight Loss and the Impact on Cardiovascular Risk Factors: A Systematic Review and Meta-Analysis. *Obes. Rev.* **2016**, *17*, 1001–1011. [CrossRef] [PubMed]

50. Verma, H.; Garg, R. Effect of Magnesium Supplementation on Type 2 Diabetes Associated Cardiovascular Risk Factors: A Systematic Review and Meta-Analysis. *J. Hum. Nutr. Diet.* **2017**. [CrossRef] [PubMed]

51. Humalda, J.K.; Keyzer, C.A.; Binnenmars, S.H.; Kwakernaak, A.J.; Slagman, M.C.; Laverman, G.D.; Bakker, S.J.; de Borst, M.H.; Navis, G.J. Concordance of Dietary Sodium Intake and Concomitant Phosphate Load: Implications for Sodium Interventions. *Nutr. Metab. Cardiovasc. Dis.* **2016**, *26*, 689–696. [CrossRef] [PubMed]

52. Joosten, M.M.; Gansevoort, R.T.; Mukamal, K.J.; van der Harst, P.; Geleijnse, J.M.; Feskens, E.J.; Navis, G.; Bakker, S.J.; PREVEND Study Group. Urinary and Plasma Magnesium and Risk of Ischemic Heart Disease. *Am. J. Clin. Nutr.* **2013**, *97*, 1299–1306. [CrossRef] [PubMed]

53. Chang, A.R.; Grams, M.E. Serum Phosphorus and Mortality in the Third National Health and Nutrition Examination Survey (NHANES III): Effect Modification by Fasting. *Am. J. Kidney Dis.* **2014**, *64*, 567–573. [CrossRef] [PubMed]

54. Palomino, H.L.; Rifkin, D.E.; Anderson, C.; Criqui, M.H.; Whooley, M.A.; Ix, J.H. 24-Hour Urine Phosphorus Excretion and Mortality and Cardiovascular Events. *Clin. J. Am. Soc. Nephrol.* **2013**, *8*, 1202–1210. [CrossRef] [PubMed]

55. Ritz, E.; Hahn, K.; Ketteler, M.; Kuhlmann, M.K.; Mann, J. Phosphate Additives in Food—A Health Risk. *Dtsch. Arzteblatt Int.* **2012**, *109*, 49–55.

56. Kieneker, L.M.; Bakker, S.J.; de Boer, R.A.; Navis, G.J.; Gansevoort, R.T.; Joosten, M.M. Low Potassium Excretion but Not High Sodium Excretion is Associated with Increased Risk of Developing Chronic Kidney Disease. *Kidney Int.* **2016**, *90*, 888–896. [CrossRef] [PubMed]

57. Meuleman, Y.; Hoekstra, T.; Dekker, F.W.; Navis, G.; Vogt, L.; van der Boog, P.J.M.; Bos, W.J.W.; van Montfrans, G.A.; van Dijk, S.; ESMO Study Group. Sodium Restriction in Patients with CKD: A Randomized Controlled Trial of Self-Management Support. *Am. J. Kidney Dis.* **2017**, *69*, 576–586. [CrossRef] [PubMed]

58. Van Zuilen, A.D.; Bots, M.L.; Dulger, A.; van der Tweel, I.; van Buren, M.; Ten Dam, M.A.; Kaasjager, K.A.; Ligtenberg, G.; Sijpkens, Y.W.; Sluiter, H.E.; et al. Multifactorial Intervention with Nurse Practitioners does Not Change Cardiovascular Outcomes in Patients with Chronic Kidney Disease. *Kidney Int.* **2012**, *82*, 710–717. [CrossRef] [PubMed]

59. Smits, K.P.J.; Sidorenkov, G.; Navis, G.; Bouma, M.; Meulepas, M.A.; Bilo, H.J.G.; Denig, P. Prescribing Quality and Prediction of Clinical Outcomes in Patients with Type 2 Diabetes: A Prospective Cohort Study. *Diabetes Care* **2017**, *40*, e83–e84. [CrossRef] [PubMed]

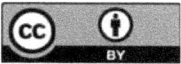

nutrients

MDPI

Article

Butyrate Reduces HFD-Induced Adipocyte Hypertrophy and Metabolic Risk Factors in Obese LDLr-/-.Leiden Mice

Charlotte E. Pelgrim [1,†], Bart A. A. Franx [1,†] (ORCID), Jessica Snabel [2], Robert Kleemann [2] (ORCID), Ilse A. C. Arnoldussen [1] and Amanda J. Kiliaan [1,*]

[1] Donders Institute for Brain, Cognition and Behaviour, Preclinical Imaging Centre, Department of Anatomy, Radboud University Medical Center, 6525 EZ Nijmegen, The Netherlands; charlottepelgrim@gmail.com (C.E.P.); bart.franx@gmail.com (B.A.A.F.); ilse.arnoldussen@radboudumc.nl (I.A.C.A.)

[2] Department of Metabolic Health Research, Netherlands Organisation for Applied Scientific Research (TNO), 2301 CE Leiden, The Netherlands; jessica.snabel@tno.nl (J.S.); robert.kleemann@tno.nl (R.K.)

* Correspondence: Amanda.Kiliaan@radboudumc.nl; Tel.: +31-24-361-4378

† Authors contributed equally to this work.

Received: 10 May 2017; Accepted: 4 July 2017; Published: 7 July 2017

Abstract: Adipose tissue (AT) has a modulating role in obesity-induced metabolic complications like type 2 diabetes mellitus (T2DM) via the production of so-called adipokines such as leptin, adiponectin, and resistin. The adipokines are believed to influence other tissues and to affect insulin resistance, liver function, and to increase the risk of T2DM. In this study, we examined the impact of intervention with the short-chain fatty acid butyrate following a high-fat diet (HFD) on AT function and other metabolic risk factors associated with obesity and T2DM in mice during mid- and late life. In both mid- and late adulthood, butyrate reduced HFD-induced adipocyte hypertrophy and elevations in leptin levels, which were associated with body weight, and cholesterol and triglyceride levels. HFD feeding stimulated macrophage accumulation primarily in epididymal AT in both mid- and late life adult mice, which correlated with liver inflammation in late adulthood. In late-adult mice, butyrate diminished increased insulin levels, which were related to adipocyte size and macrophage content in epididymal AT. These results suggest that dietary butyrate supplementation is able to counteract HFD-induced detrimental changes in AT function and metabolic outcomes in late life. These changes underlie the obesity-induced elevated risk of T2DM, and therefore it is suggested that butyrate has potential to attenuate risk factors associated with obesity and T2DM.

Keywords: obesity; T2DM; high-fat diet; butyrate; adipose tissue; macrophages; adipokines

1. Introduction

In line with the rise of type 2 diabetes mellitus (T2DM) the global prevalence of obesity has more than doubled since 1980 [1]. Moreover, obesity is a major risk factor for T2DM, accounting for 80–85% of the overall risk [2]. Weight or fat loss has the strongest effect on reducing the risk of developing T2DM [3]. It has been suggested that the relationship between obesity and T2DM exists already at a young age [4–6]. In addition, obesity is suggested to exaggerate aging processes [7], and aging is associated with impaired insulin signaling [8], which causes an increase in blood glucose levels. Over time, high blood glucose concentrations combined with high blood pressure and high cholesterol levels affect vascular function, and may evolve into cardiovascular disease, kidney failure, and subsequent cognitive deficits [9,10].

Accumulating evidence suggests that adipose tissue dysfunction—with adipocyte hypertrophy as a first manifestation—may play a role in the development of obesity-induced metabolic conditions that increase the risk for T2DM [11]. Adipocyte hypertrophy results in an elevated recruitment of macrophages surrounding dead or dying adipocytes, which is referred to as crown-like structures (CLS)—an important hallmark of adipose tissue dysfunction— [12]. Macrophages are believed to be major sources of inflammatory cytokines with detrimental effects on insulin signaling in obesity [13]. In addition, adipocyte hypertrophy may lead to the altered production and secretion of adipokines like leptin, resistin, serum amyloid A (SAA), and adiponectin [14–16]. These adipokines play important roles in insulin signaling and the development of a chronic low-grade inflammatory state, which is characteristic for obesity. Overall, amelioration of these obesity-induced and adipose tissue-related changes may provide an important approach to attenuate the risk of developing T2DM.

There is a growing interest in short-chain fatty acids—such as butyrate—as dietary intervention for obesity and related metabolic diseases [17,18]. Butyrate is one of the fatty acids produced during bacterial fermentation in the distal gut of nondigestible carbohydrates like dietary fiber and resistant starch. Both intake of butyrate and dietary fibers have shown positive effects on body weight and insulin sensitivity [17,19–22]. In addition, butyrate has anti-inflammatory properties and affects lipogenesis [17]. A decreased concentration of butyrate-producing bacteria has been observed both in patients with obesity [23] and T2DM [24]. Butyrate may therefore play an essential role in the maintenance of an optimal metabolic state.

It is acknowledged that obesity may differentially affect various organs and tissues, like the brain and cardiovascular system, during midlife as opposed to late life [18,25–27]. Recently, we demonstrated that butyrate is able to restore high-fat diet (HFD)-induced neuroinflammation and changes in brain function in low-density-lipoprotein receptor knockout (LDLr-/-).Leiden mice in mid-adulthood [18]. In addition, mid-adult mice seem to be more susceptible to the development of HFD-induced cardiovascular damage as compared to late-adult mice [18]. However, it has not been elucidated whether diet-induced obesity affects adipose tissue function and its metabolic outcomes differentially during mid- and late adulthood. As follow-up of the previous published study [18], we investigated in the current study the effects of a therapeutic butyrate intervention on adipose tissue function and adipokine levels in the context of manifested HFD-induced obesity in both mid- and late-adult LDLr-/-.Leiden mice.

2. Materials and Methods

2.1. Animals and Diets

The adipose tissues and plasma samples analyzed in this experiment originate from a previously described study [18]. LDLr-/-.Leiden mice were selected because of their high sensitivity to developing HFD-induced obesity and subsequent complications like vascular damage and fatty liver [28–30]. Briefly, male LDLr-/-.Leiden mice (TNO Metabolic Health Research, Leiden, The Netherlands) were housed in individually ventilated cages in a conventional animal room situated in the preclinical imaging center (PRIME) at the central animal laboratory, Radboudumc Nijmegen, the Netherlands. A maximum of five mice were housed per cage with ad libitum access to acidified tap water and food (temperature 21 °C; relative humidity 50–60%; light-dark cycle 7 a.m.–7 p.m.). The experiments were approved by an independent ethical committee on animal care and experimentation (Zeist, The Netherlands), approval project number DEC3682 [18] and carried out in accordance to the ARRIVE guidelines [31].

The intervention regimen of the study [18] is schematically presented in Figure 1. A total group of $n = 60$ LDLr-/-.Leiden mice were divided into a mid- and late-adult cohort ($n = 30$ each). Both cohorts consisted of three diet groups. For the cohort representing mid-adulthood, the first group received a chow diet from birth until the end of the study (Chow). The second group switched to a HFD at three months of age (HFD). The third group switched to a HFD when three months old (m.o.) as well, but this HFD was subsequently enriched with 5% w/w butyrate from seven months of age until the end of the study (HDFB) (Figure 1a). The cohort representing late adulthood was subdivided in the same manner, but mice were switched to HFD at six months of age and butyrate intervention started at 10 months of age (Figure 1b).

(a) Mid-adulthood

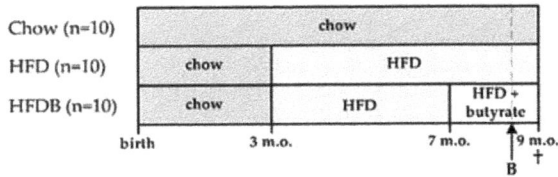

(b) Late adulthood

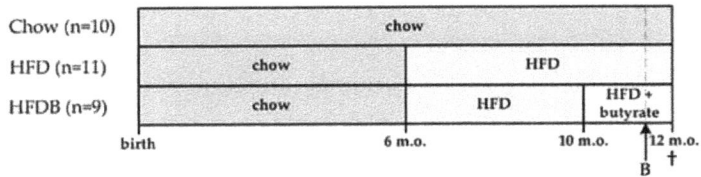

Figure 1. Schematic overview of the study design. (**a**) Mid-adulthood, exposure of the high-fat died HFD started at 3 m.o. in the HFD and HFDB groups. At 7 months of age, the butyrate intervention (HFD supplemented with 5% *w/w* butyrate) started in the HFDB group; (**b**) Late adulthood, exposure to the HFD started at 6 months of age in the HFD and HFDB groups, and a butyrate intervention initiated at 10 months of age in the HFDB group. Body weight (individual) and food intake (cage level) were monitored weekly. Blood samples were taken after five hours of fasting. At 9 m.o. and 12 m.o., mice were sacrificed and both liver and adipose tissues were harvested. These tissues were subsequently processed for immunohistochemical staining. B = blood sample collection; HFD = high-fat diet; HFDB = high fat diet enriched with butyrate; m.o. = months old.

2.2. Plasma Analyses

Blood was collected after five hours of fasting (8 a.m. to 1 p.m.). Plasma cholesterol, triglyceride and insulin levels were measured using standardized ELISA kits as previously described [18]. Moreover, ELISA kits (Quantikine, R&D systems, Inc., Minneapolis, MN, USA) were used to define plasma leptin (DY498), adiponectin (DY1119), resistin (DY1069) and interleukin-6 (IL-6; M6000B) levels. SAA plasma levels were determined by an ELISA kit as well (KMA0021, Invitrogen, Carlsbad, CA, USA).

2.3. (Immuno)histochemistry

Mice were sacrificed by transcardial perfusion with 0.1 M phosphate buffered saline (PBS) after being anesthetized with isoflurane (3.5%, Nicholas Primal (I) limited, London, UK), as described in Arnoldussen et al. [18]. Directly thereafter, the liver and two different adipose tissue depots were harvested and post-fixed in 4% paraformaldehyde for 24 h. Fat depots seem to be differentially active and affected by a HFD and, therefore, we dissected in addition subcutaneous (inguinal) and visceral (epididymal) adipose tissue depots [32,33]. Liver outcomes used for correlation analyses were obtained from a previous experiment [18].

Both epididymal and inguinal adipose tissues were processed for immunohistochemistry on 5 μm paraffin embedded sections. Briefly, paraffin sections were first deparaffinized in xylene and rehydrated in a series of ethanol followed by endogenous peroxidase blocking with 0.3% H_2O_2 in 0.1 M PBS. Antigen retrieval was achieved by treating the tissue in hot 0.05 M sodiumcitrate with a constant temperature of 85 °C. After pre-incubation with 0.1% bovine serum albumin in 0.1 M PBS

(PBS-B), the tissue was incubated overnight at room temperature with primary macrophage (MAC-3) antibodies (1:100; eBioscience, 14-1072) [34]. Next, sections were incubated with secondary donkey anti-rat IgG antibodies (1:200; Jackson ImmunoResearch) in 0.1 M PBS-B at room temperature. Staining was visualized using the ABC method with a Vectastain kit (Vector Laboratories, Burlingame, CA, USA) and diaminobenzidine imidazole solution as chromogen. Finally, sections were dehydrated in a series of ethanol, cleared in xylene, and mounted.

Two entire sections per animal were visualized using a VisionTek live digital microscope (Sakura Finetek, Torrance, CA, USA) at a $10\times$ magnification. Sampling of these sections was carried out with Adobe Illustrator CC 2016 (Adobe, San Jose, CA, USA) using a template with three randomly placed artboards (592.7×886.2 mm). Adipocyte cell size (μm^2) and the number of CLS were determined in a total of six samples—three samples per section—per animal. Analyses to determine these measures were performed using CellProfiler [35] version 2.3.0 together with Ilastik version 0.5 [36] for pixel classification. Separate pipelines and classifiers for epididymal and inguinal adipose tissue analyses were used. In order to verify the reliability of these relatively novel analyses, we included an established analysis to determine adipocyte size using ImageJ software as previously described [37]. CLS were determined based on intensity of the cell edge, and total numbers of CLS per animal were calculated per 1000 adipocytes.

2.4. Statistical Analyses

A random and blinded selection procedure was maintained throughout the study. Group means were compared using univariate analysis of variance (ANOVA) with Bonferroni correction for multiple testing with a statistical program, SPSS 24 (IBM SPSS Statistics 24, IBM Corporation, Armonk, NY, USA). Parameter correlation tests were performed using Pearson correlations. Nonparametric tests were used when assumptions of normality and homogeneity of variance were not met. p-values lower than 0.05 were considered significant. Data are presented as mean $\pm$ SEM.

3. Results

3.1. Adipocyte Size

Adipocyte size—measured as area (μm^2)—of both epididymal and inguinal adipose tissue depots were determined to assess morphological adaptations. A HFD increased the average epididymal adipocyte size in both mid- and late-adult mice (mid: $p < 0.001$; $F(1,18) = 26.05$, late: $p < 0.02$; $F(1,19) = 7.01$) (Figure 2a). Butyrate intervention significantly reduced adipocyte size in both age cohorts (mid: $p = 0.001$; $F(1,18) = 14.95$, late: $p < 0.02$; $F(1,18) = 7.14$).

Similarly, inguinal adipocyte size was increased by HFD in both mid- and late adulthood ($p = 0.001$; mid: $F(1,18) = 20.49$, late: $F(1,19) = 14.25$) (Figure 2b). After HFD exposure, inguinal adipocyte size was reduced due to butyrate intervention in mid-adult mice ($p < 0.001$; $F(1,18) = 25.69$), but not in late-adult mice. Mean inguinal adipocyte size was significantly larger in late adult as compared to mid-adult high fat diet enriched with butyrate (HFDB) mice ($p < 0.01$; $F(1,18) = 11.28$).

In addition, we compared the number of adipocytes as an additional indication of adipose tissue function. Our analysis indicated that the epididymal adipose tissue contained a lower number of adipocytes than inguinal adipose tissue. The mean adipocyte number in epididymal adipose tissue was higher in mid-adult Chow mice as compared to HFD mice (Table 1). Butyrate intervention increased epididymal adipocyte number solely in mid-adulthood. In both age cohorts, inguinal adipocyte numbers were significantly higher in Chow mice as opposed to HFD mice (Table 1). Only in mid-adulthood did butyrate intervention increase the inguinal adipocyte numbers.

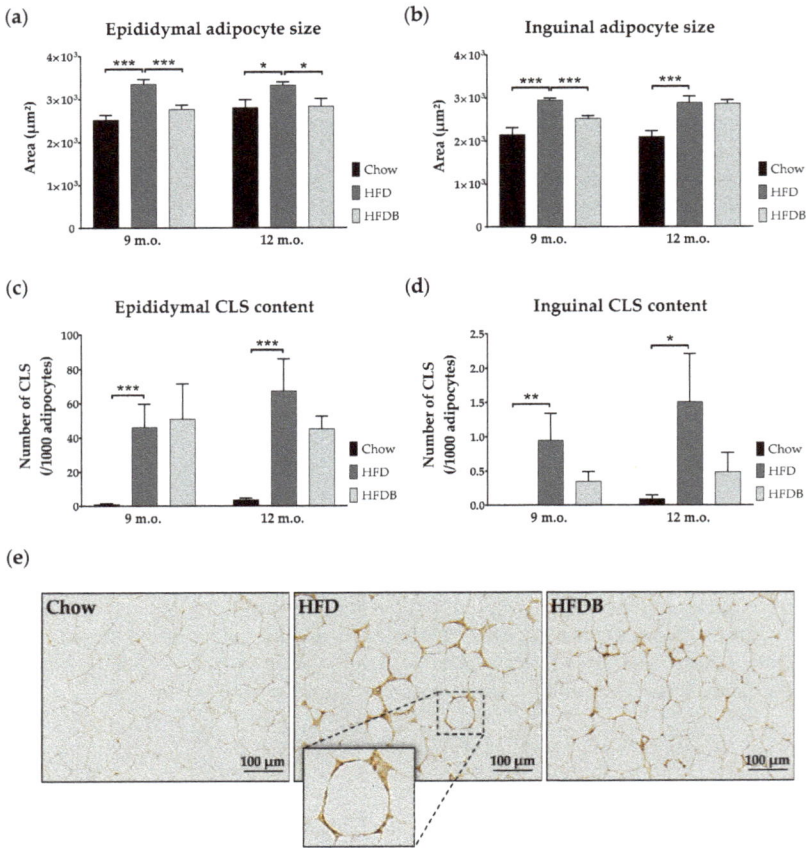

Figure 2. Adipose tissue cell sizes and macrophage infiltration. Mean adipocyte sizes in epididymal (**a**) and inguinal (**b**) adipose tissue depots in both mid- (9 m.o.) and late- (12 m.o.) adult mice. (**c,d**) Mean number of crown-like structures (CLS) in epididymal (**c**) and inguinal (**d**) adipose tissue. (**e**) Representative photomicrographs of epididymal adipose tissue stained with antibodies against macrophages (MAC-3) in late-adult mice. In addition, a magnification (40×) of a CLS is represented. These examples are comparable to those observed in mid-adulthood. Data are presented as mean ± standard error of mean (SEM). * $p < 0.05$; ** $p < 0.01$; *** $p \leq 0.001$.

In mid- and late adulthood, both epididymal and inguinal adipocyte size were positively associated with body weight, and cholesterol and triglyceride plasma levels (Tables 2 and 3). In addition, only inguinal adipocyte size was positively correlated with inguinal adipose tissue weight (mid: $p < 0.01$; $R = 0.55$, late: $p < 0.001$; $R = 0.64$). Solely in late adulthood, epididymal adipocyte size correlated positively with plasma insulin levels ($p < 0.01$; Table 3).

Moreover, body weight, cholesterol and triglyceride levels revealed significant and positive inter correlations (Tables 2 and 3). Finally, insulin levels correlated positively with these outcomes in late-adult mice (Table 3).

Table 1. Adipocyte numbers. Represented are the combined mean numbers of two slides.

Adipocyte Numbers Per 10^6 μm^2 (Mean ± SEM)				
Epididymal				
Chow vs. HFD	mid	468 ± 34 vs. 376 ± 31	$0.05 < p < 0.08$	$F(1,18) = 3.95$
	late	452 ± 40 vs. 410 ± 21	$p = 0.02$	$F(1,18) = 6.54$
HFD vs. HFDB	mid	376 ± 31 vs. 496 ± 35	ns	
	late	410 ± 21 vs. 481 ± 47	ns	
Inguinal				
Chow vs. HFD	mid	665 ± 59 vs. 449 ± 16	$p < 0.01$	$F(1,18) = 12.61$
	late	659 ± 44 vs. 474 ± 41	$p < 0.01$	$F(1,19) = 9.54$
HFD vs. HFDB	mid	449 ± 16 vs. 522 ± 15	$p < 0.01$	$F(1,18) = 11.27$
	late	474 ± 41 vs. 446 ± 18	ns	

ns = not significant.

Table 2. Correlation coefficients among mid-adult mice.

	BW		Chol		Trigl		eAS		iAS		eCLS		iCLS		Leptin		SAA
BW	x																
Chol	0.80^R	+	x														
Trigl	0.58^R	+	0.69^R	+	x												
eAS	0.53^R	+	0.64^R	+	0.57^R	+	x										
iAS	0.55^R	+	0.57^R	+	0.37^R	+	NE		x								
eCLS	$0.53^{\tau b}$	+	$0.49^{\tau b}$	+	$0.15^{\tau b}$	+	$0.24^{\tau b}$	+	NE		x						
iCLS	$0.31^{\tau b}$	+	$0.29^{\tau b}$	+	$0.10^{\tau b}$	+	NE		$0.37^{\tau b}$	+	NE		x				
Leptin	0.78^R	+	0.87^R	+	0.62^R	+	0.76^R	+	0.67^R	+	$0.52^{\tau b}$	+	$0.37^{\tau b}$	+	x		
SAA	$0.56^{\tau b}$	+	$0.50^{\tau b}$	+	$0.13^{\tau b}$	+	$0.17^{\tau b}$	+	$0.24^{\tau b}$	+	$0.69^{\tau b}$	+	$0.28^{\tau b}$	+	NE		x

Either the Pearson's (^{R}) or Kendall's tau ($^{\tau b}$) test was used. Not significant. + = positive correlation; Adi = adiponectin; BW = body weight; Chol = cholesterol; eAS = epididymal adipocyte size; eCLS = epididymal CLS; iAS = inguinal adipocyte size; iCLS = inguinal CLS; LI = liver inflammation; NE = not estimated; SAA = serum amyloid A; Trigl = triglycerides.

Table 3. Correlation coefficients among late-adult mice.

	BW	Insulin	Chol	Trigl	eAS	iAS	eCLS	iCLS	LI	Leptin	Adi	SAA
BW	x											
Insulin	+ 0.66 ^{R}	x										
Chol	+ 0.87 ^{R}	+ 0.66 ^{R}	x									
Trigl	+ 0.79 ^{R}	+ 0.77 ^{R}	+ 0.81 ^{R}	x								
eAS	+ 0.52 ^{R}	+ 0.49 ^{R}	+ 0.57 ^{R}	+ 0.53 ^{R}	x							
iAS	+ 0.47 ^{R}	+ 0.31 ^{R}	+ 0.54 ^{R}	+ 0.50 ^{R}	NE	x						
eCLS	+ 0.43 $^{\tau b}$	+ 0.30 $^{\tau b}$	+ 0.55 $^{\tau b}$	+ 0.34 $^{\tau b}$	+ 0.23 $^{\tau b}$	NE	x					
iCLS	+ 0.45 $^{\tau b}$	+ 0.21 $^{\tau b}$	+ 0.38 $^{\tau b}$	+ 0.33 $^{\tau b}$	NE	+ 0.37 $^{\tau b}$	NE	x				
LI	+ 0.41 $^{\tau b}$	+ 0.33 $^{\tau b}$	+ 0.45 $^{\tau b}$	+ 0.30 $^{\tau b}$	+ 0.15 $^{\tau b}$	+ 0.22 $^{\tau b}$	+ 0.57 $^{\tau b}$	+ 0.21 $^{\tau b}$	x			
Leptin	+ 0.88 ^{R}	+ 0.69 ^{R}	+ 0.91 ^{R}	+ 0.87 ^{R}	+ 0.65 ^{R}	+ 0.64 ^{R}	+ 0.49 ^{R}	+ 0.41 $^{\tau b}$	+ 0.46 $^{\tau b}$	x		
Adi	− 0.56 ^{R}	− 0.48 ^{R}	− 0.68 ^{R}	− 0.47 ^{R}	− 0.25 ^{R}	− 0.25 ^{R}	− 0.19 $^{\tau b}$	− 0.30 $^{\tau b}$	− 0.28 $^{\tau b}$	NE	x	
SAA	+ 0.42 $^{\tau b}$	+ 0.29 $^{\tau b}$	+ 0.57 $^{\tau b}$	+ 0.46 $^{\tau b}$	+ 0.19 $^{\tau b}$	+ 0.53 $^{\tau b}$	+ 0.58 $^{\tau b}$	+ 0.30 $^{\tau b}$	+ 0.44 $^{\tau b}$	NE	NE	x

Either the Pearson's (^{R}) or Kendall's tau ($^{\tau b}$) test was used. Not significant. + = positive correlation; − = negative correlation; Adi = adiponectin; BW = Body weight; Chol = cholesterol; eAS = epididymal adipocyte size; eCLS = epididymal CLS; iAS = inguinal adipocyte size; iCLS = inguinal CLS; LI = liver inflammation; NE = not estimated; SAA = serum amyloid A; Trigl = triglycerides.

3.2. Inflammation in Adipose Tissue and Liver

To assess the degree of inflammation in adipose tissue, the number of adipocytes infiltrated by macrophages—known as crown-like structures (CLS)—has been determined. Both mid- and late-adult mice on HFD showed higher numbers of CLS in epididymal adipose tissue as opposed to Chow-fed mice (Kruskal Wallis: $p < 0.001$; mid: $\chi^2(1) = 13.50$, late: $\chi^2(1) = 13.02$) (Figure 2c). No effects of butyrate on CLS number in epididymal adipose tissue were observed. In inguinal adipose tissue, the number of CLS was increased after HFD exposure in both mid- (Kruskal-Wallis: $p < 0.01$; $\chi^2(1) = 7.30$) and late- (Kruskal-Wallis: $p < 0.02$; $\chi^2(1) = 6.16$) adult mice (Figure 2d). No significant differences in the number of CLS in inguinal adipose tissue were observed between HFD and HFDB mice (Figure 2d). As scales differ between Figure 2c,d, caution should be taken when interpreting these results. In Figure 2e, examples of epididymal adipose tissue stained for macrophages are shown.

In late adulthood, the number of CLS in epididymal adipose tissue correlated significantly with body weight ($p = 0.001$), and plasma triglyceride ($p < 0.02$), cholesterol ($p < 0.001$) and insulin ($p < 0.05$) levels (Table 3). In mid-adulthood, epididymal adipose tissue CLS content showed only significant correlations with body weight ($p < 0.001$) and plasma cholesterol levels ($p < 0.001$) (Table 2).

In addition to CLS in adipose tissue, data including inflammatory aggregates were used [18] to examine potential relationships to inflammation in the liver, which is another crucial organ regulating insulin sensitivity. Liver inflammation was increased after HFD exposure only in late-adult mice [18]. No significant changes were observed after butyrate intervention. In this age cohort, the number of inflammatory aggregates in the liver was positively correlated with the number of CLS in epididymal adipose tissue ($p < 0.001$) (Table 3).

3.3. Adipokine Plasma Levels

Adipokine plasma levels were determined at either nine or 12 months of age. HFD exposure strongly increased leptin plasma levels in both age cohorts ($p < 0.001$; mid: $F(1,18) = 50.10$, late: $F(1,19) = 44.87$) (Figure 3a). Late-adult HFD-fed mice showed higher leptin levels as compared to mid-adult mice fed a HFD ($p < 0.02$; $F(1,19) = 7.71$). Subsequent butyrate intervention resulted in reduced plasma leptin levels, almost reaching control levels in Chow mice ($p < 0.001$; mid: $F(1,18) = 26.49$, late: $F(1,19) = 32.88$). HFD did not affect plasma resistin levels (Figure 3b). Adiponectin plasma levels were reduced after HFD exposure in late-adult mice ($p < 0.001$; $F(1,19) = 17.57$) and were moderately increased after butyrate intervention ($p = 0.053$; $F(1,18) = 4.29$) (Figure 3c). An age effect was observed in both Chow and HFD animals ($p < 0.05$; $F(1,18) = 4.60$ and $F(1,19) = 4.55$, respectively). Serum amyloid A (SAA) plasma levels were increased in mice fed a HFD when compared to Chow-fed mice in both age cohorts (Kruskal-Wallis: $p \leq 0.001$; mid: $\chi^2(1) = 10.14$, late: $\chi^2(1) = 14.46$) (Figure 3d). Plasma levels of interleukin-6 (IL-6) were below detectable levels in all animals in the absence of abnormal positive and negative controls.

In both mid- and late adulthood, plasma leptin levels were positively correlated with body weight ($p < 0.001$), both epididymal and inguinal adipocyte size ($p < 0.001$), and epididymal CLS content ($p < 0.001$) (Tables 2 and 3). Solely in late-adult mice, plasma leptin levels positively correlated with insulin levels ($p < 0.001$) and liver inflammation ($p = 0.001$) (Table 3). Only in late adulthood plasma adiponectin levels showed a negative correlation with body weight ($p < 0.01$), insulin plasma levels ($p < 0.02$), and liver inflammation ($p < 0.05$) (Table 3).

Plasma SAA levels were positively correlated with body weight (mid: $p < 0.001$, late: $p < 0.01$) and the number of CLS in epididymal adipose tissue ($p < 0.001$) in both mid- and late adulthood (Tables 2 and 3). Whereas, SAA plasma levels were positively correlated with insulin levels ($p < 0.05$), inguinal adipocyte size ($p < 0.001$), and liver inflammation ($p < 0.01$) only in late adulthood (Table 3).

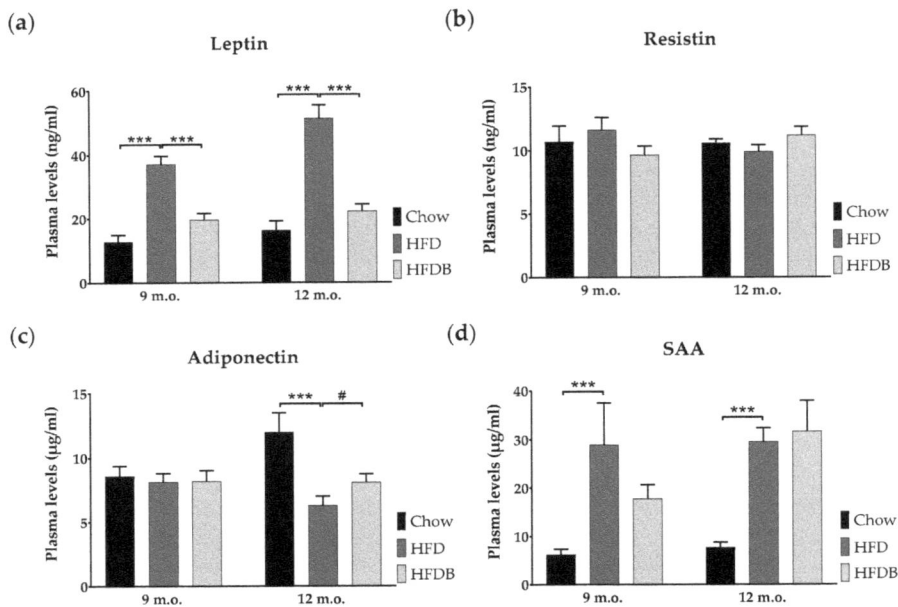

Figure 3. Adipokine plasma levels. Mean plasma levels of leptin (**a**), resistin (**b**), adiponectin (**c**), and serum amyloid A (SAA) (**d**) are represented in both mid- (9 m.o.) and late- (12 m.o.) adult mice as mean ± SEM. *** $p \leq 0.001$; # $p = 0.053$.

4. Discussion

This study describes the detrimental effects of a six-month HFD exposure in mid-adult and late-adult mice, and examined potential health effects of butyrate administered during the last two months of HFD feeding. In this study, HFD exposure caused adipocyte hypertrophy and inflammation, as well as an increase in the plasma levels of proinflammatory adipokines (leptin, SAA) in mid- and late life. Butyrate attenuated HFD-evoked effects, though the effects of butyrate varied in mice that were exposed to HFD in mid-life as compared to late life.

In our study, HFD treatment increased body weight and adiposity, and subsequent butyrate intervention diminished these changes in the LDLr-/-.Leiden mice [18]. Moreover, these changes were observed without significant differences in calorie intake, suggesting that energy intake was similar between the dietary interventions. Other rodent research has shown that a HFD increases body weight and adiposity [38–40], and similar effects of butyrate have been reported in obese mice [38,41]. The LDLr-/-.Leiden mouse model was chosen for this study because of its high sensitivity to develop vascular complications and obesity when fed a HFD even with modest fat content. We found that 12 m.o. LDLr-/-.Leiden mice on standard Chow show a disposition towards pronounced weight gain and are approximately 32% heavier than Chow-fed male C57BL/6 mice of the same age [42], supporting the obesity-prone condition of the model chosen. It is unclear why these mice are susceptible to obesity development, and comparative molecular analysis to C57BL/6 mice have not been made. In our experimental design, a control group of wild-type mice was not included due to restrictions in mice per experiment and time. Therefore, a generalization of the results cannot be made, the more so because the interaction between the LDLr-/- genotype and HFD are still not fully understood. A detailed comparison with wild-type mice and other obesity models would be required to elucidate the role of the LDLr in obesity.

In a previous study, insulin levels were significantly increased in late-adult mice after HFD feeding, whereas no changes in glucose levels were observed [18]. Plasma insulin levels are extremely high due to the experimental conditions employed in this disease model (>20 ng/mL) and much higher than in wild-type mice fed the same diet (<5 ng/mL) [18,30], indicating insulin resistance but no overt T2DM because glucose levels are not elevated and seem to be controlled. Interestingly, butyrate supplementation restored insulin levels to values found in Chow-fed mice, suggesting an improvement in insulin signaling [18]. Previous research described similar effects of butyrate on insulin levels and sensitivity in HFD-fed mice [38,43]. It is not clear whether this effect of butyrate is mediated by improvement of insulin signaling in liver, in peripheral organs, or both. It is possible that both organs are involved, given the time frame in which insulin resistance develops under the conditions employed. For instance, a time resolved clamp study using C57BL/6 mice that were treated with the same HFD as used in the current study showed that the adipose tissue develops insulin resistance after about six to 12 weeks of HFD feeding [44]. Second, the development of insulin resistance in the liver requires longer periods of HFD feeding (about 24 weeks), i.e., a period that is comparable to the duration of HFD exposure herein [44].

Even in the absence of obesity, metabolic dysfunction in adipose tissue induced by adipocyte hypertrophy has consistently been related to insulin resistance and may serve as a predictor for T2DM [45,46]. We observed increased adipocyte size in both epididymal and inguinal adipose tissue depots after HFD feeding. Adipocyte hypertrophy was reduced by butyrate with the exception of inguinal adipose tissue in late-adult mice. Epididymal adipocyte sizes were associated with insulin levels in late adulthood suggesting that epididymal, as opposed to inguinal, adipose tissue may be important in mediating the effects on insulin. Previous studies have demonstrated the significant role of visceral fat in mediating insulin sensitivity in rats [47,48], which may be attributed to the higher degree of metabolic activity of visceral fat as opposed to subcutaneous fat [16,49,50]. The beneficial effects of butyrate on adipocyte size in epididymal adipose tissue have been demonstrated before [51]. Although our knowledge about the exact mechanisms is incomplete, it is likely that butyrate may reverse adipocyte hypertrophy by promoting fatty acid oxidation in adipose tissue [38]. In particular, butyrate may induce a shift from lipid synthesis to utilization resulting in decreased fat storage in white adipose tissue [43]. Our data confirm this hypothesis as adipocyte sizes were significantly associated with both cholesterol and triglyceride levels. Dyslipidemia is a regularly observed condition in T2DM patients [52]. HFD-induced elevations in cholesterol and triglycerides were diminished by butyrate in LDLr-/-.Leiden mice [18], suggesting a mitigation of hyperlipidemia that is not related to enhanced clearance, suggesting effects on very-low-density lipoprotein (VLDL) production. For instance, butyrate may affect hyperlipidemia as it can induce a switch from lipid synthesis to utilization [53]. Unfortunately, our study is limited with respect to functional analyses such as glucose transport, insulin signaling, lipogenesis, and adipogenesis in adipose tissue. Therefore, it would be valuable to investigate these aspects in future studies. The effects of butyrate supplementation on key regulators of adipogenesis in mid-adult versus late-adult mice may provide insight into the pathways by which butyrate may modulate adiposity. It has been shown that butyrate may reduce body weight and improve insulin sensitivity via the modulation of peroxisome proliferator-activated receptor-γ (PPAR-γ) [43], which is a key regulator of adipogenesis [54]. Consistent with this, we recently showed that specific activation of PPAR-γ in adipose tissue attenuates CLS development and, related to this, the development of nonalcoholic fatty liver disease/nonalcoholic steatohepatitis [55]. Anti-inflammatory effects in adipose tissue may attenuate the release of inflammatory mediators and may also affect the development of diseases in other organs such as the liver [56,57]. A notion which is further supported by the coordinated and interactive expression of inflammatory genes in adipose tissue and liver during metabolic overload [58].

It is well established that a correlative and causative relation exists between chronic inflammation and both insulin resistance and T2DM in humans and rodents [13,59]. More specifically, a reduction of macrophage infiltration in adipose tissue can improve insulin sensitivity in diet-induced obese mice by reducing the expression of inflammatory cytokines in adipose tissue [11]. As shown in the present study, HFD feeding results in increased macrophage infiltration mainly in epididymal adipose tissue associated with body weight and insulin levels. Epididymal adipose tissue was characterized by an abundance of CLS, whereas CLS were almost absent in inguinal adipose tissue, which is consistent with previous studies investigating adipose tissue inflammation of various adipose tissue depots in the context of their expandability and maximal storage capacity [30,57]. It is possible that visceral fat may excrete higher amounts of inflammatory proteins and fatty acids affecting insulin signaling, and that macrophages play an important role in this [56,60]. CLS formation in epididymal adipose tissue was not affected by butyrate supplementation in mid-adult mice, whereas a mean reduction of almost 33% was observed in late-adult mice. Consistent with the inflammatory cross-talk between epididimal adipose tissue and liver, medial lobular inflammation was not affected in mid-adult mice, whereas the number of inflammatory aggregates in the liver was reduced by 44% after dietary butyrate intervention in late-adult mice [18]. Furthermore, liver inflammation in late-adult mice, indicated by inflammatory aggregates in the medial lobe [18], correlated significantly with the number of CLS in epididymal adipose tissue in this study. It is not known via which pathways butyrate can affect inflammation, and future studies may examine the expression of inflammatory mediators at tissue level, in both adipose tissue and the liver. In addition, mechanistic studies examining the expression of transcription factors, such as nuclear factor κB, support the notion that the activation of inflammatory processes in adipose tissue and liver are necessary.

Both the increase in pro-inflammatory and the reduction in anti-inflammatory adipokine secretion by adipose tissue can contribute to systemic and tissue-specific inflammation. In this study, HFD exposure results in increased levels of leptin and serum amyloid A (SAA). These findings are accompanied by a reduction in adiponectin in late adulthood, whereas it remains unclear why adiponectin was not affected by HFD or butyrate treatment in mid-adult mice. An exaggerated metabolic load in adipocytes and inflammatory state may underlie the effects of a HFD on leptin, adiponectin, and SAA levels [16]. Both leptin and SAA are suggested to be pro-inflammatory adipokines, whereas adiponectin has anti-inflammatory properties [61]. Leptin contributes to the inflammatory state in obesity by modulating TNF-α and activating macrophages [62], and butyrate reduced leptin levels in mid-adult and late-adult mice. Leptin can also affect insulin sensitivity by modulating pancreatic β-cells [60]. It thereby contributes to the observed reduction in plasma insulin by butyrate in late-adult mice the more, because butyrate reduced leptin levels nearly to those of Chow-fed mice. Our finding that leptin levels were significantly related to insulin levels in late-adult mice further supports this notion. Although current evidence for the role of SAA in insulin signaling is contradictory [63–65], SAA levels have been correlated with insulin resistance and T2DM [66], which may be related to the pro-inflammatory properties of SAA [14]. Interestingly, adiponectin plasma levels were only affected by HFD feeding in late-adult mice. It is possible that the circulating SAA is mainly released from adipose tissue and that butyrate reduced CLS only in adipose tissue of late-adult mice. Low adiponectin levels may add to an impaired insulin signaling via polarization towards M1 macrophages in adipose tissue [67]. Butyrate intervention reduced changes in both leptin and adiponectin levels, which may in part be attributed to its effect on adipocyte size and its differential effects on CLS, i.e., adipose tissue inflammation, in mid-and late-adult mice.

5. Conclusions

This study provides evidence that dietary supplementation with butyrate constitutes a strategy to counteract features of HFD-induced adipose tissue dysfunction and accompanying metabolic disturbances. These metabolic adaptations often affect insulin signaling and may therefore indicate an increased risk of developing T2DM. Late-adult mice are particularly sensitive to HFD-evoked metabolic risk factors and adaptations. The findings of the current study provide novel insights about the attenuating effects of butyrate on adipose tissue dysfunction and inflammation. Overall, dietary interventions with butyrate may constitute means to ameliorate the risk of developing metabolic disorders such as T2DM in people with obesity.

Acknowledgments: The authors would like to thank Bram Geenen, Jos Dederen, Peter Wielinga and Tim Emmerzaal for their valuable scientific support. In addition, we would like to acknowledge the biotechnicians at TNO Leiden and Preclinical Imaging Centre (PRIME) Radboud university medical center for taking outstanding care of the animals.

Author Contributions: I.A.C.A. and A.J.K. conceived and designed the experiments; C.E.P., B.A.A.F. and J.S. performed the experiments; C.E.P. and B.A.A.F. analyzed the data; J.S. and R.K. contributed reagents/materials/analysis tools; C.E.P., B.A.A.F., I.A.C.A. and A.J.K. wrote the paper.

Conflicts of Interest: The authors declare no conflict of interest.

References

1. World Health Organization. Fact Sheet 311: Obesity and Overweight. 2016. Available online: http://www.who.int/mediacentre/factsheets/fs311/en/ (accessed on 28 February 2017).
2. Diabetes UK. Facts and Stats. 2016. Available online: https://www.diabetes.org.uk/Documents/Position%20statements/DiabetesUK_Facts_Stats_Oct16.pdf (accessed on 27 February 2017).
3. Hamman, R.F.; Wing, R.R.; Edelstein, S.L.; Lachin, J.M.; Bray, G.A.; Delahanty, L.; Hoskin, M.; Kriska, A.M.; Mayer-Davis, E.J.; Pi-Sunyer, X. Effect of weight loss with lifestyle intervention on risk of diabetes. *Diabetes Care* **2006**, *29*, 2102–2107. [CrossRef] [PubMed]
4. Molnar, D. The prevalence of the metabolic syndrome and type 2 diabetes mellitus in children and adolescents. *Int. J. Obes.* **2004**, *28*, S70–S74. [CrossRef] [PubMed]
5. Schwartz, M.S.; Chadha, A. Type 2 diabetes mellitus in childhood: Obesity and insulin resistance. *J. Am. Osteopath. Assoc.* **2008**, *108*, 518–524. [PubMed]
6. Wabitsch, M.; Hauner, H.; Hertrampf, M.; Muche, R.; Hay, B.; Mayer, H.; Kratzer, W.; Debatin, K.; Heinze, E. Type ii diabetes mellitus and impaired glucose regulation in caucasian children and adolescents with obesity living in germany. *Int. J. Obes.* **2004**, *28*, 307–313. [CrossRef] [PubMed]
7. Pérez, L.M.; Pareja-Galeano, H.; Sanchis-Gomar, F.; Emanuele, E.; Lucia, A.; Gálvez, B.G. 'Adipaging': Ageing and obesity share biological hallmarks related to a dysfunctional adipose tissue. *J. Physiol.* **2016**, *594*, 3187–3207. [CrossRef] [PubMed]
8. Fink, R.I.; Kolterman, O.G.; Griffin, J.; Olefsky, J.M. Mechanisms of insulin resistance in aging. *J. Clin. Investig.* **1983**, *71*, 1523. [CrossRef] [PubMed]
9. Inzucchi, S.E.; Bergenstal, R.M.; Buse, J.B.; Diamant, M.; Ferrannini, E.; Nauck, M.; Peters, A.L.; Tsapas, A.; Wender, R.; Matthews, D.R. Management of hyperglycemia in type 2 diabetes: A patient-centered approach. *Diabetes Care* **2012**, *35*, 1364–1379. [CrossRef] [PubMed]
10. Arvanitakis, Z.; Wilson, R.S.; Bienias, J.L.; Evans, D.A.; Bennett, D.A. Diabetes mellitus and risk of alzheimer disease and decline in cognitive function. *Arch. Neurol.* **2004**, *61*, 661–666. [CrossRef] [PubMed]
11. Jung, U.J.; Choi, M.S. Obesity and its metabolic complications: The role of adipokines and the relationship between obesity, inflammation, insulin resistance, dyslipidemia and nonalcoholic fatty liver disease. *Int. J. Mol. Sci.* **2014**, *15*, 6184–6223. [CrossRef] [PubMed]
12. Cinti, S.; Mitchell, G.; Barbatelli, G.; Murano, I.; Ceresi, E.; Faloia, E.; Wang, S.; Fortier, M.; Greenberg, A.S.; Obin, M.S. Adipocyte death defines macrophage localization and function in adipose tissue of obese mice and humans. *J. Lipid Res.* **2005**, *46*, 2347–2355. [CrossRef] [PubMed]
13. Olefsky, J.M.; Glass, C.K. Macrophages, inflammation, and insulin resistance. *Annu. Rev. Physiol.* **2010**, *72*, 219–246. [CrossRef] [PubMed]
14. Poitou, C.; Divoux, A.; Faty, A.; Tordjman, J.; Hugol, D.; Aissat, A.; Keophiphath, M.; Henegar, C.; Commans, S.; Clément, K. Role of serum amyloid a in adipocyte-macrophage cross talk and adipocyte cholesterol efflux. *J. Clin. Endocrinol. Metab.* **2009**, *94*, 1810–1817. [CrossRef] [PubMed]
15. Skurk, T.; Alberti-Huber, C.; Herder, C.; Hauner, H. Relationship between adipocyte size and adipokine expression and secretion. *J. Clin. Endocrinol. Metab.* **2007**, *92*, 1023–1033. [CrossRef] [PubMed]
16. Bays, H.E.; González-Campoy, J.M.; Bray, G.A.; Kitabchi, A.E.; Bergman, D.A.; Schorr, A.B.; Rodbard, H.W.; Henry, R.R. Pathogenic potential of adipose tissue and metabolic consequences of adipocyte hypertrophy and increased visceral adiposity. *Expert Rev. Cardiovasc. Ther.* **2008**, *6*, 343–368. [CrossRef] [PubMed]

17. Canfora, E.E.; Jocken, J.W.; Blaak, E.E. Short-chain fatty acids in control of body weight and insulin sensitivity. *Nat. Rev. Endocrinol.* **2015**, *11*, 577. [CrossRef] [PubMed]

18. Arnoldussen, I.A.; Wiesmann, M.; Pelgrim, C.E.; Wielemaker, E.M.; van Duyvenvoorde, W.; Santos, P.A.; Verschuren, L.; Keijser, B.J.; Heerschap, A.; Kleemann, R.; et al. Butyrate restores hfd induced adaptations in brain function and metabolism in mid-adult obese mice. *Int. J. Obes.* **2017**, *41*, 935–944. [CrossRef] [PubMed]

19. Khan, S.; Jena, G. The role of butyrate, a histone deacetylase inhibitor in diabetes mellitus: Experimental evidence for therapeutic intervention. *Epigenomics* **2015**, *7*, 669–680. [CrossRef] [PubMed]

20. Weickert, M.O.; Möhlig, M.; Schöfl, C.; Arafat, A.M.; Otto, B.; Viehoff, H.; Koebnick, C.; Kohl, A.; Spranger, J.; Pfeiffer, A.F. Cereal fiber improves whole-body insulin sensitivity in overweight and obese women. *Diabetes Care* **2006**, *29*, 775–780. [CrossRef] [PubMed]

21. Weickert, M.O.; Pfeiffer, A.F. Metabolic effects of dietary fiber consumption and prevention of diabetes. *J. Nutr.* **2008**, *138*, 439–442. [PubMed]

22. Marlett, J.A.; McBurney, M.I.; Slavin, J.L. Position of the american dietetic association: Health implications of dietary fiber. *J. Am. Diet. Assoc.* **2002**, *102*, 993–1000. [CrossRef]

23. Elli, M.; Colombo, O.; Tagliabue, A. A common core microbiota between obese individuals and their lean relatives? Evaluation of the predisposition to obesity on the basis of the fecal microflora profile. *Med. Hypotheses* **2010**, *75*, 350–352. [CrossRef] [PubMed]

24. Qin, J.; Li, Y.; Cai, Z.; Li, S.; Zhu, J.; Zhang, F.; Liang, S.; Zhang, W.; Guan, Y.; Shen, D. A metagenome-wide association study of gut microbiota in type 2 diabetes. *Nature* **2012**, *490*, 55–60. [CrossRef] [PubMed]

25. Kivipelto, M.; Ngandu, T.; Fratiglioni, L.; Viitanen, M.; Kåreholt, I.; Winblad, B.; Helkala, E.L.; Tuomilehto, J.; Soininen, H.; Nissinen, A. Obesity and vascular risk factors at midlife and the risk of dementia and alzheimer disease. *Arch. Neurol.* **2005**, *62*, 1556–1560. [CrossRef] [PubMed]

26. Boitard, C.; Etchamendy, N.; Sauvant, J.; Aubert, A.; Tronel, S.; Marighetto, A.; Layé, S.; Ferreira, G. Juvenile, but not adult exposure to high-fat diet impairs relational memory and hippocampal neurogenesis in mice. *Hippocampus* **2012**, *22*, 2095–2100. [CrossRef] [PubMed]

27. Emmerzaal, T.L.; Kiliaan, A.J.; Gustafson, D.R. 2003–2013: A decade of body mass index, alzheimer's disease, and dementia. *J. Alzheimers Dis.* **2015**, *43*, 739–755. [PubMed]

28. Ma, Y.; Wang, W.; Zhang, J.; Lu, Y.; Wu, W.; Yan, H.; Wang, Y. Hyperlipidemia and atherosclerotic lesion development in ldlr-deficient mice on a long-term high-fat diet. *PLoS ONE* **2012**, *7*, e35835. [CrossRef] [PubMed]

29. Radonjic, M.; Wielinga, P.Y.; Wopereis, S.; Kelder, T.; Goelela, V.S.; Verschuren, L.; Toet, K.; van Duyvenvoorde, W.; Stroeve, J.H.; Cnubben, N. Differential effects of drug interventions and dietary lifestyle in developing type 2 diabetes and complications: A systems biology analysis in ldlr−/− mice. *PLoS ONE* **2013**, *8*, e56122. [CrossRef] [PubMed]

30. Morrison, M.C.; Mulder, P.; Salic, K.; Verheij, J.; Liang, W.; Van Duyvenvoorde, W.; Menke, A.; Kooistra, T.; Kleemann, R.; Wielinga, P. Intervention with a caspase-1 inhibitor reduces obesity-associated hyperinsulinemia, non-alcoholic steatohepatitis and hepatic fibrosis in ldlr-/-.Leiden mice. *Int. J. Obes.* **2016**, *40*, 1416–1423. [CrossRef] [PubMed]

31. Kilkenny, C.; Browne, W.J.; Cuthill, I.C.; Emerson, M.; Altman, D.G. Improving bioscience research reporting: The arrive guidelines for reporting animal research. *PLoS Biol.* **2010**, *8*, e1000412. [CrossRef] [PubMed]

32. Gesta, S.; Tseng, Y.-H.; Kahn, C.R. Developmental origin of fat: Tracking obesity to its source. *Cell* **2007**, *131*, 242–256. [CrossRef] [PubMed]

33. Caesar, R.; Manieri, M.; Kelder, T.; Boekschoten, M.; Evelo, C.; Müller, M.; Kooistra, T.; Cinti, S.; Kleemann, R.; Drevon, C.A. A combined transcriptomics and lipidomics analysis of subcutaneous, epididymal and mesenteric adipose tissue reveals marked functional differences. *PLoS ONE* **2010**, *5*, e11525. [CrossRef] [PubMed]

34. Wielinga, P.Y.; Harthoorn, L.F.; Verschuren, L.; Schoemaker, M.H.; Jouni, Z.E.; van Tol, E.A.; Kleemann, R.; Kooistra, T. Arachidonic acid/docosahexaenoic acid-supplemented diet in early life reduces body weight gain, plasma lipids, and adiposity in later life in apoe* 3leiden mice. *Mol. Nutr. Food Res.* **2012**, *56*, 1081–1089. [CrossRef] [PubMed]

35. Carpenter, A.E.; Jones, T.R.; Lamprecht, M.R.; Clarke, C.; Kang, I.H.; Friman, O.; Guertin, D.A.; Chang, J.H.; Lindquist, R.A.; Moffat, J. Cellprofiler: Image analysis software for identifying and quantifying cell phenotypes. *Genome Biol.* **2006**, *7*, R100. [CrossRef] [PubMed]

36. Sommer, C.; Straehle, C.; Koethe, U.; Hamprecht, F.A. Ilastik: Interactive learning and segmentation toolkit. In Proceedings of the 2011 IEEE International Symposium on Biomedical Imaging: From Nano to Macro, Chicago, IL, USA, 30 March–2 April 2011; pp. 230–233.

37. Arnoldussen, I.A.; Zerbi, V.; Wiesmann, M.; Noordman, R.H.; Bolijn, S.; Mutsaers, M.P.; Dederen, P.J.; Kleemann, R.; Kooistra, T.; van Tol, E.A. Early intake of long-chain polyunsaturated fatty acids preserves brain structure and function in diet-induced obesity. *J. Nutr. Biochem.* **2016**, *30*, 177–188. [CrossRef] [PubMed]

38. Gao, Z.; Yin, J.; Zhang, J.; Ward, R.E.; Martin, R.J.; Lefevre, M.; Cefalu, W.T.; Ye, J. Butyrate improves insulin sensitivity and increases energy expenditure in mice. *Diabetes* **2009**, *58*, 1509–1517. [CrossRef] [PubMed]

39. Jakobsdottir, G.; Xu, J.; Molin, G.; Ahrne, S.; Nyman, M. High-fat diet reduces the formation of butyrate, but increases succinate, inflammation, liver fat and cholesterol in rats, while dietary fibre counteracts these effects. *PLoS ONE* **2013**, *8*, e80476. [CrossRef] [PubMed]

40. Bocarsly, M.E.; Fasolino, M.; Kane, G.A.; LaMarca, E.A.; Kirschen, G.W.; Karatsoreos, I.N.; McEwen, B.S.; Gould, E. Obesity diminishes synaptic markers, alters microglial morphology, and impairs cognitive function. *Proc. Natl. Acad. Sci. USA* **2015**, *112*, 15731–15736. [CrossRef] [PubMed]

41. Lin, H.V.; Frassetto, A.; Kowalik, E.J., Jr.; Nawrocki, A.R.; Lu, M.M.; Kosinski, J.R.; Hubert, J.A.; Szeto, D.; Yao, X.; Forrest, G. Butyrate and propionate protect against diet-induced obesity and regulate gut hormones via free fatty acid receptor 3-independent mechanisms. *PLoS ONE* **2012**, *7*, e35240. [CrossRef] [PubMed]

42. Bondolfi, L.; Ermini, F.; Long, J.M.; Ingram, D.K.; Jucker, M. Impact of age and caloric restriction on neurogenesis in the dentate gyrus of c57bl/6 mice. *Neurobiol. Aging* **2004**, *25*, 333–340. [CrossRef]

43. Den Besten, G.; Bleeker, A.; Gerding, A.; van Eunen, K.; Havinga, R.; van Dijk, T.H.; Oosterveer, M.H.; Jonker, J.W.; Groen, A.K.; Reijngoud, D.J. Short-chain fatty acids protect against high-fat diet–induced obesity via a ppary-dependent switch from lipogenesis to fat oxidation. *Diabetes* **2015**, *64*, 2398–2408. [CrossRef] [PubMed]

44. Mulder, P.; van den Hoek, A.M.; Kleemann, R. The ccr2 inhibitor propagermanium attenuates diet-induced insulin resistance, adipose tissue inflammation and non-alcoholic steatohepatitis. *PLoS ONE* **2017**, *12*, e0169740. [CrossRef] [PubMed]

45. Wang, Y.; Rimm, E.B.; Stampfer, M.J.; Willett, W.C.; Hu, F.B. Comparison of abdominal adiposity and overall obesity in predicting risk of type 2 diabetes among men. *Am. J. Clin. Nutr.* **2005**, *81*, 555–563. [PubMed]

46. Hammarstedt, A.; Graham, T.E.; Kahn, B.B. Adipose tissue dysregulation and reduced insulin sensitivity in non-obese individuals with enlarged abdominal adipose cells. *Diabetol. Metab. Syndr.* **2012**, *4*, 42. [CrossRef] [PubMed]

47. Gabriely, I.; Ma, X.H.; Yang, X.M.; Atzmon, G.; Rajala, M.W.; Berg, A.H.; Scherer, P.; Rossetti, L.; Barzilai, N. Removal of visceral fat prevents insulin resistance and glucose intolerance of aging. *Diabetes* **2002**, *51*, 2951–2958. [CrossRef] [PubMed]

48. Barzilai, N.; She, L.; Liu, B.Q.; Vuguin, P.; Cohen, P.; Wang, J.; Rossetti, L. Surgical removal of visceral fat reverses hepatic insulin resistance. *Diabetes* **1999**, *48*, 94–98. [CrossRef] [PubMed]

49. Arner, P. Obesity and the adipocyte. Regional adipocity in man. *J. Endocrinol.* **1997**, *155*, 191–192. [CrossRef] [PubMed]

50. Tan, G.D.; Goossens, G.H.; Humphreys, S.M.; Vidal, H.; Karpe, F. Upper and lower body adipose tissue function: A direct comparison of fat mobilization in humans. *Obes. Res.* **2004**, *12*, 114–118. [CrossRef] [PubMed]

51. Khan, S.; Jena, G. Sodium butyrate reduces insulin-resistance, fat accumulation and dyslipidemia in type-2 diabetic rat: A comparative study with metformin. *Chem. Biol. Interact.* **2016**, *254*, 124–134. [CrossRef] [PubMed]

52. Mooradian, A.D. Dyslipidemia in type 2 diabetes mellitus. *Nat. Clin. Pract. Endocrinol. Metab.* **2009**, *5*, 150–159. [CrossRef] [PubMed]

53. Den Besten, G.; van Eunen, K.; Groen, A.K.; Venema, K.; Reijngoud, D.J.; Bakker, B.M. The role of short-chain fatty acids in the interplay between diet, gut microbiota, and host energy metabolism. *J. Lipid Res.* **2013**, *54*, 2325–2340. [CrossRef] [PubMed]

54. Camp, H.S.; Ren, D.; Leff, T. Adipogenesis and fat-cell function in obesity and diabetes. *Trends Mol. Med.* **2002**, *8*, 442–447. [CrossRef]

55. Mulder, P.; Morrison, M.C.; Verschuren, L.; Liang, W.; van Bockel, J.H.; Kooistra, T.; Wielinga, P.Y.; Kleemann, R. Reduction of obesity-associated white adipose tissue inflammation by rosiglitazone is associated with reduced non-alcoholic fatty liver disease in ldlr-deficient mice. *Sci. Rep.* **2016**, *6*, 31542. [CrossRef] [PubMed]

56. Morrison, M.C.; Kleemann, R. Role of macrophage migration inhibitory factor in obesity, insulin resistance, type 2 diabetes, and associated hepatic co-morbidities: A comprehensive review of human and rodent studies. *Front. Immunol.* **2015**, *6*, 308. [CrossRef] [PubMed]

57. Mulder, P.; Morrison, M.C.; Wielinga, P.Y.; van Duyvenvoorde, W.; Kooistra, T.; Kleemann, R. Surgical removal of inflamed epididymal white adipose tissue attenuates the development of non-alcoholic steatohepatitis in obesity. *Int. J. Obes.* **2016**, *40*, 675–684. [CrossRef] [PubMed]

58. Liang, W.; Tonini, G.; Mulder, P.; Kelder, T.; van Erk, M.; van den Hoek, A.M.; Mariman, R.; Wielinga, P.Y.; Baccini, M.; Kooistra, T.; et al. Coordinated and interactive expression of genes of lipid metabolism and inflammation in adipose tissue and liver during metabolic overload. *PLoS ONE* **2013**, *8*, e75290. [CrossRef] [PubMed]

59. Xu, H.; Barnes, G.T.; Yang, Q.; Tan, G.; Yang, D.; Chou, C.J.; Sole, J.; Nichols, A.; Ross, J.S.; Tartaglia, L.A. Chronic inflammation in fat plays a crucial role in the development of obesity-related insulin resistance. *J. Clin. Investig.* **2003**, *112*, 1821–1830. [CrossRef] [PubMed]

60. Hajer, G.R.; van Haeften, T.W.; Visseren, F.L. Adipose tissue dysfunction in obesity, diabetes, and vascular diseases. *Eur. Heart J.* **2008**, *29*, 2959–2971. [CrossRef] [PubMed]

61. Antuna-Puente, B.; Feve, B.; Fellahi, S.; Bastard, J.P. Adipokines: The missing link between insulin resistance and obesity. *Diabetes Metab.* **2008**, *34*, 2–11. [CrossRef] [PubMed]

62. Loffreda, S.; Yang, S.; Lin, H.; Karp, C.; Brengman, M.; Wang, D.; Klein, A.; Bulkley, G.; Bao, C.; Noble, P. Leptin regulates proinflammatory immune responses. *FASEB J.* **1998**, *12*, 57–65. [PubMed]

63. De Oliveira, E.M.; Ascar, T.P.; Silva, J.C.; Sandri, S.; Migliorini, S.; Fock, R.A.; Campa, A. Serum amyloid a links endotoxaemia to weight gain and insulin resistance in mice. *Diabetologia* **2016**, *59*, 1760–1768. [CrossRef] [PubMed]

64. Ahlin, S.; Olsson, M.; Olsson, B.; Svensson, P.A.; Sjöholm, K. No evidence for a role of adipose tissue-derived serum amyloid a in the development of insulin resistance or obesity-related inflammation in hsaa1+/− transgenic mice. *PLoS ONE* **2013**, *8*, e72204. [CrossRef] [PubMed]

65. Den Hartigh, L.J.; Wang, S.; Goodspeed, L.; Ding, Y.; Averill, M.; Subramanian, S.; Wietecha, T.; O'Brien, K.D.; Chait, A. Deletion of serum amyloid a3 improves high fat high sucrose diet-induced adipose tissue inflammation and hyperlipidemia in female mice. *PLoS ONE* **2014**, *9*, e108564. [CrossRef] [PubMed]

66. Leinonen, E.; Hurt-Camejo, E.; Wiklund, O.; Hultén, L.M.; Hiukka, A.; Taskinen, M.R. Insulin resistance and adiposity correlate with acute-phase reaction and soluble cell adhesion molecules in type 2 diabetes. *Atherosclerosis* **2003**, *166*, 387–394. [CrossRef]

67. Yamauchi, T.; Kamon, J.; Minokoshi, Y.A.; Ito, Y.; Waki, H.; Uchida, S.; Yamashita, S.; Noda, M.; Kita, S.; Ueki, K. Adiponectin stimulates glucose utilization and fatty-acid oxidation by activating amp-activated protein kinase. *Nat. Med.* **2002**, *8*, 1288–1295. [CrossRef] [PubMed]

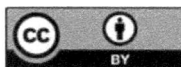

MDPI

St. Alban-Anlage 66

4052 Basel

Switzerland

Tel. +41 61 683 77 34

Fax +41 61 302 89 18

www.mdpi.com

Nutrients Editorial Office

E-mail: nutrients@mdpi.com

www.mdpi.com/journal/nutrients